Thoracic Surgery

Thoracic Surgery

50 Challenging Cases

Edited by

Wickii T. Vigneswaran
Loyola University Health System
Maywood, Illinois

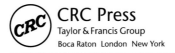

CRC Press
Taylor & Francis Group
Boca Raton London New York

CRC Press is an imprint of the
Taylor & Francis Group, an **informa** business

CRC Press
Taylor & Francis Group
6000 Broken Sound Parkway NW, Suite 300
Boca Raton, FL 33487-2742

International Standard Book Number-13: 978-0-367-40832-9 (Hardback)
978-1-138-03565-2 (Paperback)

Visit the Taylor & Francis Web site at
http://www.taylorandfrancis.com

and the CRC Press Web site at
http://www.crcpress.com

To Rupy, Yalini, Hari, and Janani
who give relevance to everything that is good and worth a struggle

CONTENTS

Contents

PREFACE

Surgical morbidity and mortality are the direct result of incorrect decisions. Correct diagnosis, appropriate procedure(s), the ability of the patient to tolerate the procedure, and the limitations of the surgeon and team performing it are equally important. On occasion, the surgeon must alter a procedure due to unexpected findings or events, and the success may depend how the surgeon adapts to the situation. In this book, we present 50 cases contributed by thoracic surgeons, describing patients with diagnostic challenges and unconventional and innovative solutions, adapting to unexpected findings, or describing new techniques to treat an old problem, and more often than not, all while sweating it out under the glare of the operating room lights. Each case may bring out a teachable moment for working out a diagnostic challenge, a therapeutic expertise that may help the novice or an experienced surgeon in their clinical practice, or an interesting and entertaining reading at leisure. The discussions after each case make no pretense at being exhaustive, and the references provide a mere starting point for further inquiry.

ACKNOWLEDGMENTS

I wish to thank the entire group of contributors in making this venture a success. This book initially started as a single-author book, but it evolved over time inviting other contributors not because of lack of cases, but to have an infusion of varied training and practice backgrounds. I am particularly indebted to Drs. Thomas, Seder, Reddy, Opitz, Parekh, Long, Blakmon, and Podbielski, who not only collected their cases, but also encouraged colleagues to contribute their experience. I extend a special thanks to Adrian Gonzales, MD, who wrote some of the cases with me but, more importantly, assisted me in organizing the chapters. Without Miranda Bromage of Taylor & Francis Group, I would not have been able to complete this work. Her encouragement throughout the process is very much appreciated. I thank Samantha Cook of Taylor & Francis Group for her patience with me and her expert editorial assistance. Finally, to all the patients who consented to have their stories told in this book, without them this contribution would have been impossible.

EDITOR

Professor Wickii T. Vigneswaran, MD, MBA, was born in northern Sri Lanka. After graduating from Faculty of Medicine, University of Peradeniya, Sri Lanka, he trained in many prestigious institutions in the United Kingdom and the United States. Following his advanced fellowship training in cardiothoracic surgery at the Mayo Clinic in Rochester, Minnesota, he started his clinical and academic practice in Chicago, holding academic appointments at University of Illinois at Chicago, Loyola University Stritch School of Medicine, and the University of Chicago Pritzker School of Medicine. He served as chief of Thoracic Surgery at Loyola University Medical Center, associate chief of Cardiac and Thoracic Surgery at University of Chicago Medical Center, and currently serves as director of Thoracic Surgery at Loyola University Health System and systems director of Edward and Elmhurst Health. He is a fellow of the American College of Surgeons, Royal College of Surgeons and Physicians of Canada, Royal College of Surgeons of Edinburgh, and American College of Chest Physicians. He is a past president of the International College of Surgeons of the U.S. Section and a former trustee of the Chest Foundation of the American College of Chest Physicians. He is well-respected for his expertise in treating patients with end-stage lung disease, including lung transplantation, robotic thoracic surgery, and treatment of malignant pleural mesothelioma. He has authored more than 150 manuscripts and edited three books covering lung transplantation and thoracic surgery.

CONTRIBUTORS

Raed Abdulkareem
Department of Surgery
University of Illinois at Chicago
Chicago, Illinois

John Agzarian
Division of General Thoracic Surgery
Department of Surgery
Mayo Clinic
Rochester, Minnesota

Gillian Alex
Department of Cardiovascular and
    Thoracic Surgery
Rush University Medical Center
Chicago, Illinois

Betty Allen
Division of General Surgery
Department of Surgery
University of Wisconsin
Madison, Wisconsin

Eric P. Anderson
Department of Cardiovascular and Thoracic
    Surgery
Rush University Medical Center
and
Department of Cardiothoracic Surgery
John H. Stroger Hospital of Cook County
Chicago, Illinois

Evgeny V. Arshava
Division of Cardiothoracic Surgery
Department of Surgery
Carver College of Medicine
University of Iowa
Iowa City, Iowa

Adnan Al Ayoubi
Division of Cardiothoracic Surgery
Department of Surgery
Carver College of Medicine
University of Iowa
Iowa City, Iowa

Curtis S. Bergquist
Department of Surgery
University of Michigan
Ann Arbor, Michigan

Shanda H. Blackmon
Division of General Thoracic Surgery
Department of Surgery
Mayo Clinic
Rochester, Minnesota

Alexander A. Brescia
Department of Surgery
University of Michigan
Ann Arbor, Michigan

Claudio Caviezel
Department of Thoracic Surgery
University Hospital Zürich
Zürich, Switzerland

Gary W. Chmielewski
Department of Cardiovascular and
    Thoracic Surgery
Rush University Medical Center
Chicago, Illinois

Alison Coogan
Department of Cardiovascular and
    Thoracic Surgery
Rush University Medical Center
Chicago, Illinois

Julia Coughlin
Department of Cardiovascular and
    Thoracic Surgery
Rush University Medical Center
Chicago, Illinois

Brett Curran
Stritch School of Medicine
Loyola University Medical Center
Maywood, Illinois

Kate Gallo
Department of Cardiovascular and Thoracic
  Surgery
Rush University Medical Center
Chicago, Illinois

Nicole M. Geissen
Department of Cardiovascular and Thoracic
  Surgery
Rush University Medical Center
and
Department of Cardiothoracic Surgery
John H. Stroger Hospital of Cook County
Chicago, Illinois

Bastian Grande
Institute of Anesthesiology
University Hospital of Zürich
Zürich, Switzerland

Benjamin Haithcock
Division of Cardiothoracic Surgery
University of North Carolina School of
  Medicine
Chapel Hill, North Carolina

John Hallsten
Stritch School of Medicine
Loyola University Medical Center
Maywood, Illinois

James B. Hendele
Department of Surgery
Jesse Brown VA Medical Center
Chicago, Illinois

Reilly Hobbs
Department of Surgery
University of Michigan
Ann Arbor, Michigan

Ilhan Inci
Department of Thoracic Surgery
University Hospital Zürich
Zürich, Switzerland

Taylor Jaraczewski
Stritch School of Medicine
Loyola University Health System
Maywood, Illinois

Lia Jordano
Department of Cardiovascular and Thoracic
  Surgery
Rush University Medical Center
Chicago, Illinois

John Keech
Division of Cardiothoracic Surgery
Department of Surgery
Carver College of Medicine
University of Iowa
Iowa City, Iowa

Danuel V. Laan
Division of General Thoracic Surgery
Department of Surgery
Mayo Clinic
Rochester, Minnesota

Max Lacour
Department of Thoracic Surgery
University Hospital Zürich
Zürich, Switzerland

Kiran H. Lagisetty
Department of Surgery
University of Michigan
Ann Arbor, Michigan

Grant Lewin
Department of Cardiovascular and Thoracic
  Surgery
Rush University Medical Center
Chicago, Illinois

Michael J. Liptay
Department of Cardiovascular and Thoracic
  Surgery
Rush University Medical Center
Chicago, Illinois

Jason Long
Division of Cardiothoracic Surgery
University of North Carolina School
   of Medicine
Chapel Hill, North Carolina

James L. Lubawski Jr.
Department of Thoracic and Cardiovascular
   Surgery
Loyola University Health System
Maywood, Illinois

Yulia N. Matveeva
Department of Family Medicine
Carver College of Medicine
University of Iowa
Iowa City, Iowa

Hiroko Nakahama
Department of Surgery
Loyola University Health System
Maywood, Illinois

Isabelle Opitz
Department of Thoracic Surgery
University Hospital Zürich
Zürich, Switzerland

Anita Ong
Mercy Medical Center
Loyola University Health System
Chicago, Illinois

Mark B. Orringer
Department of Pathology
University of Michigan
Ann Arbor, Michigan

Albert Pai
Division of Cardiothoracic Surgery
Department of Surgery
Carver College of Medicine
University of Iowa
Iowa City, Iowa

Kalpaj R. Parekh
Division of Cardiothoracic Surgery
Department of Surgery
Carver College of Medicine
University of Iowa
Iowa City, Iowa

Francis J. Podbielski
Department of Surgery
University of Illinois at Chicago
Chicago, Illinois

Ashish Pulikal
Division of Cardiothoracic Surgery
University of North Carolina School of
   Medicine
Chapel Hill, North Carolina

Samine Ravanbakhsh
Department of Cardiovascular and
   Thoracic Surgery
Rush University Medical Center
Chicago, Illinois

Rishindra M. Reddy
Department of Surgery
University of Michigan
Ann Arbor, Michigan

Amber Redmond
Department of Cardiovascular and
   Thoracic Surgery
Rush University Medical Center
Chicago, Illinois

Christian Renz
Loyola University Medical Center
Maywood, Illinois

Adrian E. Rodrigues
Department of Thoracic and Cardiovascular
   Surgery
Loyola University Medical Center
Maywood, Illinois

Phillip G. Rowse
Division of General Thoracic Surgery
Department of Surgery
Mayo Clinic
Rochester, Minnesota

Didier Schneiter
Department of Thoracic Surgery
University Hospital Zürich
Zürich, Switzerland

Christopher W. Seder
Department of Cardiovascular and
    Thoracic Surgery
Rush University Medical Center
and
Department of Cardiothoracic Surgery
John H. Stroger Hospital of Cook County
Chicago, Illinois

Kimberly Song
Department of Cardiovascular and
    Thoracic Surgery
Rush University Medical Center
Chicago, Illinois

Mathew Thomas
Mayo Clinic
Jacksonville, Florida

Lambros Tsonis
Department of Thoracic and Cardiovascular
    Surgery
Mercy Medical Center
Loyola University Health System
Chicago, Illinois

Ozuru Ukoha
Department of Cardiovascular and
    Thoracic Surgery
Rush University Medical Center
and
Division of Cardiothoracic Surgery
John H. Stroger Jr. Hospital of Cook County
Chicago, Illinois

Wickii T. Vigneswaran
Department of Thoracic and Cardiovascular
    Surgery
Loyola University Health System
Maywood, Illinois

Tessa Watt
Department of Surgery
University of Michigan
Ann Arbor, Michigan

Walter Weder
Department of Thoracic Surgery
University Hospital Zürich
Zürich, Switzerland

Stephanie G. Worrell
Department of Surgery
University of Michigan
Ann Arbor, Michigan

Poorani Sekar, MD
Clinical assistant professor
Division of Infectious Diseases
Department of Internal Medicine
University of Iowa Hospitals and Clinics
Iowa City, IA

Hiroko Nakahama and Wickii T. Vigneswaran

 Key Words

- Robotic-assisted thoracoscopic surgery
- Fibrous dysplasia
- Chest wall tumor

Introduction

Fibrous dysplasia is a skeletal disorder that replaces medullary bone with benign fibrous connective tissue. These tumors are typically asymptomatic but can present as a painful mass or with pathologic fractures. Radiographically, they appear as a fibrous bone deformity with fusiform expansion and cortical thinning [1,2]. Surgical resection is indicated for symptomatic lesions or lesions suspicious for malignant disease.

Traditionally, chest wall tumors are resected with a large thoracotomy, often necessitating reconstruction for large defects. Video-assisted resection has also been described in case reports; however, their use is limited by the bony chest wall anatomy [3–6]. The robotic system has the advantage of high-definition three-dimensional reconstruction of the dissection plane with fine motor maneuverability through small port sites. Here, we report successful robotic-assisted thoracoscopic resection of fibrous dysplasia of the ribs.

Case Report

A 68-year-old female with fibrous dysplasia of the ribs presented with right-sided chest pain and difficulty breathing. She was diagnosed with fibrous dysplasia over 30 years ago and was clinically followed for the progression of the disease. With a serial computed tomography (CT) scan, she was found to have an interval increase in size of her tumors; the lateral third rib tumor measured 7 cm by 6 cm, and the 10th rib tumor measured 4 cm by 2.6 cm compared to 6 cm by 4.5 cm and 3.1 cm by 1.1 cm, respectively, 8 years prior (Figure 1.1). On physical exam, she did not have any palpable masses in her chest wall. Due to the expansile nature of the enlarging tumors, surgical intervention to exclude malignant degeneration was recommended to her.

The patient was given anesthesia and a double-lumen endotracheal tube was inserted for lung isolation. She was placed in a left-lateral decubitus position. A camera port incision was made in the subscapular area, and the second and third thoracoports were placed under direct visualization in the sub-mammary area and paravertebral area and the utility port in the ninth intercostal space at the anterior area of the second tumor. The robotic da Vinci Si surgical system was docked in the appropriate position.

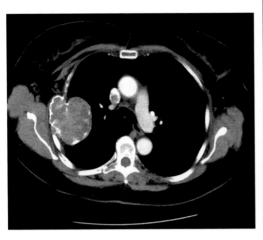
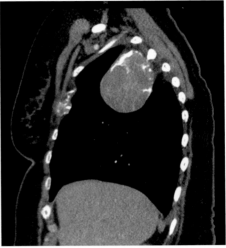

Figure 1.1 Preoperative CT scan with axial (left) and sagittal (right) view of fibrous dysplasia of the third rib

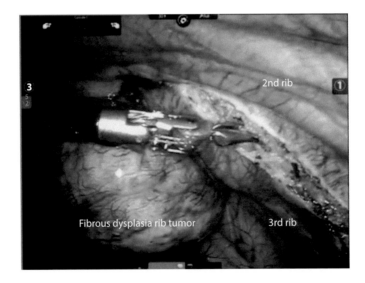

Figure 1.2 Intrathoracic view of the fibrous dysplasia tumor of the third rib during robotic dissection

First, the resection of the large tumor on the third rib was performed (Figure 1.2). The intercostal resection was performed using bipolar and unipolar electrocautery. The ribs were divided on both ends using Dennis rib shears for an en-bloc resection of the tumors, preserving the chest wall muscles while removing adequate margin and mobilization of the tumor. The large mass on the third rib was then placed in an Endo-bag.

Next, the tenth rib intercostal space and neurovascular bundle was dissected with a similar technique using electrocautery. After the tenth rib was sheared, video-assisted thoracoscopic technique was utilized for resection of the remaining tumor on the tenth rib. Through a 3 cm skin incision over the tenth rib, the second tumor was removed and extracted through the incision site. The third rib tumor contained within the Endo-bag was then extracted through the same incision that was made to remove the tumor on the tenth rib.

The patient recovered well from surgery and was discharged home on the following day. The large tumor on the third rib and the tumor on the tenth rib measured 9 cm and 5 cm, respectively, at their greatest dimension. The pathology report confirmed fibrous dysplasia for both tumors, and the edges showed increased cellularity resembling giant-cell reparative granuloma. There was no atypia or increased mitotic figures identified. At the one-week and two-month follow-ups, the patient remained without pain or signs of recurrent disease (Figure 1.3).

Comments

Fibrous dysplasia comprises approximately 30%–50% of benign bone tumors [1]. Fibrous dysplasia can be divided into two types: monostotic with one bone involvement and polyostotic with multiple bone involvement. Monostotic fibrous dysplasia occurs in approximately 70%–80% of cases and arises most commonly in the ribs, proximal femur, tibia, and skull [1,7]. Polyostotic fibrous dysplasia involves more than one bone and is closely associated with McCune-Albright syndrome [1]. Fibrous dysplasia arises sporadically and affects the ribs in approximately 6%–20% of cases [8]. Surgical resection is indicated when lesions become symptomatic and cause significant deformation, or when malignant disease is in question. Malignant degeneration occurs in approximately 0.5%–4% of cases [8–10].

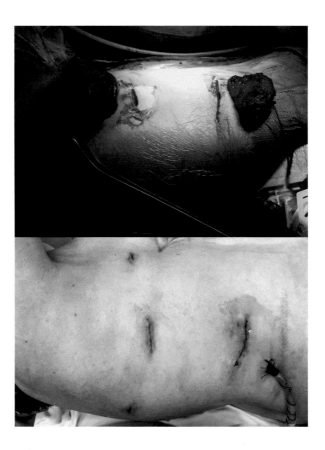

Figure 1.3 Image of specimen and incision on patient in left-lateral decubitus position

Surgical management of chest wall tumors has traditionally been performed with a thoracotomy with wide local excision and chest wall reconstruction for defects greater than 5 cm [2]. This approach is associated with high morbidity caused by altered respiratory mechanics due to deformed chest wall architecture and perioperative pain. More recently, video-assisted thoracoscopic rib resection has been reported for various chest wall tumors [3–6]. Although this approach decreases the pain associated with a large thoracotomy and can preserve chest wall structure, the instrumentation is largely limited by chest wall anatomy and dependent on the location of the tumors.

Robotic-assisted thoracoscopic surgery for use in chest wall tumor resection has not been well described in literature. Robotic-assisted resection of the first rib for Paget-Schroetter syndrome has been reported [11,12]. A series of cases have demonstrated low rates of neurovascular complications in the setting of superior visualization of the operative field, minimized pain, and long-term patency of the subclavian vein [11,12].

Robotic-assisted thoracoscopic resection of chest wall tumors is a good alternative to thoracotomy or video-assisted thoracoscopic resection. This approach has the advantage of high-definition three-dimensional reconstruction with fine motor maneuverability for dissection through confined spaces. This method preserves the underlying muscular architecture of the chest wall, limiting the need for subsequent reconstructive procedures. The small incision and limited rib retraction significantly reduces perioperative pain and shortens the length of the hospital stay. The disadvantage of this approach is the cost of the robotic system, which is shared amongst multiple disciplines at our institution, and may also be offset by the decreased hospital stay and reduced use of analgesic medications. Although this case took 499 minutes to complete, as this was the first robotic chest resection case done at our institution, we anticipate the operative time can be significantly reduced with subsequent cases and training of ancillary staff.

Here, we describe the first robotic-assisted resection of fibrous dysplasia tumors of the rib with excellent results (Figure 1.4). This method can be applied for any benign lesion of the ribs and should be considered to reduce perioperative pain and morbidity associated with the traditional methods.

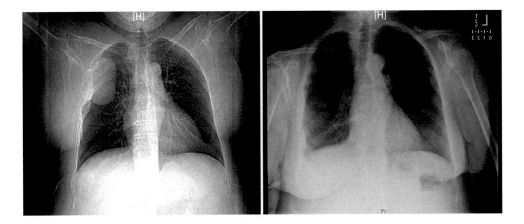

Figure 1.4 Chest X-ray before (left) and after (right) robotic resection of fibrous dysplasia of the ribs

REFERENCES

1. Smith, S., Keshavjee, S. Primary chest wall tumors. *Thorac Surg Clin.* 2010;20(4):495–507. doi:10.1016/j.thorsurg.2010.07.003.
2. Thomas, M., Shen, K. Primary tumors of the osseous chest wall and their management. *Thorac Surg Clin.* 2017;27(2):181–193. doi:10.1016/j.thorsurg.2017.01.012.
3. Shim, J., Chon, S., Lee, C., Heo, J. Polyostotic rib fibrous dysplasia resected by video-assisted thoracoscopic surgery with preservation of the overlying periosteum. *J Thorac Cardiovasc Surg.* 2010;140(4):938–940. doi:10.1016/j.jtcvs.2010.03.010.
4. Kara, H., Keenan, J., Balderson, S., D'Amico, T. Video assisted thoracic surgery with chest wall resection. *Video-Assist Thorac Surg.* 2018;3:15–15. doi:10.21037/vats.2018.03.07.
5. Gera, P., Hei, E., Cummins, G., Harvey, J. Thoracoscopy in chest wall Ewing's sarcoma. *J Laparoendosc Adv Surg Tech.* 2006;16(5):509–512. doi:10.1089/lap.2006.16.509.
6. Rocco, G., Fazioli, F., Martucci, N., Cicalese, M., La Rocca, A., La Manna, C., De Chiara, A. Video-assisted thoracic surgery rib resection and reconstruction with titanium plate. *Ann Thorac Surg.* 2011;92(2):744–745. doi:10.1016/j.athoracsur.2011.03.019.
7. Rubin, A., Byrns, K., Zhou, D., Freedman, L. Fibrous dysplasia of the rib: AIRP best cases in radiologic-pathologic correlation. *Radiographics.* 2015;35(7):2049–2052. doi:10.1148/rg.2015140335.
8. Traibi, A., El Oueriachi, F., El Hammoumi, M., Al Bouzidi, A., Kabiri, E. Monostotic fibrous dysplasia of the ribs. *Interact Cardiovasc Thorac Surg.* 2011;14(1):41–43. doi:10.1093/icvts/ivr048.
9. O'Connor, B., Collins, F. The management of chest wall resection in a patient with polyostotic fibrous dysplasia and respiratory failure. *J Cardiothorac Vasc Anesth.* 2009;23(4):518–521. doi:10.1053/j.jvca.2008.09.009.
10. DiCaprio, M., Enneking, W. Fibrous dysplasia. Pathophysiology, evaluation, and treatment. *J Bone Joint Surg Am.* 2005;87(8):1848–1864. doi:10.2106/jbjs.d.02942.
11. Kocher, G., Zehnder, A., Lutz, J., Schmidli, J., Schmid, R. First rib resection for thoracic outlet syndrome: The robotic approach. *World J Surg.* 2018;42(10):3250–3255. doi:10.1007/s00268-018-4636-4.
12. Gharagozloo, F., Meyer, M., Tempesta, B., Gruessner, S. Robotic transthoracic first-rib resection for Paget–Schroetter syndrome. *Eur J Cardiothorac Surg,* doi: 10.1093/ejcts/ezy275.

Mathew Thomas

 Key Words
- Aneurysmal bone cyst
- Rib resection
- Minimally invasive surgery

Introduction

Primary bony tumors arising from the chest wall are uncommon tumors and can be either benign or malignant in nature. Surgical resection plays a major role in the management of most bony chest wall tumors as the primary modality of treatment. However, resection of the chest wall is often a morbid procedure that commonly involves large incisions and extensive division of both soft tissues and bone. Minimally invasive chest wall resection (MICR) and reconstruction is not commonly performed either due to lack of suitable thoracoscopic instruments or tumor characteristics such as size and location that would require a large incision for access and removal. In this report, we describe our innovative approach to resection of an aneurysmal bone cyst (ABC) of the second rib using video-assisted thoracoscopy, along with a laparoscopic balloon dissector to assist with subpectoral dissection.

Case Report

A 62-year-old female presented with gradually worsening right-sided anterior chest wall pain that had been present over several months. Imaging with chest X-ray and computed tomography (CT) scan showed an expansile 3 cm mass along the anterolateral aspect of the right, second rib (Figure 2.1). A percutaneous core needle biopsy was performed and reported to be consistent with ABC. Her comorbidities included hypothyroidism, obesity, and hypertension.

On our examination, she was noted to have generalized central obesity with large breasts. The edge of the tumor was barely palpable under the lateral part of the pectoralis muscle in the axilla and was fixed to the bony chest wall. Due to her symptoms, surgical resection using a video-assisted approach to resect the second rib was recommended.

After induction of general anesthesia, a double-lumen endotracheal tube was placed for single, left-lung ventilation. The patient was then positioned in a sloppy lateral thoracotomy position with the right arm draped overhead on a padded arm board (Figure 2.2). The right breast was retracted to the left side using adhesive tapes. The entire right chest from the sternum to the posterior axillary line was then prepared and draped in a sterile fashion.

In addition to the standard thoracoscopic instruments, we used a laparoscopic balloon dissector (Spacemaker Plus Dissector System, Covidien, USA), commonly used for minimally

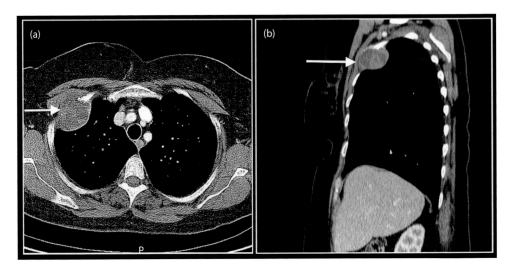

Figure 2.1 (a) Axial and (b) lateral preoperative CT scan images showing second rib aneurysmal bone cyst (arrows) with internal septations

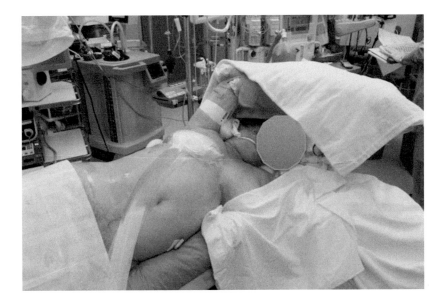

Figure 2.2 Intraoperative photo showing positioning of patient for thoracoscopic second rib resection

invasive repairs of inguinal hernias. Other special instruments used in this case were the Kerrison bone punch and the Giertz-Stille rib shears, also known as the Guillotine rib cutter.

To begin with, the right lung was deflated and a 1.2 cm thoracoscopic port was placed in the seventh intercostal space in the midaxillary line. The right thoracic cavity was examined with a 10 mm thoracoscopic camera showing the rib mass arising from the second rib. Pneumothorax was obtained using CO_2 gas insufflation to a pressure of 8 mm Hg to assist with exposure.

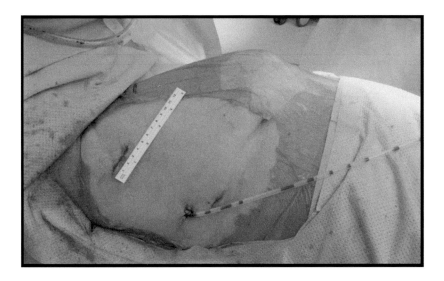

Figure 2.3 Intraoperative photo showing 3.5 cm axillary access incision and other port sites at completion of the operation

A 3.5 cm access incision (Figure 2.3) was then made in the right axilla in line with the second rib exposing the lateral edge of the pectoralis muscle. An attempt was made to elevate the pectoralis muscle off the chest wall to expose the mass on the rib using a combination of blunt and electrocautery dissection. However, this was limited due to the thickness of the patient's chest wall. The laparoscopic balloon dissector was then used to complete the dissection along the avascular subpectoral plane by inserting it under the muscle, gradually inflating it and progressing medially, as seen in the video. Once the plane had been developed, the medial edge of the mass could be assessed by digital palpation.

A second 5 mm thoracoscopic port was placed in the fifth intercostal space in the midaxillary line. A laparoscopic hook cautery was used through this port to incise the pleura circumferentially around the tumor and divide the intercostal vessels. The lateral margin of resection of the rib and intercostal muscles was developed with cautery through the access incision. The medial aspect of the rib was then divided with the Kerrison bone punch that was advanced directly through the superior port site, and the lateral division was performed with a Guillotine rib cutter through the utility incision. The remaining soft tissue attachments of the rib were completely divided by cautery. The medial margin of the specimen was marked with clips for orientation before removal from the chest cavity. Since only a segment of one rib had been resected and was well covered by the breast, reconstruction was not necessary. A 19Fr soft intrapleural drain was placed through the lower port site and was removed the next day. Final surgical pathology was consistent with ABC, and margins were negative.

The patient tolerated the procedure well and was discharged from the hospital on day 3. She was off all pain medications three weeks later and returned to her desk job one month after surgery.

Comments

ABC is a very rare, benign tumor of unclear pathogenesis in which osteolytic expansion of the medullary cavity of the bone occurs, leading to severe pain and occasionally pathological fractures. ABC typically occurs in the long bones, spine, and pelvis and has been occasionally reported to occur in the ribs [1]. Histopathology of ABCs is characterized by blood-filled non-endothelialized cystic spaces separated by fibroblastic connective tissue septa. They are most commonly seen in the first three decades of life and rarely occur after that. Differential diagnoses of ABC include telangiectatic osteosarcoma [2] and giant cell tumor. ABCs have been reported to undergo changes such as spontaneous involution or malignant degeneration into sarcoma. The treatment of ABCs may include radiation and curettage with bone grafting, although these interventions themselves have been associated with malignant degeneration. Intracystic injections with sodium amidotrizoate and selective arterial embolization have also been used to treat ABCs but, because they have been associated with high rates of systemic and cerebral embolization, they are not considered as a first line of treatment. Surgical resection with wide margins is curative and has the lowest reported rate of local recurrence [3].

The traditional, more common open approach to chest wall resection involves large incisions and the division of multiple chest wall muscles, which can be very painful and often cosmetically unappealing. Although chest wall resection using minimally invasive techniques has been reported before, it is not commonly employed for primary tumors of the chest wall and is mostly reported in combination with lung resection for lung tumors invading the chest wall [4,5]. MICR is often limited by the challenges in maneuvering rigid instruments around tight angles within the chest from fixed thoracoscopic ports. To the best of our knowledge, there are no instruments specifically designed for MICR and reconstruction, although certain surgical instruments from the orthopedic or neurosurgery repertoire can be useful for this purpose. One such instrument is the Kerrison bone punch, which has a slim profile that allows it to be advanced through a minimally invasive incision for the division of the ribs.

Minimally invasive approaches should be considered for small- to medium-sized benign or low-grade malignant lesions of the chest wall that do not require large margins of resection and have less risk of local recurrence. Although this does not preclude MICR for malignant tumors that require more radical resection [6], this may best be done in a clinical trial setting since long-term outcomes including recurrence have not yet been reported with this approach. It is critical to adhere to the principles of surgical oncology when resecting any chest wall tumor, taking care to ensure that adequate margins are obtained and to avoid contamination of normal tissue by malignant cells. Reconstruction of the chest wall is not always necessary when resection is limited and should be determined on an individual basis. Minimally invasive reconstruction of the chest wall via thoracoscopy is also feasible and has been described by other authors [7].

REFERENCES

1. Medina, M., Paul, S. Aneurysmal bone cyst arising from the first rib: A rare cause of thoracic outlet syndrome. *Thorac Cardiovasc Surg Rep*. 2016;5(1):74–76.
2. Saguem, I., Ayadi, L., Kallel, R., et al. Telangiectatic osteosarcoma of the rib: A rare entity and a potential diagnostic pitfall. *Pathologica*. 2016;108(4):175–178.
3. Cottalorda, J., Bourelle, S. Current treatments of primary aneurysmal bone cysts. *J ediatr Orthop B*. 2006;15(3):155–167.

4. Bourgeois, D.J., III, Yendamuri, S., Hennon, M., et al. Minimally invasive rib-sparing video-assisted thoracoscopic surgery resections with high-dose-rate intraoperative brachytherapy for selected chest wall tumors. *Pract Radiat Oncol.* 2016;6(6):e329–e335.

5. Demmy, T.L., Nwogu, C.E., Yendamuri, S. Thoracoscopic chest wall resection: What is its role? *Ann Thorac Surg.* 2010;89(6):S2142–S2145.

6. Hennon, M.W., and Demmy, T.L. Thoracoscopic resection and re-resection of an anterior chest wall chondrosarcoma. *Innovations (Phila).* 2012;7(6):445–447.

7. Demmy, T.L., Yendamuri, S., Hennon, M.W., Dexter, E.U., Picone, A.L., and Nwogu, C. Thoracoscopic maneuvers for chest wall resection and reconstruction. *J Thorac Cardiovasc Surg.* 2012;144(3):S52–S57.

HYBRID APPROACH TO REPAIR OF ACQUIRED THORACIC DYSTROPHY IN AN ADULT PATIENT AFTER FAILED CHILDHOOD RAVITCH PROCEDURE

Mathew Thomas

 Key Words

- Acquired thoracic dystrophy
- Pectus excavatum
- Ravitch procedure

Introduction

Acquired thoracic dystrophy (ATD), also sometimes called asphyxiating thoracic dystrophy or thoracic insufficiency syndrome, is an uncommon condition in which the growth of the thoracic cage is limited, leading to varying degrees of restriction in cardiopulmonary function [1]. This condition is most commonly associated with prior open repair of congenital pectus excavatum at a young age, during which extensive resections of costal cartilages were performed. Most patients with ATD require correction before adulthood, and only a small fraction present as adults. Management of ATD in adults is extremely challenging with limited evidence available on how best to correct the deformity and reconstruct the chest wall in these patients.

We describe our management of an adult patient with ATD using a hybrid approach combining a minimally invasive and open resection technique followed by complex reconstruction of the chest wall.

Case Report

A 38-year-old, otherwise healthy, never smoker, male patient in a physically demanding occupation presented with a two-year history of severe episodic palpitations, light-headedness, and progressive feeling of restricted breathing with intolerance to moderate to severe effort. His medical history included severe congenital pectus excavatum that recurred shortly after open surgical repair (modified Ravitch) done at the age of 15. He underwent an extensive evaluation including a 24-hour Holter monitoring by his primary physician and cardiologist. He was noted to have occasional premature atrial and ventricular contractions, along with brief supraventricular tachycardia lasting approximately one minute that were associated with palpitations. No specific cardiac pathology could be identified as the etiology for his arrhythmias. He was treated with beta-blockers (metoprolol), which did not give him any significant relief. After ruling out other possible causes for his arrhythmias and other symptoms, he was referred to us for correction of his pectus excavatum deformity.

On our examination, he was noted to be a tall male (190 cm, 88 kg) with a severe pectus excavatum deformity (Figure 3.1) and features suggestive of ATD (narrow shoulders, narrow anterior-posterior diameter, and wide transverse diameter of the lower chest). A transverse

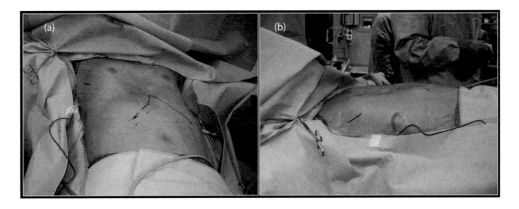

Figure 3.1 (a) Front and (b) lateral pictures of the patient showing severe recurrent pectus excavatum

anterior scar was visible at approximately the level of the fifth costal cartilage. A treadmill stress test was performed during which he developed a hypotensive response and incomplete right bundle branch block features on EKG.

A CT scan of the chest with our standard pectus protocol was obtained (Figure 3.2). His Haller index on inspiration was 4.2 and increased to 5.4 with expiration; the correction index was 42.1. Sternal tilt to the right and extensive calcification with hypertrophy of the costal cartilages on both sides were present. Pulmonary function tests showed mild to moderate restrictive findings: total lung capacity 86% of predicted; vital capacity 81% of predicted; and 1 minute forced expiratory volume at 82% of predicted. Echocardiogram showed the estimated left ventricle ejection fraction was 55%–60% of normal but was otherwise unremarkable.

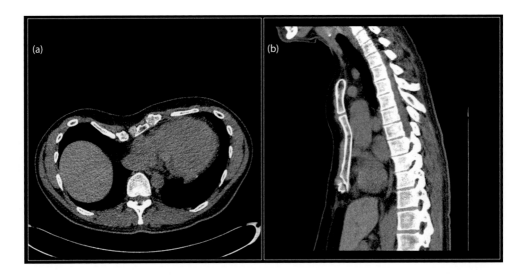

Figure 3.2 Preop CT of the chest: (a) axial and (b) sagittal sections, showing severe pectus excavatum with calcified costochondral junctions and sternal angulation

After evaluation and multidisciplinary discussion between thoracic surgery, cardiology, and pulmonology specialists, he was given the recommendation to undergo correction of his pectus excavatum via a hybrid approach using both open and minimally invasive techniques. He provided his informed consent.

The entire operation was done under general anesthesia and with intermittent single lung ventilation via a double-lumen tube. The patient was positioned supine with both arms extended outward at approximately 75 degrees and supported on well-padded arm boards. The entire chest and abdomen were sterilely prepared and draped. Intraoperative transesophageal echocardiogram was used to evaluate the cardiac function and to rule out cardiac injury by observing for pericardial effusion.

After deflating the right lung, a 5 mm thoracoscope placed through the fifth intercostal space in the midaxillary line was used to evaluate the thoracic cavity. Internally, the right sternocostal junctions were severely depressed, displaced, and angulated. Significant compression of the anterior wall of the right ventricle by the sternum was also observed. The left chest was evaluated with a 5 mm thoracoscope in a similar manner.

A 4 cm incision was then made on each side, extending from the midaxillary line to the anterior axillary line along the fifth intercostal space. Through this incision, the subpectoral space was developed bluntly using a finger. The right fifth intercostal space was opened along the incision, through which an endoscopic vein harvester (VirtuoSaph Plus, Terumo, USA) was advanced in the chest and used to create a substernal tunnel across to the left pleural cavity. The thoracoscope was also used simultaneously to observe the endoscopic vein harvester during creation of the substernal tunnel. Once the thoracoscopic dissection of the substernal plane had been completed from the second rib to the xiphoid process, the previous anterior transverse incision was opened, and subcutaneous flaps were raised cephalad to the level of the second rib. The midline fascia was incised vertically, and the pectoralis muscle flaps were raised bilaterally from the third rib to the xiphoid process and laterally to midclavicular lines. Following this, 2 cm segments of the calcified costochondral junctions (CCJ) of the fourth–sixth ribs on the right were resected using a micro sagittal oscillating bone saw. The right internal mammary vessels were identified and spared. Vertical wedge osteotomies of the left third–fifth CCJs without resection were used to correct the sternal angulation. Multiple wedge osteotomies of the anterior table of the sternum (3 transverse and 2 vertical) were created using the oscillating bone saw, which we have named the "waffling technique" (Figure 3.3).

Using the principles of minimally invasive technique of pectus repair, we then placed three curved bars under the ribs, equidistant from one another, and secured them using a stabilizer bar and multipoint fixation to the ribs with FiberWire (Arthrex Inc, Naples, USA). By placing the bars, we were able to elevate the anterior chest wall and distract the ribs from the sternum. An absorbable polyglactin 910 mesh was placed under the resected segments and anchored to the ribs above and below using absorbable sutures. The removed calcified segments of bone were placed back into the gaps caused by distraction and held in place using rib and sternal plates (RibFix and SternaBlu, Biomet Microfixation, USA) (Figure 3.3). Commercially prepared bone graft putty was applied to the remaining defects on the right side and on the wedge osteotomies. The underlay polyglactin mesh acted as a scaffold for the bone graft and prevented it from falling into the chest. At the end of the procedure, bilateral thoracoscopy was again performed to rule out any intrathoracic or mediastinal injury. The pectoralis muscle flaps were brought back to the midline over the sternum. 15Fr Jackson-Pratt drains were placed in subpectoral space, and 24Fr chest tubes were placed bilaterally (Figure 3.4). The entire operation

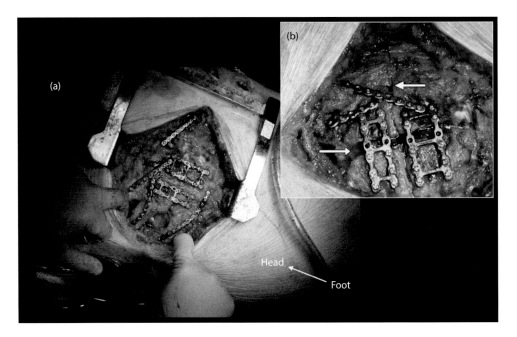

Figure 3.3 Intraoperative pictures showing multiple sternal vertical and horizontal osteotomies (arrows) along with rib and sternal plating

lasted approximately eight hours, and the patient was transferred to the intensive care unit where he was extubated shortly afterwards.

He had significant postoperative pain, which was managed initially with epidural analgesia and multimodality pain therapy. His chest tubes were removed three days later, and he was discharged home nine days later. He returned to work after three months and has had periodic follow-ups since. Two years later he has had no further symptoms and reported active participation in gym activities and in his job without any significant limitations compared to his peers. He is scheduled for removal of the pectus bars three years after surgery.

Comments

Surgical correction of congenital pectus excavatum in adults is usually performed using either an open technique with subperichondrial resection of multiple bilateral costal cartilages or a minimally invasive approach using multiple curved rigid bars inserted through axillary incisions. The reported recurrence rate after open repair ranges from 2% to 20% but may be higher if all patients including those who had late recurrences and those who followed up elsewhere, other than the primary hospital, were taken into account [2].

ATD does not result when the initial pectus repair occurred in adulthood or if the patient presents with a recurrence soon after open repair or after removal of pectus bars. In such cases, the chest wall is often pliable, and the sternum can be reelevated without much effort. Reoperation in these patients can often be successfully completed with minimally invasive repair alone in expert hands [3].

Various innovative techniques for the management of ATD have been used in children and range from distraction osteogenesis [4] to hybrid techniques, often done in stages. Very few

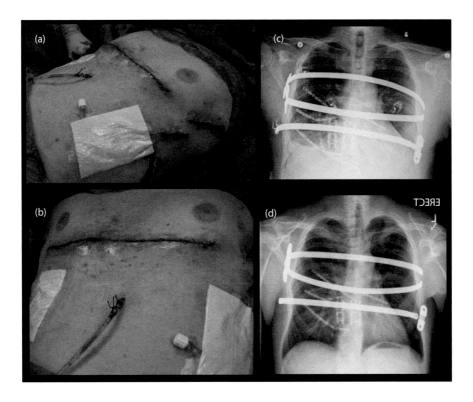

Figure 3.4 (a) and (b): Immediate postoperative pictures after repair of recurrent pectus excavatum. (c) Immediate postoperative chest X-ray and (d) chest X-ray at two-year follow-up visit

groups [2,5] have reported the management of ATD in adults since the problem tends to require correction before the patient reaches adulthood.

ATD in adults presents as a nonpliable chest with malunion and ossification of the sterno-costal junctions in addition to reduced intrathoracic volume. The goal of surgical correction is to increase the intrathoracic volume, achieved by elevating the fixed sternum and increasing the circumference of the anterior chest wall using osteotomies and distraction techniques.

Jaroszewski et al from the Mayo Clinic in Arizona and Phoenix Children's Hospital reported using the hybrid operation in nine adult patients with ATD, all of who had subjective improvement in symptoms over the long-term but without objective measurements to corroborate [5]. The same group later described their experience with the repair of recurrent pectus excavatum in 73 adults [3]. The hybrid approach was required in 34 patients (71%), including 14 patients with ATD. Patients with ATD had more complications including prolonged respiratory failure requiring tracheostomy (21% vs. 0%) compared to those without ATD.

In our practice, the hybrid approach is used in adults when preoperative imaging shows severe calcification of the costal cartilages and when the sternum fails to elevate during minimally invasive repair of pectus excavatum. The open component may not be as extensive, as in the current case, when only few ribs are involved and may consist of limited anterior osteotomies alone without resection.

Repair of recurrent pectus excavatum with or without ATD is a complex operation that often involves significant perioperative risk of morbidity and mortality. Patients undergoing surgical repair of recurrent pectus excavatum, regardless of the technique, have considerable amount of postoperative pain and require long periods of recovery before becoming fully functional. Careful patient selection is important in ensuring successful outcomes after surgery.

REFERENCES

1. Phillips, J.D., and van Aaist, J.A. Jeune's syndrome (asphyxiating thoracic dystrophy): congenital and acquired. *Semin Pediatr Surg.* 2008;17(3):167–72.
2. Johnson, K.N., Jaroszewski, D.E., Ewais, M., Lackey, J.J., McMahon, L., Notrica, D.M. Hybrid technique for repair of recurrent pectus excavatum after failed open repair. *Ann Thorac Surg.* 2015;99(6):1936–1943.
3. Croitoru, D.P., Kelly, R.E., Jr, Goretsky, M.J., Gustin, T., Keever, R., Nuss, D. The minimally invasive Nuss technique for recurrent or failed pectus excavatum repair in 50 patients. *J Pediatr Surg.* 2005;40(1):181–186.
4. Piper, M.L., Delrosario, L., Hoffman, W.Y. Distraction osteogenesis of multiple ribs for the treatment of acquired thoracic dystrophy. *Pediatrics.* 2016;137(3):e20152053.
5. Jaroszewski, D.E., Notrica, D.M., McMahon, L.E., et al. Operative management of acquired thoracic dystrophy in adults after open pectus excavatum repair. *Ann Thorac Surg.* 2014;97(5):1764–1770.

Wickii T. Vigneswaran

Key Words
• Fibrous dysplasia • Aneurysmal bone cyst • Sternal tumor

Introduction

Primary chest wall tumors are often asymptomatic and can affect both the bone and the soft tissue. They can be malignant or benign, and diagnosis is made clinically due to a palpable mass and chest pain or when incidentally detected on imaging. Almost half of the chest wall tumors are benign and frequently encountered types are osteochondroma, chondroma, and fibrous dysplasia [1,2]. The common primary malignant tumors include chondrosarcoma, osteosarcoma, myeloma, and malignant lymphoma. Those affecting the sternum alone are rare. The treatment for cure is wide resection, but in practice, the inability to reconstruct large chest wall defects may compromise curative resection. Improvements in reconstruction techniques using musculocutaneous flaps for soft tissue coverage and titanium mesh and bars prosthetic material for rigid reinforcement make coverage of wide defects more reliable [3,4].

Case Report

A 48-year-old female was seeing a chiropractor for chest wall pain. The patient was lifting her elderly sick mom, who was bedridden, and felt she injured her chest cage. Initially "felt like the muscles were very tight under the breasts, right across". She went to see a chiropractor who made "some adjustments," and the discomfort went away. She was feeling well for almost six months, but it "flared-up" again causing pain in the left upper chest. She has seen her chiropractor weekly since, but it has been getting worse. It hurts when sneezing, bending forward, twisting, or when making any fast movement. It is "super tender" to touch, localized to the left-upper parasternal area. Taking Advil and icing helps. A diagnosis of costochondritis was made, and the chiropractor ordered a chest X-ray, which was reported normal.

The past medical history of the patient is significant and includes an ACL reconstruction 14 years previously, a salpingectomy for hydrosalpinx 13 years before, a needle biopsy of the left breast mass, which was negative for malignancy 12 years before. She is known to have a multinodular goiter.

On clinical exam, she was 1.645 meters tall, weighed 68.5 kg (BMI 25.32 kg/m^2). The pulse was regular at 67/min, blood pressure was 129/70 mmHg in the left arm and patient sitting, her oral temperature was 36.5°C, and her respiratory rate was 18/min. She was tender in the left parasternal area. No obvious masses.

At this point, a diagnosis of costochondritis was made, and she was treated with a lidocaine patch and referred for a possible cortisol injection. A CT scan was ordered during this visit.

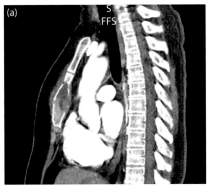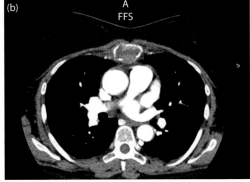

Figure 4.1 Preoperative CT scan. a) sagital and b) axial views

The CT scan revealed a heterogeneous lytic and soft tissue expansion of the sternum with cortical breakthrough posteriorly and anteriorly (Figure 4.1a,b). The report suggested that this is statistically most likely to represent metastatic disease, myeloma, or plasmacytoma. A percutaneous interventional radiology biopsy of this sternal lesion was ordered.

Core needle biopsy showed changes of the type seen in aneurysmal bone cyst, including proliferation of bland fibroblastic cells, osteoclastic giant cells, and streamers of an osteoid-like matrix. It was also reported that a spindle cell giant cell tumor could not be excluded. The appearances most likely represents a secondary aneurysmal bone cyst as much of this lesion shows radiographic features of fibrous dysplasia. However, areas of fibrous dysplasia were not present in the biopsy. An outside second opinion was requested and confirmed the diagnosis of aneurysmal bone cyst. The patient obtained an oncology consultation followed a thoracic surgery consultation. In view of the painful large sternal aneurysmal cyst, excision of the mass was recommended.

A transverse submammary skin incision was made, and the skin flaps with the pectoralis muscle and breast were raised to expose the sternum. A further assessment confirmed that the mass was occupying the whole body of the sternum. A lateral dissection was carried out on the ribs. Then the cartilage-rib junction was divided using a knife starting from the third to the sixth ribs on both sides. On the left-side, this was done more laterally as there was concern that the mass was extending laterally in this area. Using a sternal oscillating saw, the attachment to the xiphisternum and manubrium were divided. The mass was then removed (Figure 4.2). After mapping the defect on sterile paper, methyl methacrylate bone cement was used to create the body of the sternum, and titanium bars were used within the cement to create neo-ribs (Figure 4.3a–c). These three "ribs" were appropriately sized and sandwiched in the bone cement. Then the "ribs" were appropriately shaped to the contour. Then a sternal plate of a narrow "ladder" was chosen and screwed to the upper end of the prosthetic "sternum." This was then brought into the operative field, and after shaping the plate fit, the upper part of the plate was screwed to the manubrium. The neo-ribs #3, 4, and 5 were attached to the anterior ends of the patient's 3, 4, and 5 ribs using screws (Figure 4.4). With satisfactory reconstruction of the rigid wall, the right pleural space and the flaps were drained using separate size 16 Blake drains, which were connected to the pleura-vac drain. The flaps were approximated using "O" Vicryl and subcutaneous tissues with two "O" Vicryl and the skin with subcuticular sutures. The patient made an uneventful recovery and was discharged home on the third postoperative day.

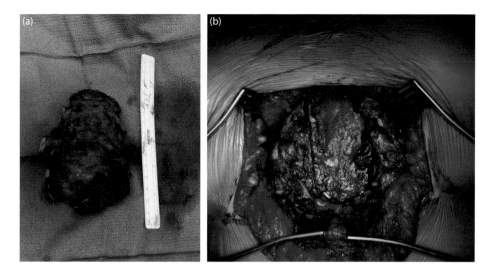

Figure 4.2 (a) Excised bone tumor. (b) Postresection bed

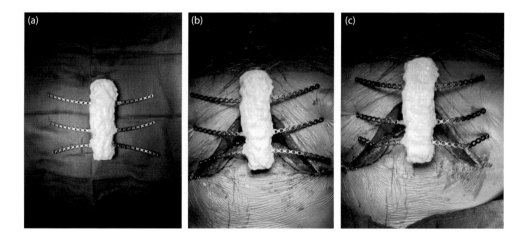

Figure 4.3 Construction of the prosthetic composite, methyl methacrylate, and titanium rib and sternal plates. a) methyl methyl methacrylate and rib composite allowed to set outside on the back table, b) in-situ c) titanium rib are bent to shape for plating

Resected sternal bone demonstrated an aneurysmal bone cyst, and focal adjacent regions showed features compatible with fibrous dysplasia (6.5 cm in maximum dimension). All inked soft tissue and bone margins were free of involvement. A single sternal lymph node showed areas of reactive sinus histiocytosis and focal fatty infiltration. There was no morphologic evidence of tissue-invasive fungal organisms, parasitic organisms, viral inclusions, epithelioid granulomas, or malignant neoplastic infiltrates.

During follow-up, the patient remained well and completed a 12-month follow-up without incident, but experienced occasional pinching pain with certain movements. She was doing clinically very well with excellent cosmetic outcome (Figure 4.5a,b).

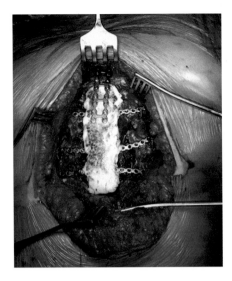

Figure 4.4 Prosthetic implantation completed

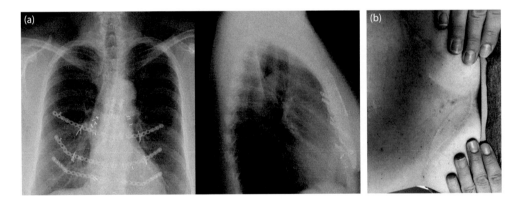

Figure 4.5 Postoperative appearance. a) Chest X-ray, b) healed appearance of incision

Comments

The three most common indications for chest wall resection and reconstructions are the primary lung cancer or recurrent lung cancer that invades the chest wall, primary chest wall tumors, and primary breast cancer with recurrence or metastasis to the chest wall [5]. When the tumor is invasive into the mediastinal structure, the sternectomy presents a major technical challenge. In these patients, the pulmonary status should be carefully evaluated to anticipate postoperative pulmonary complication. The risk of pulmonary complications are higher if associated with lung resection. If the mass is confined to the sternum, the issue following resection is the restoration of the structural integrity of the chest wall and satisfactory cosmetic results. Many synthetic materials such as polypropylene mesh, polyester mesh, polytetrafluoroethylene mesh, and expanded polytetrafluoroethylene mesh have been be used to reconstruct the chest wall defect. When it comes to the sternum, though, more rigid material is necessary for restoration of the structural integrity but also a protective shield is needed for the underlying heart. Methyl methacrylate can be used alone or incorporated between two layers of polypropylene mesh in a sandwich fashion to provide this desired feature. Methyl methacrylate is lightweight, versatile, with minimal cost, and penetrable by X-rays. Today, no consensus exists on which is the ideal prosthesis material and the optimal technique to reconstruct chest wall defects. The decision still remains the surgeon's choice. However, 3D printing technologies are currently available for titanium alloy, bringing a change in the strategy of chest wall reconstruction. Preoperative individualized modeling of the implant enables easy insertion and fixation of prosthesis. The 3D printing using the principles of biomimetics enables production of preoperative 3D-printed customized prosthesis [6]. If the cost can be contained, this would be an attractive approach as preoperative individualized modeling of the implant enables easy insertion and fixation, which reduces the operative time with excellent cosmetic outcome.

REFERENCES

1. Dahlin, D.C., Unni, K.K. *Bone Tumours: General Aspects and Data on 8,542 Case.* Springfield, IL, Charles C Thomas, 1986.
2. Martini, N., McCormack, P.M., Bains, M.S. Chest wall tumors: Clinical results of treatment. In Grillo, H.C. and Eschapasse, H., eds. *International Trends in General Thoracic Surgery.* Vol. 2. Major Challenges, Philadelphia, PA, Saunders, 1987, p. 285
3. Chapelier, A. Resection and reconstruction for primary sternal tumors. *Thorac Surg Clin.* 2010;20(4):529–534. doi:10.1016/j.thorsurg.2010.06.002
4. Zhang, Y., Li, J.Z., Hao, Y.J., Lu, X.C., Shi, H.L., Liu, Y., Zhang, P.F. Sternal tumor resection and reconstruction with titanium mesh: A preliminary study. *Orthop Surg.* 2015;7(2):155–60. doi:10.1111/os.12169
5. Mansour, K.A., Thourani, V.H., Losken, A., Reeves, J.G., Miller, J.I., Jr, Carlson, G.W., et al. Chest wall resection and reconstruction: A 25-year experience. *Ann Thorac Surg.* 2002;73:1720–1725. doi:10.1016/S0003-4975(02)03527-0.
6. Wen, X., Gao, S., Feng, J., Li, S., Gao, R., Zhang, G. Chest-wall reconstruction with a customized titanium-alloy prosthesis fabricated by 3D printing and rapid prototyping. *J Cardiothorac Surg.* 2018;13(1):4. doi:10.1186/s13019-017-0692-3.

Mathew Thomas

Key Words
• Sternoclavicular joint
• Osteomyelitis
• Septic arthritis, bone infection

Introduction

Septic arthritis involving the sternoclavicular joint (SCJ) is an uncommon but challenging problem to manage. We present the unusual case of a patient with spontaneous and recurrent infection of both SCJs that required multiple aggressive surgical debridement and resections before complete resolution.

Case Report

A 70-year-old white female presented to us for a second opinion regarding chronic sternoclavicular joint infection. Six months before her visit with us, she had developed right chest cellulitis after an episode of pneumonia. Although blood cultures were negative, she was treated with multiple antibiotics targeting methicillin-resistant *Staphylococcus aureus* (MRSA). Eventually, incision and drainage with resection of the right SCJ and partial manubriectomy were performed. Pathology was consistent with osteomyelitis, but tissue culture was negative. She was treated intermittently at different time periods with prolonged courses of intravenous vancomycin, linezolid, daptomycin, and doxycycline without relief. She was then referred to us. Her comorbidities included a history of hypertension, chronic obstructive pulmonary disease, multinodular goiter, Sjögren's syndrome, and recurrent shingles of the right neck.

At the time our initial evaluation, she complained mainly of right arm and shoulder pain. On examination, a chronic sinus in the right SCJ region (Figure 5.1a) with purulent greenish-colored drainage was seen. The rest of her examination was unremarkable. A computerized tomography (CT) scan of the chest showed evidence of chronic osteomyelitis of the right SCJ (Figure 5.2a).

We discussed radical debridement including resection of all the involved bone. She consented and underwent resection of the sinus tract along with the surrounding skin and soft tissues, down to the bone (Figure 5.1b–c). The right SCJ and right edge of the manubrium were resected completely, while the costochondral cartilages of the right first and second ribs were resected leaving the posterior perichondrium intact (Figure 5.1c). The wound was packed open and dressed twice daily with gauze soaked in a double antibiotic solution (DBS) containing bacitracin and polymyxcin B. A planned reexploration with further debridement and bone resection was performed two days later. The tissue culture grew methicillin-sensitive *Staphylococcus*

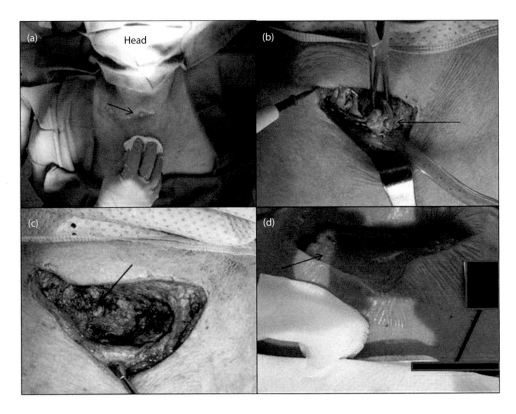

Figure 5.1 (a) and (b) Initial operative images showing chronic sinus tract (arrows) to the right SCJ. (c) Intraoperative image showing wound bed after initial operation following resection of right SCJ joint (arrow) and hemi-manubrium. (d) Wound bed prior to delayed primary closure after five months of NPWT showing good granulation tissue

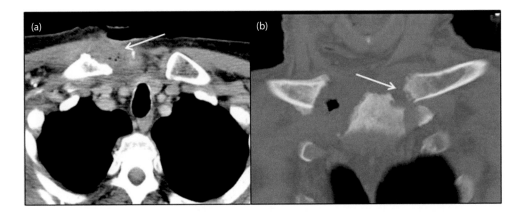

Figure 5.2 (a) CT scan showing initial osteomyelitis of the right SCJ (arrow); and (b) MRI scan showing subsequent infection of the left SCJ (arrow)

aureus. She was later discharged home with negative pressure wound therapy (NPWT) and intravenous (IV) antibiotics for about three months before discontinuing NPWT because of severe discomfort. One month later, she returned with swelling and redness of the contralateral SCJ. An MRI scan confirmed osteomyelitis and destruction of the left SCJ (Figure 5.2b). We performed another extended radical resection, removing the entire manubrium, medial one-third of both clavicles, and heads of both first ribs (Figure 5.3). The wound was left open and multiple reoperations for debridement were performed. Her cultures now grew *Pseudomonas aeruginosa.* A course of multiple IV antibiotics were given for eight weeks followed by oral antibiotics for three months. Soon after completing her antibiotics, her infection reoccurred and required surgical debridement. Her wound now measured 10 cm × 12 cm. Cultures now grew methicillin-resistant *Staphylococcus aureus* and IV antibiotics were resumed. NPWT was reinitiated and resulted in good granulation tissue after five months of therapy (Figure 5.1d) with shrinkage of the wound size, and the wound was closed primarily in a delayed manner. She then developed a deep venous thrombus in the right internal jugular vein and was started on anticoagulation. Two months after delayed primary closure was performed, she sustained a fall resulting in a hematoma over the right SCJ region and was found to have supratherapeutic international normalized ratio (INR > 8.0). This required reexploration, washout of the hematoma, and additional debridement. The wound was closed primarily, and a bulb drain was placed and removed a week later. Interestingly, the cultures from the hematoma showed *Candida glabrata*, but she recovered well.

The patient underwent a total of eight operations over a twelve-month period. Three years later, she remains without symptoms and is on chronic antibiotic suppression therapy with Bactrim.

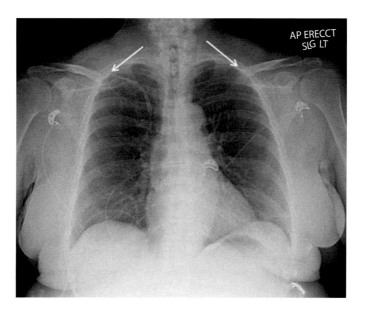

Figure 5.3 Postoperative chest X-ray at one year showing both clavicles with medial one-third resected (arrows)

Comments

Spontaneous SCJ infection is a rare condition likely caused by hematogenous spread of organisms from another source of infection. The risk factors for this infection include immunosuppression, central lines, trauma, and IV drug abuse [1], but it has also been reported to occur spontaneously in healthy adults. Although staphylococcus species appears to be the predominant organism [2], other kinds of pathogens have also been isolated from infected SCJs, and in some instances, superinfections with more than one organism may be present, as seen in our patient. The SCJ consists of not two but three bones, the manubrium, clavicle, and first rib, and as such has two capsules, one anterior and the other posterior. The reasons for the predisposition of the SCJ to infection is unclear but may be related to its composition of fibrocartilage rather than hyaline cartilage [3]. The typical presentation for spontaneous SCJ osteomyelitis is localized or diffuse upper chest wall pain [2], with tenderness and swelling over the affected joint; systemic manifestations may not be present in most patients.

SCJ infections can be quite difficult to manage due to the persistent but destructive process in a region of the chest wall that is in close proximity to the great vessels. The management typically involves systemic IV antibiotics along with radical debridement of all involved tissues including resection of the bone and cartilage [1]. The infection is localized in only a minority of patients and often involves the adjacent clavicle and sternum [1]; it can also spread to the adjacent lung and may lead to a lung abscess. The costoclavicular ligament between the first rib and clavicle maintains stability and prevents any significant disability after resection of the SCJ and medial aspect of the clavicle. The extent of the infection can be evaluated preoperatively either with CT or MRI scans to allow proper surgical planning.

Following debridement, a large anterior chest wall defect is typically left behind and different strategies have been used to manage the wound. These include immediate or delayed closure, either of which can be done with or without the use of a well-vascularized muscular flap (typically the pectoralis major) [2,4,5]. Delayed primary closure after NPWT appears to be a reasonable way to manage even large wounds as in our patient [4]. In most patients with such extensive open wound, a muscle flap closure would typically be required to close the defect. We deferred from using a muscle flap due to the recurrent nature of the infection, which made it important to preserve as much healthy tissue as possible for future contingencies. In a Cleveland Clinic retrospective study comparing patients who had primary closure with those who had delayed closure with NPWT [2], the authors noted that there was no difference in functional outcome between the two strategies and recurrences were similar. In a smaller study from Washington University by Puri et al., 10 patients who underwent immediate closure with flap after SCJ resection were compared with 10 others who had open wound care [4]. The open group had fewer wound complications and a shorter length of stay, but all required much longer wound care (median 12 weeks) when compared to the flap group. This is consistent with our experience.

In summary, SCJ infections are rare but are best managed with aggressive surgical debridement and systemic antibiotics. Primary or delayed closure strategies for the chest wall defect are both effective and should be tailored to the individual patient. If any doubt about possible recurrence or need for additional debridement is present, the open wound strategy with NPWT should be strongly considered.

REFERENCES

1. Kuhtin, O., Schmidt-Rohlfing, B., Dittrich, M., Lampl, L., Hohls, M., Haas, V. Treatment strategies for septic arthritis of the sternoclavicular joint. *Zentralbl Chir.* 2015;140 Suppl 1:S16–S21.

2. Kachala, S.S., D'Souza, D.M., Teixeira-Johnson, L., Murthy, S.C., Raja, S., Blackstone, E.H., et al. Surgical management of sternoclavicular joint infections. *Ann Thorac Surg.* 2016;101(6):2155–2160.

3. Schipper, P. and Tieu, B.H. Acute chest wall infections: Surgical site infections, necrotizing soft tissue infections, and sternoclavicular joint infection. *Thorac Surg Clin.* 2017;27(2):73–86.

4. Puri, V., Meyers, B.F., Kreisel, D., Patterson, G.A., Crabtree, T.D., Battafarano, R.J., et al. Sternoclavicular joint infection: A comparison of two surgical approaches. *Ann Thorac Surg.* 2011;91(1):257–261.

5. Al-Mufarrej, F., Martinez-Jorge, J., Carlsen, B.T., Saint-Cyr, M., Moran, S.L., Mardini, S. Use of the deltoid branch-based clavicular head of pectoralis major muscle flap in isolated sternoclavicular infections. *J Plast Reconstr Aesthet Surg.* 2013;66(12):1702–1711.

CASE 6: MALIGNANT SOLITARY FIBROUS TUMOR OF THE PLEURA

Amber Redmond, Eric P. Anderson, Christopher W. Seder, and Nicole M. Geissen

	Key Words
	• Malignant • Solitary fibrous tumor • Pleural-based mass

Introduction

Solitary fibrous tumors (SFTs) are rare neoplasms that arise from tissue with mesenchymal origin [1]. Although relatively rare, the number of patients being diagnosed with SFTs is on the rise. While the majority of SFTs arising from the pleura are benign, 13%–23% are classified as malignant [1]. After a complete resection, recurrence of a malignant solitary fibrous tumor (MSFT) has been reported as late as 16 years after initial presentation [2]. Given the unpredictable nature and variable clinical behavior of the disease, long-term surveillance after resection is recommended. This is a report of a 61-year-old female who presented with a left pleural-based mass with boney invasion found to have a MSFT of the pleura.

Case Report

A 61-year-old African American female, nonsmoker, with a history of hypertension, presented to the emergency department with a two-month history of worsening left shoulder pain. She denied recent trauma, chest wall pain, or constitutional symptoms. A chest X-ray was notable for a left-sided chest wall mass (Figure 6.1). A computed tomography (CT) scan of the chest was completed, and it showed a 39 mm × 48 mm hyperattenuating pleural-based mass with local osseous invasion of the left eighth rib (Figure 6.2). There was no evidence of axillary, mediastinal, or hilar lymphadenopathy.

The patient was admitted to the hospital for pain control. An ultrasound-guided fine needle aspiration (FNA) was completed with findings of an anechoic density with Doppler color flow consistent with vascularity. The aspirate had the appearance of liquefied hematoma, and cytology only revealed rare histiocytes. A nuclear medicine bone scan and CT scan of the abdomen and pelvis showed no evidence of distant disease.

With a nondiagnostic FNA, the patient was referred to thoracic surgery for surgical resection. Given the radiographic appearance, our differential diagnosis included schwannoma, sarcoma, hemangioma, and a solitary fibrous tumor of pleura. She was taken to the operating room for exploratory thoracoscopy. A vascular appearing mass was identified arising from the eighth intercostal space. The seventh and eighth intercostal arteries were directly entering the mass. The mass was excised with a circumferential rim of pleura. There was no obvious osseous invasion of the eighth rib. Final pathology demonstrated a 5.1 cm malignant

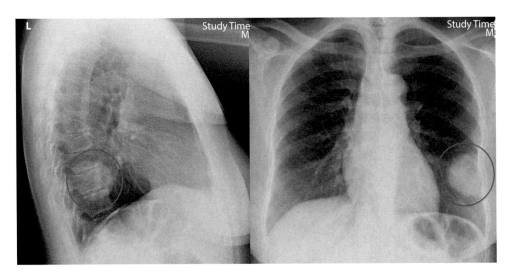

Figure 6.1 PA/Lateral CXR on presentation. Circle identifies the SFT

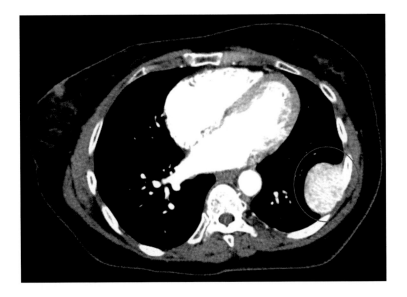

Figure 6.2 Axial cut of CT scan of the chest. Circle identifies the SFT as a parietal pleural-based lesion at the level of the left seventh and eighth ribs

solitary fibrous tumor with a mitotic index of 2–5 mitoses per 10 high-power field (hpf) and a focally-positive inked margin. There was no evidence of lymphovascular or perineural invasion. Final pathology was consistent with malignant solitary fibrous tumor of the pleura. Given the positive margin, a wide chest wall resection was performed of ribs 7 and 8, and a polytetrafluoroethylene mesh was used for reconstruction. Her postoperative course was uneventful. Surveillance will be initiated with a CT chest six months postoperatively.

Comments

The presentation, clinical features, clinical outcomes, and treatment of SFTs have largely been derived from case reports and retrospective studies. While our patient presented with vague symptoms of progressive shoulder pain, symptoms at the time of diagnosis of pleural SFTs are variable. Approximately 40%–60% of patients present with symptoms including cough, shortness of breath, or chest pain, with rare instances of hemoptysis or obstructive pneumonitis. SFTs may be associated with immune-mediated syndromes such as Bierre-Marie-Bamberger syndrome (hypertrophic pulmonary osteoarthropathy) and Doege–Potter syndrome (non-islet cell tumor hypoglycemia). The majority of pleural SFTs arise from the visceral pleura and have a pedicled stalk containing the vasculature. Parietal pleural-based tumors tend to have a broad-based sessile attachment.

On chest X-rays, SFTs of the pleura have a well-defined and rounded appearance, as seen in this case. CT imaging of the chest frequently demonstrates a well-circumscribed lesion arising from the pleura with displacement, rather than invasion, of surrounding structures. Magnetic resonance imaging (MRI) is usually not indicated in the workup of pleural-based SFTs. FNA rarely makes the diagnosis of SFTs due to inadequate cellularity of the specimen. Core needle biopsy may provide enough tissue to diagnose SFTs but may be inadequate to assess histopathologic high-risk tumor characteristics.

The surgeon must achieve negative margins when resecting SFTs from any location. An R0 resection of pleural-based SFTs is most often accomplished via a wedge resection of the lung but may require lobectomy, bilobectomy, pneumonectomy, chest wall resection, or diaphragm resection. There are no established guidelines for adjuvant radiation therapy or chemotherapy; however, generally no additional therapy is recommended if an R0 resection is achieved. Likewise, there are no established guidelines for adjuvant therapy for incompletely resected (R1 or R2) or recurrent SFTs. The use of adjuvant radiation therapy and/or chemotherapy in these instances should be considered on a case-by-case basis by a multidisciplinary team. In this patient, because an R0 resection was not achieved at the initial operation, she underwent reoperation with formal chest wall resection. There were no signs of residual tumor on the final pathology.

While pleural SFTs are generally benign and indolent in nature, 10%–25% recur locally or distantly. Findings associated with an increased risk of recurrence (malignant characteristics) include high mitotic index (≥4 mitosis per 10 hpf), necrosis, increased cellularity, nuclear pleomorphism, stromal or vascular invasion, or large tumor size (≥10 cm) [3–5]. Pleural-based SFTs are unique in that morphology (pedunculated vs. sessile) and derivation (visceral vs. parietal pleura) are predictive of the risk of recurrence. Sessile and parietal lesions are associated with a higher risk of recurrence. Our patient has several characteristics of an aggressive SFT with increased risk of recurrence, including a high mitotic index, sessile-based lesion, and derivation from the parietal pleura.

Several malignancy risk assessment algorithms have been published in the literature with regards to pleural SFTs. England et al. reviewed 223 cases of SFTs of the pleura that underwent resection [3]. Patients who had one or more of the following tumor characteristics, >4 mitoses/hpf, hypercellularity, pleomorphism, necrosis, hemorrhage, tumor size >10 cm, sessile lesion, or parietal pleural location, had a 55% risk of recurrence. If a patient's SFT had none of these characteristics, the risk or recurrence was 0%. De Perrot et al. proposed classifying pleural SFTs based on tumor characteristics (pedunculated vs. sessile/inverted tumors) and histologic risk factors (>4 mitoses/hpf, hypercellularity, pleomorphism, necrosis, and stromal/vascular invasion) [4]. Patients with pedunculated tumors without any histologic risk factors had a 2% recurrence rate; while sessile, or inverted, tumors and at least one histologic sign of malignancy had the highest recurrence rate at 63%. Finally, Tapias et al. proposed a scoring system for SFTs of the pleura composed of six factors (≥4 mitoses/hpf, hypercellularity, necrosis/hemorrhage, size >10 cm, sessile lesion, and parietal pleura origin) with a patient receiving one point for each factor that was present [5]. A score of ≥3 was considered high-risk for recurrence. Patients with low-risk SFTs had a risk of recurrence between 0% and 3.5%, while high-risk SFTs were associated with a 28%–77% recurrence rate.

There are no specific guidelines regarding the optimal timing or duration for surveillance. Based on a natural history of the lesion, long-term follow-up should be performed on all patients with SFTs, since even patients with low-risk features have been reported to have a recurrence over a decade after the initial operation. In general, patients with low-risk features can be followed annually with a CT chest, while patients with high-risk features should be followed with CT scans twice a year for the first 2–3 years and then annually thereafter. It is unclear if surveillance should be continued lifelong or discontinued after 10, 15, or 20 years.

REFERENCES

1. Langman, G. Solitary fibrous tumor: A pathological enigma and clinical dilemma. *J Thorac Dis.* 2011;3(2):86–87.
2. Gholami, S., Cassidy, M.R., Kirane, A., et al. Size and location are the most important risk factors for malignant behavior in resected solitary fibrous tumors. *Ann Surg Oncol.* 2017;24:3865.
3. England, D.M., Hochholzer, L., McCarthy, M.J. Localized benign and malignant fibrous tumors of the pleura. A clinicopathologic review of 223 cases. *Am J Surg Pathol.* 1989;13:640.
4. de Perrot, M., Fischer, S., Bründler, M.A., et al. Solitary fibrous tumors of the pleura. *Ann Thorac Surg.* 2002;74:285.
5. Tapias, L.F., Mino-Kenudson, M., Lee, H., et al. Risk factor analysis for the recurrence of resected solitary fibrous tumours of the pleura: A 33-year experience and proposal for a scoring system. *Eur J Cardiothorac Surg.* 2013;44:111.

Mathew Thomas

 Key Words

- Solitary fibrous tumors
- Pleura
- Chest wall

Introduction

Solitary fibrous tumors (SFTs) of the pleura are uncommon, slow growing tumors of mesenchymal origin that usually have a benign course. About up to 40% of these tumors may undergo malignant degeneration over time [1]. These tumors are often asymptomatic for years and can reach large sizes before being detected. In the majority of cases, SFTs are often well encapsulated and can be completely resected without major resection of adjacent structures. Chest wall invasion by SFTs is uncommon, and major resection of the chest wall for such cases has not been reported widely.

We report the case of a patient with a large malignant solitary fibrous tumor (MSFT) with chest wall and pericardial invasion, requiring extensive resection and reconstruction of the chest wall.

Case Report

A 41-year old female patient with an anterior mediastinal mass presented for a thoracic surgical opinion at our institution. Her symptoms started two years before when she first noted swelling and pain along the left side of her upper chest after a cat jumped on her. She was treated by her primary care doctor for costochondritis. Her pain persisted over the next year, leading to further workup with a chest X-ray and CT scan of the chest, which showed a large anterior mediastinal mass measuring 16 cm in the largest dimension. The CT scan showed displacement of the heart and compression of the left lung as well as a tumor invasion into the left half of the manubrium and the sternomanubrial junction. She then underwent an incisional biopsy through a left anterior thoracotomy in the third intercostal space (Chamberlain-McNeil approach) at her local hospital. Pathology revealed a SFT. She was treated at first with bevacizumab and temozolomide for about three months with no notable reduction in the size of the tumor. She was then referred to our hospital for further management. Her medical history included hemochromatosis for which she underwent phlebotomy every 2–3 months at her local Red Cross and was otherwise negative.

On our evaluation, she was stable hemodynamically and local examination of the chest wall revealed a well-healed 4 cm transverse incision overlying the second and third intercostal space along the left parasternal border. The pathology slides from the initial biopsy were reviewed at our institution and reported to be consistent with dedifferentiated SFT. An MRI

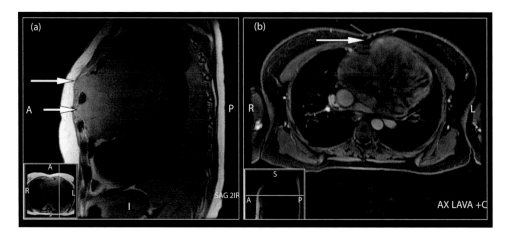

Figure 7.1 (a) Lateral and (b) Axial MRI scan views of the chest showing tumor invasion (arrows) through the upper left intercostal spaces

scan of the chest was obtained and showed tumor invasion of the anterior chest wall from the second and third intercostal spaces on the left side (Figure 7.1). The tumor also caused severe displacement of the heart and compression of the left lung.

After discussion at our multidisciplinary sarcoma tumor conference, radical resection was recommended to be followed by radiation therapy, depending on the success of resection.

The operation was performed under general anesthesia with a double-lumen tube placed for single lung ventilation. A transesophageal echocardiogram was performed and showed severe right ventricle outlet tract obstruction, including extrinsic narrowing of the pulmonary valve by the tumor. A large pericardial effusion was also present. The patient was positioned supine with both arms extended outwards at approximately 75 degrees and supported on well-padded arm boards. The entire chest and abdomen were sterilely prepared and draped.

First, an elliptical incision was made around the prior biopsy incision scar and carried down to the ribs with 2 cm wide margins around the biopsy tract. Next, through bilateral sub-mammary incisions connected in the midline, subpectoral flaps were raised to the level of the fourth intercostal space. Bilateral anterior thoracotomies were made at this level and connected via a transverse sternotomy after ligating both internal mammary vessels, thereby creating a clamshell thoracotomy.

On intraoperative examination (Figure 7.2), the tumor was confirmed to be compressing both the heart and the left lung, and it had focally invaded the left second–fourth sternocostal junctions. The pericardium was opened transversely above the diaphragm and laterally just anterior to both phrenic nerves with an energy sealing device (Harmonic Scalpel) to the level of semilunar valves, allowing the tumor to be lifted off the heart en-bloc with the anterior pericardium (Figure 7.3a). There was no evidence of invasion to the cardiac structures. The left second–fourth ribs were divided 3 cm lateral to the edge of the tumor, and an oscillating saw was used to resect the adjacent involved portion of the left hemisternum. The sessile tumor appeared to originate from the left upper lobe of the lung. The entire tumor with the resected chest wall, pericardium, and wedge of the left upper lobe were removed en-bloc (Figure 7.3b). Multiple random soft tissue biopsies were taken from around the perimeter

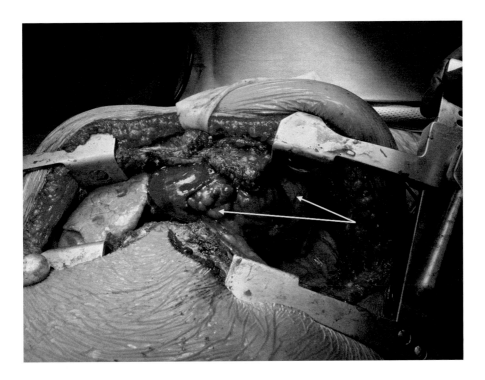

Figure 7.2 Intraoperative view of clamshell thoracotomy and anterior mediastinal tumor (arrows)

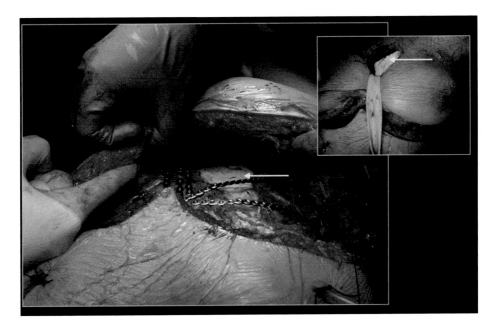

Figure 7.3 Intraoperative view of the reconstructed chest wall. The Gore-Tex patch (arrows) can be seen below the resected portion of the chest wall and through the superior defect created by resection of the prior incisional biopsy tract (inset picture)

of resection. The tumor was well encapsulated, except for the area on the anterior chest wall where it had invaded.

After placing bilateral chest tubes, the right thoracotomy portion of the clamshell incision was closed first with paracostal figure-of-eight non-absorbable braided sutures and one steel wire. Two long sternal plates (SternaLock Blu, Zimmer Biomet, USA) were then used to close the transverse sternotomy. A 2 mm thick Gore-Tex mesh measuring 10 mm × 15 mm was then placed as a taut underlay patch below the defect in the chest wall and anchored to the ribs and sternum using 0-0 non-absorbable braided sutures. Rib reconstruction plates (RibFix Blu, Zimmer Biomet, USA) were used to transfix the ends of the three divided ribs to the sternum for a rigid fixation (Figure 7.4). The pectoralis muscle and submammary incision were then closed in layers over the reconstructed chest wall. The resected biopsy tract was closed primarily.

After extubation in the operating room, the patient was observed in the ICU for three days and discharged home on day 6. Immunohistochemistry analysis on the surgical specimen showed: diffusely positive CD34; STAT6 was weakly positive in the subset of tumor cells; cytokeratin AE1/AE3 was positive with a patchy distribution; FISH for SS18 rearrangement was negative. These findings were consistent with dedifferentiated SFT. Because the margins of resection were close (<1 cm) to the ribs around the prior biopsy site, adjuvant radiation therapy was recommended. She underwent proton beam therapy to the anterior chest wall eight weeks later and continued to recover well.

She continued surveillance with CT scans of the chest abdomen and pelvis every 3 months. One year after her surgery, a small 5 mm nodule in the left-lower lobe was identified and showed continued growth to 7 mm. A uniportal video-assisted wedge resection of the nodule was performed after a CT-guided radiotracer localization, and pathology was consistent with metastatic SFT. She has had no evidence of further local or distant recurrence nine months after her second lung resection (Figure 7.5).

Comments

SFTs commonly arise from the visceral pleura and usually present with nonspecific symptoms or may be incidentally discovered in an asymptomatic patient [1]. They may not be discovered until they have achieved significant local growth and commonly tend to compress

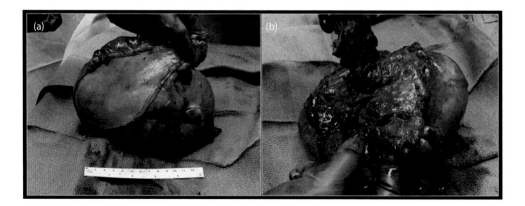

Figure 7.4 Gross views of the en-bloc surgical specimen showing: (a) Posterior surface of tumor with attached pericardium, and (b) Anterior surface with resected portion of chest wall and lung

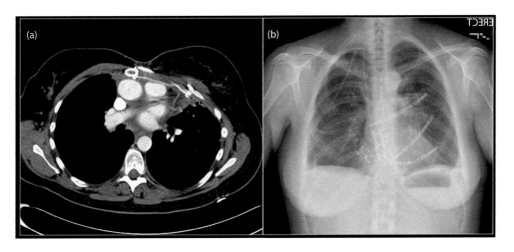

Figure 7.5 (a) CT scan-axial view and (b) Chest X-ray, at the two-year follow-up from surgery

rather than invade adjacent structures. Most SFTs are can be completely resected en-bloc, but local recurrence occurs in approximately 8%–16% of patients [2]. SFTs do not commonly invade the chest wall even when malignant degeneration is present. In a review of SFTs treated surgically over 30 years (1972–2002) at our institution, 13% (11/84) were malignant, but only 10.7% (9/84) of all SFTs required any kind of chest wall resection [3]. In another single institutional series of 157 patients with SFTs treated with surgical resection, only eight (5%) required chest wall resection [1].

MSFTs have a worse prognosis compared to benign SFTs and have been reported to have a local recurrence rate of above 60% after excision. Okike et al. reported a 12% long-term survival rate for MSFTs after resection [4], and in our institutional experience, the 5-year survival for MSFTs was 45.5% compared to 88.9% for benign SFTs [3]. De Perrot et al. classified SFTs according to tumor characteristics and prognosis as: (1) benign pedunculated tumors, 2% recurrence rate; (2) benign sessile tumors, 8% recurrence rate; (3) malignant pedunculated tumors, 14% recurrence rate; and (4) malignant sessile tumors, 63% recurrence rate and a 30% mortality, with most deaths occurring within 24 months [5].

Benign SFTs cannot be accurately differentiated from MFSTs based on radiographic imaging or percutaneous biopsies [6,7]. The role of a fluorodeoxyglucose (FDG)-positron emission tomography (PET) scan in the diagnosis and management of SFTs is not clear since these tumors are often not PET positive but may show some hypermetabolic activity with malignant degeneration [8]. In most cases where SFT has been diagnosed from radiographic imaging, tissue biopsies do not change the management and can be avoided since surgery is the standard of care for both benign and malignant SFTs. If tissue diagnosis is essential, core-needle biopsies should be considered rather than fine needle aspiration. Due to the risk of local recurrence, surgical biopsy of an intrathoracic mass suspected to be an SFT should be carefully planned in such a way to allow subsequent resection of the incision scar and tract.

Referral to a center with expertise in surgical management of complex intrathoracic tumors should be strongly considered before precluding surgery as a treatment modality. Tumor size does not appear to be related to survival if complete en-bloc resection can be performed [1].

We have found MRI scans with contrast useful in assessing resectability of large tumors of the chest, especially when vascular invasion is suspected. Although there is no supporting evidence, in our opinion, SFTs invading the chest wall should be managed as low-grade primary tumors of the chest wall, and resection should aim for wide negative margins (at least 2 cm) when possible due to the high risk of local recurrence. Complex reconstruction of the chest wall using a combination of techniques, as in our patient, may be required after resection.

The role of neoadjuvant and adjuvant chemotherapy or radiation in the management of SFTs is unclear but appears limited. Radiation therapy for incompletely resected tumors or close surgical margins has been suggested without strong evidence to support its use [7]. Proton therapy is a newer modality of delivering radiation therapy and has not been described in the treatment of SFTs of the chest before. The toxicity of proton beam therapy is reported to be less than conventional radiation therapy, thus making it more suitable to treat post-resection fields involving mediastinal and lung tissue [9].

Due to the potential for local recurrence in the long-term, monitoring with radiographic imaging should continue for at least 10 years and possibly up to 15 years after resection of SFTs.

REFERENCES

1. Lahon, B., Mercier, O., Fadel, E., et al. Solitary fibrous tumor of the pleura: Outcomes of 157 complete resections in a single center. *Ann Thorac Surg*. 2012;94(2):394–400.
2. Tapias, L.F., Mercier, O., Ghigna, M.R., et al. Validation of a scoring system to predict recurrence of resected solitary fibrous tumors of the pleura. *Chest*. 2015;147(1):216–223.
3. Harrison-Phipps, K.M., Nichols, F.C., Schleck, C.D., et al. Solitary fibrous tumors of the pleura: Results of surgical treatment and long-term prognosis. *J Thorac Cardiovasc Surg*. 2009;138(1):19–25.
4. Okike, N., Bernatz, P.E., Woolner, L.B. Localized mesothelioma of the pleura: Benign and malignant variants. *J Thorac Cardiovasc Surg*. 1978;75(3):363–372.
5. de Perrot, M., Fischer, S., Brundler, M.A., Sekine, Y., Keshavjee, S. Solitary fibrous tumors of the pleura. *Ann Thorac Surg*. 2002;74(1):285–293.
6. Gupta, A., Souza, C.A., Sekhon, H.S., et al. Solitary fibrous tumour of pleura: CT differentiation of benign and malignant types. *Clin Radiol*. 2017;72(9):796.e9–796.e17.
7. Saynak, M., Veeramachaneni, N.K., Hubbs, J.L., Okumus, D., Marks, L.B. Solitary fibrous tumors of chest: Another look with the oncologic perspective. *Balkan Med J*. 2017;34(3):188–199.
8. Yeom, Y.K., Kim, M.Y., Lee, H.J., Kim, S.S. Solitary fibrous tumors of pleura of the thorax: CT and FDG PET characteristics in a tertiary referral center. *Medicine (Baltimore)*. 2015;94(38):e1548.
9. Hoppe, B.S., Flampouri, S., Henderson, R.H., et al. Proton therapy with concurrent chemotherapy for non-small-cell lung cancer: Technique and early results. *Clin Lung Cancer*. 2012;13(5):352–358.

Raed Abdulkareem and Francis J. Podbielski

Key Words
• Empyema • Nephrostomy • Case report

Introduction

Empyema is defined as an accumulation of purulent fluid in the pleural space and is most commonly secondary to pneumonia or a lung abscess. Empyema can however arise in other conditions as well. In this case report, we discuss the development of an empyema due to percutaneous nephrostomy tube placement. In this instance, the nephrostomy tube was found to be traversing the pleural space and diaphragm resulting in bacterial tracking from a chronically infected kidney into the pleural space with resultant empyema. Nephrostomy tube placement is a common procedure employed to manage several different types of ureteral obstruction. Complications of nephrostomy tube placement are rare and most commonly include bleeding, sepsis, organ injury, and death. Multiple reports appear in the literature describing these complications, but based on our literature review, no other cases were found in which a nephrostomy tube traversing the thoracic cavity en route to the kidney resulted in an empyema.

Case Report

A 64-year-old male with a history of stage 4 chronic kidney disease, hypertension, type 2 diabetes, multiple urinary tract infections, and obstructive uropathy of the left ureteropelvic junction, for which pyeloplasty, endopyelotomy, and ureteral metal stent, which was placed eleven months ago and last exchanged two months ago, presented to us three weeks after this tube exchange with worsening renal function beyond his chronic kidney disease. A renal ultrasound showed worsening hydronephrosis of the left kidney, for which a left nephrostomy tube was placed by the interventional radiology service. Five weeks later, he was admitted with complaints of general malaise, fever, and chills. He was noted to have gross hematuria, back pain, and exertional dyspnea; he reported left-sided pleuritic chest pain.

Physical examination revealed a patient in moderate distress secondary to fever and an increased oxygen requirement. His breath sounds were diminished on the left, and there was gross blood draining from the nephrostomy tube. His blood urea nitrogen level and creatinine levels were elevated at 87 and 4.5 mg/dL, respectively, with a potassium level of 5.3 mEq/L and a white blood cell count of 13.9 K. Urinalysis was consistent with a urinary tract infection; thus, intravenous piperacillin/tazobactam was started.

A chest radiograph showed a large left-sided pleural effusion (Figure 8.1a), for which the pulmonary medicine service was consulted and a size 18 French left-sided chest tube placed

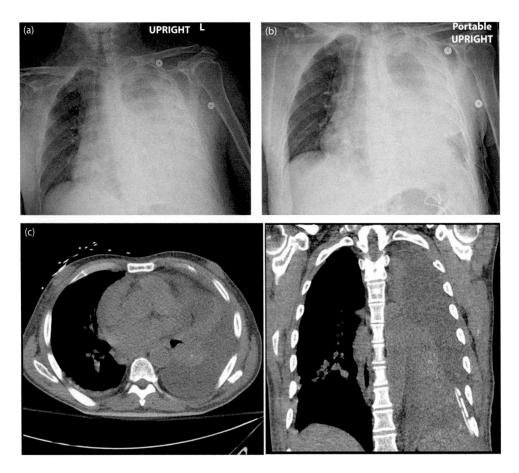

Figure 8.1 (a) Initial chest X-ray shows large left sided pleural effusion. (b) Post-chest tube placement imaging shows a persistent, large left-sided pleural effusion. (c) CT scan of the chest revealed a large left-sided pleural effusion with loculations

with drainage of 150 mL of serosanguinous fluid; there was minimal improvement on the post-procedure chest radiograph (Figure 8.1b). Given the suspicion for an underlying loculated pleural effusion, a CT scan of the chest was performed, which demonstrated a persistent moderate-sized loculated pleural effusion (Figure 8.1c).

The thoracic surgery service was consulted and upon evaluation elected to proceed with a left-sided video-assisted thoracoscopy. Upon entry to the thorax via a small incision above sixth rib at midaxillary line, an extensive yellowish-green fibrinopurulent coating over the entire surface of the left lung was found, most dense over the lower lobe and lingula. A second entry site was created in the posterior axillary line above the seventh rib, and from this site, we drained approximately 400 mL of effusion fluid. A portion of the fluid was sent for culture, and another portion for cytological examination. The empyema was definitively drained, and the surface of the lung decorticated. We were able to completely free the lung, with special attention to debridement of fluid from the left costophrenic angle. In that area, we discovered that the nephrostomy tube traversed the thorax proper for a short distance before diving into the diaphragm (Figure 8.2a and 8.2b). The nephrostomy tube was left in

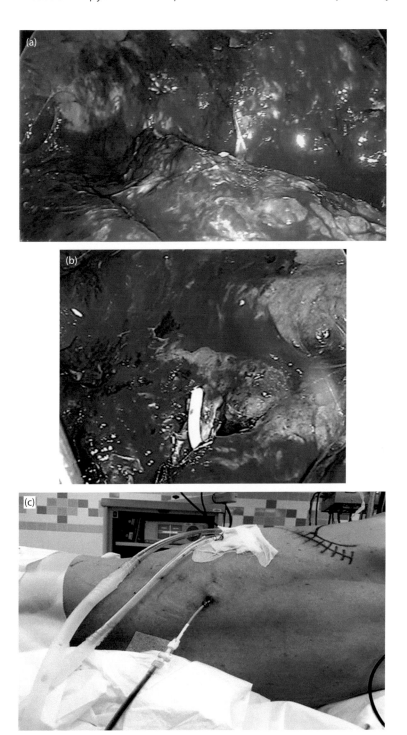

Figure 8.2 (a) Empyema observed in the upper chest. (b) Depicting the nephrostomy tube coming into the chest wall and piercing the diaphragm. (c) Left nephrostomy tube and chest tubes

place as the interventional radiology service was planning for tube removal and replacement through a separate location at the conclusion of our operative procedure. Two 28-French chest tubes were placed (Figure 8.2c).

The postoperative course was uneventful with the patient defervescing and feeling better. White blood cell count normalized to 9.4 K, and the patient returned to room air oxygen on postoperative day 2. Anterior and posterior chest tubes were removed on postoperative day 2 and 3, respectively. A chest radiograph after the chest tube removal showed marked improvement (Figure 8.3).

Comments

Urinothorax and nephropleural fistula have been reported soon after placement or removal of percutaneous nephrostomy tubes [1,2]; this complication usually resolved after simple thoracentesis or serial thoracenteses [3]. A similar case from our review is presented by Kumar et al., who described a patient who underwent percutaneous nephrolithotomy (PCNL) for the removal of kidney stones [4]. Thus, to our knowledge, the case presented here in our report is the first of its kind to be reported.

Interestingly, the pleural fluid collected during this Video Assisted Thoracoscopyic Surgery (VATS) procedure was negative on culture. A large cohort trial reported in the *American Journal of Respiratory and Critical Care Medicine* stated that negative cultures occur in approximately 42% (184 of 434) cases of thoracic empyema. In addition, the study also noted that 77 patients received antibiotics before pleural fluid sampling, and the culture was negative in 47 (61%) of these patients [5]. Similarly, our patient had received intravenous piperacillin-tazobactam for three days prior to the time of his VATS procedure.

Other studies have shown even lower yields of bacteria when pleural fluid is cultured. Jimenez et al., in a series 259 patients with a parapneumonic effusion, found that the pleural fluid

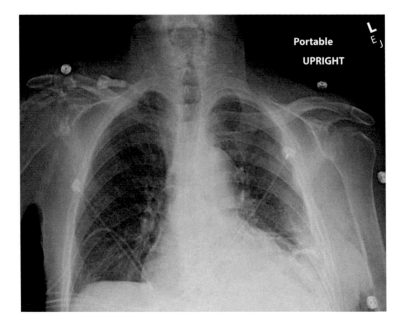

Figure 8.3 Chest radiograph after removal of chest tubes, postoperative day 4

culture revealed bacterial pathogens in only 50 (19.3%) of the cases [6]. Similarly, Po and colleagues demonstrated that a bacterial cause for the parapneumonic effusion was not found in 66 out of 91 cases [7]. Also, Wait et al. showed that 8 out of 20 loculated pleural effusions were negative for bacterial growth [8]. Thus, although one would expect to identify a bacterial etiology for an empyema, multiple sources show that a bacterial source is often elusive.

At the time of initial presentation, the patient had a urinary tract infection that was treated with antibiotics; prior to the VATS procedure a repeat urine culture was negative. Thus, a negative culture from the empyema fluid is not surprising.

This unusual case in which the nephrostomy tube actually traversed the chest proper a short distance before diving into the diaphragm and to the left kidney illustrates a rare complication. The tube provided a portal from the renal hilum to the thorax, which eventually led to an empyema. A high index of suspicion is warranted from the practitioner to aid in making the diagnosis.

REFERENCES

1. Toubes, M.E., Lama, A., Ferreiro, L., Golpe, A., Álvarez-Dobaño, J.M., González-Barcala, F.J., San José, E., et al. Urinothorax: A systematic review. *J Thorac Dis.* 2017; 9(5):1209–1218. doi:10.21037/jtd.2017.04.22.
2. Batura, D., Haylock-Vize, P., Naji, Y., Tennant, R., Fawcett, K. Management of iatrogenic urinothorax following ultrasound guided percutaneous nephrostomy. *J Radiol Case Rep.* 2014;8(1):34–40. doi:10.3941/jrcr.v8i1.1424.
3. Deel, S., Robinette, E., Jr. Urinothorax: A rapidly accumulating transudative pleural effusion in a 64-year-old man. *South Med J.* 2007;100(5):519–521.
4. Kumar, S., Gautam, S., Kumar, S., Rai, A. Chronic empyema thoracis after percutaneous nephrolithotomy. *BMJ Case Reports.* 2014;pii: bcr2014203637. doi: 10.1136/bcr-2014-203637.
5. Maskell, N.A., Batt, S., Hedley, E.L., Davies, C.W., Gillespie, S.H., Davies, R.J. The bacteriology of pleural infection by genetic and standard methods and its mortality significance. *Am J Respir Crit Care Med.* 2006;174(7):817–823.
6. Jimenez, D., Diaz, G., Garcia-Rull, S., Vidal, R., Sueiro, A., Light, R.W. Routine use of pleural fluid cultures. Are they indicated? Limited yield, minimal impact on treatment decisions. *Respir Med.* 2006;100(11):2048–2052.
7. Poe, R.H., Marin, M.G., Israel, R.H., Kallay, M.C. Utility of pleural fluid analysis in predicting tube thoracostomy/decortication in parapneumonic effusions. *Chest.* 1991;100(4):963–967.
8. Wait, M.A., Sharma, S., Hohn, J., Dal Nogare, A. A randomized trial of empyema therapy. *Chest.* 1997;111(6):1548–1551.

Evgeny V. Arshava, Adnan Al Ayoubi, and Kalpaj R. Parekh

 Key Words
- Solitary fibrous tumor of the pleura
- Doege–Potter syndrome
- Paraneoplastic hypoglycemia

Introduction

Malignant solitary fibrous tumors (MSFTs) are rare neoplasms and account for less than 5% of all the tumors arising from the pleura. Their surgical management may be difficult due to the large size at the time of the diagnosis and tendency for local recurrence. Noninsulin mediated paraneoplastic hypoglycemia (NIMH) and Doege–Potter syndrome may be rarely associated with MSFT cases.

Case Report

A 72-year-old male with an unremarkable past medical history initially presented with an altered mental status of a two-week duration secondary to new-onset hypoglycemia (serum glucose level as low as 35 mg/dL) complicated by seizures. The patient reported 12 kg weight loss over the preceding three months. The patient was a former heavy smoker (100 pack-years) with no other relevant environmental exposure. Physical examination was only remarkable for deceased breath sounds on the left and by clubbing of the fingers.

During the workup, the chest radiograph (CXR) revealed prominent opacity of the left lower chest. Chest computed tomography (CT) demonstrated 17 × 13.5 × 11 cm heterogenous mass of the left posterior pleura (Figure 9.1). While the mass effect resulted in compressive atelectasis of the adjacent lung, there was no evidence of invasion of the mass into the mediastinum or chest wall. Positron emission tomography (PET CT) showed a diffuse mild uptake of fluorodeoxyglucose (FDG) in the known large, left pleural-based mass with no evidence of metastatic disease.

The thoracentesis yielded 700 mL of serous fluid, which was negative for malignant cells on cytology. Percutaneous needle biopsy on pathology was interpreted as an epithelioid to spindle cell neoplasm consistent with solitary fibrous tumor (SFT). Immunohistochemical stains of the neoplastic cells were strongly positive for STAT6, BCL2, beta-catenin, and vimentin expression. Stains were negative for CK-OSCAR, EMA, S100, CD34, TLE-1, actin, and calretinin.

Due to intractable hypoglycemia, the patient required intravenous therapy with 10% dextrose with resolution of the mental status changes. An endocrine workup was performed with the following serum levels found: insulin 0.1 units/mL (reference range [RR] 1.9–23), proinsulin 1.6 pMole/L (RR 0–10), C-peptide 0.21 ng/mL (RR 0.78–5.19), IGF-1 159 ng/mL

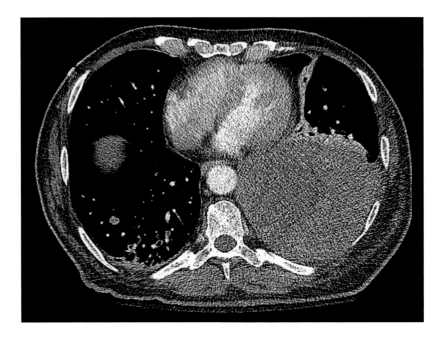

Figure 9.1 CT scan of the chest showing 17 × 13.5 × 11 cm mass (SFT) without chest wall or mediastinal invasion (arrow indicates the feeding vessels)

(RR 36–215), and IGF-2 670 ng/mL (ref range 333–967). The patient's hypoglycemia was felt to be secondary to a noninsulin-mediated paraneoplastic Doege–Potter syndrome.

After an appropriate workup, in several days the patient underwent semi-urgent resection of the mass. The operation was performed under general endotracheal anesthesia with a double-lumen endotracheal tube for selective lung ventilation. An epidural catheter was placed preoperatively. The operation was performed via a generous posterolateral thoracotomy. A multilobulated tumor was excised en-bloc with the left lower lobe wedge. The mass originated on an approximately 5 × 5 cm area of the parietal pleura on the lateral chest wall. This pedicle had prominent vascular collaterals in the extrapleural plane perfusing the tumor (Figure 9.2). Frozen sections on the residual extrapleural tissues in the areas of attachments were negative for tumor. Thorough exploration of the chest was performed. The discrete 8 mm nodule in the area of the apex was resected and on frozen section was consistent with a similar SFT. Mediastinal lymph nodes were resected and were negative on frozen section for malignancy.

Pathology of the resected specimen confirmed the core-needle biopsy, demonstrating an SFT that was 17 cm in its largest dimension (Figure 9.3). On immunohistochemistry, the tumor had a diffuse nuclear STAT6 expression. The tumor was considered malignant given its high mitotic rate (12/10 high-power field), presence of necrosis, and only weak variable expression of CD34 (Figure 9.4a and b). All surgical margins were uninvolved by the tumor 0.1 cm from the closest (pleural base) margin.

The patient had an uncomplicated postoperative course with prompt resolution of hypoglycemia on postoperative day 1, and he was discharged on postoperative day 8. At the one-year follow-up, the patient had no recurrent symptoms of hypoglycemia. A CT scan of the chest demonstrated no evidence of recurrent disease.

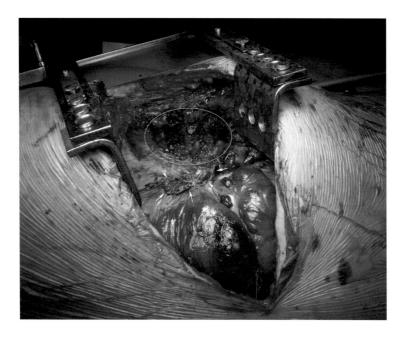

Figure 9.2 Intraoperative photograph demonstrating extrapleural dissection of the tumor base. (Arrows mark the base on the pedicle and the circle indicates the margin of the pleural resection)

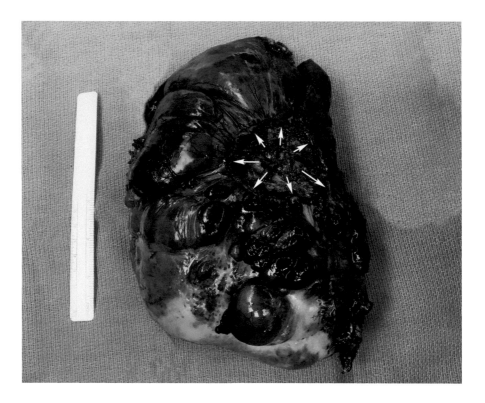

Figure 9.3 Resected surgical specimen showing pedunculated, multiloculated tumor with fibrous pseudocapsule. Arrows mark the extrapleural base

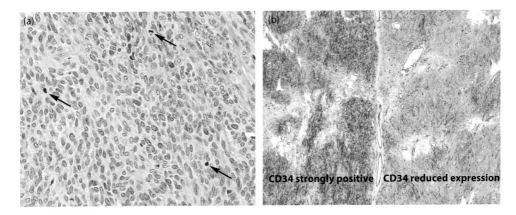

Figure 9.4 (a) Histological slide with a hematoxylin and eosin stain and magnification of 400 (1 high-power field) demonstrates a cellular spindle cell tumor with an increased mitotic activity (marked with arrows). (b) Heterogenous CD34 expression on a single immunohistochemistry slide of the resected tumor, with strongly positive staining in the left half of the field and reduced staining in the right half. (Courtesy of Andrew M. Bellizzi.)

Comments

SFTs comprise the spectrum of rare fibroblastic mesenchymal neoplasms that may arise on serosal membranes throughout the body, including chest, abdomen, brain, and soft tissues; they rarely metastasize [1]. While the exact incidence is hard to estimate, pleuropulmonary solitary fibrous tumors (PSFT) account for approximately 30% of this spectrum, while accounting for only less than 5% of all pleural-based tumors. Up until 2017, only approximately 1000 cases have been reported in the literature. PSFTs are equally distributed in males and females with the fifth decade as the medium age at diagnosis [2].

Tumors may be asymptomatic in almost half of patients at the time of diagnosis. Slow growth and an indolent course may allow tumors to reach a very large size before the diagnosis is made; this is related to their slow growth. Intrathoracic symptoms arise to mass effect or invasion and include dyspnea, chest pain, cough, and hemoptysis. Systemic symptoms may include hypoglycemia, hypertrophic osteoarthropathy (digital clubbing), weight loss, and fatigue.

NIMH in the setting of PSFT, or Doege–Potter syndrome, is present in <5% of cases of SFTs and is the result of the tumor-secreting insulin-like growth factors (IGF) 2. In NIMH, the serum levels of insulin, C-peptide, and IGF 1 are usually decreased or undetectable. In some cases, total IGF 2 level may be increased, decreased, or normal. Many IGF 2 proteins have a higher molecular weight ("big" IGF) and are not detectable by conventional immunometric assay. In such cases, including ours, while both IGF 1 and total IGF 2 may be within the reference range, the relative excess of IGF 2 over IGF 1 can bind insulin receptors and lead to hypoglycemia [3].

While PSFT were originally described in 1870 by Wagner as a "localized pleural mesothelioma," their nomenclature has changed multiple times. They have been called localized fibrous tumors, fibrous mesotheliomas, pleural fibromas, and submesothelial fibromas.

This reflected initial uncertainty about the origins of the cells. SFTs originate from the pluripotent submesothelial mesenchymal cells.

Grossly, SFTs range in size from a few centimeters to giant sizes of over 40 cm. Tumors are usually well circumscribed and surrounded by a fibrous pseudocapsule or serosal lining. Tumors are sessile, or less commonly pedunculated, and have a base that contains larger feeder vessels.

While several histologic subtypes exist, intersecting fascicles composed of bland spindle cells and thick bands of collagen, in a so-called randomly distributed "patternless pattern," are characteristic features of SFTs (a review of several slides may be required to establish this pattern). Immunohistochemistry markers CD34, Bcl2, CD99, and vimentin may be inconsistently expressed, which may lead to some difficulties in establishing the diagnosis in cases with non-classical histology. Actin, desmin, S100 protein, and epithelial markers are negative. Genetically, SFTs are characterized by a translocation and resultant fusion of the NGFI-A binding protein 2 gene (NAB2) to the signal transducer and activator of transcription 6 gene (STAT6) [4]. Thus, nuclear STAT6 expression is generally specific for SFTs.

The radiographic differential diagnosis for PSFT is broad and depends on the location of the mass. Radiograms may alert about the existence of the mass but are nonspecific. CT is the main imaging modality to characterize location, size, and relationship to adjacent structures. Characteristically, CT demonstrates well-defined and occasionally a lobulated mass of soft tissue density. PET typically shows mild diffuse uptake and an absence of distant metastasis. Magnetic resonance imaging may help to characterize involvement of the diaphragm and spine in certain cases, but otherwise it is rarely useful.

Pleural masses need to be differentiated from extrapleural hematomas and loculated pleural effusions, pleural metastases, sarcomatoid mesothelioma, and lymphoma. Intralobar fissure masses need to be differentiated from pulmonary carcinoma, carcinoid, and hamartomas. Thymic epithelial neoplasm, sarcomas, and peripheral nerve sheath tumors need to be considered in the mediastinum.

Fine-needle aspiration biopsies are often inadequately cellular and are not recommended for diagnosis. In most cases, core biopsy will provide diagnostic material to establish a diagnosis of SFT, but the limited sampling provided by core biopsy may not accurately demonstrate the histologic evidence indicative of high risk for aggressive behavior.

Biological behavior of these tumors is highly variable, and some tumors show malignant behavior leading to recurrence and/or metastasis. OF these tumors, 15%–20% demonstrate malignant behavior with a tendency to local recurrence and metastases. Malignant behavior is predicted by high mitotic rate (>4 mitoses/10 HPFs), increased pleomorphism (including nuclear size, irregularity, and prominence), high cellularity, hemorrhage and necrosis, stromal or vascular invasion, and a tumor of a size of >10 cm. Loss or reduction of CD34 expression correlates with an aggressive behavior in SFT (Figure 9.4b). Conversion of CD34-positive into CD34-negative tumors is related to malignant transformation.

Although increased expression of Ki-67 protein (a cellular marker for proliferation) has been proposed as an indicator for malignant behavior, at present there are no distinct molecular characteristics that clearly differentiate benign from malignant tumors.

Surgical resection remains the single effective treatment for the management of these tumors. Depending on the size and location of the tumor, posterolateral, clamshell thoracotomy, or sternotomy may be utilized. A video-thoracoscopic approach may be used for very small pedunculated tumors.

The principle of SFT surgery is en-bloc resection with a 1–2 cm margin for malignant variants. Such margins may be hard to obtain in the chest without major morbidity, especially for tumors near the apex, mediastinum, or diaphragm. Tumors abating the chest wall should be excised in an extrapleural plane. Adherent lung can be resected as a non-anatomic wedge resection, lobectomy, or even pneumonectomy. Occasionally, diaphragmatic or chest wall resection may be necessary. Intraoperative frozen section of the residual chest wall tissues may be helpful to assure complete (R0) resection of the tumor.

Currently, there is no data to recommend radiation or chemotherapy as adjuvant modalities for the treatment of SFT. Use of radiation therapy or chemotherapy can be considered on a case-by-case basis for patients with incompletely resected tumors, as their benefits are very controversial. Molecular agents targeting the tyrosine kinases signaling pathway that are under investigation for the treatment of SFTs include tyrosine kinase pathway inhibitors (Sunitinib, Sorafenib, Pazopanib) and are currently limited to clinical trials.

Due to the rarity of the disease, there are no established guidelines for the optimal frequency and duration of post-treatment surveillance. While up to 25% of the tumors recur at 10 years after the initial operation, the median time to recurrence may exceed 10 years, and late recurrences up to 20 years after initial treatment have been described as well.

Positive resection margins increase the rate of recurrence. Invasion of the chest wall and malignant effusion may additionally increase the risk for disease recurrence. Late recurrences even for tumors that were initially classified as benign may occur. Pathologically confirmed cases of malignant transformation of initially benign tumors have been reported as well. Recurrences carry poor prognosis and are often associated with invasion of adjacent structures.

Several prediction models have been described by de Perro, Demicco, Tapias, and Salas for risk stratification of SFTs. Different existing systems may have different ability to predict the overall and progression-free survival [5]. Overall, these models provide comparable data, indicating that a worse prognosis is predicted by the age of 55 years and above, unfavorable histology (as described above), increasing size of the tumor (usually above 10 cm), sessile shape, and metastatic and multifocal disease at presentation. Overall, analysis of patient outcomes is complicated by the rarity of these tumors.

While progression-free survival can be predicted in excess of 80% at 20 years for low-risk tumors, it may approach 50% at 5 years in high-risk tumors, as is overall survival. Prolonged survival after a SFT recurrence is possible, especially in those patients who can undergo resection. In cases of multiple synchronous metastases not amenable to resection, patients have very poor prognosis.

Follow-up of high-risk patients requires regular imaging of the chest at 6–12 month intervals. While no uniformly accepted guidelines exist, low-risk patients should be followed for up to 10 years, and higher-risk patient up to 20 years. With long-term follow-up, chest radiographs may be used in place of CT scans to decrease the overall risk of radiation exposure.

REFERENCES

1. de Perrot, M., Fischer, S., Brundler, M.A., Sekine, Y., Keshavjee, S. Solitary fibrous tumors of the pleura. *Ann Thorac Surg.* 2002;74:285–293.
2. Tapias, L. et al. Validation of a scoring system to predict recurrence of resected solitary fibrous tumors of the pleura. *Chest.* 2015;147(1):216–223.
3. Dutta, P. et al. Non-islet cell tumor-induced hypoglycemia: A report of five cases and brief review of the literature. *Endocrinol Diabetes Metab Case Rep.* 2013;2013:130046.
4. Chmielecki, J. et al. *Nat Genet.* 2013;45:131–132.
5. Reisenauer, J.S. et al. Comparison of risk stratification models to predict recurrence and survival in pleuropulmonary solitary fibrous tumor. *J Thorac Oncol.* 2018;13(9):1349–1362.

Raed Abdulkareem and Francis J. Podbielski

Key Words
• Empyema • Laproscopy • Appendectomy

Introduction

An appendectomy is one of the most commonly performed surgical procedures in the United States. As the primary treatment for acute appendicitis, most of these procedures are now performed laparoscopically. Complications most commonly include surgical wound infections, intra-abdominal abscess formation, and rarely thoracic empyema. In this case, we report a patient who developed a right thoracic empyema approximately six weeks after undergoing a laparoscopic appendectomy in treatment of a perforated appendicitis. At the time of thoracoscopy, particulate fecal material was identified in the thoracic cavity that appeared to have entered through a small defect in the diaphragm.

While most commonly secondary to pneumonia or a lung abscess, thoracic empyema can arise in other clinical conditions as well. Empyema after appendectomy has been previously described. This case discusses not only the development of empyema several weeks after a laparoscopic appendectomy, but the actual presence of fecal material inside the pleural cavity upon performing video-assisted thoracoscopy for the presumptive diagnosis of empyema.

Case Report

The patient is a 71-year-old male with past medical history remarkable for coronary artery disease, hypertension, hyperlipidemia, hiatal hernia, and fatty liver infiltration and a previous low midline exploratory laparotomy for resection of a carcinoid tumor of the small bowel causing small bowel obstruction. The patient initially presented with classic symptoms of appendicitis (low-grade fever, leukocytosis, and right-lower quadrant tenderness). He underwent laparoscopic exploration and was found to have a perforated appendix with fecal spillage into the abdomen. An appendectomy and abdominal wash-out was performed laparoscopically.

The patient needed to return to the operating room four days later for an open repair of an incarcerated left inguinal hernia. The remainder of his hospital course was uneventful, and he was discharged to home on postoperative day 9. He underwent multiple follow-up appointments after being discharged from the hospital and was doing reasonably well with no complaints of fever, except ongoing general malaise.

The patient presented once again to the hospital emergency department approximately two months after his index appendectomy with complaints of anorexia, worsening malaise, and a one-week history of non-radiating right-sided pleuritic chest pain. He denied fever, chills, or cough.

On physical examination, the patient was found to be diaphoretic and in moderate distress secondary to pleuritic chest pain and dyspnea. He was found to have had diminished breath sounds in the right lower lung field; his left lung was clear. His abdomen was soft and non-tender with a well-healed lower midline laparotomy scar as well as left groin and two laparoscopy scars. His white blood cell count was 11.6 K with the remainder of his laboratory studies being normal. A CT scan of the chest revealed a large, multiloculated right pleural effusion consistent with right thoracic empyema (Figure 10.1a and b).

A decision was made to proceed with a right video-assisted thoracoscopy for definitive management of what was strongly suspected to be an empyema. Upon entry to the chest via a two-centimeter incision in the midaxillary line above the seventh rib, 300 mL of a foul smelling yellowish-green thick fluid was drained. The fibrinous peel on the lower lobe of the lung and undersurface of the chest wall was debrided using a metal-tipped suction. On further exploration inferiorly and laterally at the junction of the diaphragm and the chest wall, there was noted to be what appeared to be fecal material present (Figure 10.2a and b). This particulate material was delivered through the chest wall in a collection; it was noted to be extremely friable and ill-formed. The right thorax was then irrigated copiously with warm saline, and on reexploration, a one centimeter defect was identified in the lateral surface of the diaphragm immediately adjacent to the chest wall. Gentle pressure on the right upper abdomen resulted in ongoing drainage of purulent secretions from the abdomen into the thorax (Figure 10.2c). A single 28-French right-angled chest tube was directed inferiorly and posteriorly, such that its tip was in the area of the diaphragmatic defect.

A CT scan of the abdomen performed after the surgical procedure showed fluid collections in the subdiaphragmatic, lateral hepatic, and right paracolic gutter areas (Figure 10.3a and b). The patient was returned to the operating room the following day in conjunction with the general surgery service. A right subcostal incision was performed to enter the abdomen. The aforementioned areas were explored with additional particulate material

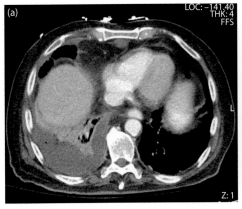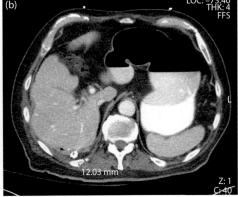

Figure 10.1 (a) CT of the chest showing right lower chest pleural effusion. (b) CT of the chest showing calcified mass nearby the diaphragm

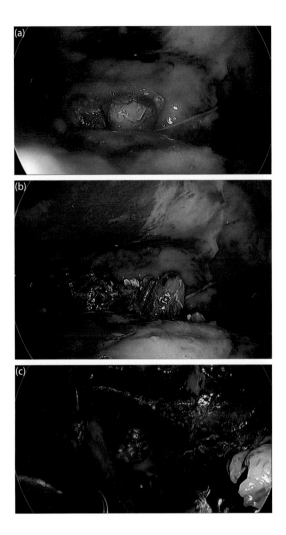

Figure 10.2 (a) Fecal material in the right thoracic cavity. (b) Another figure showing fecal material in the right thorax. (c) Showing the diaphragmatic defect from the thoracic side

and purulent debris being removed. At the conclusion of the procedure, the abdomen was irrigated copiously, and two Blake drains placed.

A culture of thoracic empyema fluid showed growth of *Escherichia coli, Enterococcus avium,* and *Bacteroides fragilis.* Directed antibiotic therapy was initiated per the recommendation of the infectious disease service.

The patient did well after these operations, and he was discharged home from the hospital on postoperative day 9 after tolerating diet and removal of the chest tube and one of the abdominal Blake drains.

Comments

Acute appendicitis is a common surgical emergency. Successful surgical appendectomy requires removal of the appendix and its contents. An ectopic appendicolith can migrate to a variety of locations and act as a nidus for infection and abscess formation. In this case, the

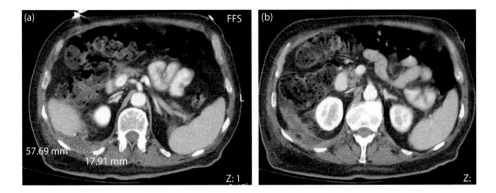

Figure 10.3 (a) CT of the abdomen showing subdiaphragmatic fluid collection. (b) CT of the abdomen showing fluid collection in the right paracolic gutter

appendicolith/fecal matter was found in the thoracic cavity along with subsequent formation of a thoracic empyema.

Betancourt et al. [1] reported a migrating or "wandering" appendicolith in the chest as well as a diaphragmatic defect in a two-year-old patient. The patient was treated with US-guided placement of chest drains, and the appendicolith removed under fluoroscopic guidance by the interventional radiology service using basket retrieval. In that case, the drainage catheter was removed five days later. The patient remained asymptomatic at a one-month follow-up.

There are several other reports in the literature with migrated appendicoliths in the peritoneal cavity, Morrison's pouch, iliopsoas compartment, gluteal region, and pelvis [2–4]. To our knowledge, this is a unique case of documented migration of an appendicolith/fecal matter to the pleural cavity in an adult patient. We hypothesize that the appendicolith/fecal material eroded through the diaphragm, causing the defect that was identified at the time of our thoracoscopy and then migrated to the thoracic cavity causing empyema. A congenital defect in the diaphragm or a defect resulting from trauma also offers a possible explanation for our finding. One might postulate that a patient with congenital diaphragmatic fenestrae would be more susceptible to developing empyema from any type of suppurative disease in the abdomen.

Symptoms and signs associated with abscess formation due to retained fecal matter/ appendicolith may present days to years after appendectomy. In our case, the patient developed malaise and pleuritic chest pain at approximately six weeks and four weeks, respectively. Management of this problem includes drainage of the abscess and extraction of the appendicolith, either via radiographic assisted means, laparoscopy, or an open approach [5]. For our patient, video-assisted thoracoscopy was performed to definitively drain the thoracic empyema and retrieve the fecal matter/appendicolith. An exploratory laparotomy was then performed to address the residual debris in the abdomen and drain the abdominal abscesses. Chest tube and abdominal closed suction drains were placed for continued drainage in the postoperative period.

A key point of focus in this case is the adequacy of irrigation of the abdomen in the presence of a perforated appendicitis using the laparoscopic approach. Given the reduction in postoperative pain and faster return to normal activity, a minimally invasive approach is generally favored for surgical procedures. This enthusiasm must however be tempered by a thorough understanding of the disease process and a sanguine appreciation for the complications that can ensue from an inadequate operation that focuses on cosmesis rather than cure.

In conclusion, a retained appendicolith after laparoscopic appendectomy is a rare complication. In our unique case report, a video-assisted thoracoscopy was done for presumptive diagnosis of empyema; during which, a migrating appendicolith/fecal matter was found in the pleural cavity and is the culprit for thoracic empyema in an adult patient.

REFERENCES

1. Betancourt, S.L., Palacio, D., Bisset, G.S., III. The "wandering appendicolith." *Pediatr Radiol.* 2015;45(7):1091–1094.
2. Kaya, B, and Eris, C. Different clinical presentation of appendicolithiasis. The report of three cases and review of the literature. *Clin Med Insights Pathol.* 2011;30(4):1–4.
3. Lambo, A., Nchimi, A., Khamis, J., Khuc, T. Retroperitoneal abscess from dropped appendicolith complicating laparoscopic appendectomy. *Eur J Pediatr Surg.* 2007; 17(2):139–141.
4. Vyas, R.C., Sides, C., Klein, D.J., Reddy, S.Y., Santos, M.C. The ectopic appendicolith from perforated appendicitis as a cause of tubo-ovarian abscess. *Pediatr Radiol.* 2008;38(9):1006–1008.
5. Singh, A.K., Hahn, P.F., Gervais, D., Vijayraghavan, G., Mueller, P.R. Dropped appendicolith: CT findings and implications for management. *AJR Am J Roentgenol.* 2008;190(3):707–711.

Lia Jordano, Christopher W. Seder, and Gary W. Chmielewski

Key Words
• Diaphragm eventration • Robotic surgery • Endostapling

Introduction

Eventration of the diaphragm is a rare congenital disorder with an incidence of less than 0.05% and constitutes a developmental defect in the muscular diaphragm, resulting in impaired caudal descent with respiration [1]. Operative repair of diaphragmatic eventration was first described in 1923 by Morrison, using an open approach and hand-sewn plication [2]. Over time, various methods including both open and minimally invasive techniques have been described [1,3,4]. Each of these techniques carry benefits as well as challenges. Presented here is a novel method for the plication of a diaphragmatic eventration using a robot-assisted thoracic approach, endostapling, and laparoscopic guidance, which capitalizes on the advantages of a minimally invasive operation while mitigating some operative risks and technical impediments.

Case Report

A 53-year-old non-smoking female presented with progressive dyspnea and symptoms of gastroesophageal reflux for the last three years. She was referred to thoracic surgery with a diagnosis of a giant paraesophageal hernia. Her medical history included chronic obstructive pulmonary disease, sleep apnea (on continuous positive airway pressure), hypertension, and hidradenitis suppurativa. She had no history of chest trauma or thoracic surgery. Physical exam revealed an obese woman (body mass index 35 kg/m²), with decreased breath sounds over the left lung base. Recent pulmonary function testing demonstrated a restrictive pattern with decreased total lung capacity (57% predicted), functional vital capacity (42% predicted), and forced expiratory volume in one second (36% predicted) (Table 11.1). A chest X-ray showed a left hemidiaphragm elevated to the level of the carina, significant volume loss of the left lung, mild left to right shift of the mediastinum, and the presence of the stomach, portions of the colon and small bowel, spleen, and pancreatic tail all within the left hemithorax (Figure 11.1). To exclude a hiatal hernia, an upper endoscopy was performed that demonstrated the gastroesophageal junction at 38 cm from the incisors and no evidence of a hiatal hernia. A sniff test was not performed, as she lacked a history of chest trauma or thoracic surgery, making diaphragmatic paralysis unlikely. She was diagnosed with left diaphragmatic eventration and was offered a combined laparoscopic and robot-assisted thoracoscopic diaphragmatic plication.

Table 11.1 **Pulmonary function tests**

	TLC (% predicted)	FVC (% predicted)	FEV1 (% predicted)
Preoperative	57	42	36
18-months postoperative	81	76	68

Abbreviations: TLC = total lung capacity, FVC = functional vital capacity, FEV1 = forced expiratory volume in one second.

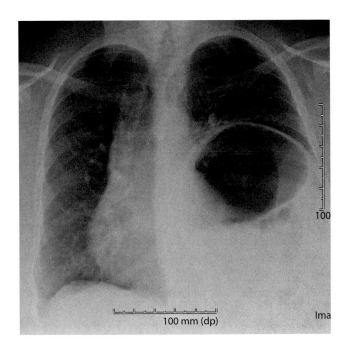

Figure 11.1 Preoperative chest X-ray

The patient was placed under general anesthesia and intubated with a double-lumen endo-tracheal tube. She was placed in the right lateral decubitus position with mild reverse Trendelenburg positioning and slightly rolled back to facilitate access to the left upper abdominal quadrant. Entry into the chest was achieved via a sixth intercostal space, 2-cm mid-chest port site. Two robotic ports were placed 8 cm apart on either side of the initial port. Visual inspection confirmed left hemidiaphragmatic eventration to the level of the carina without evidence of abdominal contents in the chest. In the left subcostal region, a Veress needle was placed at Palmer's point and gentle pneumoperitoneum was established, after which the abdomen was entered using a 10-mm Visiport™ (Medtronic, Dublin, Ireland) and a 30-degree scope was used to visualize the relationship of the abdominal organs to the left hemidiaphragm. The area directly under the left hemidiaphragm was cleared of abdomi-nal viscera. From the thorax, the diaphragm was grasped and gathered up by utilizing two robotic arms with fenestrated bipolar graspers beginning at the lateral aspect and work-ing medially. This redundant diaphragmatic tissue was sequentially stapled using an Endo GIA™ (Medtronic, Dublin, Ireland) with thick tissue (black) stapler, moving from lateral to medial aspect with the stapler passing through the posterior port site. Revisualization via the laparoscope ensured no impingement of abdominal viscera in the staple line. In order to pro-vide increased durability to the staple line, horizontal mattress sutures were placed and tied robotically with number 1 Ethibond (Ethicon Inc, Somerville, NJ) non-absorbable suture. The lung was re-expanded over a 24-French chest tube placed through one of the anterior port sites. The total console time was 120 minutes.

The patient was admitted for observation and recovered well without any short- or long-term complications. Her chest tube was removed on postoperative day 1, and she was deemed appropriate for discharge home. At 18 months, her chest X-ray displayed marked improvement in the elevation of the left hemidiaphragm (Figure 11.2), her dyspnea on exertion has resolved, and she is able to tolerate a normal diet without reflux. Follow-up pulmonary function testing revealed significant improvement: TLC 81% of predicted, FVC 76% of predicted, and FEV1 68% of predicted (Table 11.1).

Comments

Operative repair of diaphragmatic eventration is indicated for symptomatic cases. The surgical literature is limited by the relative rarity of this condition. A variety of techniques exist including both hand-sewn and stapled repairs performed via open, thoracoscopic, and laparoscopic approaches. In our technique, we describe a robotic-assisted approach with the simultaneous use of laparoscopy. A minimally invasive technique offers the benefits of reduced postoperative pain and shorter length of stay relative to an open operation [5]; however, maneuvering with only six degrees of freedom in the restricted workspace afforded by the elevated diaphragm can render video-assisted thoracoscopic surgery (VATS) repair problematic. A robotic approach addresses these challenges posed by a VATS and allows for more technical precision with enhanced articulation (seven degrees of freedom) and three-dimensional visualization. A disadvantage of a robotic approach is the loss of tactile feedback, which may increase the risk of inadvertent injury, particularly to abdominal viscera, which are not directly visualized. To ameliorate this, we employed the simultaneous use of laparoscopy. The addition of a single abdominal port allows for visualization of both sides of the diaphragm and reduces the risk of injury. This technique has demonstrated safety and efficacy with good mid-term results at 18 months.

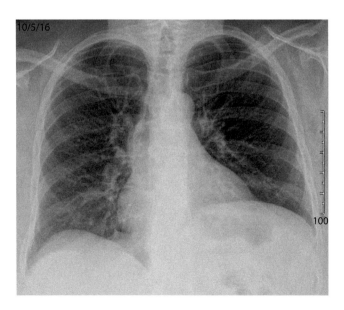

Figure 11.2 Postoperative chest X-ray at 19 months

REFERENCES

1. Groth, S., Andrade, R.S. Diaphragm plication for eventration or paralysis: A review of the literature. *Annal Thorac Surg.* 2010;89(6):S2146–S2150.
2. Morrison, J.M. Eventration of diaphragm due to unilateral phrenic nerve paralysis. *Arch Radiol Electrother.* 1923;28:72–75.
3. Groth, S., Rueth, N.M., Kast, T., D'Cunha, J. Laparoscopic diaphragmatic plication for diaphragmatic paralysis and eventration: An objective evaluation of short-term and midterm results. *J Thorac Cardiovasc Surg.* 2010;139(6):1452–1456.
4. Kwak, T., Lazzaro, R., Pournik, H., Ciaburri, D., Tortolani, A., Gulkarov, I. Robotic thoracoscopic plication for symptomatic diaphragm paralysis. *J Robotic Surg.* 2012;6(4):345–348.
5. Bendixen, M., Jørgensen, O.D., Kronborg, C., Andersen, C., Licht, P.B. Postoperative pain and quality of life after lobectomy via video-assisted thoracoscopic surgery or anterolateral thoracotomy for early stage lung cancer: A randomised controlled trial. *Lancet Oncol.* 2016;17(6):836–844.

Brett Curran and Wickii T. Vigneswaran

 Key Words
- Diaphragmatic hernia
- Hepatic resection
- Hernia repair

Introduction

A DH is the movement of abdominal contents into the chest cavity through a defect or opening in the diaphragm. DHs can be either primary or acquired. A primary DHs is rare, arising in 1 in 2,500 births, and is associated with congenital diaphragmatic defects that arise during embryogenesis [1]. These primary DHs, such as a Bochdalek hernia, can lead to lung hypoplasia and are typically identified in infancy [1]. Acquired DHs are also rare and are commonly associated with trauma. It has been found that 1%–5% of hospitalized automobile accident victims and 10%–15% of victims of penetrating trauma to the lower chest experience DHs [2]. Trauma induced hernias are associated with direct injury to the diaphragm or high abdominal pressure that leads to the herniation of abdominal contents into the chest cavity [2]. These traumatic DHs almost exclusively arise on the left side because of the protective effect of the liver on the right side [2]. Acquired DHs can also arise by iatrogenic mechanisms, albeit much less encountered than those occurring as a result of trauma. These iatrogenic DHs most commonly occur after surgical procedures [3]. Specifically, there has been a limited number of documented cases of iatrogenic DHs following hepatic resection. These post-hepatic resection DHs are typically small and present with a wide variation of symptoms from months to years after hepatic resection [3].

Case Report

A 27-year-old Caucasian female presented with shortness of breath lasting a few months. She believed this was caused by her asthma. Her guardian also reported that the patient had occasional episodes of diarrhea and spontaneous emesis without any associated abdominal pain. She denied any fever, chills, or nausea. Upon physical exam, the patient was found to have a blood pressure of 120/60 mmHg, heart rate (HR) of 72 bpm, respiratroy rate 16/min, and body mass index (BMI) of 38 kg/m^2. A chest X-ray was followed by a computed tomography (CT) scan that demonstrated herniation of the abdominal contents including the small bowel and colon into the right hemithorax, virtually filling the right thoracic cavity (Figure 12.1). Her past medical history was complex with cerebral palsy, developmental delay, asthma, seizures, and an atrial septal defect repair when she was two years old. The patient also underwent a right hepatectomy for a 9-cm benign adenoma in the right hepatic lobe 32 months previously (Figure 12.2). Her post-hepatectomy recovery was complicated by repeated respiratory failure requiring reintubation and sepsis of pulmonary origin. Her

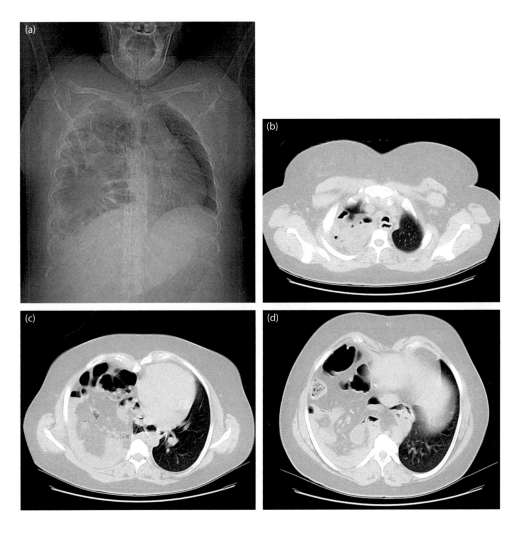

Figure 12.1 (a–d) MRI of the liver with contrast, well-circumscribed 9-cm diameter lobulated mass with possible encapsulation within the right hepatic lobe

recovery since discharge was uncomplicated until a few months ago when she developed the above symptoms. Her previous CT scan, two months post-hepatic resection, demonstrated normal regrowth of her liver and a normal chest scan.

After completing a thoracic surgical evaluation, she underwent a right thoracic approach. A right muscle sparing thoracotomy was performed. It was noted that the major part of the small bowel and the transverse colon was completely filling the right pleural space. The right lower lobe was completely atelectatic. The right upper lobe was partially ventilating but was compressed by the abdominal contents. After careful inspection, it was noted that there was a 6 × 5 cm central defect in the diaphragm through which most of the bowel and omentum had migrated into the pleural space. The diaphragm itself was of good quality, but the defect was large requiring a prosthetic repair. With systematic dissection and mobilization, the edges of the defect were defined. The adhesions to the edges of the defect were taken down carefully using electrocautery. Then the bowel and omentum in the chest

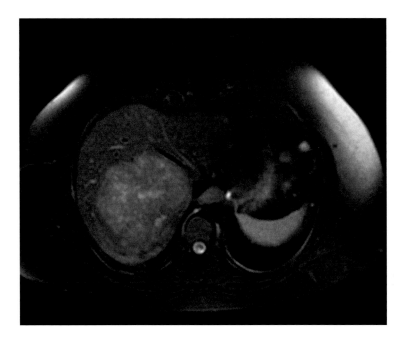

Figure 12.2 CT scan of the chest showing herniation of small bowel and colon into the right hemithorax, virtually filling the right thoracic cavity with near total atelectasis of the right lung

were slowly replaced into the abdominal cavity. A 1-mm thick 10 × 15 Gore-Tex patch was selected and trimmed to fit the defect and then sewn on to the edges of the diaphragm defect using a #1 Polypropylene suture. The chest was closed in the routine fashion with a single chest tube.

The patient was discharged on postoperative day 3. On the day of discharge, the patient was ambulating well with appropriate oral intake, on a regular diet, and her pain was well controlled on oral pain medication. At the follow-up appointment four months later, she was doing well without any shortness of breath. She denied any pain, had a good appetite, was eating well, and went back to normal activities. An X-ray showed mild elevation of the right hemidiaphragm but was otherwise unremarkable (Figure 12.3).

Comments

An iatrogenic DH following hepatic resection is rare, with studies finding an incidence rate of 1% and 2.3% [3,4]. Although uncommon, DH after hepatic resection should still be considered a potential serious adverse effect. A majority of the hernias that arise following hepatic resection are small, right-sided, and typically patients are asymptomatic for months to years after the operation [3]. When symptoms do arise, most patients present with respiratory distress, abdominal pain, or bowel obstruction symptoms [3].

Previous reports indicate that the main factors placing patients at risk for DH following hepatic resection is tumor size and diaphragmatic resection during hepatic resection [3]. Patients who develop DH after hepatic resection have an average tumor size of 9.2 cm, which was similar to the size seen in our patient [3]. Tumor size appears to be a risk factor for DHs. This may be due to multiple factors including stretching of diaphragm musculature by the

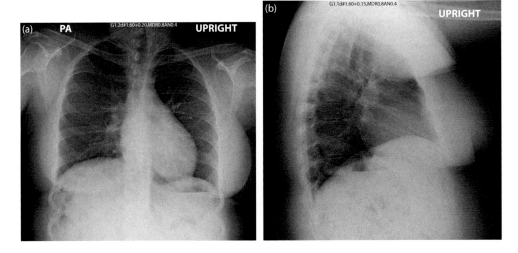

Figure 12.3 Chest X-ray a) PA and b) lateral. Four months following DH repair

tumor, causing thinning and extensive dissection that might be required during liver mobilization [4]. DHs can also be attributed to the use of electrocautery as it is used to mobilize the liver from the diaphragm, which may increase the risk for diaphragm injuries and devascularization [4]. Nearly all diaphragmatic injuries that are caused during surgery are identified intraoperatively and repaired by the surgeon, although some may go unnoticed and eventually result in complications. A small diaphragmatic injury from surgery can be exacerbated because of the inability of the diaphragm to heal and due to any increased intra-abdominal pressure eventually resulting in a notable DH [5].

Our patient presented with shortness of breath and diarrhea more than two years after surgical removal of the benign adenoma. During the hepatic resection, no diaphragmatic resection or repair was performed in our patient. Her postoperative scan at two months did not show any DH. The patient presented with symptoms more than two years after the hepatic resection. The slow development of her hernia is likely to be multifactorial. A chest X-ray that prompted a CT scan found that the patient had a large DH with almost complete right lung atelectasis. This patient had one of the largest DHs documented following hepatic tumor resection. This further elucidates that a DH should be considered a significant adverse effect that can present from months to years following hepatic resection. The severity of such occurrence can vary and can, as seen in our patient, require urgent repair to prevent potentially life-threatening complications.

REFERENCES

1. Yagmur, Y., Yiğit, E., Babur, M., Gumuş, S. Bochdalek hernia: A rare case report of adult age. *Ann Med Surg.* 2016;5:72–75.
2. Crandall, M., Popowich, D., Shapiro, M., West, M. Posttraumatic hernias: Historical overview and review of the literature. *Amer Surg.* 2007;73(9):845–850.

3. Tabrizian, P., Jibara, G., Shrager, B., Elsabbagh, A.M., Roayaie, S., Schwartz, M.E. Diaphragmatic hernia after hepatic resection: Case series at a single western institution. *J Gastrointest Surg.* 2012;16(10):1910–1914. doi:10.1007/s11605-012-1982-7.

4. Esposito, F., Lim, C., Salloum, C., Osseis, M., Lahat, E., Compagnon, P., Azoulay, D. Diaphragmatic hernia following liver resection: Case series and review of the literature. *Ann Hepato-Biliary-Pancreat Surg.* 2017;21(3):114–121. doi:10.14701/ahbps.2017.21.3.114.

5. Elikplim, N.Y., Mustapha, O., Zahra, L.F., Laila, J. Diaphragmatic hernia following a liver resection: A rare cause of bowel obstruction. *Int J Case Rep Imag.* 2018;9. Article ID 100915Z01NE2018.x

Christian Renz and Wickii T. Vigneswaran

 Key Words
- Case report
- Diaphragmatic hernia
- Cirrhosis
- Hernia repair

Introduction

Diaphragmatic hernias can be categorized as either acquired or congenital. Acquired diaphragmatic hernias are typically secondary to a traumatic event. The diaphragmatic injury may be missed in the initial evaluation and may present late with worsening of the diaphragmatic defect. These hernias are often on the left side in part because the liver tends to impede a right-sided hernia from developing [1].

A chest X-ray can show evidence of herniation of abdominal contents into the chest. This requires repair to prevent complications. A computed tomography (CT) is helpful to evaluate the extent of the diaphragmatic defect, the contents of the hernia sac, evaluate any complications [2].

Diaphragmatic hernias are currently being repaired via laparotomy, laparoscopy, or thoracoscopy [3]. When there is little surrounding diaphragmatic tissue destruction, a primary repair without the use of mesh is preferred. When there is excess tissue loss or an excessively large diaphragmatic defect, the use of nonabsorbable prosthetic mesh should be considered [4].

Case Report

A 53-year-old man presented to his primary care physician with a non-productive cough, wheezing, and shortness of breath worsening over time. He initially felt better after the visit but represented with fever, chills, productive cough, and tightening of his chest with the cough. On arrival, a clinical examination revealed no fever, pulse 97/min, saturations 96% on room air, and body mass index (BMI) 31.7 kg/m². A chest X-ray was obtained that showed elevated right diaphragm (Figure 13.1). A CT scan was obtained the same day that demonstrated a large diaphragmatic defect on the right side with the entire liver, portions of the right colon, and portions of the distal stomach extending into the chest causing a leftward mediastinal shift (Figure 13.2). The liver showed a nodular appearance raising concern for mild or early cirrhosis. The spleen was also enlarged raising suspicion for portal hypertension. Significant past medical history included an umbilical hernia repair, and a remote history of trauma secondary to a motor vehicle accident. He presented with a 35-pack-year smoking history and drank eight beers during the weekends and some during the weekdays. He was referred for further evaluation and treatment of his diaphragmatic hernia to thoracic surgery service.

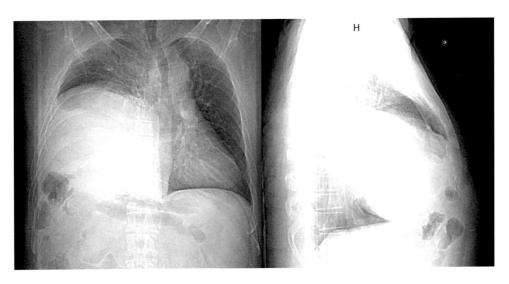

Figure 13.1 Preoperative chest X-ray

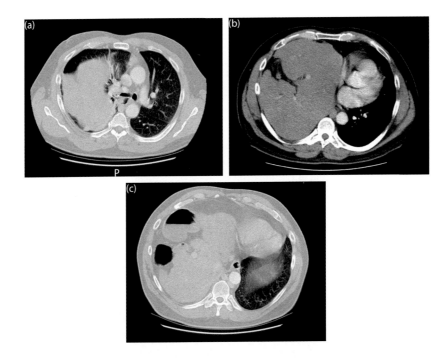

Figure 13.2 Preoperative CT scan of the chest (a) upper chest, (b) mid chest, (c) lower chest

At his initial office visit, the patient's physical exam was unremarkable, with no abdominal tenderness or distention, but reduced air entry to the right chest. A review of his chest X-ray and the CT scan confirmed the findings reported. The patient was deemed a candidate for elective repair, but he was counseled on the cessation of smoking leading up to surgery. As he had not followed up with a physician in many years, he required an additional workup for suspected cirrhosis, and his blood tests showed ALT 355 u/l, AST 368 u/l, alkaline phosphate 84 u/l, and total bilirubin 2.8 mg/dl.

Approximately one month after his initial clinic visit, the patient underwent a right thora-cotomy. The liver appeared cirrhotic and was rotated on its axis. There was also large amount of small bowel and transverse colon in the right chest cavity. The diaphragmatic defect mea-sured 10×15 cm. The diaphragmatic edges of the defect were identified, after slight posterior enlargement of the defect the herniating organs were gently reduced into the intraabdominal space. Because of the large defect, the dome of the liver was contained in the abdominal cavity by a Gore-Tex that measuring 20×15 cm that was sewn onto the edges of the defect using interrupted and running sutures of a #1 polypropylene suture. The lung required par-tial decortication, and a nodule in the middle lobe was wedged out. The nodule was a benign scar on pathology. At the end of the surgical procedure, a single chest tube was placed in the posterior mediastinum, and the chest was closed.

On postoperative day 4, there was noted an erythematous wound and purulent drainage from the incision site. The patient was started on empiric antibiotics, and cultures eventually showed growth of *Streptococcus milleri*. He was initially treated conservatively with continued anti-biotic therapy and a wound VAC but soon underwent re-exploration and debridement of the chest wound in the operating room. It was noted the infection was confined to the superficial layers of the chest wound only. After debridement, two Jackson-Pratt drains were placed on suc-tion, and the wound was closed with appropriate antibiotic treatment. The patient's subsequent hospital course had no further complications, and he was discharged home shortly after the wound healed well. His liver function studies showed, at the time of discharge from hospital, ALT 11 u/l, AST 21 u/l, Alkaline phosphate 95 u/l, and total bilirubin 0.5 mg/dl. At six months follow-up, the patient remained symptom free, and a chest X-ray showed mildly elevated dia-phragm without any herniation and fully expanded lungs on both sides (Figure 13.3).

Comments

This case describes a right-sided diaphragmatic defect with herniation of the entire liver and portions of the right colon, which is significant for various reasons. Right-sided diaphragmatic hernias are quite rare, partly because the liver occupies a majority of the space under the

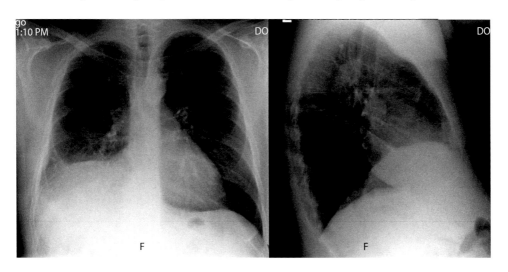

Figure 13.3 Chest X-ray six months postoperative

diaphragm on the right side, making it difficult for herniation to occur there [1]. However, in the above case, we see that our patient experienced complete herniation of the liver through the right-sided diaphragmatic defect. The etiology of his herniation is unclear; however, the remote history of the motor vehicle accident may have played a role in its development over the years. A tension-free repair of the hernia is mandatory for the repair to be successful. When there is a significant defect, it is necessary to repair the defect with a prosthetic material. The ideal material for repair is debatable. Many factors should be considered including cost and user handling properties. A tissue prosthetic such as a homograft or similar should be considered if there is any concern of infection. In our patient, in retrospect, we could postulate that he may have had a recent infection in his pleural space that might have necessitated the decortication and the middle lobe lung wedge resection. Fortunately, the wound infection appeared superficial layers and cleared with superficial debridement and vacu-dressing. If this involved deeper layers, it would have been necessary to remove the prosthetic material.

A complete herniation of the liver through the diaphragmatic defect is very rare. In an acquired hernia for this to occur, the liver needs to rotate on its axis as observed in our patient. The axial rotation can result in twisting of the vascular structures, thereby affecting the forward flow or the venous drainage. Some of the features were observed in the preoperative CT scan such as the nodular liver and enlarged spleen that is suggestive that this may have been the case in our patient. The CT finding of nodular liver was confirmed during the surgery, and additionally the patient showed some decrease in the liver function blood tests during his presentation. Initially, it was not clear if the cirrhotic-appearing liver and associated derangement in function was due to his excessive alcohol consumption or the malrotation of the liver. His liver functions normalized after the surgery and that is indicative that there was some contribution to the derangement from his liver herniation, even though any contribution from his alcohol consumption cannot be ruled out. At short term follow-up, his liver function remained normal supporting the former.

REFERENCES

1. Feliciano, D.V., Cruse, P.A., Mattox, K.L., Bitondo, C.G., Burch, J.M., Noon, G.P., Beall, A.C., Jr. Delayed diagnosis of injuries to the diaphragm after penetrating wounds. *J Trauma*. 1988;28(8):1135–1144. doi:10.1097/00005373-198808000-00005.
2. Testini, M. et al. Emergency surgery due to diaphragmatic hernia: Case series and review. *World J Emerg Surg*. 2017;12:23.
3. Takaichi, S. et al. Laparoscopic repair of an incarcerated diaphragmatic hernia after right hepatectomy for hepatic injury: A case report. *Surg Case Rep*. 2018;4(1):135. doi:10.1186/s40792-018-0542-0.
4. Edington, H.D., Evans, S., Sindelar, W.F. Reconstruction of a functional hemidiaphragm with use of omentum and latissismus dorsi flaps. *Surgery*. 1989;105(3):442–445.

Adrian E. Rodrigues and Wickii T. Vigneswaran

Key Words
• Diaphragmatic hernia • Diaphragm rupture • Blunt trauma • Viscera herniation • Viscus reduction

Introduction

Diaphragmatic hernias aren't novel maladies; thus, much about them is extensively known. These are congenital or acquired. Congenital occur through the foramen of Morgagni or Bochdalek, while another congenital form, not a hernia, diaphragmatic eventration develops as a result of an elevated diaphragm with limited connective tissue [1]. If a step in the diaphragmatic growth process is disrupted, congenital diaphragmatic hernias can develop and will depict a discernible smooth border encompassing the defect [2]. The acquired hernias are also well recognized and are categorized as either iatrogenic or traumatic, with traumatic subdivided into penetrating or blunt. Although these conditions are well documented, what remains provoking is how blunt force diaphragmatic ruptures can be easily missed during their acute phase, and more so, how some slowly progress into diaphragmatic hernias once the defect is present. The process driving the viscera upward, slowly, and at times with limited symptoms may be multifactorial; but it undoubtedly includes opposite physiological influences of both the abdominal and thoracic cavities that the diaphragm, under healthy conditions, helps separate [3].

Those induced by blunt trauma, however, will show jagged borders with local inflammation and may induce symptoms [4]. Unfortunately, not all those induced by blunt force will herniate or show symptoms acutely. For this reason, many are difficult to diagnose, and some cases have lasted several months before they're detected [5–7].

According to Kumar et al., cases that go undetected are more likely to develop visceral strangulation; therefore, adequate clinical workup tethered with epidemiological knowledge can aid the diagnosis. Most acquired diaphragmatic hernias result from motor vehicle accidents [7]. Only 5% of people who endure thoracoabdominal blunt forces will develop a hernia, with 80% of them developing on the left side and 13% on the right. They are also more frequent in males, and the viscera most commonly herniated is the omentum, stomach, colon, and spleen—in that order [8]. The absence of herniation with limited symptoms will make a diagnosis challenging, even with a computed tomography (CT). It is therefore prudent to examine asymmetric contours, hemidiaphragm levels, and if available, fluoroscopic diaphragmatic motion, all of which will support a clinicians' degree of suspicion.

Case Report

We encountered a 40-year-old male who was involved in a motor vehicle accident with unknown seatbelt use. The patient was driving a vehicle, and while stopped at an intersection, an oncoming car collided with his vehicle from behind at an unknown speed. The patient's ventral thoracoabdominal wall subsequently struck the failed airbag-deployed steering wheel of his vehicle. He then made his way to the emergency department by unknown transportation.

While in the emergency department, the patient was in no acute distress with vitals within the normal limits. His past medical history was non-contributory, but his social history revealed moderate exercise with running, occasional alcohol, and previous tobacco use of one pack-per-day for five years. A physical exam failed to reveal any findings aside from thoracoabdominal ecchymosis cause by striking the steering wheel. A chest X-ray was ordered and showed only effusion on the left side. He was discharged the same day and told to follow-up with a pulmonologist.

Two months after the motor vehicle accident, the patient was seen by a pulmonologist. Clinical findings revealed post-accident shortness of breath with moderate walking and an inability to run. Left chest tightness was also present. Meals produced dysphagia with prolonged esophageal clearing, heartburn, and excessing bloating and belching. Bowels were regular, and he denied a history of fever, chills, light-headedness, or palpitations. Vitals revealed a blood pressure of 140/76, pulse of 70, and a respiratory rate of 16. His body mass index was 28. A chest X-ray was obtained followed by a diagnostic CT and it revealed a large left-sided diaphragmatic hernia (Figure 14.1a–d). Given the finding, the patient was referred for surgical evaluation.

Surgical treatment was recommended after the patient's initial clinical visit with the Department of Thoracic Surgery. The patient agreed with the treatment and was scheduled for surgery shortly thereafter.

In the operating room, the patient was prepared for a transthoracic robotic surgical procedure in a reverse Trendelenburg position. During robotic camera inspection, large bowel, small bowel, abundant omentum, and part of the liver's left lobe was present in the pleural space, with the herniating contents occupying up to the apex. Under carbon dioxide insufflation, attempts were made to reduce the viscus but were unsuccessful. Additionally, the lack of pleural space created insufficient room to manipulate the robotic instruments safely. Consequentially, the robotic approach was aborted, and instead, a low lateral thoracotomy with muscle sparing procedure was used to enter the pleural space.

Upon entering, the left lung appeared normal, while the herniating viscus and ruptured diaphragm showed diffuse adhesions. Systematic electrocautery followed by blunt dissection was used to free adhesions and identify the edges of the ruptured diaphragm. Once the diaphragmatic rupture was identified, it revealed a 20-cm tear with good quality edges. However, the abundant herniating viscus was incarcerated around the diaphragmatic defect. We therefore followed with a 3-cm lateral diaphragmatic extension. After liberating the incarceration, we continued with adhesion takedown between the defect and the viscus until the tear's edges were completely free.

Once the diaphragmatic opening was free, systematic reduction of the herniating viscus ensued. During this process, the hepatophrenic ligament of the left lobe was observed to be attached to both ends of the diaphragmatic tear. The ligament was therefore divided, and the hepatic lobe was mobilized away from the under surface of the diaphragm to provide a surface for sutures. After successful viscus reduction, the diaphragmatic borders were approximated and closed with sutures.

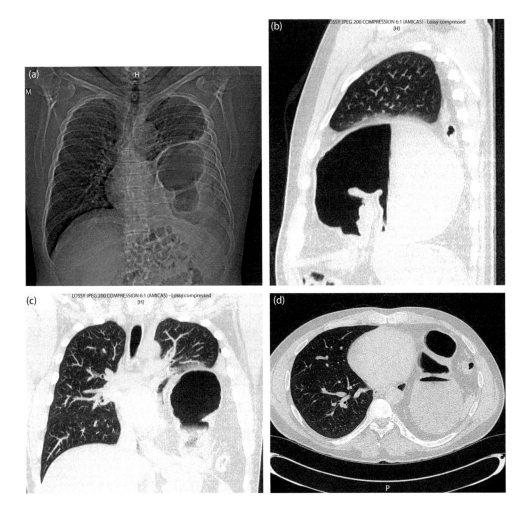

Figure 14.1 (a–d) Large left-sided hernia

Upon completing the surgical procedure, liposomal bupivacaine was infiltrated around the incisional sites, and a single chest tube was placed in the posterior mediastinum. Once all external incisions were closed, the patient was extubated and transferred to the intensive care unit. The patient recovered well and was discharged in stable condition a few days after the surgical procedure.

During a postoperative clinical follow-up, a chest X-ray showed a small left pleural effusion, which decreased with subsequent visits (Figure 14.2a and b). After two months of follow-up, the patient was referred to his pulmonologist for continued care.

Comments

Different surgical approaches exist for the treatment of diaphragmatic hernias. The list includes thoracotomies, laparotomies, and thoraco-laparotomies, with midline laparotomies being the most common [9]. Once inside the thoracic or abdominal cavity, the diaphragm can be repaired with sutures, and if necessary, a Gore-Tex patch may be used in cases with

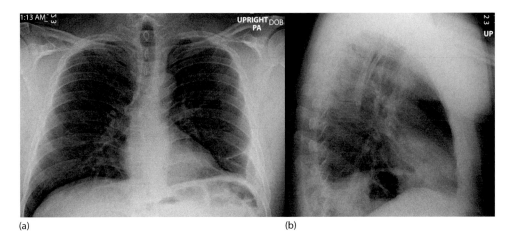

(a)   (b)

Figure 14.2 (a, b) Postoperative chest X-ray

incomplete viscus reduction. In this case, we initially attempted a robotic thoracic approach, but after camera inspection, we observed a collapsed left lung with herniating viscus overwhelming the pleural space. Physical attempts were made to create more space under carbon dioxide insufflation, but such efforts proved unsuccessful. The robot was therefore aborted, and instead, a thoracotomy was used to enter the pleural space and to reduce the herniating viscus.

Although the start of the viscus moving upward in this patient is not known, the period between the motor vehicle accident and the resulting diagnosis is known: a time of two months exactly. Fortunately, this patient's post-accident follow-up care resulted favorably, but this isn't always so. In the absence of herniating contents, some clinicians have found ruptured diaphragms incidentally during surgical procedure. This begs the question, why do some ruptures result in herniation while others don't? Clinical outcomes can generate more questions than answers, but the reason cases do herniate result from opposite physiological forces. The intraabdominal cavity generates a positive pressure that varies with meals, body position, bowel movements, and comorbidities to name a few; while the intrathoracic area produces a negative pressure [2]. In the presence of a diaphragmatic defect, the barrier separating these two compartments is lost, thereby allowing the viscera to vector cranially. The development of herniation is therefore straightforward, but the lack of symptomatology is more complex.

The sensory innervation to the diaphragm is notoriously unreliable. Some cases with blunt force ruptured diaphragms will present with vague pain, while in other cases pain is absent. Like the lack of visceral pain, some ruptures seldomly impact the respiratory mechanics enough to alter ventilation, leaving respiratory rate and saturation unimpeded. And worse yet, in the presence of a herniating viscus, the cardiothoracic and gastrointestinal physiologies adapt to the new compartment, further masking symptoms. In our case, all these findings were present, most noticeably in our patient's left lung, which collapsed from the herniating viscus but retained its ventilatory mechanics after reduction.

This lack of symptoms likely stems from evolutionary adaptations. If these adaptations weren't present, breathing would become difficult due to pain, abundant inflammation, and a faulty diaphragm; likewise, gastrointestinal, and worse yet, cardiothoracic homeostasis wouldn't be maintained. Evolutionary adaptations work toward prolonging survival in times of stress, but such mechanisms make diagnosing these maladies more difficult. It may seem that our clinical expertise forms a paradox with natures adaptations, but without evolution, we wouldn't survive a diaphragmatic rupture, and without modern medicine, the rupture wouldn't be closed. It seems both must be embraced and appreciated.

REFERENCES

1. Kansal, A.P., Chopra, V., Chahal, A.S., Grover, C.S., Singh, H., Kansal, S. Right-sided diaphragmatic eventration: A rare entity. *Lung India*. 2009;26(2):48–50. doi:10.4103/0970-2113.48898.

2. Mirensky, T.L., Warner, B.W. Congenital diaphragmatic hernia masquerading as traumatic diaphragm rupture. *J Pediatr*. 2014;165(6):1269.e1. doi:10.1016/j.jpeds.2014.08.026.

3. Hanna, W., Ferri, L. Acute traumatic diaphragmatic injury. *Thorac Surg Clin NA*. 19:485–489. doi:10.1016/j.thorsurg.2009.07.008.

4. Ouazzani, A., Guerin, E., Capelluto, E., et al. A laparoscopic approach to left diaphragmatic rupture after blunt trauma. *Acta Chir Belg*. 109(2):228–231.

5. Corbellini, C. Diaphragmatic rupture: A single-institution experience and review of the literature. *Turkish J Trauma Emerg Surg*. 2017. doi:10.5505/tjtes.2017.78027.

6. Asakage, N. Delayed left traumatic diaphragmatic hernia repaired by laparoscopic surgery. *Asian J Endosc Surg*. 2011;4(4):192–195. doi:10.1111/j.1758-5910.2011.00101.x.

7. Adegboye, V.O., Ladipo, J.K., Adebo, O.A., Brimmo, A.I. Diaphragmatic injuries. *Afr J Med Sci*. 2002;31(2):149–153.

8. Kumar, A., Bagaria, D., Ratan, A., Gupta, A. Missed diaphragmatic injury after blunt trauma presenting with colonic strangulation: A rare scenario. *BMJ Case Rep*. 2017;2017:bcr-2017-221220. doi:10.1136/bcr-2017-221220

9. Gwely, N.N. Outcome of blunt diaphragmatic rupture. Analysis of 44 Cases. *Asian Cardiovasc Thorac Ann*. 2010;18(3):240–243. doi:10.1177/0218492310368740.

Taylor Jaraczewski and Wickii T. Vigneswaran

Key Words
• Ganglioneuroma • Mediastinal mass • Robotic resection

Introduction

Ganglioneuromas (GNs) are highly differentiated solid tumors arising from sympathetic ganglion cells [1]. Symptomatology of these tumors is diverse and ranges from asymptomatic to non-specific mass effect to, rarely, autonomic dysfunction due to hormone secretion. In general, these tumors are considered benign and are treated with complete surgical resection. We report the case of an asymptomatic female who had one incidence of dysphagia and was found to have a giant GN, which was treated with robotic-assisted mobilization and subsequent open thoracotomy and mass resection.

Case Report

A 19-year-old female with no significant past medical history presented two weeks after a recent trip to the emergency room for an incident of dysphagia. The patient denied any past history of dysphagia, chest pain, difficulty breathing, arm pain, decreased range of motion, or numbness of her upper extremities. Emergency room X-ray revealed a mass located in the right upper lung. A subsequent computed tomography (CT) scan revealed a 9.6 × 10.8 × 9.6 cm rounded mediastinal mass (Figure 15.1). An MRI of the mass revealed involvement of the T1–T3 right neural foramen and potential right dural involvement from T1–T5, suggestive of nerve root involvement (Figure 15.2). Further findings showed that the mass partially encased the superior vena cava (SVC). A CT-guided needle biopsy revealed GN. Laboratory studies did not reveal elevated urine norepinephrine or fractionated metanephrines, which ruled out catecholamine production by the GN as well as pheochromocytoma. Based on these findings, the patient underwent a staged procedure with neurosurgery and thoracic surgery at the same sitting. The patient initially underwent a right T1–T2 hemilaminectomy, T3 subtotal superior hemilaminectomy, right T1–T2 and T2–T3 total facetectomy, and a right T2 transpedicular resection of the epidural tumor with neurosurgery from a posterior approach. She then underwent right lateral robotic dissection of the intrathoracic mass and open completion resection of the tumor while monitoring the T1–T2 nerve roots. The patient tolerated the procedure well with no complications and was discharged on postoperative day 5 with the chest tube maintained due to high fluid outputs. At her one-week follow-up, the chest tube was removed, and a chest X-ray showed stable findings within her thoracic cavity and mild ptosis of the right upper eyelid. At a one-month follow-up, her ptosis has resolved.

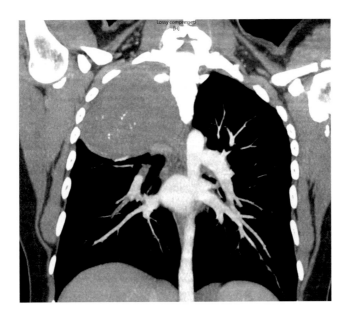

Figure 15.1 CT scan of chest

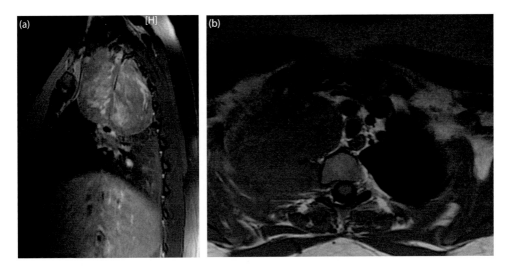

Figure 15.2 (a, b) MRI of chest, representative images, T1–T3 right neural foramen and potential right dural involvement from T1–T5, suggestive of nerve root involvement

Comments

Neurogenic tumors make up about 75% of all posterior mediastinal tumors [2]. These tumors include neuroblastoma, ganglioneuroblastoma, ganglioneuroma (GN), schwannoma, neurofibroma, neurofibrosarcoma, and paraganglioma. GNs are the most common posterior mediastinal mass in adolescents and young adults [2]. While GNs are thought to arise spontaneously, some case reports have reported them arising after chemotherapeutic treatment of neuroblastomas [3]. These findings suggest the possible etiology of some GNs as a result of neuroblastoma differentiation. Others have reported an association of these tumors with neurofibromatosis type II or multiple endocrinologic neoplasia type II [4]. Unlike neuroblastomas, however, GNs tend to be found later in life (16 vs 79 months) and are slower growing. GNs are also different than other neurogenic tumors as they microscopically consist of more benign and well-differentiated ganglion cells, neurites, Schwann cells, and perineural cells. Macroscopically, they are typically well-delineated, large, homogenous white masses that are surrounded by a fibrous capsule [2]. The most common location is in the posterior mediastinum followed by the retroperitoneal space; however, they have also been found in the neck, adrenal gland, and pelvis. Posterior lying tumors can often present with extensions into the spinal cord, such as in our patient. Many of these characteristics were exemplified in our patient. While she first presented at 19-years of age, which is later than average, given the size of the tumor, it likely existed for a number of years prior to presentation.

GNs are generally incidentalomas as they are often asymptomatic. Geoerger et al. performed an assessment of common symptoms at diagnosis and found that most patients with tumors in the abdomen had non-specific symptoms such as abdominal pain, emesis, gastroenteritis, fever, weight loss, and constipation. Thoracic tumors also were associated with non-specific mass effect symptoms such as cough, bronchitis, pneumonia, thoracic pain, and gastritis. Some patients show signs of autonomic complications from hormone secreting GN or from compression of autonomic fibers of the lumbosacral plexus. These symptoms include sweating, hypertension, and diarrhea. Other functional GNs have been reported to secrete vasoactive intestinal peptides (VIP), somatostatins, and neuropeptide Y [4]. Our patient did not show laboratory signs of a functional GN; however, it is important that surgeons understand the possibility of cholinergic crisis during surgery if the GN is functional.

Radiological assessment of GNs has been investigated and shown that, on imaging, GNs are typically well-delineated lesions that are elongated in the vertical axis [5]. They present with low internal attenuation on CTs. Tumors with a larger ratio of ganglion cells may be slightly hyperattenuating. A fine speckled pattern consistent with calcifications is found in approximately 20% of GNs. On MRI, GNs are homogenous and hypointense on T1-weighted and hyperintense on T2-weighted sequences. Occasionally, they will present with a whorled appearance. Overall, however, imaging is not entirely useful diagnostically for GN. Typically, biopsy and final surgical pathology are required for diagnosis.

Surgical resection of GNs has been shown to be sufficient for treatment. While surgery is non-emergent, tumors should be removed in a timely manner to decrease pain and compression. Further, because tumors can often extend into other areas, such as the spinal foramen in our patient, it can be necessary to involve multiple specialties for safe and successful resection.

In conclusion, we describe a patient who was found to have a ganglioneuroma in her right apical thoracic space that extended into the T1–T3 epidural space. She subsequently underwent posterior decompression as well as robotic-assisted mobilization and open completion resection of the mass. Due to the range of presentations and behaviors of GN, it is vital to have them on the differential for non-specific symptoms and incidental imaging findings. Further, it is critical to understand the workup and management of these tumors to ensure successful resection.

REFERENCES

1. Decarolis, B., Simon, T., Krug, B., Leuschner, I., Vokuhl, C., Kaatsch, P., von Schweinitz, D., et al. Treatment and outcome of ganglioneuroma and ganglioneuroblastoma intermixed. *BMC Cancer*. 2016;16:542.

2. Kizildag, B., Alar, T., Karatag, O., Kosar, S., Akman, T., Cosar, M. A case of posterior mediastinal ganglioneuroma: The importance of preoperative multiplanar radiological imaging. *Balkan Med J.* 2013;30:126–128.

3. Geoerger, B., Hero, B., Harms, D., Grebe, J., Scheidhauer, K., Berthold, F. Metabolic activity and clinical features of primary ganglioneuromas. *Cancer.* 2001;91:1905–1913.

4. Ingale, S., Goyal, P., Mohaniya, P., Patil, R., Singh, S. Ganglioneuroma: A rare neural crest tumor. *J Evol Med Dent Sci.* 2015;4:15379–15381.

5. Pavlus, J.D., Carter, B.W., Tolley, M.D., Keung, E.S., Khorashadi, L., Lichtenberger, J.P., III. Imaging of thoracic neurogenic tumors. *AJR Am J Roentgenol.* 2016;207:552–561.

Lambros Tsonis, Anita Ong, and Wickii T. Vigneswaran

Key Words
• Schwannoma • Mediastinal mass • Phrenic nerve

Introduction

Neural tumors of the mediastinum are relatively common in the posterior mediastinum, but they rarely present in other locations within the mediastinum [1,2]. Schwannomas arise from the Schwann cell of neural sheath and may affect sympathetic or parasympathetic chain, intercostal nerves, or spinal ganglia. Schwannomas are usually located in the posterior mediastinum. It is very rare for them to be localized in the middle mediastinum or arise from the phrenic nerve. Schwannomas account for between 0.5% and 7% of mediastinal tumors [3]. When they occur, they are commonly associated with von Recklinghausen's disease, with a predominance in males.

Case Report

The patient is a 40-year-old female with a past medical history of diabetes and hypercholesterolemia who initially presented with a cough, sinus congestion, and rhinitis for about a month. She presented to her primary care physician, who treated her with antibiotics when her symptoms persisted for a week and ordered a chest radiograph (Figure 16.1). The chest radiograph demonstrated a mass, and a subsequent computed tomography (CT) chest was performed (Figure 16.2). The patient's symptoms completely resolved after antibiotics, and she was asymptomatic after that point except for intermittent left shoulder pain.

The patient had no relevant findings on physical exam. Biochemical workup, including for alpha-fetoprotein (AFP), carcinoembryonic antigen (CEA), and lactate dehydrogenase (LDH) was performed, and it did not show any elevation of these antigens. The patient had a PET/CT, which demonstrated heterogeneous enhancement of the mass with a max standardized uptake value (SUV) of 4.8. A decision was made to proceed with surgical exploration and resection.

The patient was brought to the operating room and given general anesthesia. A bronchoscopy was performed, demonstrating normal anatomy and no endobronchial pathology. The patient was then positioned with her left side elevated with a "bump" under that side, and the chest was prepped and draped in a sterile manner. An initial incision was made in the axillary area. Once in the pleural space, CO_2 was insufflated into the pleural space, and additional working ports were placed in the sub-mammary line, in the left parasternal area

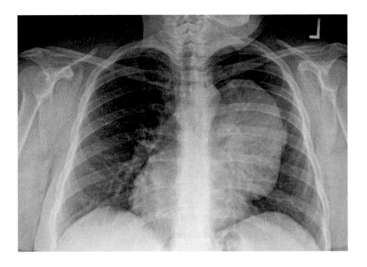

Figure 16.1 Preoperative chest X-ray

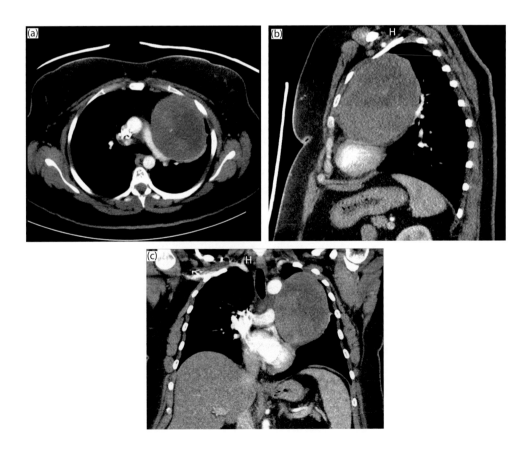

Figure 16.2 Preoperative CT scan. (a) Axial, (b) Sagital (and c) Coronal views of the tumor

midclavicular line, and the anterior axillary line above the diaphragm. A da Vinci "Si" robot was brought to the patient and docked. The dissection was initiated on the pericardium inferiorly mobilizing the pericardial fat and the tumor mass. As we proceeded cephalad, we saw that the mass was densely adherent to the superior pulmonary vein and noted the phrenic coursing into the mass. It was felt the nerve had to be sacrificed as there were no planes identified so it was divided inferiorly. The mass was dissected away from the pericardium medially, and dissection continued upwards identifying the innominate vein and the mammary vessels superiorly. As the mass was large, hard, and heavy, it was difficult to mobilize the mass robotically to expose the pulmonary hilum, superiorly. As such, we made an anterolateral thoracotomy and proceeded with an open approach. Under direct visualization, we were able to retract the mass, exposing the pulmonary hilum and separating the mass of the pulmonary artery and superior pulmonary vein. The vascular pedicle for the mass originated from the aortopulmonary (AP) window area; this was ligated and divided. The mass was then able to be separated from the remaining pericardium, and the phrenic nerve divided above the mass, using electrocautery and blunt dissection. The mass was then extracted out of the chest, and hemostasis obtained. A chest tube was placed, and the patient was closed in layers.

The mass was measured at $14.8 \times 11.3 \times 8.6$ cm and weighed 646 g (Figure 16.3a). Representative sections are shown in Figure 16.3b. These show a spindle cell tumor with an alternating compact spindle cell (Antoni A) and loosely cellular (Antoni B) areas. They form characteristic whorls and stain positive for S-100 and negative for actin and desmin; expression of Ki-67 was low (<5%). This was reported as consistent with a schwannoma of the phrenic nerve.

The patient was extubated immediately after surgery. She complained of hoarseness almost immediately. Her chest tube was removed on postoperative day 2. An ear nose and throat (ENT) consult was obtained for the hoarseness, and an indirect laryngoscopy was performed that demonstrated paralysis of the left vocal cord. This was treated with an injection of Prolaryn, and the patient's voice immediately improved. She was discharged home on postoperative day 4. Subsequent imaging nine months after surgery demonstrated no recurrence of disease. A chest X-ray performed was unremarkable except for eventration of her left hemidiaphragm (Figure 16.4).

Comments

Neural tumors most commonly arise from the structures of the posterior mediastinum; schwannomas are the most common of these tumors. Schwannomas of the chest most

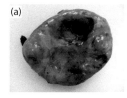 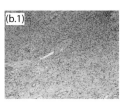 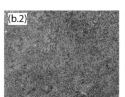 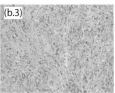

Figure 16.3 (a) Gross tumor (b) Microscopy shows spindle cell tumor with alternating compact spindle cell (Antoni A) and loosely cellular (Antoni B) areas. They form characteristic whorls and stain positive for S-100 and negative for actin and desmin; expression of Ki-67 was low (<5%)

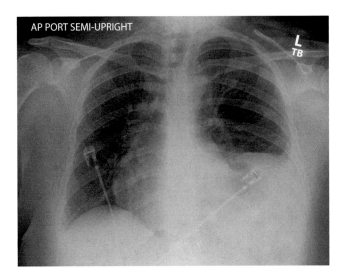

Figure 16.4 Postoperative CXR —Eventration of left hemidiaphragm

commonly arise from the intercostal nerves, although they too are uncommon. Middle mediastinal neural tumors are rare, accounting for less than 5% of cases, and have been described arising from either the phrenic, vagus, or recurrent laryngeal nerves. [4]. It is very unusual for these tumors to grow very large like in our patient unnoticed. Asymptomatic tumors are usually benign. Malignant schwannomas are even more rare. Ribet et al. reported that 9 out of 194 thoracic tumors were found to be malignant schwannomas [5]. These tumors are reported in the 20–50-year-old age group, with a female predominance [5]. They are usually described as encapsulated and well circumscribed, most often solitary. When multiple, they are associated with neurofibromatosis.

Schwannomas are most commonly benign but can be slow-growing and have the potential for malignant transformation [6]. They are frequently asymptomatic at presentation, often discovered incidentally on imaging. When they have symptoms, most commonly, it is related to paralysis of the affected nerve. CT or MRI will often demonstrate the mass, sometimes with cystic areas apparent if IV contrast is given. A PET/CT may show variable levels of uptake [7]. Histologically, schwannomas show a mixture of two distinct patterns: Antoni A and B. Antoni A areas are highly cellular consisting of spindle cells, while Antoni B areas are hypocellular in a connective tissue stroma. In addition, Antoni B areas are noted to be prone to degeneration. Immunohistochemically, schwannomas often show strong S-100 positivity [6].

While others have described doing sternotomy or thoracotomy in similar cases, in this case, we used a robotic approach to help to delineate the anatomy and perform a significant amount of the dissection. Because of the large size tumor, it was difficult to retract this mass and, as such, could not be safely mobilized from the pulmonary hilum where the vascular pedicle was located. The recurrent nerve was involved in the area of dissection and injured in the process. Despite this patient made a rapid recovery and was discharged home on fourth postoperative day. Robotic technique is a significant advance in resecting all types of mediastinal tumors, and a schwannoma is not an exception. A giant tumor in the pulmonary hilum or invasion into adjacent structures may require a thoracotomy to complete resection.

REFERENCES

1. Strollo, D.C., Rosado-de-Christenson, M.L., Jett, J.R. Primary mediastinal tumors. *Chest*. 1997;112(5):1344–1357.
2. Reeder, L.B. Neurogenic tumors of the mediastinum. *Semin Thorac Cardiovasc Surg*. 2000;12(4):261–267.
3. Marchevsky, A.M. Mediastinal tumors of peripheral nervous system origin. *Semin Diagn Pathol*. 1999;16(1):65–78.
4. Bolanos, F., et al. Schwannoma arising from the left phrenic nerve: A rare location. *Chest*. 2013;144(4_Meeting Abstracts):92A.
5. Ribet, M.E., Cardot, G.R. Neurogenic tumors of the thorax. *Ann Thorac Surg*. 1994;58(4):1091–1095.
6. Elstner K., Granger E., Wilson S., et al. Schwannoma of the pulmonary artery. *Heart Lung Circ*. 2013;22:231–233.
7. De Waele, M., Carp, L., Lauwers, P., et al. Paravertebral schwannoma with high uptake of fluorodeoxyglucose on positron emission tomography. *Acta Chirurgica Belgica*. 2005;105:537–538.

Evgeny V. Arshava, Poorani Sekar, John Keech, and Kalpaj R. Parekh

Key Words
• Histoplasmosis • Traction esophageal diverticulum • Mediastinitis • Mediastinal granuloma • Granulomatous mediastinitis

Introduction

Most infections with *Histoplasma capsulatum* are either asymptomatic or do not require treatment even in endemic regions. Acute complications of histoplasmosis requiring surgical interventions are rare but need to be diagnosed promptly and treated aggressively.

Case Report

A 20-year-old, otherwise healthy female student from the Netherlands, presented with fever, worsening chest pain, and dyspnea for several days. This was the patient's second visit to the Midwest region of the United States (US). Prior to this visit, the patient spent a year attending college in Illinois. After her return home, new symptoms of dyspepsia prompted an esophagogastroduodenoscopy (EGD) that was reported normal. There was no inflammation reported in the esophagus or stomach, and biopsies were negative for *Helicobacter pylori*. By her second visit to the US, her dysphagia has resolved.

On admission, the patient was tachycardic and hypotensive. Echocardiography showed a large pericardial effusion with moderate right atrial collapse and marked right ventricular diastolic collapse (Figure 17.1a). The patient underwent emergent pericardiocentesis with a pericardial drain placement. Four hundred milliliters of purulent fluid was removed with immediate normalization of hemodynamics. The patient required intubation for progressive respiratory failure. A repeat echocardiogram the following day showed significant residual echo-dense material (Figure 17.1b).

Contrast-enhanced computed tomography (CT) showed mediastinal lymphadenopathy and a multiloculated fluid collection with peripheral rim enhancement in the mediastinum, with the largest component measuring up to 4 cm (Figure 17.2). The middle part of the thoracic esophagus had an and thickened irregular wall with focal dilation. In retrospect, this area of dilation corresponded to the origin of the fistula. There was a moderate residual rim enhancing pericardial effusion and moderate bilateral pleural effusion and ascites.

The patient underwent flexible EGD and endoscopic ultrasonography (EUS). A small diverticulum was noted on the right lateral wall of the esophagus, 31 cm from the incisors with draining pus (Figure 17.3). A complex subcarinal mass containing multiple fluid collections was biopsied with a fine needle to rule out malignancy, and it showed necrotizing

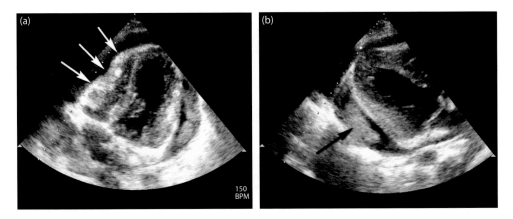

Figure 17.1 (a) Echocardiogram showing cardiac tamponade with compression of the right ventricle (arrows). (b) Echocardiogram after pericardiocentesis demonstrating residual pericardial debris (arrow)

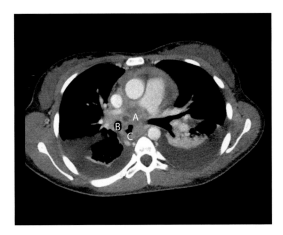

Figure 17.2 CT of the chest demonstrating showing multiloculated fluid collections with peripheral rim enhancement (A) encircling the bronchus intermedius (B). The middle part of the thoracic esophagus (C) has a thickened irregular wall with focal dilation

granulomatous inflammation and areas of liquid pus. Bronchoscopy showed no evidence of pathology in the trachea and bronchi.

The patient urgently underwent attempted thoracoscopic exploration of the right chest. This, however, required posterolateral thoracotomy due to extensive adhesions of the lung to the chest wall. Exploration of mediastinum revealed a large inflammatory mass in the mediastinum and dense fibrosis. Simultaneous EGD and flexible bronchoscopy was performed with forced transillumination under darkened operating room lights to safely identify the location of the tracheobronchial tree and esophagus. The parietal pleura and mass were incised, and the posterior mediastinum was entered between the light silhouettes of both scopes. We have not encountered description of this maneuver in the literature.

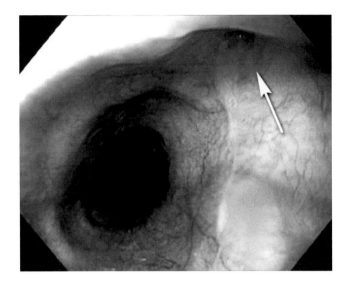

Figure 17.3 Flexible esophagogastroduodenoscopy demonstrating small traction diverticulum on the right lateral wall of the esophagus at 31 cm from the incisors (arrow). (Courtesy of Dr. Henning Gerke.)

The purulent multiloculated abscesses with liquid pus around the esophagus, bronchus intermedius, subcarinal space, and distal trachea was drained. A biopsy of chronically inflamed mediastinal lymph nodes returned as necrotizing granulomas with dense fibrosis on frozen section. One of the large lymph nodes eroded into the traction diverticulum in the mid-esophagus below the level of the carina. This node was completely removed to allow dissection of the fistula tract and appropriate mobilization of the esophageal edges. Tissues were edematous, and the esophagus was repaired with a full-thickness interrupted 2–0 absorbable suture and covered with a pleural flap.

During the same operation, the patient was repositioned, and the left pleural space was then drained via the thoracoscopic approach with a finding of fibrinous effusion. Wide pericardiotomy, effusion drainage, and removal of the extensive fibropurulent debris from the pericardial sac were performed. Pleural spaces, pericardium, and mediastinum were widely drained with surgical tubes.

Mediastinal abscess cultures were positive for *Streptococcus anginosus* and *Candida albicans*. Cultures of the pericardial fluid were positive for *Streptococcus anginosus*. Pleural fluid had no growth bilaterally.

A pathological exam of the surgical tissues showed necrotizing granulomas and, on a Grocott-Gomori's Methenamine Silver (GMS) stain, rare organisms consistent with *H. capsulatum* (Figure 17.4). A serologies study demonstrated highly elevated Histoplasma (yeast phase) and antibody titers at 1:256 (RR < 1:8). Histoplasma antigen assays in the blood and urine were negative, as were fungal cultures of the blood and surgical specimens.

The patient was weaned off vasopressors and extubated on postoperative day (POD) 4. An esophagogram on POD 7 showed no leak, and the patient was allowed to have a clear liquid diet. Thoracostomy tubes and mediastinal drains were removed once the output from them was minimal.

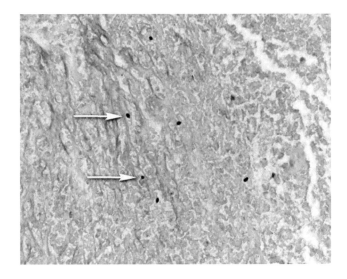

Figure 17.4 Yeast organisms (arrows) on GMS stain of the granuloma. (Courtesy of Bradley Ford.)

After two weeks of oral intake, the patient had some dysphagia and underwent a repeat EGD to rule out stenosis on POD 20, which revealed partial breakdown of the repair with a small, contained esophageal leak that could not be controlled with endoscopic clipping. The patient was further managed with a *nil per os* status and nutrition via nasogastric tube.

The patient remained without signs of systemic infection with a normal white blood cell count and no fever. On POD 32, the patient preferred to return to the Netherlands on room air, with enteral tube feeds. In Europe, the patient completed six weeks of Ertapenem and Caspofungin. Two weeks later, a repeat chest CT, EGD, and esophagram demonstrated resolution of the fistula. At 12-months follow-up, a positron emission tomography (PET) was obtained in the patient's home country and demonstrated persistent activity in the primary right upper lobe infiltrate and mediastinal lymph node, but with no residual fluid collections. The patient has been doing well clinically for over 12 months after the initial operation without signs infection or dysphagia.

Comments

Histoplasma capsulatum is a thermally dimorphic fungus that is found in soil worldwide, but particularly in North and Central America. In the US, it is particularly endemic in the Mississippi and Ohio River valleys of the Midwestern states. It is estimated that up to 3 million infections may occur in the US annually [1].

The lungs serve as a port of entry for this fungus. Until the specific cellular immunity is developed in two weeks in the lungs and mediastinal lymph nodes, infected macrophages may spread the infection hematogenously.

The diagnosis of histoplasmosis is made by morphologic examination of granulomas with findings of lymphohistiocytic aggregates and diffuse mononuclear cell infiltrates. Fungal stains may reveal ovoid yeast-phase organisms of *H. capsulatum* that need to be differentiated from *Candida glabrata*, *Cryptococcus neoformans*, and *Pneumocystis jiroveci*. Tissue and bronchoalveolar lavage (BAL) cultures produce a positive yield in the majority of chronic cases but are less sensitive in localized disease or acute disease.

Detection of antigen using the Histoplasma antigen enzyme immunoassay (EIA) in the urine, blood, or BAL fluid is possible in 60%–80% of acute infection. Complement fixation, immunodiffusion, and enzyme immunoassay are serologic tests available for antibody detection. Antibodies are typically positive during the second month after exposure and may be negative if tested during acute illness. Additionally, serologic assays may be falsely negative in immunosuppressed patients. Antibodies remain positive for several years after infection and thus may not be helpful in monitoring disease activity.

Most exposed patients are asymptomatic. Less than 1% of patients develop severe disease, and they are usually immunocompromised or they have inhaled a large inoculum. Pulmonary histoplasmosis may present in several clinical forms.

Acute, localized pulmonary histoplasmosis manifests with mild lower respiratory and systemic symptoms 2–4 weeks after exposure and resolves within several weeks. Illness is often treated as a community-acquired pneumonia, and histoplasmosis is only considered in endemic areas after there is no response to a standard therapy. Radiographs typically show focal infiltrates and mediastinal or hilar lymphadenopathy. Infiltrates clear in 2–4 months in most patients, while adenopathy may persist for years. There is insufficient data on effect of antifungal therapy on the course of mild infection or resolution of radiographic abnormalities. Retrospective diagnosis of histoplasmosis can be made as an incidental finding of calcified pulmonary and mediastinal granulomas. It takes months (in children) to years (in adults) for calcifications to form. In the absence of clinical symptoms, surveillance imaging is not recommended. PET images may remain abnormal for years after initial infection.

Acute diffuse pulmonary histoplasmosis may occur after heavy exposure to pathogens during disturbance of heavily contaminated soil or in areas with large amounts of bird or bat feces. The disease is characterized by diffuse reticulonodular pulmonary infiltrates and can progress to respiratory failure and extrapulmonary dissemination.

Chronic pulmonary histoplasmosis affects patients with underlying lung disease. Patients develop fibrotic apical infiltrates with cavitation and may present with productive cough, dyspnea, chest pain, and signs of systemic infection. The differential diagnosis must include tuberculosis, aspergilloma, atypical mycobacterial infections, and chronic or recurrent bacterial pneumonia. Such lesions typically occur in smokers and may mimic malignancy.

Mediastinal granuloma (granulomatous mediastinitis) results from progressive granulomatous inflammation, caseous necrosis, and encapsulation of the acutely inflamed mediastinal lymph nodes (mediastinal adenitis). Other causes of granulomatous mediastinitis include tuberculosis, actinomyces, aspergillus, and coccidioidomycosis. Most of these patients are asymptomatic. Some lymph nodes may enlarge up to several centimeters in size. The mass effect of these granulomas on compliant adjacent structures may lead to compression and erosion of esophagus, pulmonary vessels, and bronchi [2,3]. Small traction diverticula may develop as a result of pulling on a section of the esophageal wall by the adherent fibrotic lymph node. Traction diverticula secondary to tuberculosis were frequently seen in the past, but rarely now. Even less common, bronchoesophageal fistulae may present with infections and bleeding and require operative repair [4]. In our patient, the ongoing inflammation in the lymph node eventually led to erosion into the diverticulum, with secondary streptococcal mediastinal abscess and pericarditis. Clear goals of surgery need to be established regarding whether it is the relief of obstruction, bleeding control, or repair of fistula. General surgical principals include careful surgical planning with imaging and endoscopy, careful dissection of the inflamed planes, conservative interventions on lung parenchyma, and coverage of repaired esophageal fistula sites with vascularized tissue.

Broncholithiasis develops when calcified lymph nodes erode into adjacent bronchi. This manifests as a chronic cough, wheezing, and hemoptysis. Broncholiths usually are removed bronchoscopically. Lobectomy may be required for massive bleeding secondary to erosion of broncholith into pulmonary artery branches or recurrent pneumonias.

Fibrosing mediastinitis (FM) represents a rare delayed exaggerated fibrotic response to a prior episode of histoplasmosis that, in most cases, cannot be identified. Only a minority of patients are older than 45 years. Dense fibrosis adjacent to lymph nodes leads to diffuse entrapment and distortion of any mediastinal structures including heart and great vessels. The vast majority of granulomatous mediastinitis cases are not followed by the development of FM mediastinitis. FM is a morbid and less-amenable-to-treatment condition than granulomatous mediastinitis. Surgery is generally discouraged given limited benefits and high morbidity. Vascular obstruction is usually managed with stenting.

Antifungal treatment with itraconazole is indicated for acute pulmonary illness with duration of symptoms over four weeks, chronic cavitary pulmonary histoplasmosis, and symptomatic cases of granulomatous mediastinitis. Severe forms of acute pulmonary or disseminated histoplasmosis are treated with liposomal amphotericin B [5]. Antifungal treatment is also indicated for immunocompromised patients or those exposed to a large inoculum of histoplasma. Histoplasmosis must be excluded before treating patients with presumed sarcoidosis with immunosuppressive medications, especially in endemic areas.

REFERENCES

1. Wheat, L.J. et al. Histoplasmosis. *Infect Dis Clin North Am.* 2016;30(1):207–227.
2. Dukes, R.J., Strimlan, V., Dines, D.E., Payne, W.S., MacCarty, R.L. Esophageal Involvement with mediastinal granuloma. *JAMA.* 1976;236:2313–2315.
3. Hammoud, Z.T., Rose, A.S., Hage, C.A., Knox, K.S., Rieger, K., Kesler, K.A. Surgical management of pulmonary and mediastinal sequelae of histoplasmosis: A challenging spectrum. *Ann Thorac Surg.* 2009;88:399–404.
4. Ballehaninna, U.K., Shaw, J.P., Brichkov, I. Traction esophageal diverticulum: A rare cause of gastro-intestinal bleeding. *Springerplus.* 2012;1(1):50.
5. Hage, C., Azar, M., Bahr, N., Loyd, J., Wheat, L. Histoplasmosis: Up-to-Date evidence-based approach to Diagnosis and Management. *Semin Respir Crit Care Med.* 2015;36(5):729–745.

CASE 18: MEDIASTINAL LIPOSARCOMA AFTER REMOTE HISTORY OF RADIATION AS AN INFANT

James L. Lubawski Jr. and Wickii T. Vigneswaran

 Key Words

- Chest wall tumor
- Liposarcoma
- Mediastinal sarcoma

Introduction

During the dawn of the radiation era, this new technology was tried as a potential cure for a wide range of disease. Not just cancer, but a diverse set of problems from asthma to acne were targets for this revolutionary new form of therapy. Time has shown us that these treatments were of no benefit. However, those who underwent them may only now be experiencing the repercussions. Certainly, we know that radiation can increase the chances of thyroid cancer and that radiation for breast cancer can lead to chest wall sarcomas [1]. But what of these infrequent, short-lived treatments that have been cast off to the dusty corners of medical history? Have they lead to any long-term consequences? This case suggests that there may have been negative effects for this patient.

Case Report

A 65-year-old man with no significant past medical history presented to his primary care physician with a three-month history of progressively worsening cough and wheezing. This was worse when he would lie flat. He saw his primary care physician who ordered a chest X-ray, which showed a large, perihilar soft tissue mass. The chest X-ray was then followed by a computed tomography (CT) scan of the chest with contrast, which showed a large anterior mediastinal mass measuring at least 21 cm at its greatest dimension (Figure 18.1). The mass density was predominantly of fat. A core-needle biopsy showed a well-differentiated liposarcoma, and he was referred for surgical resection. An in-depth history done on surgical consultation revealed that the patient had undergone radiation therapy of the chest as an infant. At that time, it was believed that he had an "enlarged thymus." He underwent several radiation treatments at six months of age. No records exist of how much radiation was given. The patient was otherwise healthy, other than symptoms of allergic rhinitis.

A PET scan and MRI chest scan were done to ensure that his disease was localized and was not invading any of the nearby bones or great vessels. It was not, and an operation was planned. A left hemi-clamshell incision was made. A thymectomy was done, with all fatty tissue taken from the left phrenic to the right. The tissue did not appear to be invading the innominate vein or pericardium, and these structures were left intact. The left mediastinal pleural was stretched by the tumor and was removed. No invasion of the tumor past the mediastinal pleura into the left or right chest could be seen. Mediastinal lymph nodes were included in the dissection, and the area was skeletonized of all fatty tissue. Postoperative recovery was unremarkable.

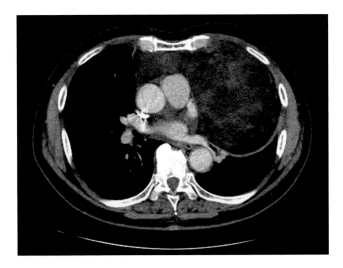

Figure 18.1 Representative CT scan demonstrating the giant anterior mediastinal mass

Final pathology was described with 26 × 15 × 13 cm, 2 kg, grade 1, well-differentiated lipo-sarcoma. Sixteen lymph nodes were negative, and no invasion into surrounding fat or pleura was noted. Preoperative pulmonary symptoms had resolved, and no signs of recurrence were noted on initial scans during the first year of surveillance.

Comments

The practice of giving radiation therapy to infants with an "enlarged thymus" began in the early twentieth century. During this time, the normal size range of the infant thymus was not well understood, and it was believed that an enlarged thymus would put an infant at risk for status lymphaticus and suffocation [2]. Thousands of infants were irradiated due to this misconception. It is unknown what dose this patient got, but regimens ranged from 0.03–10 Gy [7]. In 1950, the first paper was published that established a link between thymic and tonsilar radiation and subsequent development of thyroid cancer [3]. After this, it took several years for the practice to die out. That was not soon enough for the patient who presented in this case as his date of birth was 1953. After this first link, additional tumors began appearing in this population. Breast cancer in males, osteochondromas, lymphomas, salivary gland tumors, and brain tumors have all been associated with juvenile radiation [4–6].

This case represents the first reported case of mediastinal liposarcoma in a patient who had undergone thymic radiation as an infant. Mediastinal liposarcomas are very rare. They represent 0.13%–0.75% of all mediastinal tumors. Certainly, a causal relationship cannot be confirmed without additional cases, but the history is suggestive. We know from studying this population that their cancer risk, particularly for thyroid cancer, does not go away with time, but persists over 50 years later [7]. Certainly for this patient, and for all who have had juvenile radiation exposure, a heightened level of suspicion for cancer should be maintained when considering any symptom, lump, or bump. Given the low doses that many of these children were exposed to, practitioners today, during a time in which we are becoming increasingly dependent on imaging, should take radiation dosing into account for our youngest and most vulnerable patients.

REFERENCES

1. Curtin, C.T., McHeffy, B., Kolarsick, A.J. Thyroid and breast cancer following childhood radiation. *Cancer.* 1977;40:2911–2913.
2. Friedlander, A. Status lymphaticus and enlargement of the thymus with report of a case being successfully treated by x-ray. *Arch Pediatr.* 1907;24:491–501.
3. Duffy, B.J., Fitzgerald, P.J. Cancer of the thyroid in children. A report of 28 cases. *J Clin Endocriol Metab.* 1950;10:1296–1308.
4. Janower, M., Niettinen, O. Neoplasms after childhood irradiation of the thymus gland. *JAMA.* 1971;215:753–756.
5. Hempelmann, L.H., et al. Neoplasms in persons treated with x-rays in infancy for thymic enlargement. A report of the third follow up study. *J Natl Cancer Inst.* 1967;38:317–341.
6. Modan, B., et al. Radiation induced head and neck tumors. *Lancet.* 1974;303:277–279.
7. Adams, M.J., et al. Thyroid cancer risk 40+ years after irradiation for an enlarged thymus: An update of the Hempelmann cohort. *Radiat Red.* 2010;174(6):753–762.

Wickii T. Vigneswaran

Key Words
• Esophageal perforation • Intrathoracic stomach • Aortic pseudoaneurysm • TEVAR

Introduction

Paraesophageal hernias cause few or no symptoms and remain undiagnosed for years until they are recognized on imaging or symptoms resulting from mechanical consequences of an intrathoracic stomach. The potential complications include bleeding, incarceration, perforation and strangulation. The common symptoms are due to obstruction, such as post prandial pain, vomiting and dysphagia. Similarly an aortic aneurysm can remain asymptomatic for years, remaining undiagnosed until it's incidentally found on imaging, or until it ruptures and triggers symptoms. Both conditions most often affect the elderly, a group who regularly harbor additional comorbidities. Therefore, diagnosis and management of these two rare and potentially lethal conditions is challenging, often requiring advanced skills.

Case Report

A 91-year-old female was referred from an outside hospital with 4 days of vomiting and difficulty of eating. Two months previously she had undergone a colon resection for adenocarcinoma with good recovery and prior to that she was independently living with no limitations. She underwent a chest X-ray and a CT scan in the outside institution on admission, and the findings were suspicious for gastric obstruction at the gastroesophageal (GE) junction as well as extra-luminal air and fluid in posterior mediastinum (Figure 19.1). A diagnosis of intrathoracic stomach with perforation was made and the referral for transfer and possible surgical intervention was requested. On admission to the outside hospital, the patient was started on broad spectrum antibiotic coverage with intravenous Vancomycin and Zosyn, a nasogastric tube, and intravenous fluid therapy. No oral contrast study was performed at the outside institution. According to previous medical records, the patient was suspected to have a hiatal hernia and history of coronary artery disease and previous stents placement. Her medications were metoprolol, atorvastatin, 81 mg aspirin, furosemide, quetiapine, and miralax.

On arrival to our institution the patient was alert, with a temperature of 98.9°F, SpO2 94%, pulse at 93/min with rhythm in atrial fibrillation, and a blood pressure (BP) of 125/91 mmHg. The abdominal examination was unremarkable and clinically stable. Basic laboratory tests revealed, hemoglobin (Hb) 10.3 g/dL, white blood cell count (WBC) 18,700 cells/mcL, sodium (Na) 134 mEq/L, potassium (K) 3.6 mEq/L, Creatinine 0.93 mg/dL, Blood urea nitrogen

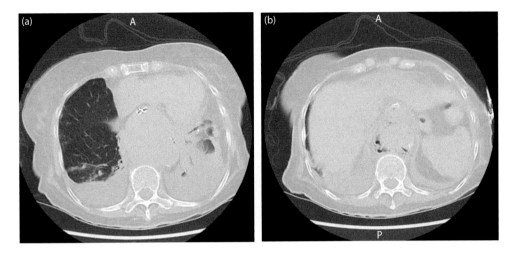

Figure 19.1 (a, b) Non-contrast CT scan showing posterior mediastinal mass with bilateral effusions and mediastinal air

(BUN) 33. After discussion with the radiologist, we repeated the CT scan with oral contrast, and the findings were reported as follows:

> Complex posterior mediastinal collection of fluid and air immediately posterior to the esophagus with evidence of pneumomediastinum raises the concern for organized collection secondary to esophageal perforation. No evidence of active oral contrast extravasation. On this noncontrast study, it is difficult to delineate the distal thoracic aortic lumen from the posterior mediastinal collection, and a contrast-enhanced CT chest scan would better exclude acute aortic pathology if clinically indicated. Enteric tube coils seen within the distal esophagus at the level of the GE junction. Repositioning is recommended. Moderate bilateral pleural effusions. (Figure 19.2).

There was concern that this was a contained esophageal perforation with an intrathoracic stomach. Following resuscitations during the night, the patient was taken to the operating room the following morning. A left thoracotomy was performed, and on entry, we encountered a serous pleural effusion with no surrounding purulent material. After additional entry, a pulsatile posterior mediastinal mass consistent of an aortic aneurysm was revealed. The chest was closed with a posterior mediastinal tube. An aortogram was obtained, and the thoracic vascular team was consulted immediately. The patient underwent a CT angiogram, which demonstrated marked dilatation of the intrahiatal aorta, up to 7.3 cm, and likely an aneurysm or pseudoaneurysm, accounting for a previously described posterior mediastinal mass (Figure 19.3). That evening, the patient underwent treatment of the pseudoaneurysm percutaneously with thoracic endovascular aortic repair (TEVAR) using Cook Alpha 26 × 26 × 105 mm endovascular prosthesis (Figure 19.4). Four days later, the patient was discharged home ambulating well and on full oral intake. The laboratory values at discharge were Hb 8.6 g/dL, WBC 7,800 cells/mcL, Na 142 mEq/L, K 4.2 mEq/L, Creatinine 0.68 mg/dL, BUN 23.

Comments

An intrathoracic stomach is the end stage of a hiatal hernia and is often a disease of the elderly, with a very low incidence. Frequently, the diagnosis is made incidentally by radiographic

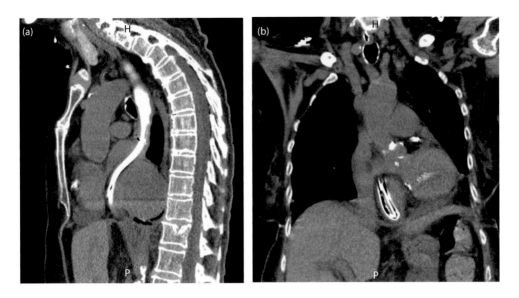

Figure 19.2 (a, b) CT scan with oral contrast, posterior mediastinal mass with curled up nasogastric (NG) tube in distal esophagus and calcified mediastinal lymph nodes and aortic calcification

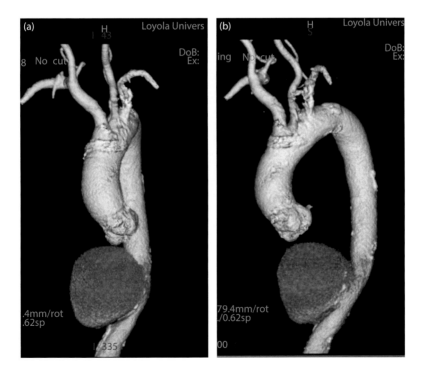

Figure 19.3 (a, b) CT angiogram, 3D reconstruction of aorta showing descending aortic pseudoaneurysm

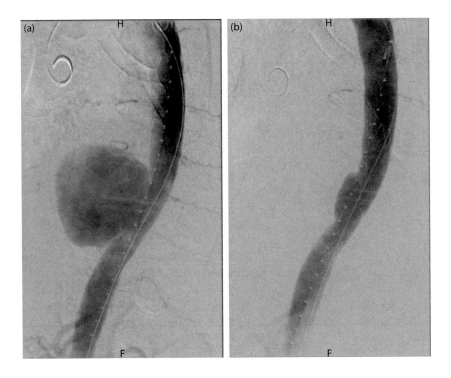

Figure 19.4 (a) Aortic angiogram pseudoaneurysm of the descending aorta pre-TEVAR (b) Post-TEVAR

investigations. There could be no clinical symptoms; however, complications associated with an intrathoracic stomach could be life threatening [1,2]. It is not unusual to maintain the GE junction in the normal anatomical location where the stomach has migrated along the side into the chest occupying the posterior mediastinum. When a patient is asymptomatic or presents with nonspecific symptom, a high index of suspicion is necessary to make the diagnosis [3]. In our case, the location and mediastinal air pointed the diagnosis towards a perforated intrathoracic stomach. As often taught, that all mediastinal masses are vascular until proven otherwise, is an important lesson when working up a mediastinal mass. An intravenous contrast scan would have helped us make the correct diagnosis early in our patient. However, the recent vomiting and dysphagia, along with the laboratory findings and the non-contrast CT scan from the outside institution, directed us away from an aortic pathology.

Pseudoaneurysm of the thoracic aorta results from transmural disruption of the aortic wall, with the leak contained by surrounding mediastinal structures. They can be secondary to trauma, infection or previous cardiac surgery, being the most frequent cause. It affects the descending thoracic aorta in about 10% of cases [4]. Endovascular approaches are being increasingly utilized to treat a variety of thoracic aortic pathologies, including aneurysms, dissections, and transections. Advances in the stent designs make this a successful approach [5]. Endovascular techniques have been considered superior in terms of postoperative morbidity. In situations of a contaminated field, a percutaneous stent graft provides enough window to control an infection and would be a preferred approach, as was suspected initially in our case. Further intervention may be necessary after controlling the infection in this circumstance. In an elderly patient, an endovascular approach would still be the preferred treatment choice.

REFERENCES

1. Naunheim, K.S., Edwards, M. Paraesophageal hiatal hernia. In *General Thoracic Surgery* (7th edition), Shields T.W., Locicero, J., Reed, C.E., Feins, R.H. (Eds). Lippincott Williams & Wilkins, Philadelphia, PA, 2009, pp 1951–1959.

2. Allen, M.S., Trastek, V.F., Deschamps, C., Pairolero, P.C. Intrathoracic stomach: Presentation and results of operation. *J Thorac Cardiovasc Surg.* 1993;105:253–258.

3. Bawahab, M., Mitchell, P., Church, N., Debru, E. Management of acute paraesophageal hernia. *Surg Endosc.* 2009;23:255–259. doi: 10.1007/s00464-008-0190-8.

4. Atik, A.F., Navia, J.L., Svensson, L.G, et al. Surgical treatment of pseudoaneurysm of the thoracic aorta. *J Thorac Cardiovasc Surg.* 2006;132(2):379–385.

5. Lu, Q., Jing, Z., Bao, J., Pei, Y. Endovascular repair of a distal aortic arch pseudo-aneurysm with use of a scallop-edged stent-graft. *J Vasc Interventional Radiol.* 2009;20(11):1500–1502.

CASE 20: TRACHEAL CHONDROSARCOMA

Alison Coogan, Lia Jordano, Michael J. Liptay, and Christopher W. Seder

 Key Words

- Tracheal chondrosarcoma
- Tracheal resection
- Primary tracheal tumor
- Case report

Introduction

Malignant tumors of the trachea only represent 0.2% of respiratory tract cancers [1]. Tracheal chondrosarcomas are among the rarest tracheal tumors with only 20 cases reported in the English literature, to date. They are slow-growing tumors that, unlike the present case, typically present with obstructive symptoms [2]. Metastases are uncommon and, after complete resection, recurrence is rare [3]. Herein, a case of tracheal chondrosarcoma is reported, and the presentation and natural history are examined.

Case Report

A 67-year-old morbidly obese male was referred for evaluation of a tracheal nodule that was identified on chest computed tomography (CT) (Figure 20.1). He was a never-smoker and had a past medical history significant for hypertension, hyperlipidemia, gastroesophageal reflux disease, prostate cancer treated with prostatectomy, diabetes mellitus, stage III chronic kidney disease, and obstructive sleep apnea. At time of presentation, he reported fatigue and a productive cough, with clear sputum, but denied fever, chills, shortness of breath, chest pain, or unintentional weight loss. His pulmonary function tests were normal.

Flexible bronchoscopy revealed a non-ulcerative 5-mm lesion on the left lateral wall of the cartilaginous trachea, approximately 5 rings above the carina (Figure 20.2). An endobronchial ultrasound-guided fine needle aspiration of the lesion was performed; however, the aspirate was non-diagnostic. Therefore, rigid bronchoscopy was used to resect the entire endobronchial portion of the lesion. Pathologic analysis revealed increased cellularity and atypical cytology, consistent with a low-grade chondrosarcoma.

Given the incomplete resection, the decision was made to proceed with a formal resection of the tracheal chondrosarcoma. Relative contraindications to tracheal resection include (1) preoperative steroid use, (2) mechanical ventilation, and (3) prior irradiation. Inability to perform a tension-free anastomosis is an absolute contraindication to surgery. The length of trachea that can be safely resected varies by patient but is generally less than 5 rings.

The patient was placed in the left lateral decubitus position, and a single lumen endotracheal tube was advanced into the left main stem bronchus to provide right-sided lung isolation.

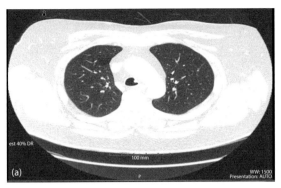
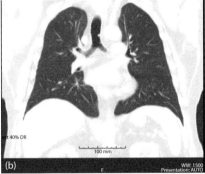

Figure 20.1 CT scan showing the tracheal tumor at presentation in (a) axial and (b) coronal views

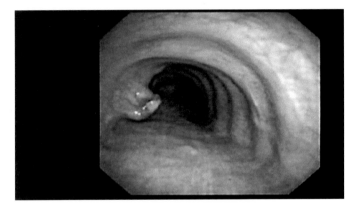

Figure 20.2 Bronchoscopic view of the tracheal tumor at presentation

Other strategies for ventilation during transthoracic tracheal resection include the use of oscillator jet ventilation, cardiopulmonary bypass, and cross-field ventilation into the left mainstem bronchus. We chose to use a size 7.0 single-lumen endotracheal tube advanced from the mouth into the left mainstem bronchus as it represented the simplest, least morbid option that did not obstruct the operative field.

A right fourth intercostal space posterolateral thoracotomy provided adequate visualization of the trachea. The distal half of the trachea can be accessed via a high right thoracotomy, while the proximal ½–⅔ of the trachea can be accessed from a cervical collar incision with neck extension. The entire trachea can be accessed through a sternotomy. The lung was reflected inferiorly, and the azygos vein was divided. The tumor was visualized with a bronchoscope, and a stitch was placed on the external trachea to mark the tumor. A 25-guage needle can be advanced through the trachea and visualized with bronchoscopy to identify the extent of endolumenal lesions.

While encircling the distal trachea, it is important not to injure the left recurrent laryngeal nerve that runs in the opposite tracheoesophageal groove. Three rings of trachea on the left and one ring on the right were resected, with proximal and distal margins negative on frozen section.

Lateral dissection of the trachea should be limited to only the portion to be resected, as the blood supply runs laterally. 2-0 vicryl traction sutures were placed laterally 1 ring above and 1 ring below, and the anastomosis was performed using interrupted 4-0 vicryl sutures placed 3–4 mm apart. The knots can be tied on the inside or outside of the trachea. The traction sutures were tied together at the end to minimize tension.

Achieving a tension-free anastomosis is paramount in tracheal surgery. Extension and flexion of the neck allows the most length of trachea into the field. The trachea can be mobilized anteriorly and posteriorly with a finger, without concern for compromising the blood supply. Although not required in this case, a right hilar release can be performed to minimize anastomotic tension, as it allows the lung to shift cephalad 1–2 cm. This maneuver is performed by dividing the inferior pulmonary ligament and incising the pericardium inferiorly in a U-shape, with care not to injure the phrenic nerve anteriorly.

The lung was re-expanded over a 24-French chest tube, and the patient was extubated in the operating room. He was discharged on postoperative day 8 without complication. Final pathology confirmed grade I chondrosarcoma. No evidence of disease recurrence has been identified on flexible bronchoscopy or serial CT scans 24 months postoperatively.

Comments

Primary tracheal cancers are very rare, making up only 0.2% of cancers of the respiratory tract and 0.03% of all reported cancers [1]. Unlike tracheal squamous cell carcinomas, tracheal chondrosarcomas typically present with a long history of dyspnea that is often misdiagnosed as asthma [2]. Patients with an asymptomatic presentation typically have tumors that occlude less than 50% of the trachea, while dyspnea generally occurs only after 60%–75% of the trachea is occluded [2].

Diagnosis of tracheal chondrosarcoma is best done by CT scan followed by flexible and rigid bronchoscopy [3,4]. A chest CT provides information regarding the size and extent of the tumor but may underestimate tracheal wall involvement [5]. Bronchoscopy allows better visualization of and ability to biopsy the tumor.

Complete surgical resection with negative margins followed by end-to-end anastomoses is the standard treatment for tracheal chondrosarcoma [3]. Most reported cases of tracheal chondrosarcoma undergo an R0 resection with no reported recurrence [3]. Endoscopic resection is a palliative treatment option to restore the airway for patients who are unable or choose not to undergo surgery [6]. However, the ability to provide a complete resection endoscopically is limited, leading to a high rate of recurrence [5,6]. More recently, patients who have elected to have endoscopic resection have received endoscopic laser debulking in combination with radiotherapy [6].

Tracheal chondrosarcomas are typically unresponsive to chemotherapy and radiotherapy due to the slow growth rate [3,6]. Radiotherapy should be considered as adjuvant therapy in situations when a complete surgical resection is not possible or as a palliative treatment.[5] Chemotherapy has not been shown to be effective for treating chondrosarcomas but it may be used if there is lymph node metastasis [4].

Tracheal chondrosarcomas are very rare, typically slow-growing tumors with 90% five-year survival rate after appropriate resection [3]. CT scan followed by flexible and rigid bronchoscopy is the standard for diagnosis. To date, all reported patients who have received an R0 resection with negative margins have had no reported recurrence [6]. For patients with contraindications to surgery, endoscopic resection and radiotherapy should be considered.

REFERENCES

1. Nouraei, S.M., Middleton, S.E., Nouraei, A.R., Virk, J.S., George, P.J., Hayword, M., Sandhu, G.S. Management and prognosis of primary tracheal cancer: A national analysis. *Laryngoscope.* 2014;124(1):145–150.
2. Allen, M.S. Surgery of the trachea. *Korean J Thorac Cardiovasc Surg.* 2015;48:231–237.
3. Andolfi, M., Vaccarilli, M., Crisci, R., Puma, F. Management of tracheal chondrosarcoma almost completely obstructing the airway: A case report. *J Cardiothorac Surg.* 2016;11(1):101.
4. Sherani, K., Vakil, A., Dodhia, C., Fein, A. Malignant tracheal tumors: A review of current diagnostic and management strategies. *Curr Opin Pulm Med.* 2015;21(4):322–326.
5. Maia, D., Elharrar, X., Laroumagne, S., Maldonado, F., Astoul, P., Dutau, H. Malignant transformation of a tracheal chondroma: The second reported case and review of the literature. *Rev Port Pneumol.* 2016;22(5):283–286.
6. Kutzner, E.A., Park, J.S., Salman, Z., Inman, J.C. Tracheal chondrosarcoma: Systematic review of tumor characteristics, diagnosis, and treatment outcomes with case report. *Case Rep Oncol Med.* 2017;2017:4524910.

Mathew Thomas

 Key Words

- Tracheoesophageal fistula
- Trachea
- Esophagus
- Fistula

Introduction

Tracheoesophageal fistulas (TEFs) can be extremely challenging to manage and have a high risk of recurrence after surgical repair [1,2]. Despite modern advancements in surgical techniques and technology, adult TEFs remain among some of the most difficult problems encountered by thoracic surgeons, with mortality rates of up to 23% reported after surgery [3]. The majority of literature on recurrent or persistent TEF refers to the pediatric population, with little evidence derived from adult patients. In this report, we describe our evaluation and management of a persistent iatrogenic TEF in an adult patient with achalasia managed successfully with surgical repair after laparoscopic myotomy. We highlight the diagnostic and technical challenges encountered and describe an innovative technique to repair the TEF using a full thickness button of the anterior esophageal wall, which has not been reported before.

Case Report

A 56-year-old male with a history of chronic end-stage renal failure on hemodialysis presented for an evaluation to undergo renal transplantation at our institution. He had a significant medical history of severe hypertension, gastroesophageal reflux, and a chronic TEF acquired four years before following percutaneous tracheostomy. He had undergone two operations to repair the fistula via transverse cervical approach, both of which incorporated the use of neck strap muscles as pedicle flaps. Despite this, he continued to have coughing and aspiration when drinking fluids, leading to frequent respiratory infections. He also developed moderate hoarseness after his second operation. Direct laryngoscopy did not show any evidence of vocal cord weakness and generalized laryngeal inflammation suspected to be secondary to chronic reflux. A video swallow evaluation with oral contrast at our institution showed a persistent TEF at the level of the thoracic inlet, confirmed by bronchoscopy and upper gastrointestinal endoscopy (Figure 21.1a and b). This was considered a contraindication for renal transplantation, and he was referred to Gastroenterology for endoscopic management of the TEF.

He underwent endoscopic closure of the TEF with over-the-scope (Ovesco) clips after the fistula tract was deepithelialized with a microbrush. On follow-up three months later, the patient continued to be symptomatic, and there was a persistent TEF seen on radiographic imaging.

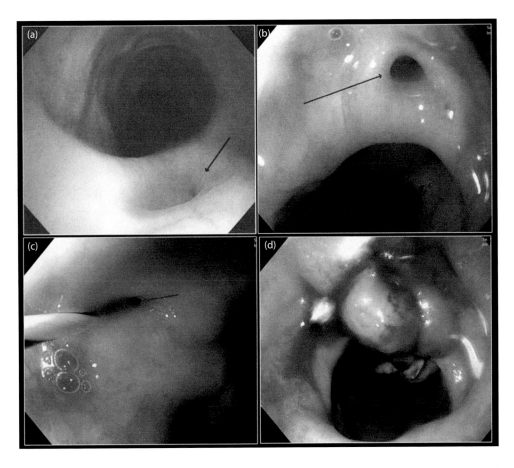

Figure 21.1 Tracheoesophageal fistula (arrows) seen on (a) initial bronchoscopy, (b) initial upper endoscopy, (c) upper endoscopy done three months after first endoclip application, with reduction in size of fistula noted, and (d) upper endoscopy after re-application of endoclips

Endoscopy showed the TEF to be smaller and clips were reapplied (Figure 21.1c and d). He was then referred to Thoracic Surgery for further management.

As part of our evaluation, a complete barium esophagram (Figure 21.2) was obtained showing a dilated esophagus with "bird-beak-like" appearance, typical of achalasia and delayed emptying of the esophagus. The obstruction in the distal esophagus was considered to be one of the reasons for repeated failure of the fistula to close. He underwent laparoscopic Heller myotomy and partial anterior fundoplication with percutaneous gastrotomy tube placement, which were recommended to improve emptying of the esophagus. He recovered uneventfully and was kept on gastric tube feeds alone with nothing by mouth to allow the fistula to heal. After six months, a contrast esophagram was repeated and showed the fistula to be still present. Surgical repair was recommended. The esophageal clips were removed by endoscopy the day prior to surgery.

Under general anesthesia, the patient was positioned supine with a posterior thyroid pillow and the neck extended. Flexible bronchoscopy was performed initially through a laryngeal mask airway (LMA). We identified a crater-like area with a pinhole fistula on the posterior tracheal membrane at level of sternal notch. The LMA was then exchanged for a single lumen

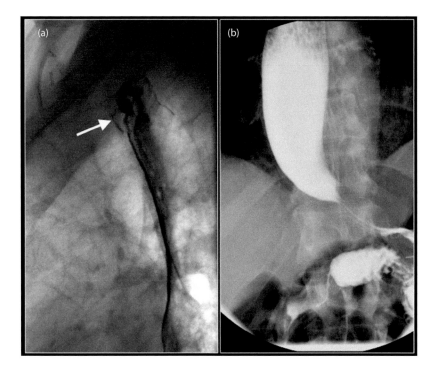

Figure 21.2 Preoperative contrast esophagram showing (a) persistent TEF (arrow) and (b) bird-beak-like appearance of the lower esophageal sphincter with dilated esophagus characteristic of achalasia

endotracheal tube, and flexible upper endoscopy was performed; granulation tissue without an obvious fistula was seen on the anterior wall of the esophagus located 21–23 cm from the incisors. The endoscope was used to insufflate the esophagus with air while simultaneously visualizing the trachea with the bronchoscope. The presence of air bubbling on the tracheal side confirmed the location of the TEF.

The surgical field included the entire neck and the chest, from the ear lobes to below the xiphoid process. The prior U-shaped cervical incision was re-incised and subplatysmal flaps were raised to the level of the thyroid cartilage superiorly and to the sternoclavicular joints inferiorly. The fascia over the trachea was incised longitudinally in the midline and then elevated away from the trachea on the left side using fine-tipped scissors. This sharp dissection was then carried posteriorly towards the tracheoesophageal groove, staying on the tracheal wall. The pedicled strap muscle flap created during the previous operation was identified and divided from its attachment to the trachea and preserved for later use. The left carotid sheath was palpated, but due to severe scarring, no attempt was made mobilize it.

At this point, intraoperative bronchoscopy was repeated, and the transilluminated light from the bronchoscope was used as a guide to determine the location of the TEF through the neck incision. The light was seen just below the sternal notch, and a partial upper sternotomy was then performed to the level of the sternomanubrial junction to expose the upper thoracic trachea. The right innominate artery was mobilized laterally to the right using a vessel loop. The esophagus could not be separated from the posterior tracheal membrane immediately cephalad to the fistula site due to severe scarring, which prevented us from dissecting out the fistula tract. Caudad to the fistula, there was minimal scarring and the esophagus and trachea could be bluntly dissected away from each other.

A full thickness incision was then made on the left lateral wall of the esophagus at the level of the TEF and extended circumferentially around the TEF as a 1.5-cm-wide anterior esophageal wall button (Figure 21.3a). The esophagus could now be separated from the posterior tracheal membrane. Because of chronic dilation from achalasia, the esophagus was redundant, and a two-layered transverse closure of the esophageal defect was performed without tension using absorbable sutures. The base of the fistula tract was obliterated with running 4-0 absorbable sutures, and the excised esophageal wall button with the fistula tract was then folded caudad on to the posterior trachea and sutured to the edge of tracheal wall with interrupted 4-0 absorbable sutures (Figure 21.3b). The preserved pedicled strap muscle flap was placed between the trachea, and the esophagus and tacked to the edge of the trachea with 4-0 absorbable sutures. A 3-cm × 3-cm bioprosthetic patch (Surgimend, Integra Lifescience, USA) was placed between the muscle flap and the esophageal suture line, followed by

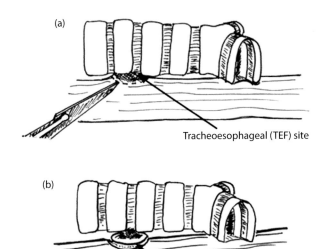

(a)

Tracheoesophageal (TEF) site

(b)

Full thickness anterior esophageal wall button

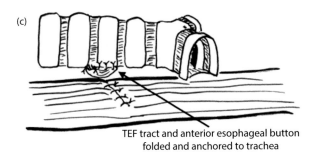

(c)

TEF tract and anterior esophageal button folded and anchored to trachea

Figure 21.3 Illustration of anterior esophageal wall technique for closure of TEF: (a). & (b). Excision of anterior esophageal wall button at the level of the fistula; (c). plication of the TEF tract and esophageal button to the trachea, with transverse closure of esophageal wall defect

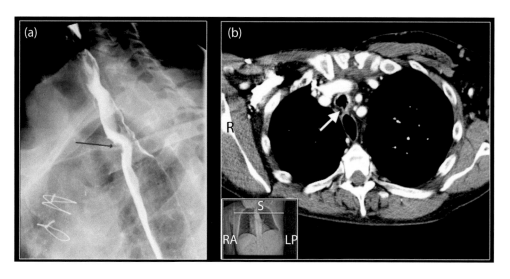

Figure 21.4 Post-operative images at 6 months with (a). contrast esophagram and (b). CT scan showing closed TEF (arrows)

application of fibrin glue. A 15-Fr drain was placed in the mediastinum and brought out laterally through the neck. The partial sternotomy was closed with two sternal wires.

The patient was extubated in the operating room and discharged home 1 week later after drain removal, without any immediate complications. However, 2 weeks later he developed staphylococcal infection of the sternal wound, requiring washout, curettage of the edges of the sternum and negative pressure therapy. He was kept on gastric tube feeds for another eight weeks, and further radiographic evaluation showed the fistula to have healed completely (Figure 21.4). He was then started on oral feeds, which he tolerated well. After showing no signs of TEF recurrence on clinical or radiographic evaluation nine months later, he was placed on the renal transplant waiting list.

Comments

Regardless of their etiology, TEFs can be extremely difficult to manage and often present a dilemma regarding the best approach for permanent closure. While open surgery still remains the standard for most primary TEFs [3,4], this approach can be technically challenging in cases of recurrent or persistent TEF. The difficulties in reoperation have opened up avenues for endoscopic closure [5,6], which may involve multiple interventions over extended periods of time. Yet when endoscopic closure is either not feasible or unsuccessful, open surgery may be the last resort to permanently close the fistula.

Nonmalignant recurrent TEFs require meticulous evaluation to determine the reasons for failure to close. It is important to rule out underlying malignancy, granulomatous disease, foreign bodies, or distal obstruction, all of which can prevent healing of the fistula. In the case of our patient, achalasia was identified as a contributing factor for failure of closure of the TEF after two surgical attempts. The delayed esophageal emptying likely elevated the intraluminal esophageal pressure, which was presumed to contribute to the patency of the fistula. We believe that the probability of closure with subsequent repair increased after relieving the distal obstruction by Heller myotomy.

Surgical repair of TEF requires separation of the trachea and esophagus, division and ligation of the fistula tract, followed by interposition of viable tissue between the esophagus and trachea. However, when reoperating for TEF, the trachea-esophageal plane may be nonexistent, leading to the risk of creating a severe defect along the posterior tracheal membrane if aggressive dissection is performed. In addition, there is an increased risk of injury to the recurrent laryngeal nerves, which may not be easily visible due to scar tissue. In such cases, where the esophagus and the trachea cannot be separated without significant risk, the anterior esophageal wall button technique, as described above, should be considered. The remaining segments of the esophagus can often be mobilized enough to facilitate primary transverse closure. The risks of this approach include esophageal suture line dehiscence, esophageal leaks, pseudo-esophageal diverticulum formation, or even recurrence of the TEF. The use of multiple adjunct techniques such as bioprosthetics and fibrin glue applied between the tracheal and esophageal suture lines is important to decrease the risk of these potential complications and recurrence of TEF. This technique may not be suitable for large TEFs where resection of a large portion of the esophageal wall would make primary closure of the esophageal defect difficult.

Other open techniques to repair complex TEFs include transtracheal closure with or without tracheal resection; primary resection and closure of the esophagus, esophageal diversion, and the use of vascularized pedicle interposition grafts [1,2,7]. We recommend that the anterior esophageal wall button technique should be added to the armamentarium of any surgeon who deals with TEFs.

REFERENCES

1. Shen, K.R., Allen, M.S., Cassivi, S.D., et al. Surgical management of acquired nonmalignant tracheoesophageal and bronchoesophageal fistulae. *Ann Thorac Surg.* 2010;90(3):914–918; discussion 919.
2. Muniappan, A., Wain, J.C., Wright, C.D., et al. Surgical treatment of nonmalignant tracheoesophageal fistula: A thirty-five year experience. *Ann Thorac Surg.* 2013;95(4):1141–1146.
3. Foroulis, C.N., Nana, C., Kleontas, A., et al. Repair of post-intubation tracheoesophageal fistulae through the left pre-sternocleidomastoid approach: A recent case series of 13 patients. *J Thorac Dis.* 2015;7(Suppl 1):S20–S26.
4. Downey, P., Middlesworth, W., Bacchetta, M., Sonett, J. Recurrent and congenital tracheoesophageal fistula in adults dagger. *Eur J Cardiothorac Surg.* 2017;52(6):1218–1222.
5. Gregory, S., Chun, R.H., Parakininkas, D., et al. Endoscopic esophageal and tracheal cauterization for closure of recurrent tracheoesophageal fistula: A case report and review of the literature. *Int J Pediatr Otorhinolaryngol.* 2017;98:158–161.
6. Lelonge, Y., Varlet, F., Varela, P., et al. Chemocauterization with trichloroacetic acid in congenital and recurrent tracheoesophageal fistula: A minimally invasive treatment. *Surg Endosc.* 2016;30(4):1662–1666.
7. Macchiarini, P., Verhoye, J.P., Chapelier, A., Fadel, E., Dartevelle, P. Evaluation and outcome of different surgical techniques for postintubation tracheoesophageal fistulas. *J Thorac Cardiovasc Surg.* 2000;119(2):268–276.

Wickii T. Vigneswaran

 Key Words
- Tracheal fistula
- Congenital T-E fistula
- Repair of T-E fistula

Introduction

Congenital trachea-esophageal fistula present at birth or soon thereafter. Less commonly found *H-type* congenital tracheoesophageal fistula without concomitant esophageal atresia is often high in the trachea and usually small in diameter can present with coughing especially after ingestion of fluid [1]. Patient with persistent fistula growing to adolescent without any symptom is unusual. A large fistula often requires tracheal resection and closure of the fistula [2].

Case Report

A 20-year-old female presented to the emergency room with sudden onset right-sided chest pain that was made worse with deep breathing. She denied any cough, shortness of breath, or any hemoptysis. She has been receiving treatment with bronchodilators for asthma, which was well-controlled with medication. She has been on birth control pills. Her last menstrual period (LMP) was two days previously. Her past medical history was significant for removal of an ovarian cyst at age 19. Clinical examination revealed a regular pulse rate of 78/min, temporal temperature of 37.3°C, left arm blood pressure of 130/76 mmHg, and respiratory rate was 16/min. She weighed 62.1 kg with a height 5'10", (body mass index [BMI] 19.37 kg/m²), and her was SpO2 99%. The lung examination was clear, but with pleuritic chest pain under the right breast and right lateral ribs that was not reproducible to palpation.

A posterior-anterior (PA) and lateral chest X-rays were obtained. There were previous chest x-ray to compare. The lung examination showed no focal consolidation vascularity was normal. There was a 1.1-cm nodular density partially projecting over the anterior right third rib and the right posterior lateral sixth rib suggesting either a pulmonary nodule or an artifact. Cardiac size and silhouette were normal as well as the mediastinum and pleura. Instead of a repeat chest X-ray (CXR), the patient underwent a CT scan with intravenous contrast to evaluate nodule and look for pulmonary emboli. There was no significant pulmonary pathology, but there was scaring in the right upper lobe abutting the lateral aspect of the major fissure and the lateral chest wall pleura with slight thickening of the major fissure. Diffuse air filling of the esophageal lumen was noted. There was a communication between the trachea and esophagus in the upper third (Figure 22.1).

Repeat CT scan of the chest three months later showed a significant decrease in the size of the pleural-based density seen on the previous CT examination. Residual linear configuration

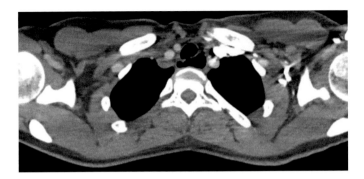

Figure 22.1 CT scan preoperative demonstrating the tracheal-esophageal connection

suggested scarring from an infectious or inflammatory process. Resolved aspiration pneumonia cannot be excluded given the findings of the trachea/esophagus. A single contrast (Isovue-300) esophagram showed a small trachea-esophageal fistula in upright, right posterior oblique view. A small amount of contrast spill into the trachea/fistulous track and the fistulous opening was seen (Figure 22.2a and b).

Patient was referred to Thoracic Surgery for consult. On direct questioning during her visit, the patient admitted that, since becoming aware of the fistula, she has noticed that she cannot drink a lot of water right after exercising because it will cause her to cough. She denied coughing up any food particles. She also denied fever, chills, chest pain, and shortness of breath. A repeat CT scan now six months after the initial diagnosis showed gas-filled and dilated esophagus throughout to the level of the gastroesophageal (GE) junction. Approximately a 2 × 5 mm defect between the anterior wall of the proximal thoracic esophagus and the posterior wall of the trachea was again observed.

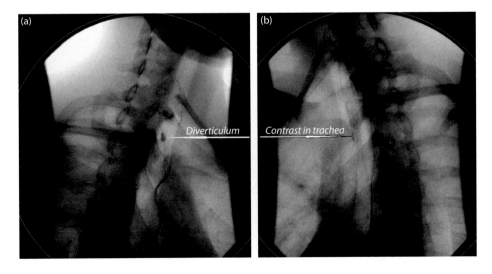

Figure 22.2 (a) Esophagram showing the esophageal diverticulum; (b) Oral contrast in trachea

Bronchoscopy and an esophagoscopy were performed. It showed on the proximal part, a defect in the membranous part of the trachea, about 5 mm wide and about 8 mm in length at the 17 cm from the incisors. Esophagoscopy examination performed simultaneously showed a diverticular opening identified at 19 cm from the incisor, and an obvious communication could not be demonstrated. This was not probed due to the concern that probing might make the fistula bigger.

Endoscopic closure was considered, but the lesion appeared high for manipulation of suture device. Therefore, an open approach was recommended to the patient, and the patient consented to a cervical approach. Bronchoscopy and esophagoscopy confirmed the fistula between 17 cm and 19 cm, respectively, from the incisor. A left cervical incision along the anterior border of the lower sternoclavicular muscle was made, and the esophagus was approached. The bridge between the esophagus and trachea was located, assisted by the pediatric esophagoscope in the esophagus. A small fistulous connection was identified in the mediastinum. A division of the fistula was considered, but as there was not much access to perform repair, a simple suture ligation of the tract was performed with nonabsorbable monofilament suture. A bronchoscopy performed following ligation confirmed obliteration of fistula opening on the tracheal side. Patient recovered well and discharged home on a soft diet on postoperative day 2. The oral intake was advanced to a normal diet one week later.

Patient was asymptomatic at a four-month visit. A repeat Bronchoscopy/esophagoscopy showed a small persistent "diverticulum" in the upper esophagus. On the tracheal examination, a persistent but a smaller tract below the visible suture was observed with small amount of granulation tissue around it. The tract was not probed due to the risk of "re-opening." A repeat CT scan was performed to further evaluate, which showed a persistent connection, although smaller than what was noticed before the intervention (Figure 22.3). The patient was asymptomatic again at a 12-month follow-up.

Comments

Congenital trachea-esophageal fistula presents at birth or soon thereafter. Patient with persistent fistula growing to adolescent without any symptom is unusual [2]. Our patient had been treated for asthma and reported to be well-controlled on medication. It is possible her "asthma" may be due to aspiration through the small trachea esophageal fistula. The CT finding suggest that there is all possibility that the patient would aspirate, but she only became aware of the aspiration after informing her of the diagnosis of the fistula suggesting this was not clinically significant. We postulate the food bolus as it travels close to the fistula preventing the patient having any symptoms. This can be hypothetically supported by our

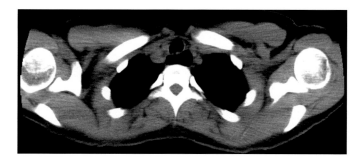

Figure 22.3 Postoperative CT scan at four-month follow-up

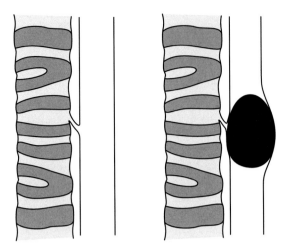

Figure 22.4 Possible mechanism of closure of small congenital fistula during the passage of food bolus due to the angle of the fistula

endoscopic finding that the distance of the tracheal opening was higher than the esophageal opening, and the bridge may be on a downward slope from the trachea to the esophagus (Figure 22.4).

The ideal operative procedure would have been to divide the fistulous tract and close both ends [3]. This, however, would have required detailed dissection that would require more exposure. In our patient, the fistulous tract was observed at 19 cm from the incisor in the esophagus and was noted at 17 cm in the trachea. The angulation perhaps prevented aspiration during swallowing, as when the food bolus travels it compress the esophagus against the trachea and narrows the fistulous track, closing it for practical purposes (Figure 22.4). This can explain why the patient was relatively asymptomatic even before the operative procedure. She also perhaps learnt to tuck her chin while swallowing, making the angulation longer and facilitating this mechanism.

The fistula track was relatively high in our patient and is not easily approached from the neck. There are many ways to approach a high trachea-esophageal fistula [4]. Better exposure can be obtained for a fistula that cannot be reached from the neck is from an anterior approach including a sternotomy and closure trans-tracheal. This was considered prior to the operative intervention and discussed with the patient including the risks and benefits and the approach we took from the lateral aspect. As the patient had minimal symptoms and not any notable complication due the fistula, we choose the less invasive approach as we did not think the risk associated with trans-tracheal approach, including short- and long-term tracheal complication due to the tracheal division, was justified.

REFERENCES

1. Evans, J.A., Greenberg, C.R., Erdile, L. Tracheal agenesis revisited: Analysis of associated anomalies. *Am J Med Genet.* 1999;82(5):415–422.
2. Acosta, J.L., Battersby, J.S. Congenital tracheoesophageal fistula in the adult. *Ann Thrac Surg.* 1974;17:51–57.

3. Albuquerque, K.V., Deshpande, R.K., Desai, P.B. Cervical approach for repair of congenital trachea-esophageal fistula presenting in an adult. *J Postgrad Med.* 1993;39(4):216–217. Review.

4. Grillo, H.C. Acquired tracheoesophageal and bronchoesophageal fistula. In *Surgery of the Trachea and Bronchi*, Grillo H.C. (Ed). BC Decker Inc., Hamilton, Canada, 2004, pp. 341–356.

CASE 23: REPAIR OF A NEAR FULL-LENGTH MALIGNANT TRACHEAL-ESOPHAGEAL FISTULA—A 17-YEAR SUCCESS STORY

Wickii T. Vigneswaran

 Key Words
- Tracheal esophagus fistula
- Malignant fistula
- Repair of tracheal esophageal fistula

Introduction

Malignant esophago-respiratory fistulae are an uncommon complication of esophageal or lung cancer that is secondary to tumor invasion through the walls of the esophagus and airway associated with tumor necrosis. The incidence is reported 5%–10% of esophageal and 1% of lung cancer [1]. Tumor necrosis is often the result of treatment using radiation and/or chemotherapy. When a fistula develops, it leads to contamination of the lung and, if untreated, is fatal. When there is distal obstruction of the esophagus, the contamination is worse. Sealing the fistula with a covered stent can reduce respiratory contamination and relieve obstruction, if present, allowing the patient to swallow better and improve their quality of life.

The mean survival of patients developing malignant esophago-respiratory fistulae are generally calculated in weeks or months due to the advanced stage of the underlying malignancy and pulmonary infection. Endoscopic therapy using covered stents in the esophagus or airway, or both, are sometimes used. Biologic glues also have been effectively used in sealing small fistula [2]. Surgical treatments to exclude or bypass the fistula are useful when endoscopic intervention is not available. Esophageal bypass with stomach or colon has been used in patients otherwise in good general condition [3,4]. If the fistula is effectively treated, it is the underlying malignancy that determines the outcome. We report one of the longest survivors of a malignant trachea-esophageal fistula who underwent radical surgical treatment.

Case Report

A 52-year-old man was transferred from an outside institution with acute respiratory distress to the emergency room. He was stridulous and was visibly having difficulty breathing. His past medical history was significant for squamous carcinoma of the upper third of the esophagus that was treated with chemo-radiation. Subsequently, he developed a tracheal esophageal fistula, which was treated with an endoscopic placement of a covered wire stent. After a brief period of relief, the patient developed recurrent signs of aspiration. Esophagostomy confirmed an extension of the trachea-esophageal fistula, and he underwent a second straddling stent covering the upper end of the previous stent, offering brief symptomatic relief. He was brought to the emergency room of the outside institution because of symptoms of significant respiratory distress and then transferred to our institution for further care.

On arrival, he was distressed with audible stridor. Hemodynamically stable, O_2 saturations were in the high eighties on room air. As part of the workup, a CT scan of the chest and upper abdomen, obtained immediately in the emergency room, showed the esophageal stent extending from the level of the clavicle to the sub-carinal region measuring 11.5 cm in length and eroding into the trachea 4 cm bellow the clavicle without any evidence of membranous portion of the distal trachea (Figure 23.1). The distal esophagus bellow the stent was dilated. There was no evidence of any local tumor on the imaging. Multiple ill-defined densities in the lung consistent with infection, but metastasis could not be excluded.

A bronchoscopy examination revealed a prolapsing stent into the tracheal lumen obstructing 90% of the lumen. The patient was referred to thoracic surgery for treatment consideration, and he was taken to the operating room emergently with the aim of repairing the trachea. After placement of arterial and venous access and monitoring lines, the patient was intubated with a single-lumen endotracheal tube with bronchoscopic guidance. A bronchial blocker was placed into the right main bronchus, then the patient was placed in a left lateral position, and through a posterolateral a right thoracotomy incision, the serratus anterior muscle was harvested on

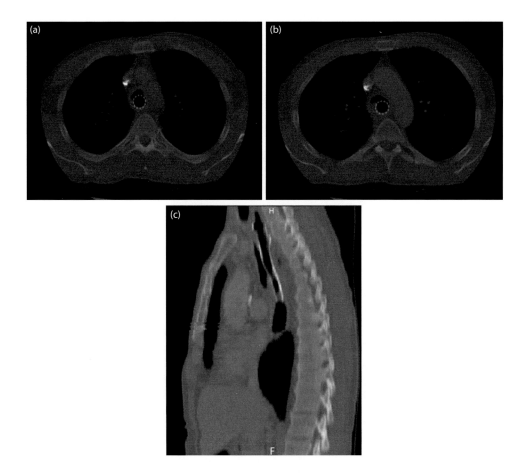

Figure 23.1 Preoperative CT imaging show the prolapse of the straddling esophageal stent into the tracheobronchial tree with destruction of posterior tracheal wall. (a) Mid-trachea, (b) Carina, and (c) Sagittal view demonstrate the straddling stents

its vascular pedicle. Then the pleural space was entered through the fourth intercostal space. The esophagus was isolated bellow the carina. The trachea and esophagus appeared one structure above the carina. The esophagus was separated from the trachea and bronchus, paying attention not to damage the cartilage part of the trachea. There was very little membranous portion of the trachea, and clearly the endo-tracheal tube was visible in the field. The defect extended from thoracic inlet to the left main bronchus. The bronchial blocker was withdrawn, the left main bronchus was intubated with a separate endo-tracheal tube in the field, and ventilation of left lung established. The incision was extended up, and the stents removed. A large defect was noted between the trachea and the esophagus. A small part of the esophageal wall was salvaged circumferentially all the way. Following the separation, the posterior wall of the trachea was absent from thoracic inlet to the proximal left main bronchus. After separating the esophagus from the posterior wall of trachea, a preserved bovine pericardium was trimmed to fit the tracheal defect and, using interrupted polydioxanone (PDS) and 4 "O" polypropylene sutures, the patch was sutured taught replacing the posterior wall of the trachea from proximal end of left main bronchus to the thoracic inlet. Before completion of the repair, the endotracheal intubation of the left main bronchus was established from above after the tube from the operating field was removed. Then, the serratus anterior muscle with the vascular pedicle was transferred into the pleural cavity, brought through the window created between second and fourth ribs in the chest wall [5]. The muscle was then sutured onto the edges of the tracheal defect covering the bovine pericardium from the inlet to the left main bronchus. The excess muscle was anchored with additional sutures. The partially circumferential remnant of esophagus was sutured to the posterior aspect of the muscle around an nasogastric tube maintaining esophageal continuity. After closure of the thoracotomy, the patient was then turned supine, and a feeding jejunostomy and a draining gastrostomy were performed. The patient recovered from this surgery well and was discharged home.

Three weeks postoperatively he complained of cough and altered breathing. A repeat CT scan with contrast revealed a residual fistula approximately measuring 1.5 cm in craniocaudal dimension at the level of great vessels. A bronchoscopy revealed that the superior repair had become loose, and an esophagoscopy confirmed a corresponding defect in the esophagus. After a period of conservative observation, but with radiological evidence of abscess formation in the posterior mediastinum, he was returned to the operating room, and a subtotal esophagectomy via repeat right thoracotomy and retrosternal gastric bypass and left-sided esophago-gastric cervical anastomosis was performed in the neck. He recovered well form this procedure and was discharged home. Six weeks later he complained of fluttering in his trachea whenever he coughed, but otherwise he is doing well. He was electively brought in for a bronchoscopy. A flexible bronchoscopy was performed under general anesthesia, and noted, the pericardial patch had partially separated from the trachea, where absorbable sutures were used. However, the muscle patch underneath has healed well, providing solid support to the posterior trachea. The patient underwent a rigid bronchoscope, and the remaining sutures holding the pericardial patch was divided by long endo-scissors and the whole patch extracted through the rigid scope. He was discharged home the following day. In the follow-up period, he required proximal dilation three times of the esophagogastric anastomosis during the next six months. Bronchoscopy during these visits showed a completely healed posterior tracheal wall. The only observation was the muscle repair was redder than the remaining trachea. The patient remained well without further intervention. He was cancer-free for the next 17 years and passed due to an unrelated cause at the age of 69. During his life, he was involved in counseling other cancer survivors through "Smart Patients Esophageal Cancer Community" (https://www.smartpatients.com/communities/esophageal-cancer) and the "Gilda's Club."

Comments

When a malignant fistula develops between esophagus and trachea, the underlying primary cancer is invariably of an advanced stage and is incurable. The frequent complication of this fistula is non-resolving aspiration pneumonia, either from ingestion or from backward flow of gastric contents into the esophagus. Life expectancy is measured in months, if the fistula can be effectively sealed, and if continued contamination is present with a persistent fistula, it is measured in days to weeks. To stop repeated episodes of aspiration and septic pneumonia, stenting of the esophagus or airway alone or double stenting of the esophagus and trachea to cover the fistula is often palliative treatment. When stenting is not possible or in failed surgical bypass, exclusion techniques are useful to reduce the contamination and maintain nutrition, although this is major surgery [6]. Staged operation to stop the contamination and later a procedure to restore alimentary continuity has been described in the past, with short-term survival advantage.

Radiation alone or in combination with chemotherapy is used for patients with locally advanced carcinoma of the esophagus. When the cancer invades the full thickness of the esophagus and tracheal-bronchial tree, the risk of developing a fistula is high. Chemotherapy alone has been reported to have a 6% rate of fistula and the risk following radiotherapy is reported as high as 73.9% [7]. Although the advances in radiation techniques have improved, still the risk remains high. Current guidelines recommend multimodality treatment for locally advanced esophageal cancer [8]. The benefit of surgical resection in improving survival compared to definitive chemo radiation for esophageal squamous cell carcinoma has been questioned [9]. These tumors often affect the upper esophagus and, when locally advanced, are likely to involve the airway. Radiation-induced tumor necrosis depends on inherent radio sensitivity of the primary cancer, the radiation dose, and how it is delivered. If it is too radio-sensitive, then the risk for fertilization by necrosis will also be high. The concomitant use of chemotherapy with radiation therapy may further increase radio sensitivity and the tumor response and necrosis. It is speculated that patients who developed a tracheo-esophageal fistula after radiation therapy would have done so in any case. However, it is probable that radiotherapy may hasten the development of a fistula by lysing the tumor. The risk is greatest in those patients with bulky tumors that indent or impinge the trachea.

Our case further confirms that the underlying tumor determines the ultimate outcome of the patient. Effective and aggressive treatment including radical surgery should be considered in a patient who can undergo surgery regardless of esophago-respiratory fistula, and if it can be demonstrated that the underlying primary malignancy has been effectively treated.

REFERENCES

1. Balazs, A., Kupcsulik, P.K., Galambos, Z. Esophagorespiratory fistulas of tumourous origin. Non-operative management of 264 cases in 20-year period. *Eur J Cardiothorac Surg.* 2008;345:103–107.
2. Sarper, A., OZ, N., Cihangir, C., Demircan, A., Isin, E. The efficacy of selfexpanding metal stents for palliation of malignant esophageal strictures and fistulas. *Eur J Cardiothorac Surg.* 2003;23(5):794–798.
3. Takeshi, H., Masaru, M., Shigematsu, Y., Takenaka, M., Oka, S., Nagata, Y., et al. Esophageal bypass using a gastric tube for a malignant tracheoesophageal/bronchoesophageal fistula: A report of 4 cases. *Int Surg.* 2011;96:189–193.

4. Shamji, F.M., Inculet, R. Management of malignant tracheoesophageal fistula. *Thorac Surg Clin*. 2018;28(3):393–402.

5. Arnold, P.G., Pairolero, P.C. Intrathoracic muscle flaps: An account of their use in the management of 100 consecutive patients. *Ann Surg*. 1990;211:656–660; discussion 660–662.

6. Meunier, B., Stasik, C., Raoul, J.L., Spiliopoulos, Y., Lakehal, M., Campion, J.P., Meunier, B., et al., Gastric bypass for malignant esophagotracheal fistula: a series of 21 cases. *Launois B Eur J Cardiothorac Surg*. 1998;13(2):184–188; discussion 188–189.

7. Martini, N., Goodner, J.T., D'Angio, G.J., et al: Tracheoesophageal fistula due to cancer. *J Thorac Cardiovasc Surg*. 1970;59:319.

8. Berry, M.F. Esophageal cancer: Staging system and guidelines for staging and treatment. *J Thorac Dis*. 2014;6(3):S289–S297.

9. Castoro, C., Scarpa, M., Cagol, M., Alfieri, R., Ruol, A., Cavallin, F., Michieletto, S., Zanchettin, G., Chiarion-Sileni, V., Corti, L., Ancona, E. Complete clinical response after neoadjuvant chemoradiotherapy for squamous cell cancer of the thoracic oesophagus: Is surgery always necessary? *J Gastrointest Surg*. 2013;17(8):1375–1381.

CASE 24: GASTROBRONCHIAL FISTULA AND CENTRAL DIAPHRAGMATIC HERNIA AFTER SLEEVE GASTRECTOMY

Mathew Thomas

 Key Words

- Fistula
- Gastric
- Bronchus
- Sleeve resection
- Diaphragm
- Hernia

Introduction

Gastrobronchial fistula (GBF) is a very rare complication after bariatric surgery, occurring in 0.2% of patients after laparoscopic sleeve gastrectomy (LSG) [1]. We describe a case of chronic GBF with a central diaphragmatic hernia after gastric sleeve resection and our management strategy.

Case Report

A 47-year-old female patient was referred to us from another facility for a chronic GBF of a 2-year duration. She had initially undergone a laparoscopic adjustable gastric band placement for morbid obesity, which failed, and had LSG six years later after removal of the band. Her postoperative course was complicated by a staple line leak leading to a 2-month hospitalization. This was managed by endoscopic gluing. Four months later, she developed a fistula between the stomach and the left lower lobe (LLL) of lung through the diaphragm, leading to multiple hospitalizations for pneumonia. Multiple endoscopic procedures including glue application and clip placement were performed in an attempt to close the fistula but failed. Two years later, she was seen at our institution for a second opinion. Her co-morbidities included HIV, morbid obesity, and diabetes. Following her sleeve resection, she had achieved a weight loss of 100 lbs. She was a former smoker of 28-pack-years.

Her main symptoms at presentation included chronic cough with bilious sputum, hoarseness of voice, and complaints of severe reflux despite high-dose proton pump inhibitor in addition to H2 blockers.

Her examination was unremarkable except for a body mass index of 34. Air entry was equal bilaterally with few crackles heard at the left base of the chest posteriorly.

Barium esophagram did not show a fistula, but the clips from prior endoscopic closure were visible (Figure 24.1). A CT scan of the abdomen and chest revealed a fistulous communication between the remnant stomach and the left lobe of the lung (Figure 24.2a and b). There was confluent heterogeneous airspace opacity in the medial inferior aspect of the LLL with small airway disease involving the lingula and in the left lower lobe.

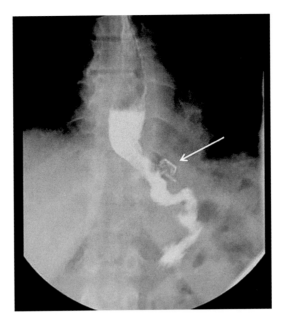

Figure 24.1 Barium esophagram showing endoscopic clips (arrow) but no fistula

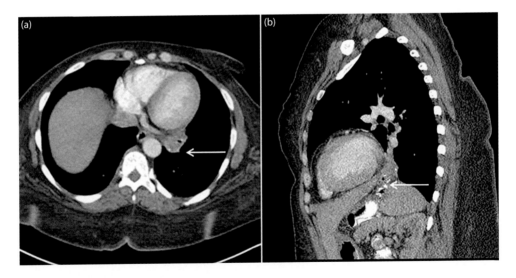

Figure 24.2 Axial (a) and sagittal (b) CT scan images showing fistula (arrow) between the stomach and left lower lobe of the lung

We recommended a left thoracotomy with lower lobectomy, total gastrectomy, and conversion to a Roux-en-Y esophagojejunostomy. She provided her informed consent.

In the operating room, the patient underwent a bronchoscopy, which showed abundant bilious secretions in the left main stem bronchus. After clearing the secretions, the fistula was visualized in medial basal segmental bronchus along with suture material. A standard posterolateral thoracotomy was then performed through the seventh intercostal space. After extensive adhesiolysis, a diaphragmatic hernia through the tendinous portion of the left hemidiaphram was identified and was adherent to the LLL. A fistula tract from the herniated stomach to the LLL could be palpated and was transected to allow mobilization of the lung. On closer examination, the superior segment of the LLL was noted to be normal while the basilar segments were consolidated. We decided to perform a basilar segmentectomy instead of a lobectomy. The anterior aspect of the interlobar fissure was dissected until the basal segmental pulmonary vessels were identified, which were then ligated and divided. This allowed the LLL bronchus to be exposed, and the fistula tract could be seen communicating with a large medial basilar bronchus through the lung parenchyma. This segmental bronchus was divided with a stapler, and the other segmental bronchi were divided en-bloc with the lung parenchyma using medium thickness stapler. The posterior aspect of the fissure was left intact to prevent torsion of the superior segment. There was no air leak from the staple line, and the superior segment inflated well.

Next, the esophagus was mobilized circumferentially from just above the level of the inferior pulmonary vein to below the diaphragmatic hiatus. The sac of the central diaphragmatic hernia was excised to reveal part of the stomach, omentum, staple line with the fistula tract, and suture material within the hernia. The hernia was freed up completely from the edges of diaphragm defect and reduced back into the abdomen. The defect measured 3 cm × 1 cm and was closed primarily with interrupted horizontal sutures of 0-Prolene and then reinforced with a single running 0-Prolene suture. After closure of the thoracotomy incision, the abdominal team proceeded with a total gastrectomy with Roux-en-Y esophagojejunostomy and feeding jejunostomy tube placement via a laparotomy.

The patient had an uneventful immediate postoperative course and had a barium contrast esophagram on postoperative day 5. A clear liquid diet was started and advanced to a postgastrectomy diet. She was discharged home after 9 days in the hospital, which included 1 day in intensive care unit. She was readmitted two weeks later with left thoracotomy pain, and CT showed a subcutaneous collection suspicious for a seroma. This was drained percutaneously, and cultures were positive for *Staphylococcus aureus*. She was treated with antibiotics and discharged one week later. Her jejunostomy feeding tube was eventually removed after she tolerated a bariatric diet. Her postoperative chest X-ray showed a well-expanded left lung with expected postoperative changes (Figure 24.3).

Comments

Enteropulmonary fistulas are rare conditions and most are caused by malignancy, trauma, or postsurgical complications. Fistulas occurring between the lung or airway and gastric conduit in the chest are well-known complications after esophagectomies. On the other hand, GBFs are extremely rare, and to the best of our knowledge, less than 40 cases caused as a complication of bariatric surgery have been reported in literature [2,3]. The pathology appears to be the sequelae of a subphrenic abscess following a staple line leak that erodes its way into the pleural cavity and lung. A case of a spontaneous GBF in an immunocompromised patient due to an invasive fungal infection has been reported and was treated with thoracic window and thoracomyoplasty [4].

GBF is a serious complication with a reported mortality rate of 6% [3] and can be extremely difficult to manage. The fistula rarely occurs in isolation and is either associated with gastric pouch stricture [5] or hernia, as in our patient. Patients are often malnourished or have severe comorbidities related to their morbid obesity such as diabetes, which contribute to poor wound healing. As a result of chronic lung contamination and the preceding gastric

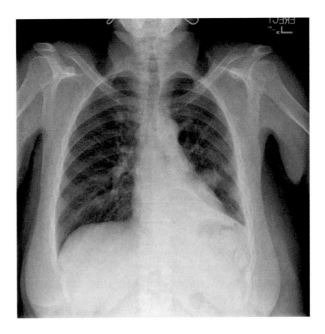

Figure 24.3 Postoperative chest X-ray at two weeks showing well expanded left lung

leak, they have recurring lung infections or abdominal abscesses and poor quality of life. Unless an emergent operation is necessary due to sepsis or bleeding, it is important to optimize the nutritional status of the patient before managing the fistula. If the patient is severely malnourished, nasojejunal feeding or parenteral nutrition should be considered before operating. The workup should include professional nutritional assessment and a CT scan of the chest and abdomen with contrast to evaluate the fistula. Endoscopy is helpful to understand the location of the fistula with regard to the gastroesophageal junction and help determine the amount of stomach to be resected. Similarly, bronchoscopy is essential to locate the fistula and plan lung resection.

The recommendations for the management of GBF are based on anecdotal evidence since this is a rare condition. The most common definitive surgical approach described in literature appears to include some form of lung resection along with gastrectomy or gastric diversion with gastrojejunostomy. In a systematic literature review of 11 studies that comprised 36 cases of post-bariatric surgery GBF [5], the mean time to diagnosis was 7.2 months (range: 1–30 months). The most common bariatric operation was a sleeve gastrectomy (n = 24), followed by Roux-en-Y Gastric Bypass (RYGB) (n = 12) with 42% of patients diagnosed with a gastric leak prior to the GBF. The main presenting symptoms were productive cough and subphrenic abscesses. Endoscopic treatment was successful in 18 out of 20 patients, with 2 complications reported. In eight patients, endoscopic treatment of pouch stricture was sufficient, while among the other twelve patients who had stents, two also had fibrin glue injection but failed and required surgery. The fistula successfully resolved in all 17 surgical patients, but this included some major complications including 1 patient who had a cervical esophagostomy following anastomotic breakdown. The majority of surgical patients (14/17) had aggressive operations, while the remaining three had thoracic or abdominal drainage procedures only. The authors concluded that GBF can be effectively treated with both endoscopy and surgery, but the latter was associated with more complications. In our opinion, the small number of cases and the variability of the surgeries performed in this study preclude a true assessment of surgical management of GBF, but the endoscopic approach with stents appear to be less variable and successful in the majority of reported cases.

In a French multicentric study [3], 13 cases of GBF after LSG were analyzed and only 2 patients were treated without surgery. In addition to all 11 patients undergoing thoracic operations, 3 splenectomies, 1 total gastrectomy, and 5 gastrojejunostomies were also performed. Six out of eight patients classified as late GBF (>30 days presentation after LSG) required lung resection and repair or reconstruction of the diaphragm. No patients died, and GBF completely resolved in all patients.

In summary, GBF is a complex and rare complication after bariatric surgery, with high mortality and morbidity rates. Endoscopic management with stents can be attempted, but most patients will likely require some kind of thoracic or abdominal surgery either for drainage of complex abscesses or definitive management of the fistula.

REFERENCES

1. Rebibo, L., Dhahri, A., Berna, P., Yzet, T., Verhaeghe, P., Regimbeau, J.M. Management of gastrobronchial fistula after laparoscopic sleeve gastrectomy. *Surg Obes Relat Dis.* 2014;10(3):460–467.
2. Nguyen, D., Dip, F., Hendricks, L., Lo Menzo, E., Szomstein, S., Rosenthal, R. The surgical management of complex fistulas after sleeve gastrectomy. *Obes Surg.* 2016;26(2):245–250.
3. Guillaud, A., Moszkowicz, D., Nedelcu, M., Caballero-Caballero, A., Rebibo, L., Reche, F., et al. Gastrobronchial fistula: A serious complication of sleeve gastrectomy results of a french multicentric study. *Obes Surg.* 2015;25(12):2352–2359.
4. Janilionis, R., Lukoseviciute, L., Beisa, V., Jotautas, V., Petrauskaite, R., Peceliunas, V., et al. Successful management of gastropulmonary fistula due to invasive fungal infection after chemotherapy and autologous stem cell transplantation: A case report. *Acta Med Litu.* 2016;23(3):169–174.
5. Silva, L.B., Moon, R.C., Teixeira, A.F., Jawad, M.A., Ferraz, A.A., Neto, M.G., et al. Gastrobronchial fistula in sleeve gastrectomy and Roux-en-Y gastric bypass: A systematic review. *Obes Surg.* 2015;25(10):1959–1965.

Stephanie G. Worrell, Kiran H. Lagisetty, and Rishindra M. Reddy

 | **Key Words**
--- | ---

* Case report
* Bronchogenic cyst
* Paraesophageal hiatal hernia

Introduction

Mediastinal masses are often found incidentally after imaging for other reasons. They may cause symptoms based on both size and location. Bronchogenic cysts are the most common primary cyst of the mediastinum and account for 5%–10% of all mediastinal masses. They often present in childhood, however, and can be identified later in life. If they contain a patent communication with the tracheobronchial tree then patients can present with recurrent upper respiratory tract infections. Since these cysts frequently lead to complications, such as compression, infection, and hemoptysis, they should be removed if possible when identified [1].

Case Report

A 62-year-old Caucasian female presented to her primary care physician with worsening shortness of breath with exertion over the prior three weeks. She had a history of recurrent upper respiratory tract infections and a cough over the prior 30 years. She was otherwise healthy and denied any history of heartburn or regurgitation. She had a CT scan that showed a large posterior mediastinal mass, and her primary care physician suspected a paraesophageal hiatal hernia. She was referred to a thoracic surgery clinic for evaluation of this reported hernia. Her past medical history was otherwise unremarkable. She had no abnormal physical exam findings.

On re-review of her original imaging (Figure 25.1), there was no apparent connection between the esophagus and an adjacent large structure, which was felt to be cystic in nature, contrary to the original interpretation of being a portion of the stomach. A barium esophagogram was ordered to determine if the gastrointestinal tract communicated with the posterior mediastinal lesion. This showed no evidence of a paraesophageal hiatal hernia (Figure 25.2). The differential diagnosis now was focused on a bronchogenic or esophageal duplication cyst, with bronchogenic cyst being more likely based on radiologic appearance. A bronchoscopy was performed and showed a small, pin-sized, opening at the carina, confirming the likelihood of a bronchogenic cyst. Pulmonary function tests showed adequate lung function to tolerate a lobectomy if necessary.

She was taken to the operating room for a cyst excision. A thoracotomy was performed with a concurrent mobilization of an intercostal muscle flap to cover the bronchial communication. The cyst was well-incorporated in the parenchyma of the right lower lobe. Given the

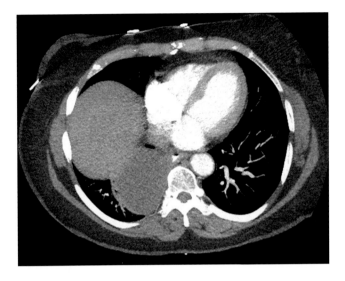

Figure 25.1 CT chest scan showing posterior mediastinal mass. White arrows show cyst and esophageal lumen

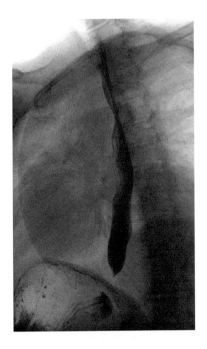

Figure 25.2 Preoperative barium esophagogram showing a normal esophageal lumen and no hernia

proximity of the cyst to the hilar structures of the lower lobe, a lobectomy was performed to completely excise the cyst (Figure 25.3). The cyst was also in close proximity to the esophagus, however, and was able to be dissected off the esophagus with no violation of the esophageal wall. The patient had an uncomplicated postoperative course and was sent home on postoperative day four. The final pathology was consistent with a benign bronchogenic cyst.

On her postoperative examination, she reported resolution of her cough and had no new respiratory infection symptoms. Her follow-up chest X-rays showed decreased lung volumes on the right, consistent with a post-lobectomy film and no other concerns. No further surveillance imaging was indicated given the benign pathology results.

Comments

Bronchogenic cysts can occur in a variety of locations but most commonly are located within the mediastinum and adjacent to the tracheobronchial tree in the subcarinal location. These cysts can also be found within the lung parenchyma, as in our case [1]. When the cysts occur within the lung parenchyma, they most commonly occur in the lower lobes (65%). However,

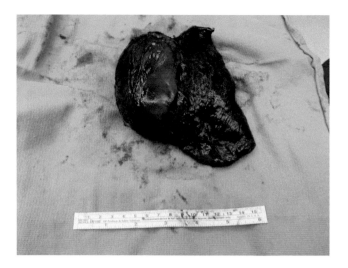

Figure 25.3 Bronchogenic cyst specimen

bronchogenic cysts have been identified within all lobes of the lung [2]. The consequence of an intraparenchymal location is the need for lung resection. Ideally, a nonanatomic resection can be performed, but if not feasible, a segmentectomy, lobectomy, and even pneumonectomies have been described [2].

When identified these cysts should be resected as they can lead to a number of minor to serious complications. Complications occur at a rate of 26%–62% [1,2]. Complications include those intrinsic to the cyst and those caused by compression of structures near the cyst. Examples of these complications include fistualization with airways, infection without fistula, hemorrhage, rupture into adjacent structures, and bronchial atresia [2,3]. Additionally, these cysts can harbor a malignancy with reports of adenocarcinoma, sarcoma, and squamous cell carcinoma [1,2,4,5].

The location of the bronchogenic cyst, in our case, led the patient's outside physician to be suspicious for a paraesophageal hernia. Although, this cyst was distinct from the esophagus, occasionally an esophageal duplication cyst can be difficult to distinguish from a bronchogenic cyst. The clues that the origin is esophageal rather than bronchial are the degree of adhesion and involvement with the esophagus. Ultimately, the histology between the two is distinct. However, one should be prepared for either when it is not clear preoperatively.

REFERENCES

1. Suen, H., Mathisen, D.J., Grillo, H.C., et al. Surgical management and radiological characteristics of bronchogenic cysts. *Ann Thorac Surg.* 1993;55:476–481.
2. St-Georges, R., Deslauriers, J., Duranceau, A., et al. Clinical spectrum of bronchogenic cysts of the mediastinum and lung in the adult. *Ann Thorac Surg.* 1991;52(1):6–13.

3. Sarper, A., Ayten, A., Golbasi, I., et al. Bronchogenic cyst. *Tex Heart Inst J.* 2003;30(2):105–108.

4. Behrend, A. and Kravitz, C.H. Sarcoma arising in a bronchogenic cyst. *Surgery.* 1951;29:142–144.

5. Moersch, H.J., Clagett, O.T. Pulmonary cysts. *J Thorac Surg.* 1947;16:179–194.

CASE 26: THE SURGICAL TREATMENT OF PULMONARY ECHINOCOCCOSIS

Gillian Alex, Christopher W. Seder, and Ozuru Ukoha

Key Words
• Echinococcosis • Hydatid • Pulmonary • Alveolar • Case report

Introduction

Echinococcosis is a zoonotic disease caused by the tapeworm *Echinococcus*. It is found throughout the world but is concentrated in Europe, the Middle East, and Asia. It carries a large societal and socioeconomic burden in the developing world and has been recently listed as a neglected treatable disease (NTD) by the World Health Organization (WHO) [1]. The following is a report of a young female who presented to a large urban county hospital in the United States with pulmonary cystic Echinococcosis.

Case Report

A 35-year-old, otherwise healthy, recently immigrated Ukrainian-born female presented with a four-month history of a chronic productive cough and low-grade fevers. She had been treated with multiple courses of antibiotic regimens without resolution of her symptoms. She had a remote five-year smoking history but quit prior to presentation. Routine laboratory investigations had been repeatedly normal without leukocytosis. A chest X-ray revealed a well-circumscribed cavitary lesion of the left lower lobe (Figure 26.1). Chest computed tomography (CT) scan demonstrated a single fluid and air-containing cystic structure (Figure 26.2). A transthoracic percutaneous needle biopsy was performed but it was nondiagnostic. The patient was referred to cardiothoracic surgery and the decision was made to proceed with a left video-assisted thoracoscopic exploration.

At the time of the operation, general endotracheal anesthesia was induced with a single-lumen tube with the patient supine in bed. Flexible fiber-optic bronchoscopy was performed showing inflammation of the left lower bronchus. The left lung was isolated using a double-lumen endotracheal tube, and the patient repositioned in the right lateral decubitus position. A 12-mm port was placed in the eight intercostal space at the anterior axillary line, through which a 10-mm 30° thoracoscope was passed into the pleural space. A utility incision was created in the fifth intercostal space at the anterior axillary line and a small Alexis Wound Protector (Applied Medical, Rancho Santa Margarita, CA) was inserted. There were no lesions other than the left lower lobe tumor identified in the chest. The inferior pulmonary ligament was divided, exposing the extent of the tumor in the lateral basal segment. A long-curved clamp was placed underneath the tumor with at least 2 cm of parenchymal margin. Serial application of Endo GIA 45-mm medium/thick stapling device (Medtronic,

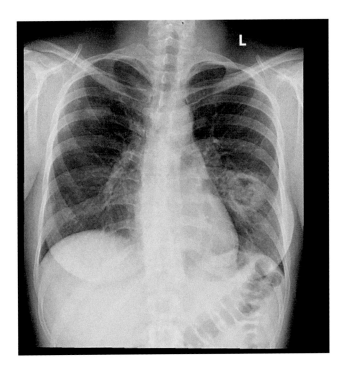

Figure 26.1 PA chest X-ray demonstrating cavitary lesion

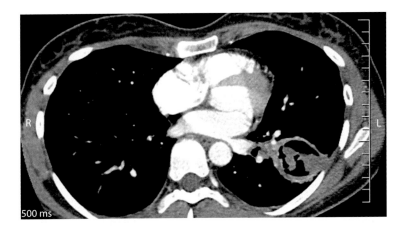

Figure 26.2 CT chest scan demonstrating cavitary lesion

Minneapolis, MN) resulted in an uneventful, single-stage, complete wedge resection of the tumor. It was opened on the back table to reveal a thick, creamy, abscess-filled cavity with organized inflammatory material lining the walls.

The patient's chest tube was removed on postoperative day (POD) 1, and she was discharged home without complication. Final pathology demonstrated a hydatid cyst infected with *E. granulosus* (Figures 26.3a and b). The patient was seen in Infectious Disease Clinic and prescribed a six-month course of the antihelminth *albendazole*. To date, she has no evidence of recurrence.

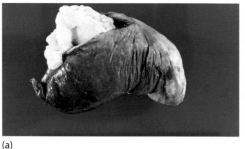

(a)

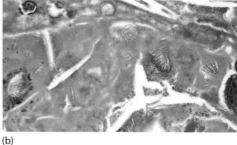

(b)

Figure 26.3 (a, b) Pathology specimen of wedge resection containing cyst

Comments

Cystic echinococcosis is relatively uncommon in the United States; however, more cases are being reported with the increase in immigrant populations. Thoracic surgeons should be familiar with the presentation and management of this disease. The presentation is dependent on the size and location of the cyst and presence of rupture. Small (<5 cm) peripherally located cysts are often asymptomatic and found incidentally on routine imaging. Larger and more centrally located cysts may present with mass effect. Complications of hydatid cysts include rupture, secondary infection, and pneumothorax. Cyst rupture most often presents with acute onset chest pain, fever, or cough. Upon rupture, the patient must be monitored for hypersensitivity reactions ranging from urticaria to anaphylaxis.

The primary treatment of pulmonary hydatid cysts is surgical. The goal of surgery is to remove the cyst while preserving lung parenchyma and avoiding spillage of cyst contents. Without a large series to rely on and a body of literature comprised primarily of case reports from various locations in the world [2], there is little consensus on the approach to surgical management with regards to timing of intervention, type of intervention, or operative approach. Most agree that patients with symptomatic disease from rupture, mass effect, or proximity to a vital structure should undergo intervention. There are, however, proponents of prophylactic intervention upon diagnosis as it is believed that the majority of hydatid cysts will eventually become symptomatic [3]. The most important surgical principle is avoidance of pleural space contamination with cyst contents, as this may cause anaphylaxis or dissemination.

The most common techniques for removal are enucleation, ectocystectomy, cystostomy, open aspiration, and formal lung resection. Enucleation removes the cyst but leaves the ectocyst behind. There is increased risk of rupture with this technique and therefore should only be used for smaller cysts [4]. Ectocystectomy involves removing the entire hydatid cyst including the outer layer. Advantages of this strategy are complete removal of all structures and therefore a possible decreased recurrence. However, as the ectocyst is actually part of the host, there is increased risk of disruption of the lung parenchyma and air leak. The most common technique is the Barrett technique, or cystectomy, which involves aspirating the fluid and removing the endocyst. This technique decreases the risk of spillage and air leak but does not damage the layers adherent to the lung parenchyma. Lobectomy is indicated when there are multiple cysts or a single cyst, those compromises >50% of the lobe. A wedge resection may be indicated when the diagnosis is in question, as it can serve both therapeutic and diagnostic purposes. Placing hypertonic saline-soaked gauzes or towels around the surgical site during any of the above procedures can reduce intraoperative spillage and contamination.

There are a variety of surgical techniques that can be used in the management of echinococcosis. The central tenant of hydatid management is safe, complete removal without intrathoracic contamination. The surgical approach should be dictated by the characteristics of the cyst and surgeon experience.

REFERENCES

1. Budke, C.M., Casulli, A., Kern, P., Vuitton, D.A. Cystic and alveolar echinococcosis: Successes and continuing challenges. PLoS *Negl Trop Dis.* 2017;11(4): e0005477. doi:10.1371/journal.pntd.0005477.
2. Rossi, P., Tamarozzi, F., Galati, F., Pozio, E., Akhan, O., Cretu, C. M, ... Casulli, A. The first meeting of the European Register of Cystic Echinococcosis (ERCE). *Parasit Vectors.* 2016;9:243 DOI 10.1186/s13071-016-1532-3.
3. Gottstein, B. and Reichen, J. Hydatid lung disease (echinococcosis/hydatidosis). *Clin Chest Med.* 2002;23:397–408.
4. McManus, D.P., Zhang, W., Li, J., Bartley, P.B. Echinococcosis. *Lancet.* 2003;362:1295–1304.

James B. Hendele and Francis J. Podbielski

 Key Words

- Pulmonary ossification
- FDG PET
- Lung mass

Introduction

Pulmonary ossification was first described by Luschka in 1856. It occurs most commonly in men in their 50s and 60s and consists of metaplastic osseous formations within the interstitium of the lung which include elements such as osteoblasts, osteoclasts, and marrow. An example of pulmonary ossification—a benign lesion—which is also fluorodeoxyglucose (FDG)-avid on positron emission tomography (PET) scan has not been previously described.

Pulmonary ossification differs from other benign lung tumors such as pulmonary calcifications, which do not contain organized bone and marrow elements, and hamartomas, which are composed of tissue elements native to the lung. Pulmonary ossification is usually diagnosed at autopsy and tends not to cause symptoms in life. A history of recurrent pulmonary insults such as pneumonia, anthracosis, fibrosis, and edema in the context of congestive heart failure or mitral stenosis is usually present. A retrospective analysis of the largest autopsy series published found an incidence of 1.63 cases of pulmonary ossification per 1,000 subjects [1].

Scattered reports of pulmonary ossification diagnosed during life do exist in the literature. Symptomatic pulmonary ossific lesions have been found independently in patients presenting with shortness of breath and pneumothorax. Asymptomatic lesions have been found within areas of colorectal carcinoma metastases. The lesions are uniformly benign, even when extensive disease is present [2–4].

Case Report

A 69-year-old male was referred to our thoracic surgery clinic with a suspicious lesion in the left upper lobe of the lung as seen on a CT scan performed after a screening X-ray was obtained to evaluate his history of weight loss. The lesion measured 9.0 × 4.1 × 2.7 cm and was 18F-fluorodeoxyglucose (18F-FDG)-avid on PET with a maximum standardized uptake value of 5.7 (Figure 27.1). His medical history was significant for a 40-pack-year history of tobacco use and a prior coronary artery bypass graft surgery (CABG) with left internal mammary artery (LIMA) conduit in 2003. He had no symptoms of congestive heart failure or fibrotic lung disease.

A transbronchial biopsy of the lesion revealed pulmonary elements with organized bone and marrow without evidence of carcinoma. Based on current recommendation for the management

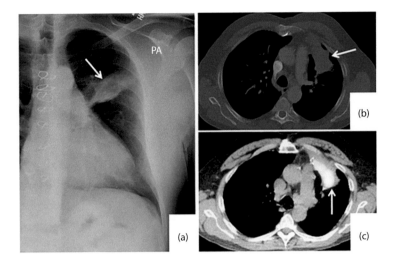

Figure 27.1 Initial radiology of the thorax. (a) The screening X-ray demonstrates a large left upper lobe mass with hazy, ill-defined borders. (b) Computed tomography (CT) of the chest reveals a homogenous, anterior upper lobe soft tissue mass abutting the parietal pleura with irregular borders. (c) 18F-FDG avidity on PET scan raised concerns for a malignant lung tumor

of solitary pulmonary nodules, the lesion was removed by left upper lobectomy using a muscle-sparing left thoracotomy [5]. Dissection of the lesion from the internal mammary artery pedicle was challenging. Postoperative recovery was uneventful, and the patient was discharged to home on postoperative day number 11. The patient did develop postoperative hoarseness and paresis of the left vocal cord, most likely secondary to traction on the recurrent laryngeal nerve during the tedious dissection of the lung parenchyma from the LIMA pedicle.

Final pathology on the specimen was returned as osteogenic metaplasia with trilineage hematopoietic elements within one of the left upper lobe bronchioles. No evidence of carcinoma was present (Figure 27.2).

Comments

We report an unusual case of asymptomatic pulmonary ossification diagnosed in life. Literature review reveals only case reports describing this phenomenon, which is generally found in autopsy specimens.

Dendriform pulmonary ossification demonstrates a branching structure with bone spicules within the interstitium and alveolar septa. Marrow elements are often present, and alveoli are intact. The process is most commonly associated with restrictive lung disease and fibrosis. Nodular pulmonary ossification is more common than its dendriform counterpart. Lesions of the latter type are more compact with smooth borders with osseous formation occurring within the alveolar spaces; marrow elements are usually not found. Associated conditions include congestive heart failure and alveolar bleeding. Each of the subtypes is composed of mature lamellar bone with osteoblast or osteoclast activity [6].

Diffuse pulmonary ossification results from multiple factors stemming from tissue injury. Alveolar bleeding results in interstitial deposits of metal (usually iron), which in turn attracts

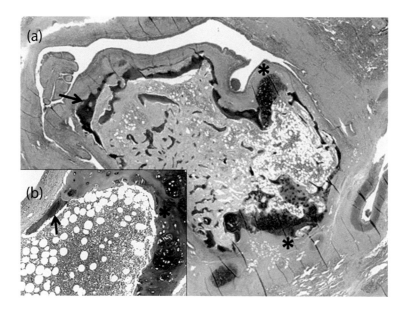

Figure 27.2 (a) Hematoxylin and eosin staining of the specimen shows pulmonary ossification and marrow elements occluding the lumen of a segmental bronchus. Note, the plates of hyaline cartilage present in the periphery of the bronchus and marked with asterisks. Arrows mark lamellar bone, although woven elements are also present. Active marrow elements and adipocytes can be seen with the bronchial lumen. Magnification x40. (b) Inset is a detail of the ossifying tumor with adipocytes and active marrow elements, lamellar bone (arrow), and hyaline cartilage (asterisk) magnification x100

multinucleated giant cells. This milieu promotes inflammation, fibrosis, and hyalinization of the alveolar wall. An alkaline environment promotes calcium salt precipitation and alkaline phosphatase and transforming growth factor beta (TGF-β) activity. This, in turn, promotes osteoblast activity, collagen type II, proteoglycan and fibronectin production, and possibly osteoblast proliferation via TGF-β's structural similarity to bone morphogenetic proteins [7]. It is hypothesized that the etiology of this patient's pulmonary ossification resulted from an initial insult at the time of his CABG procedure. Incidental damage to the left upper lobe during that surgery resulted in alveolar bleeding, which initiated the cascade of events causing the formation of his pulmonary ossific lesion.

The management of solitary pulmonary nodules is a frequently reviewed topic with a detailed, systematic, and widely known management algorithm. The Brock University cancer prediction equation assigned our patient a 60%–67% chance of his lesion being cancer. Furthermore, the American College of Chest Physicians practice guidelines for solitary pulmonary nodules suggest excision for any nodule greater than 8 mm. High clinical suspicion should be tempered by preoperative biopsy, when available, especially in situations such as our patient's case in whom preoperative pathology and positron emission tomography suggested contradictory tumor biology, respectively. Additionally, higher suspicion of pulmonary ossification should be given to patients with a history of lung insult, such as iatrogenic injury during prior surgeries, as was the case in our patient.

REFERENCES

1. Lara, J.F., et al., Dendriform pulmonary ossification, a form of diffuse pulmonary ossification: Report of a 26-year autopsy experience. *Arch Pathol Lab Med.* 2005;129(3): 348–353.
2. Gielis, J.F., et al., Pulmonary ossifications seen centrally in a lung tumor. *Ann Thorac Surg.* 2012;93(6):e153–e154.
3. Gielis, J., et al., Nodular pulmonary ossifications in differential diagnosis of solitary pulmonary nodules. *Eur Respir J.* 2011;37(4):966–968.
4. Fernandez-Fernandez, F.J., et al., Pulmonary ossification: An unusual incidental finding of a transthoracic CT guided needle biopsy of a lung lesion. *Postgrad Med J.* 2010; 86(1021):682–683.
5. Gould, M.K., et al., Evaluation of individuals with pulmonary nodules: When is it lung cancer? Diagnosis and management of lung cancer, 3rd ed: American College of Chest Physicians evidence-based clinical practice guidelines. *Chest.* 2013;143(5 Suppl): e93S–e120S.
6. Desai, H.M. and G.P. Amonkar, Florid bronchial cartilage ossification: A case report with literature revisited. *Am J Forensic Med Pathol.* 2013;34(2):125–126.
7. Konoglou, M., et al., Lung ossification: an orphan disease. *J Thorac Dis.* 2013;5(1): 101–104.

Julia Coughlin and Christopher W. Seder

 | **Key Words**
- Intralobar bronchopulmonary sequestration
- Congenital pulmonary malformation

Introduction

Bronchopulmonary sequestration (BPS) is a rare congenital malformation that consists of a nonfunctioning segment of pulmonary tissue that does not normally communicate with the tracheobronchial tree [1]. The sequestration receives its perfusion from an aberrant vascular supply [2]. Intralobar sequestration, located within the visceral pleura of the lung, commonly presents as a recurrent infection, while extralobar sequestration, which is separated from the lung by its own pleura, is commonly diagnosed in early childhood [1,3]. We report the case of a patient with an intralobar sequestration with aberrant venous drainage to the hemiazygous system who was treated with video-assisted thoracoscopic surgery (VATS) lobectomy.

Case Report

A 33-year-old Iranian female with glucose-6-phosphate dehydrogenase (G6PD) deficiency presented with two weeks of fever, cough, shortness of breath, and left-side pleuritic chest pain. She denied smoking, sick contacts, recent travel, or tuberculosis exposure. On exam, she was afebrile, and her lungs were clear to auscultation bilaterally. She did not have a leukocytosis. Chest X-ray demonstrated patchy opacities in the left lower lobe; therefore, she was diagnosed with pneumonia and treated with antibiotics. Chest computed tomography (CT) demonstrated a bronchopulmonary sequestration with two arterial feeding vessels from the thoracic aorta and venous drainage into the hemiazygous vein (Figure 28.1a and b). Upon exploration, it was found that the sequestration was invested within the pleura of the left lower lobe but had venous drainage to the hemiazygous system. She was treated with a VATS left lower lobe lobectomy (Figure 28.2). The systemic arterial and venous vessels were individually identified and ligated using standard Endo GIA staplers. Surgical pathology demonstrated a bronchopulmonary sequestration with necrotizing granulomatous inflammation. She was discharged on postoperative day 2 without complication and has been free of pulmonary infections since surgery.

Comments

BPS is a rare congenital anomaly, comprising roughly 0.15%–6.4% of congenital pulmonary malformations [2]. Intralobar pulmonary sequestration (ILS) accounts for 75% of cases, while extralobar pulmonary sequestration (ELS) accounts for the remainder [2]. Multiple embryologic theories for the development of BPS have been proposed, including developmental insult, vascular insufficiency, acquired pathology after infection, and vascular traction [3]. The most widely accepted of these theories is that, between weeks four and eight of gestation,

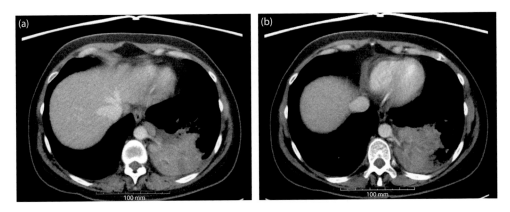

Figure 28.1 (a) Chest CT demonstrating one of two arterial feeding vessels from the thoracic aorta; (b) Chest CT demonstrating one arterial feeding vessel and aberrant venous drainage to hemiazygous system

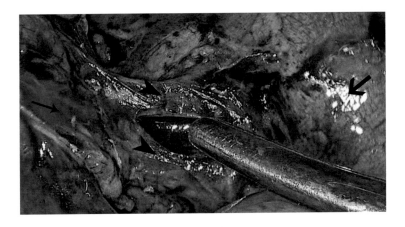

Figure 28.2 Intraoperative photo of two arterial feeding vessels (arrow heads), aorta (thick arrow), and left lung (narrow arrow)

a supernumerary lung bud arises caudal to the normal lung bud and migrates caudally with the esophagus during foregut development. Intralobar sequestration forms if the supernumerary lung bud develops prior to the pleura; it subsequently will be invested by the pleura and will lack its own visceral pleura. Extralobar sequestration forms if the lung bud develops after pleura formation; thus, it forms its own pleura, separating it from the primitive lung [3].

ILS develops within the left lower lobe in 66% of cases, a majority of which originate in the posterior basal segment, as seen in the current case [2]. ILS typically receive their blood supply from the thoracic aorta and drain via the pulmonary veins. Comparatively, 90% of ELS develop in the left lung and present in the newborn period [2]. Frequently, the child will have concurrent esophageal, vascular, or intestinal congenital anomalies. Half of newborns with ELS also have diaphragmatic defects [2]. Arterial supply is typically from the thoracic aorta; however, 10%–15% of cases are supplied by the abdominal aorta [1]. Venous drainage is usually to the systemic system via the vena cava, azygous, or hemiazygous veins [2].

Chest X-ray and CT scan are noninvasive modalities that aid in the diagnosis of pulmonary sequestration. In the current case, a chest X-ray demonstrated the typical findings of ILS: pneumonia in the medial basal posterior left lower lobe. However, the contrast-enhanced CT scan demonstrated an arterial and venous blood supply pattern generally seen in ELS, making the diagnosis unclear. Savic et al. conducted an analysis of the characteristics of intralobar and extralobar sequestrations and found more variation in the venous return of ELS than ILS. Over 95% of ILS cases demonstrated venous return via the pulmonary vein. In the remaining few cases, venous return was supplied by the azygous (1%), hemiazygous (1%), inferior vena cava (1%), superior vena cava (0.75%), and intercostal vein (0.75%) [2]. Although the majority of ELS drained via the superior vena cava, 52 of the 133 ELS cases were drained by alternative routes, such as the hemiazygous vein (15%), pulmonary vein (8%), inferior vena cava (4%), azygous vein (3%), portal vein (3%), intercostal vein (0.75%), and superior renal vein (0.75%) [2]. Thus, although imaging serves as helpful diagnostic tool, only surgical exploration allows the establishment of an accurate diagnosis.

Posterolateral thoracotomy has been the conventional approach to resection; however, VATS has been shown to be a feasible and safe alternative. Liu et al. compared VATS lobectomy with posterolateral thoracotomy for resection of pulmonary sequestration in 42 patients and concluded that there was no significant difference in terms of duration of operation, blood loss, postoperative hospital stay, and complication occurrence [4]. In addition, Sihoe et al. reported the first case in which uniportal VATS lobectomy was successful in resecting a right lower lobe ILS with three anomalous arteries [5]. Both authors stressed the importance of preoperative imaging to aid in the careful dissection and identification of aberrant vessels to prevent catastrophic hemorrhage. Thus, not only is VATS a feasible and safe alternative to thoracotomy for resection of BPS, skilled and experienced surgeons are continuing to develop advanced minimally invasive approaches.

In summary, we describe a patient with an infected intralobar pulmonary sequestration with aberrant venous drainage to the hemiazygous system. She underwent a VATS left lower lobectomy, which was both diagnostic and therapeutic. Recognition of this uncommon anatomic variant is critical for surgical management of BPS.

REFERENCES

1. Landing, B.H., Dixon, L.G. Congenital malformations and genetic disorders of the respiratory tract (larynx, trachea, bronchi, and lungs). *Am Rev Respir Dis.* 1979;120:151.
2. Savic, B., Birtel, F.J., Tholen, W., Funke, H.D., Knoche, R. Lung sequestration: Report of seven cases and a review of 540 published cases. *Thorax.* 1979;34:96–101.
3. Correia-Pinto, J., Gonzaga, S., Huang, Y., Rottier, R. Congenital lung lesions: Underlying molecular mechanisms. *Semin Pediatr Surg.* 2010;19:171.
4. Liu, C., Pu, Q., Ma, L., Mei, J., Xiao, Z., Liao, H., Liu, L. Video-assisted thoracic surgery for pulmonary sequestration compared with posterolateral thoracotomy. *J Thorac Cardiovasc Surg.* 2013;146:557–561.
5. Sihoe, A.D., Luo, Q., Shao, G., Li, Y., Li, J., Pang, D. Uniportal thoracoscopic lobectomy for intralobar pulmonary sequestration. *J Cardiothorac Surg.* 2016;11:27.

CASE 29: PULMONARY DOGWORM (*DIROFILARIA IMMITIS*) INFECTION PRESENTING AS A SOLITARY PULMONARY NODULE

Mathew Thomas

Key Words
• Lung infection • Nematode • Pulmonary • Dirofilaria • Lung nodule

Introduction

Pulmonary nematode infections are well-known entities and have been reported from all parts of the world. There are different varieties of worms that cause pulmonary infections, with some being more common than others depending on endemic nature of the parasite. Pulmonary dirofilariasis is a rare zoonotic nematode infection that can be mistaken for a malignant neoplasm. We describe a rare case of a patient with *Dirofilaria immitis* (*D. immitis*) in the lung presenting as a solid nodule.

Case Report

A 50-year-old female patient with a 35-pack-year smoking history presented with a new left lower lobe (LLL) pleural-based lesion measuring 2.4 × 2.0 cm (Figure 29.1), which was identified on a CT scan done for follow-up for a 6-mm nodule in the right lower lobe (RLL). On comparison to the previous CT chest done four years earlier, the LLL nodule was not seen and the RLL nodule was noted to be stable. The PET scan was negative. She was otherwise in excellent health and had normal pulmonary function tests. A CT-guided needle biopsy was performed that showed predominantly necrotic tissue with scant fibrous tissue and necrotic neoplasm could not be excluded.

Due to the risk factors for malignancy and indeterminate cytology, we recommended a diagnostic video-assisted thoracoscopic surgery (VATS) wedge resection with immediate conversion to robotic left lower lobectomy if malignancy was identified on frozen section.

At the time of surgery, the lesion was easily identified, but severe adhesions were noted between the lung, diaphragm, and posterior chest wall adjacent to the nodule. After adhesiolysis, a wedge resection was performed with negative margins. Frozen section revealed a benign-appearing lesion with central necrosis and surrounding histiocytes, compatible with granulomatous inflammation. The microscopic margins were uninvolved. A lobectomy was therefore not performed. She tolerated the procedure well and was discharged home after two days. Final pathology confirmed the lesion to be consistent with *Dirofiliaria immitis*, with the fragments of the dead larva seen on microscopy (Figure 29.2).

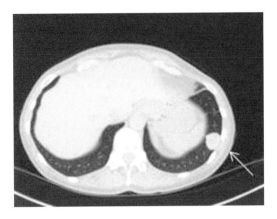

Figure 29.1 CT image of the chest showing solitary pulmonary nodule (arrow) in the left lower lobe of lung

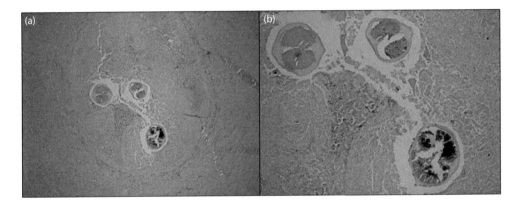

Figure 29.2 Low power (a) and High power (b) microscopic images showing *Dirofiliaria immitis* with the fragments of the dead larva seen on

Comments

The genus Dirofilaria consists of over 40 species of filarioid nematodes, but only two species, *D. repens* and *D. immitis*, have been known to affect humans. Canines are the primary hosts for Dirofilaria. *D. immitis* is commonly called dog heartworm, or dogworm, and has been reported more often in humans than *D. repens* on the American continent, but the reverse is true in other parts of the world [1]. The term heartworm is related to the residence of the adult worm in the right ventricle and pulmonary artery in dogs. *D. immitis* infection in the United States is more prevalent in the Eastern and Southeastern states [2].

D. immitis is transmitted to humans from dogs by mosquito bites when the larvae are injected into the subcutaneous tissue where they usually die and may present as a local reaction. If the larvae are directly injected into the blood stream or survive in the subcutaneous tissue, they are then transported to the heart where they are killed and can form pulmonary microemboli. Once in the lungs, these either cause an infarct or dense granulomatous inflammation with central necrosis. The resulting lesion can be easily mistaken for a neoplasm with the appearance of a well-defined peripheral coin lesion on a chest X-ray or solid nodule on

CT scans. PET scans are equivocal for the diagnosis since the lesion may show no activity, as was noted in our patient, or mild hypermetabolic activity [3]. Needle biopsy is not often diagnostic because the nodule consists mostly of necrotic tissue. Surgical biopsy as a wedge resection is the most definitive diagnostic method where the encapsulated parasite can be seen on microscopy. Dense vascularized pleural adhesions, as seen in our patient, have been reported by other authors and, in one instance, was reported to cause severe bleeding that required reoperation.

Dirofilariasis can be diagnosed by an ELISA test for a Df-specific antibody, but the test is not widely available. The pulmonary lesions do not appear to cause any symptoms in the majority of patients, and there is no current treatment recommended for *D. immitis* in asymptomatic humans. Nonspecific symptoms such as cough, chest pain, fever, and hemoptysis related to the death of the parasite in the blood stream or pulmonary infarction have been reported in a minority of patients in a large series of human pulmonary dirofilariasis [2].

In summary, pulmonary dirofilariasis is rare but should be considered in the differential diagnosis of solitary pulmonary nodules in patients who present from parts of the world where the disease is endemic.

REFERENCES

1. Dantas-Torres, F., Otranto, D. Dirofilariosis in the Americas: A more virulent Dirofilaria immitis? *Parasit Vectors.* 2013;6(1):288.
2. Asimacopoulos, P.J., Katras, A., Christie, B. Pulmonary dirofilariasis. The largest single-hospital experience. *Chest.* 1992;102(3):851–855.
3. Stone, M., Dalal, I., Stone, C., Dalal, B. 18-FDG uptake in pulmonary dirofilariasis. *J Radiol Case Rep.* 2015;9(4):28–33.

Kate Gallo, Gillian Alex, and Christopher W. Seder

🔍 | **Key Words**

- Extralobar pulmonary sequestration
- Congenital diaphragmatic hernia
- Pulmonary malformation
- Congenital anomaly
- Celiac artery

Introduction

Bronchopulmonary sequestration (BPS) is a rare pulmonary malformation, accounting for 1%–6% of all congenital abnormalities [1,2]. By definition, a BPS is a portion of nonfunctioning lung tissue that lacks communication with the tracheobronchial tree and has aberrant systemic arterial inflow [1–3]. Sequestrations are categorized as either an intralobar pulmonary sequestration, which does not have its own pleural investment, or an extralobar pulmonary sequestration (EPS), which has a pleural lining [1,2]. EPSs are more commonly associated with other malformations and are associated with congenital diaphragmatic hernias [4–6]. The relationship between these two anomalies remains incompletely understood. We report a case of a 45-year-old male diagnosed with a concurrent congenital diaphragmatic hernia and EPS. The patient was treated with a combined laparoscopic repair of the diaphragmatic hernia and resection of the pulmonary sequestration.

Case Report

A 45-year-old non-smoking male presented with complaints of food getting stuck in his mid-chest, significant postprandial abdominal and left chest pain, nausea, early satiety, postprandial emesis, and dyspnea. His past medical history was significant for hyperlipidemia and *H. pylori* gastritis, for which he had undergone treatment. The patient was a Jehovah's Witness with refusal to accept blood. A chest-abdomen-pelvis computed tomography (CT) scan demonstrated a predominantly calcified left-sided pulmonary sequestration with an associated moderate to large mid-diaphragmatic hernia. Arterial blood supply to the sequestration originated from the celiac axis and coursed cephalad into the chest (Figures 30.1 through 30.4).

The patient was taken to the operating room for repair of his diaphragmatic hernia and BPS. Upon laparoscopic inspection of the abdomen, the left diaphragmatic hernia appeared to originate in the mid-to-posterior tendinous portion of the left hemidiaphragm and was completely separate from the esophageal hiatus. We began dissection around the edges of the hernia, reducing its contents and separating it from the underlying pulmonary structures. Continued dissection freed the abdominal contents from the chest; however, the

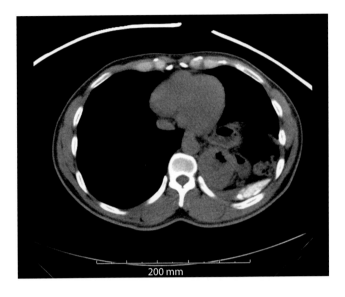

Figure 30.1 CT chest image without contrast, mediastinal view

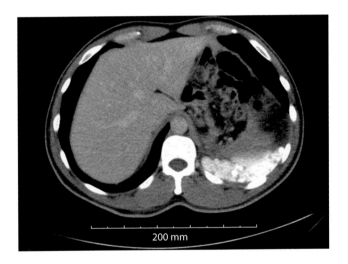

Figure 30.2 CT chest image without contrast, mediastinal view (arrow indicates calcifications within sequestration)

sequestration could not be adequately visualized due to its posterior location. Therefore, the laparoscopic ports were closed, and a small, left anterolateral thoracotomy was performed. The sequestration had a distinct separation from the other lung tissue with a pleural covering, confirming the diagnosis of extralobar BPS. An Endo GIA vascular load stapler was used to divide the arterial vessel coursing from the celiac axis, and the diaphragmatic defect was repaired primarily using interrupted, heavy permanent suture. There was no disruption of the phrenoesophageal ligament making a fundoplication unnecessary. The patient was discharged on postoperative day 2 and has had an uncomplicated postoperative course.

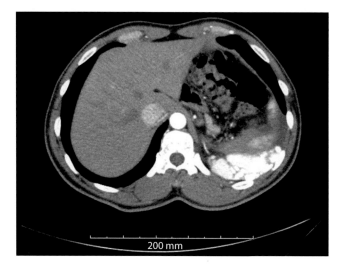

Figure 30.3 CT chest image with IV contrast (arrow indicates sequestration arterial supply)

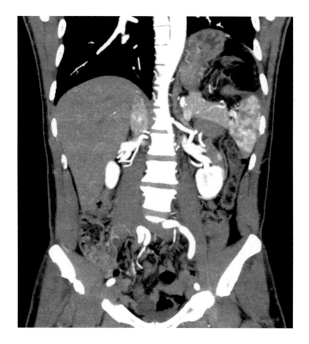

Figure 30.4 CT chest image with IV contrast

Comments

The simultaneous diagnosis of two congenital anomalies in an adult is rare. Congenital diaphragmatic hernias (CDHs) are most commonly diagnosed during gestation by prenatal ultrasound [5]. These hernias occur from improper development, or muscularization, of the diaphragm [4,5]. CDHs most often present in the left posterolateral position (Bochdalek hernias) [4]. Because of this improper diaphragmatic development, abdominal viscera can pass into the chest causing symptoms such as dyspnea, chest pain, and vomitting [5]. In the current patient, an EPS was identified when investigating his symptomatic diaphragmatic hernia. According to an analysis of 540 cases of pulmonary sequestration by Savic and colleagues, 27.6% of EPS cases had synchronous diaphragmatic hernias [3]. While described as associated anomalies in the literature, there is no clear evidence linking their simultaneous development.

The overall incidence of pulmonary sequestration is small and only represents 0.15%–6.4% of all pulmonary anomalies [3]. Of the two forms of sequestration (intralobar and extralobar), extralobar is the least common representing only 19% of sequestrations [1]. The cause of BPS is not clearly understood, which makes understanding its relationship to other intrathoracic anomalies difficult. There are two working theories that have been proposed to explain the development of EPS. The first theory suggests that the embryonic lung bud detaches and isolates from normal developing lung tissue allowing separate pleura to form [6]. The second theory involves an anomaly in foregut bud formation [6]. Unfortunately, neither of these theories explain the association between CDH and EPS.

When a congenital anomaly is identified, there should be a high level of suspicion that additional anomalies may be present. Congenital anomalies can, and often do, present in adulthood, and physicians working with adults should maintain a working knowledge of prenatal and pediatric pathologies.

REFERENCES

1. Alsumrain, M., Ryu, J.H. Pulmonary sequestration in adults: A retrospective review of resected and unresected cases. *BMC Pulmonary Med.* 2018;18:97.
2. Polaczek, M., Baranska, I., Szolkowska, M., Zych, J., Rudzinski, P., Szopinski, J., Orlowski, T., Roszkowski-Sliz, K. Clinical presentation and characteristics of 25 adult cases of pulmonary sequestration. *J Thorac Dis.* 2017;9(3):762–767.
3. Savic, B., Birtel, F.J., Tholen, W., Funke, H.D., Knoche, R. Lung sequestration: Report of seven cases and review of 540 published cases. *Thorax.* 1979;34:96–101.
4. Harris, K. Extralobar sequestration with congenital diaphragmatic hernia: A complicated case study. *Neonatal Network.* 2004;23(6):7–24.
5. Kawamura, N., Bhandal, S. Coexistent congenital diaphragmatic hernia with extrapulmonary sequestration. *Can Respir J.* 2016; Article ID 1460480; 1–4.
6. Arslanian, A., Leflour, N., Hernigou, A., Danel, C., Riquet, M., Complex extralobar sequestration in a 24-year-old woman. *Ann Thorac Surg.* 2003;76:2077–2078.

John Hallsten, Adrian E. Rodrigues, and Wickii T. Vigneswaran

---

🔍 **Key Words**

- Colloid carcinoma
- Primary lung cancer

Introduction

Colloid carcinomas of the lung are a very rare subset of lung adenocarcinomas. Historically, these neoplasms have existed under different nomenclatures including "mucinous cystadenoma," "mucinous cystic tumor," and "cystic mucinous adenocarcinoma." Grossly, these tumors vary in size from 1 to 15 cm and generally appear uni- or multilocular, gelatinous, and mucoid. Cystic changes may not be seen without microscopy. On microscopy, these tumors appear scantily solid with the majority of the tumor often appearing as pools of mucin, in which fragments of alveoli and mucous-producing tumor cells float [1]. Appropriate management of a primary colloid carcinoma includes proper staging and surgical resection. We report a case of an extremely rare giant colloid carcinoma of the right lower and middle lung lobes that was resected successfully.

Case Report

A 55-year-old male with chronic renal dysfunction was referred to the thoracic surgery service at an academic institution after a right lung mass was incidentally found during evaluation for possible renal transplantation (Figure 31.1). The CT scan was performed that demonstrated a large mass within the right lower lobe, which is well marginated measuring 12.4 × 12.5 × 9.3 cm. The differential diagnosis included bronchogenic cyst, pulmonary sequestration, primary lung neoplasm, drowned lung, chronic infection/fungal disease. An MRI scan was performed reported, "A large mass occupying much of the right lower lobe that demonstrates high T2, low T1 signal measures approximately 11.8 × 9.4 cm in the axial plane and 13.1 cm craniocaudally. Numerous septations are noted. This extends into the right hilum and subcarinal region. On this noncontrast exam there is no definite evidence of invasion involving the pericardium." At a multidisciplinary tumor board, it was decided the patient would benefit from resection of the lung mass if he was to proceed with renal transplantation (Figure 31.2).

Prior to surgery, bronchoscopy revealed significant narrowing of the intermediate bronchus just after the right main bronchus with endobronchial disease consistent with tumor, suggesting that the tumor was involving both right lower lobe and right middle lobe. A bilobectomy would be necessary to remove the tumor completely from the endobronchial examination. Initially, in view of the vascular nature of the tumor appearances on the CT scan, the plan was made to control vascular structures at the hilum, and the microscopic instrumentation of robotic technique was considered advantageous, even though it was considered that thoracotomy was inevitable because of the size of the tumor. Therefore, the

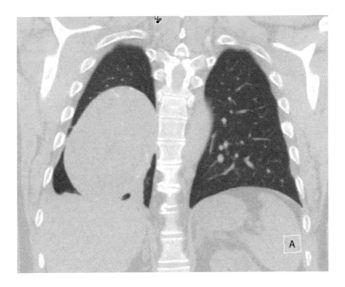

Figure 31.1 Chest imaging showing a large well-defined mass in the right chest

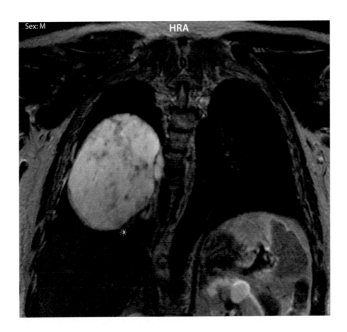

Figure 31.2 MRI of chest and a large mass occupying the right lower lobe is identified again. This demonstrates high T2 along with a low T1 signal and numerous septations

surgery was initiated with the da Vinci robotic system with the main aim of hilar vascular control. The inferior pulmonary vein was identified and isolated. However, the exposure of the pulmonary artery was not possible in view of the massive size of the tumor. The operation was converted to an open technique at this point. A standard bilobectomy was performed following the thoracotomy uneventfully with mediastinal lymph node dissection. The gross specimen resected measured 21.2 × 15.2 × 6.5 cm with clear margins, and the tumor measured 15.5 × 12.2 × 6.5 cm. A gelatinous mass grossly invaded into the bronchus. The histological examination showed pools of mucin with islands of immunohistochemical staining that revealed CK7 and CDX2 positive and negative for cytokeratin 20 (CK20) and TTF-1. The pathologic diagnosis was colloid carcinoma of the lung with no evidence of lymph node metastasis.

Postoperatively, he developed ileus and briefly rising creatinine but did not require intervention as his urine output remained adequate. He was discharged home on postoperative day 9. His six-month scan showed no evidence of tumor recurrence, and he has been considered for renal transplantation (Figure 31.3).

Comments

Colloid carcinoma of the lung is a very rare primary lung tumor but is similar to its counterpart in other body sites. These tumors are normally evident in breast tissue or in the gastrointestinal tract [2]. As there is higher prevalence of this tumor in other body sites, it is important to make sure the lung tumor is not a distant metastasis.

Colloid carcinoma of the lung represents an entity with two distinct clinic-pathologic and immune-phenotypic variants: (1) the goblet cell-type, presenting a more indolent clinical behavior and frequently co-expressing markers of intestinal and pulmonary differentiation; (2) the more aggressive signet-ring cell-type, which retains only markers of pulmonary origin. On morphologic and immunohistochemical grounds, these are easily distinguishable from mucinous bronchioloalveolar carcinoma. Since goblet cell-type strongly stains with CDX2, MUC2, and CK20, differential diagnosis with metastatic colorectal carcinoma is very challenging and requires appropriate clinical correlation. Patients with goblet cell-type tend to follow a more indolent course, while the signet-ring cell-type can follow an aggressive course [3].

In our case, it was important to rule out distant metastasis because of the patient's potential renal transplantation status. The patient's tumor demonstrated both CK7 and CDX2 positive immunohistochemical staining, suggestive of a more indolent nature of this colloid

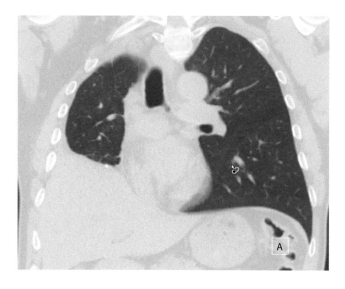

Figure 31.3 Chest imaging six months following resection

carcinoma of the lung [3]. Nevertheless, regular surveillance is still required in this patient. Since goblet cell-type strongly stains with CDX2, MUC2, and CK20, differential diagnosis with metastatic colorectal carcinoma is very challenging [4].

To our knowledge, our case represents one of the largest colloid carcinomas of the lung ever documented [5]. Our patient's tumor measures 15.5 cm at the largest diameter. Our case is extraordinary in many ways. The patient presented with a potentially unprecedented manifestation of an already rare tumor despite its large size with no pulmonary symptoms indicating its presence. Lastly, the tumor was directly invasive with multilobar involvement, but did not demonstrate any metastases to the lymph nodes [6].

REFERENCES

1. Moran, C.A., Hochholzer, L., Fishback, N., Travis, W.D., Koss, M.N. Mucinous (so-called colloid) carcinomas of lung. *Modern Patho.* 1992;5(6):634–638.
2. Ou, S.H., Kawaguchi, T., Soo, R.A., Kitaichi, M. Rare subtypes of adenocarcinoma of the lung. *Exp Rev Anticancer Ther.* 2011;11(10):1535–1542.
3. Rossi, G., Murer, B., Cavazza, A., Losi, L., Natali, P., Marchioni, A., Migaldi, M., Capitanio, G., Brambilla, E. Primary mucinous (so-called colloid) carcinomas of the lung: A clinicopathologic and immunohistochemical study with special reference to CDX-2 homeobox gene and MUC2 expression. *Am J Surg Pathol.* 2004;28(4):442–452.
4. Zenali, M.J., Weissferdt, A., Solis, L.M., Ali, S., Tang, X., Mehran, R.J., Wistuba, I.I., Moran, C.A., Kalhor, N. An update on clinicopathological, immunohistochemical, and molecular profiles of colloid carcinoma of the lung. *Human Pathol.* 2015;46(6):836–842.
5. Gao, Z.H., Urbanski, S.J. The spectrum of pulmonary mucinous cystic neoplasia: A clinicopathologic and immunohistochemical study of ten cases and review of the literature. *Am J Clin Pathol.* 2005;124(1):62–70.
6. Masai, K., Sakurai, H., Suzuki, S., Asakura, K., Nakagawa, K., Watanabe, S.I. Clinicopathological features of colloid adenocarcinoma of the lung: A report of six cases. *J Surg Oncol.* 2016;114(2):211–215.

Albert Pai, Kalpaj R. Parekh, and Evgeny V. Arshava

 Key Words
- Pulmonary mucormycosis
- Mucormycosis co-infection
- Lung resection for mucormycosis

Introduction

Mucormycosis is commonly associated with an immunosuppressed state, active malignancy, uncontrolled diabetes, and iron-overloaded states [1]. In patients with hematological malignancies, mucormycosis most commonly affects the lungs. Due to the angioinvasive nature of *Mucor*, there is an overall mortality of 70%–80% associated with delayed diagnosis and treatment of pulmonary infection [2,3].

Case Report

An 80-year-old male with a history of diabetes and chronic lymphocytic leukemia (CLL) was admitted to our facility with a one-month history of small-volume hemoptysis and productive cough refractory to antibiotic therapy. An outpatient computed tomography (CT) of the chest one month prior to admission showed an overall normal-appearing right lung without concern for focal infiltrates or masses (Figure 32.1a). Chest CT on admission (Figure 32.1b and c) showed rapid progression of an enlarging cavitary lesion in the right upper lobe (RUL). A bronchoscopy with bronchoalveolar lavage of the RUL was performed, and the samples were submitted for microbiologic stains and culture. The results showed fungal hyphae consistent with mucormycocis and Gram-positive cocci consistent with *Staphylococcus*. Due to concerns of pulmonary angioinvasion, an urgent lobectomy was performed.

In the operating room, a standard right-sided serratus-sparing posterolateral thoracotomy through the fifth intercostal space was performed. There were no adhesions of the RUL to the chest wall, but prominent inflammatory changes were noted at the hilum. A firm (5.8 cm × 8.0 cm) palpable mass was felt in the center of the RUL (Figure 32.2). An aberrant middle lobe vein was also noted to arise from the inferior pulmonary vein, but there were otherwise no difficulties in dividing the bronchovascular structures or fissures.

Pathology of the specimen demonstrated extensive parenchymal necrosis of the lung with *Mucor* and co-infecting *Staphylococcus epidermidis*. The patient recovered without any adverse events, and he was discharged on postoperative day 24. He was treated with ampicillin-sulbactam and a two-week course of liposomal amphotericin B followed by two weeks of posaconazole. At the six-month follow-up, the patient had resumed his normal activities,

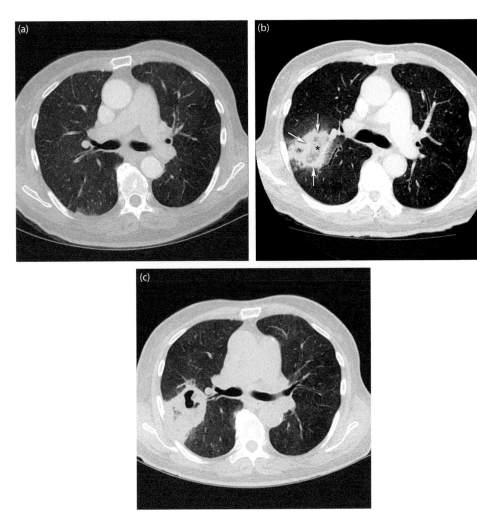

Figure 32.1 (a) Initial chest CT without focal infiltrates. (b) Chest CT one month later demonstrating RUL infiltrate with a "reverse halo" sign. The asterisk indicates central ground glass opacity and arrows point at the peripheral consolidation. (c) Chest CT one week later showing rapidly developing cavitation in the area of prior ground glass opacity

and his hemoptysis had resolved. The surveillance chest CT showed normal appearance of the remaining lung parenchyma.

Comments

Mucormycosis, previously known as zygomycosis, is an opportunistic fungal infection that commonly affects immunosuppressed patients, diabetics, patients with active malignancy, and those with iron-overloaded states [1,3]. Its involvement in patients without a predisposing factor

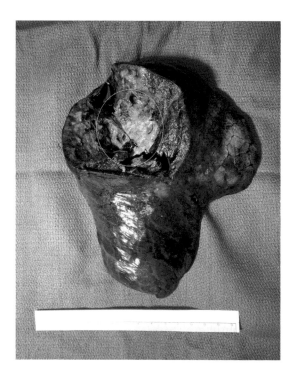

Figure 32.2 Incised right upper lobectomy specimen with a cavitary lesion (circled)

is rare. Pulmonary mononuclear and polymorphonuclear phagocytes are the primary defense against mucormycosis; thus, neutropenic patients are particularly susceptible to infection [4]. There are five clinical forms of the disease: rhinocerebral, gastrointestinal, disseminated, cutaneous, and pulmonary mucormycosis. The latter is the most common cause of morbidity and mortality in the immunocompromised host [3]. Fungal spores are introduced to the airway by inhalation, resulting in rapid development of endobronchial disease or pneumonia.

The typical presentation of pulmonary mucormycosis is nonspecific, and this makes the infection difficult to differentiate from other pathogens. These symptoms include fever refractory to broad-spectrum antibiotics, cough, pleuritic chest pain, rapidly progressive dyspnea, and hemoptysis. Approximately 30% of pulmonary infections are associated with bacterial pneumonia, which can further obscure the diagnosis and delay treatment. This can result in a lethal clinical course of fungal sepsis, respiratory failure, or hemoptysis [2]. The pathogenesis of hemoptysis is related to bronchial penetration by hyphae and angioinvasion with eventual vessel thrombosis and tissue necrosis [3,4]. Hyphae have also been known to dissect between the internal elastic membrane and media of large pulmonary arteries, resulting in severe or fatal hemoptysis [3].

Chest X-ray is usually abnormal in most patients, but findings are rarely suggestive of fungal disease. Chest CT will demonstrate consolidation, nodules, masses, cavitation, lymphadenopathy, or pleural effusions without specific lobar predilection. Radiographic signs suggestive of mucormycosis include the "reversed halo sign" (central ground-glass opacity) with peripheral consolidation; Figure 32.1b, the "perilesional halo sign" (central consolidation with surrounding rim of ground-glass opacity), or the "air crescent sign" (rim of air between radiodense lesion and normal parenchyma) [4]. Although this latter finding can be observed in lung abscesses, tuberculomas, hematomas, echinococcal cysts, and cavitating neoplasms, its presence in immunocompromised hosts is strongly suggestive of an opportunistic fungal pathogen [3].

Tissue biopsy is the gold standard for obtaining a diagnosis because radiographic signs and sputum culture are not reliable. Transbronchial biopsy is the most commonly employed technique; however, surgical excision, transthoracic lung biopsy, and percutaneous needle biopsy have also been effective [3]. Histopathologic findings of broad, nonseptate, ribbon-like hyphae, with right-angled branching in a sample with routine hematoxylin and eosin staining, are diagnostic [2].

Survival beyond two weeks is unusual if untreated, and the survival approaches 3% [2,4]. The optimal strategy is bimodal therapy with IV liposomal amphotericin B and aggressive surgical resection of the involved lung. Oral posaconazole or isavuconazonium are used as step-down antifungals for responders of amphotericin B or for salvage therapy, but either type of medication is ineffective without surgical intervention. Surgery may range from wedge resection to anatomic resections including segmentectomy, lobectomy, or pneumonectomy [2,3]. The extent of resection is ultimately dependent on the amount of diseased lung with an ultimate goal to prevent contamination of the contralateral lung [4]. Video-assisted thoracoscopic surgery (VATS) or thoracotomy are acceptable approaches based on the amount of anticipated chest wall involvement or on the functional status of the patient. Surgery should be performed as soon as possible after diagnosis in order to minimize the risk of dissemination and erosion into the pulmonary vessels. Finally, reversal of host impairment is recommended to maximize recovery.

Pulmonary mucormycosis has a poor prognosis mainly due to the difficulty in making an early diagnosis and to the limited activity of current antifungal agents. When confined to the lungs, the overall mortality rate is 65% compared to 70%–80% in other organ systems [2,3]. Patients with mucormycosis limited to the lungs demonstrate clear benefit from surgery. For pulmonary involvement, survival of 70% has been reported when both lung resection and antifungal therapy were used compared to antifungal therapy alone (61%) or to surgery alone (57%) [4,5].

Mucormycosis is a rapidly fatal fungal illness that commonly affects immunocompromised patients. The clinical presentation is nonspecific, but a delay in diagnosis and in treatment could result in poor clinical results, including dissemination and angioinvasion of the pulmonary vasculature. The recommended treatment includes initial intravenous amphotericin B and aggressive surgical resection of the involved lung followed by continued antifungal therapy until there is clinical resolution of infection. Despite prompt treatment, this infection still carries high morbidity and mortality. As such, a high index of suspicion is required for early diagnosis in order to achieve the optimal clinical outcomes [5].

REFERENCES

1. Martin, M.S., Smith, A.A., Lobo, M., Paramesh, A.S. Successful treatment of recurrent pulmonary mucormycosis in a renal transplant patient: A case report and literature review. *Case Rep Transplant*. Volume 2017, Article ID 1925070, 5 pages http://dx.doi.org/10.1155/2017/1925070.
2. Wang, X.M., Guo, L.C., Xue, S.L., Chen, Y.B. Pulmonary mucormycosis: A case report and review of the literature. *Oncol Lett* 2016;11:3049–3053.
3. Tedder, M., Spratt, J.A., Anstadt, M.P., Hegde, S.S., Tedder, S.D., Lowe, J.E. Pulmonary mucormycosis: Results of medical and surgical therapy. *Ann Thorac Surg.* 1994;57: 1044–1050.
4. Vercillo, M.S., Liptay, M.J., Weder, C.W. Early pneumonectomy for pulmonary mucormycosis. *Ann Thorac Surg.* 2015;99:67–68.
5. Chougule, A., Muthu, V., Amanjit, B., Rudramurthy, S.M., Dhooria, S., Das, A., Singh, H. Pulmonary gangrene due to *Rhizopus* spp., *Staphylocuccus aureus*, *Klebsiella pneumoniae* and probable *Sarcina* organisms. *Mycopathologia*. 2015;180:131–136.

Evgeny V. Arshava, Yulia N. Matveeva and Kalpaj R. Parekh

🔑	Key Words
	• Pulmonary echinococcosis • Hydatid disease of the lung • Complicated echinococcosis

Introduction

Pulmonary cystic echinococcosis (CE) is common in endemic areas of the world, but it is rarely seen in other regions. Given the increase in worldwide travel and migration, all thoracic surgeons must be aware of hydatic disease (HD) and the principles of its management.

Case Report

A 28-year, patient with two previous pregnancy and 1 birth presented at 23 weeks gestation (non-smoker), with an unremarkable medical history, experienced productive cough for the duration of one month. Worsening shortness of breath and chest discomfort prompted in-patient admission at a local hospital. Her social history was remarkable for travel to Sudan for several weeks one year prior to symptoms.

Chest radiography (CXR) demonstrated right lower lobe opacification with a large ovoid collection with an air-fluid level (Figure 33.1). Laboratory studies demonstrated a white blood cell (WBC) count of 11.3 k/uL (reference range [RR] 4.5–10.8) with 54% neutrophils (RR 30–70) and elevated (+16.2%) eosinophils (RR 1–5). Her comprehensive metabolic panel including liver function tests was unremarkable, and blood cultures were negative. Sputum samples showed oral flora and subsequently negative acid-fast bacilli (AFB) cultures. Her Quantiferon tuberculosis antigen test was negative. Eosinophilia prompted a parasite panel that was negative for *Giardia, Histoplasmosis,* and *Cryptosporidium.*

Low-dose unenhanced chest computed tomography (CT) demonstrated an 8-cm air-fluid collection along the posterior medial aspect of the right lower lobe with consolidation in much of adjacent lung parenchyma (Figure 33.2). Thoracentesis demonstrated cloudy exudative fluid with a pH of 5.7, elevated WBC (3394 cells/uL [RR 0–1000]) with 55% lymphocytes and 16% polynuclear cells and no bacterial growth.

One week after treatment with broad-spectrum intravenous (IV) antibiotics, the patient was transferred to our institution due to increasing effusion on CXR. Repeat low-dose chest CT demonstrated multiloculated empyema not suitable for percutaneous drainage (Figure 33.3). The patient underwent thoracoscopy with findings typical for fibropurulent,

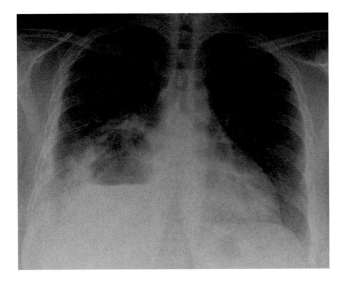

Figure 33.1 CXR demonstrates ovoid lesion with an air-fluid level in the lower lobe

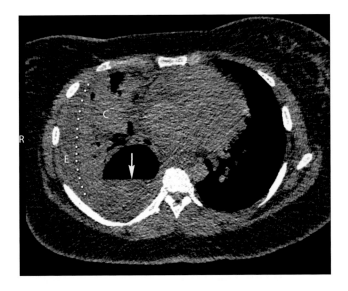

Figure 33.2 Chest CT demonstrating an 8-cm collection with an air-fluid level (arrow). Adjacent effusion (E) and lung consolidation (C) are separated by a dotted line

multiloculated empyema. Thoracoscopic drainage of empyema and decortication were performed with adequate re-expansion of the lung. Cultures of the fluid and peel were negative. Pathologic examination of the pleural peal was reported as fibrosis with mixed acute and chronic inflammation. AFB and Grocott's methenamine silver (GSM) stains were reported negative.

The patient was discharged after the chest tubes were removed on postoperative day (POD) 7 but was readmitted on POD 11 with breakdown of one of the thoracoscopic port sites and pneumo-thorax. A chest tube was placed, but the lung could not be adequately re-expanded over several

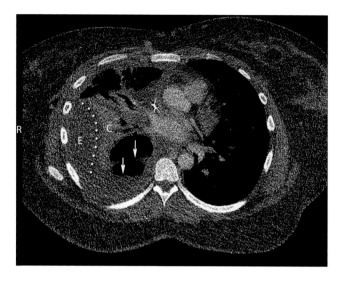

Figure 33.3 Repeat chest CT demonstrating multiloculated (arrows), enlarging effusion

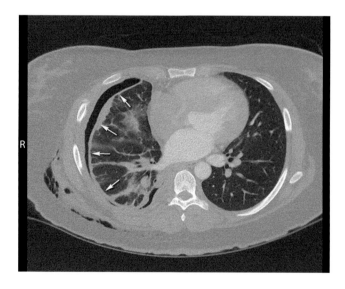

Figure 33.4 Chest CT with trapped lung and thick peel (arrows)

days. Repeat CT chest demonstrated a trapped lung with thick peel (Figure 33.4). Open decortication was then performed (Figure 33.5). Intraoperative cultures were negative. Pathology of peel was reported as fibrosis with acute, chronic, and focally granulomatous inflammation.

Perioperatively, the patient had minimal leukocytosis and low-grade fever, but she did well from a respiratory perspective. The patient was followed by obstetricians with appropriate unremarkable fetal monitoring. Prolonged air leak was present until POD 27 (open decortication).

Due to an atypical course after adequate video-assisted thoracoscopic surgery decortication (failure of lung re-expansion, ongoing inflammatory process with reformation of the fibrose

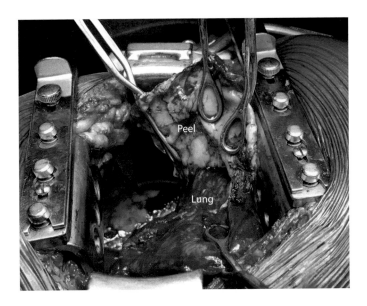

Figure 33.5 Thick fibrous peal is most prominent over the posterior medial aspect on the lower lobe in the location of the prior cystic structure

peel), and reported focal granulomatous inflammation, the clinical team requested re-review of the operative specimens. On POD 60, after initial decortication, pathologists identified the partially degenerated protoscolices and hooklets consistent with the *Echinococcus* species (Figure 33.6). *Echinococcus* Antibody IgG was 1.4 IV (RR 0.0–0.8). The patient completed a total of four weeks of albendazole 400 mg BID. A liver ultrasound was obtained and did not demonstrate any lesions. The patient had induction and uncomplicated delivery of a healthy child at 39 weeks gestational age. An interval chest CT image was obtained and demonstrated full re-expansion of the lung and absence of residual cystic lesions or effusion.

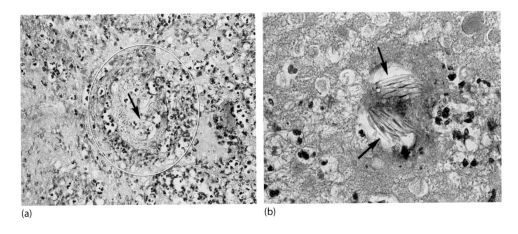

(a)   (b)

Figure 33.6 (a) Histology slide demonstrates degenerated protoscolex (circled) with hooklets (arrow), which was previously reported as focal granulomatous inflammation. (Courtesy of Bradley Ford.) (b) Magnified view of intact hooklets. (Courtesy of Bradley Ford.)

Comments

Echinococcosis, or hydatid disease, is caused by *Echinococcus* tapeworms. *Echinococcus granulosus* and *Echinococcus multilocularis* are of clinical significance causing, respectively, cystic echinococcosis (CE) and alveolar echinococcosis (AE). CE comprises over 95% of all hydatid disease cases and is endemic in pastoral areas of South America, the Mediterranean region, Eastern Europe, the Middle East, Russia, Africa, China, and Japan, with an annual incidence ranging from 1 to 200 per 100,000 inhabitants; the incidence is higher in certain endemic areas [1]. Human AE is much less common with an incidence of 0.03–1.2 per 100,000 inhabitants, with most cases occurring in China.

Adult tapeworms inhabit the small intestine of carnivores, which can be infected with thousands of worms. The tapeworms are 2–7 mm long and are composed of protoscolex ("head") with hooklets ("fangs") and proglottid segments ("body"). The tapeworm produces thousands of eggs daily that are released to the environment in the stool of the definitive host and then infect the susceptible intermediate hosts (domestic mammals or rodents). In the intermediate hosts, onchospheres hatch from the eggs and hematogenously spread to visceral organs to form hydatic cysts (HCs). When the carnivore ingests infected organs containing hydatid cysts, protoscolices attach to the intestinal mucosa and the cycle restarts. Humans are incidental hosts, as they do not transmit disease further.

E. granulosus forms a cyst containing protoscolices filled with a clear "hydatid" fluid. The cyst is made of an inner germinative (endocyst) and a distinct, white, outer acellular-laminated layer (exocyst). It is surrounded by the host inflammatory layer (pericyst). Unlike extrapulmonary cysts, pulmonary HCs do not undergo calcifications, while mediastinal, pleural, and pericardial cysts may calcify. "Daughter" vesicles of variable size may be present inside or outside the "mother" cyst, but they are rare in the lung. Over 70% of patients present with a single organ involvement by a solitary cyst. The liver-to-lung involvement ratio is approximately 5:1. In lungs, lower lobes are more frequently affected. In addition to hematogenous spread to lungs via portal circulation, parasites can bypass the liver entering the chest via the thoracic duct or the lymphatics of the diaphragm. Transdiaphragmatic rupture of liver HCs may account for some simultaneous hepatopulmonary cases. A direct route from inhalation of eggs has been described as well. Involvement of other organs is rare. Cysts of CE are unilocular and expansile, causing mass effect. Pulmonary HC doubling time is 16–20 weeks. HCs achieve 1–2 cm in diameter by the end of six months, up to 6 cm in one year, and they grow further; they may persist for years without changes. HC growth and variation in morphology depends on geographic regions, intraspecies parasite genotype variations, and host differences.

E. multilocularis cause lesions composed of numerous irregular cysts of various sizes, without clear demarcation from surrounding tissues. The cysts are composed of a thin, laminated layer with minimal or no germinative layer. The reproduction occurs by lateral budding. The lack of limiting membrane and exogenous budding allows infiltration and destruction of adjacent tissues similar to malignant processes. Central necrosis and irregular calcifications are present in 70% of cases as a result of host defense mechanisms.

The mortality rate from CE is lower (<5%). Mortality of an inadequately treated AE is >90% within 10–15 years of diagnosis. AE very rarely occurs outside of the liver (this, nor hepatic CE, will not be discussed in this chapter).

The initial phase of primary CE infection is always asymptomatic and prolonged, as symptoms are typically related to development of mass-effect on adjacent structures. Children and adolescents have weaker immune response and higher elasticity of the lung parenchyma compared to adults and may remain symptomatic despite having cysts of a very large size.

Pulmonary CE usually presents with cough, chest pain, dyspnea due to mass effect, or effusion.

Most HCs develop complications eventually. The main complication is cyst rupture through the lung parenchyma into the pleural space leading to pneumothorax, hydropneumothorax, secondary bacterial empyema, and parasitic pleural implants (hydatid thorax). Erosion in the bronchial tree may result in hemoptysis and expectoration of HC particles (hydatoptosis). Cysts can develop secondary bacterial infection resulting in abscesses. Cyst ruptures may result in acute hypersensitivity reactions to antigenic material, including anaphylaxis.

Leukopenia, thrombocytopenia, and nonspecific liver function abnormalities may be observed but are not diagnostic. Eosinophilia is observed in <15% of CE cases (usually with antigenic material leak) and >50% in AE. Hydatid disease may be diagnosed with a combination of imaging and serology. Chest radiograms may demonstrate sharp cystic opacity, effusions, and pneumothorax. Ultrasonography is an excellent modality to identify liver lesions, but its effectiveness is limited in the chest. CT has higher overall sensitivity than ultrasonography (95%–100%) and is the best modality for evaluation of extrahepatic and multiple cysts and their complications. The classic water-lily sign of a ruptured HC demonstrates floating endocyst in the cystic fluid. Magnetic resonance imaging has no major advantages over thoracic CT. Imaging allows description of the HCs as active, transitional, and inactive depending on their internal structure. Based on their type and the size, CE lesions are categorized by The World Health Organization (WHO) classification into five stages. This classification is useful for liver disease but is less practical in the management of lung lesions.

Several serologic and antigen assays are available. IgG ELISA is the preferred test, with a sensitivity of 60%–85% for lung CE lesions. Up to half of the patients with hydatid disease do not have circulating parasite antigens, which are not widely used for diagnosis. Latex agglutination and a dot-ELISA have excellent sensitivity and specificity to detect echinococcal antigens in cystic fluid; however, percutaneous aspiration should be reserved for situations when other diagnostic methods are inconclusive because of the risk of anaphylaxis and secondary spread of the infection.

While established guidelines are available for the treatment of hepatic cysts depending on the WHO stage, the presentation of pulmonary CE varies widely and no uniform consensus exists [2]. Management options for CE include observation, drug therapy, and surgery. Percutaneous management with aspiration and injection of antiparasitic agents are common for the hepatic cysts but is not recommended for pulmonary disease.

Small (<5 cm), uncomplicated cysts can be treated with pharmacotherapy (mebendazole [MBZ] and albendazole [ABZ] for 3–6 months and observation). The benefit of other agents is less clear. The WHO indicates that benzimidazoles may be administered to pregnant women in the second and third trimesters for the treatment of hydatid disease. Some reports suggest they have no increased risk of spontaneous abortions or congenital malformations in early pregnancy [3].

Surgery is the treatment of choice for symptomatic, large cysts causing mass effect or superficial cysts likely to rupture. Two-stage pleurodesis and delayed marsupialization were used in the past, but this approach has been abandoned. The objective of surgical treatment of CE is to eradicate the parasite and to maximally preserve lung tissue. Parenchymal resections are required in less than 5% of cases and usually involve en-bloc wedge resections, segmentectomy, and rarely lobectomy. Lobectomy is only indicated for replacement of the lobe with the cyst, severe pulmonary suppuration, multiple unilobar cysts, and advanced sequela of hydatid disease (bronchiectasis, fibrosis, erosion into the airway, or severe hemorrhage).

Standard posterolateral thoracotomy is the preferred approach. A thoracoscopic approach for small peripheral cysts should be limited to centers with significant experience in the treatment of hydatid disease. In bilateral cysts, the side with the unruptured cyst is operated first, and the ruptured cyst is managed as a staged operation. Median sternotomy is rarely indicated. The field surrounding the cyst is protected with 20% saline or povidone/iodine–moistened gauze.

Cysts <5 cm can be enucleated (cystectomy). Visceral pleura and pericyst are incised, exposing the obvious laminated layer. Intermittent positive pressure to the lung facilitates enucleation. Larger cysts should be managed initially with aspiration. Needle decompressions allow conversion of the tense hydatid cyst to a lax one, which can be extracted through a small parenchymal incision. Aspiration should be done slowly to prevent tears of the wall. Once the cyst is decompressed, incision of the pleura and pericyst is made in the same location, and the lax cyst removed intact. The benefits of injecting antiscolicidal agents are controversial. For deeper located cysts, initial incision of the parenchyma can be made along segmental planes. Use of negative pressure suction devices with a needle surrounded by a suction cup that fits over the convex part of the cyst can be used to prevent intraoperative spillage [4]. Incision of the laminated layer (formal cystotomy) and usage of the standard sucker inside the cyst should be avoided. Recurrence is unlikely if the intraoperative rupture or an incision of the cyst are avoided. After removal of the cyst, the pericyst cavity is explored, hemostasis assured, and visible bronchial openings are sutured with absorbable suture.

Removal of the parenchymal pericyst (pericystectomy) is rarely needed in cases of uncomplicated cysts. Obliteration of the cavity with deep absorbable suture (capitonnage) decreases air leak, infection rate, and length of hospital stay, but it carries the arguable risk of disfiguring lung parenchyma. Recurrent and daughter cysts can be treated the same way as simple cysts, but lobectomy may be required more frequently.

Ruptured and infected cysts are managed according to the same principles of complete cyst removal and maximal eradication of the parasite. Drainage of empyemas, decortication of the lung, and pericystectomy are performed as needed (as was done in our case). Closure of visible bronchial openings is performed but without capitonnage.

Rupture of liver cysts through the diaphragm into the chest comprise the most serious group of complications due to the extent of inflammation and the wide spreading of the parasite. Simple subphrenic and pleural contamination may be managed with removal of hydatid elements and wide drainage. Involvement of lung parenchyma may require limited lung resection as damage control and subsequent close follow-up. Similarly, cases of rupture into pericardium and mediastinitis require aggressive debridement and drainage.

Hydatid thorax with multiple cysts may be difficult to treat because only a few of the cysts can be removed intact.

The optimal duration of perioperative drug therapy is uncertain. Treatment should be initiated several days prior to surgery. Drugs should be avoided preoperatively in larger lung cysts because they may increase the risk of rupture. Postoperatively, ABZ should be continued for at least one month and MBZ for three months.

CE can recur after any treatment. Serology cannot be used reliably for disease follow-up after cyst resection, as antibodies may remain high many years after cyst removal with no recurrence [5]. Imaging every three to six months initially and then yearly for five years is the main method of surveillance.

REFERENCES

1. Eckert, J., Gemmell, M. A., François-Xavier, M., Pawlowski, Z. S., World Health Organization. WHO/OIE manual on echinococcosis in humans and animals : a public health problem of global concern / edited by J. Eckert et al. Paris, France : World Organisation for Animal Health, 2011. https://apps.who.int/iris/handle/10665/42427.
2. Brunetti, E. et al. Expert consensus for the diagnosis and treatment of cystic and alveolar echinococcosis in humans. *Acta Trop.* 2010;114:1–16.
3. Choi, J., Han, J., Ahn, H., Ryu, H., Koren, G. Foetal outcomes after exposure to albendazole in early pregnancy. *J Obstet Gynaecol.* 2017;37(8):1108–1111.
4. Burgos, R. et al. Pulmonary hydatidosis: Surgical treatment and follow-up of 240 cases. *European J Cardiothorac Surg.* 1999;16:628.
5. Manzano-Román, R. et al. Serological diagnosis and follow-up of human cystic echinococcosis: A new hope for the future? *Biomed Res Int.* 2015;2015.

Mathew Thomas

 Key Words

- Bronchiectasis
- Uniportal
- Lobectomy
- Lung resection
- VATS
- Thoracoscopy

Introduction

Surgical resection has been a well-established treatment for localized bronchiectasis [1]. Most operations for bronchiectasis have historically been performed through a thoracotomy because of the severe adhesions and bleeding associated with the chronic inflammation and recurrent pulmonary infections. We report a case of a bilateral sequential uniportal video-assisted thoracoscopic surgery (U-VATS) with right middle and lower bilobectomies, followed by left lower lobectomy and lingula segmentectomy for bronchiectasis.

Case Report

A 45-year-old male patient, who was a lifelong non-smoker with an underlying diagnosis of chronic non-cystic fibrosis (non-CF) bronchiectasis, was referred to us for evaluation for lung transplantation. His main symptoms included chronic bronchorrhea since birth and one episode of severe hemoptysis approximately six months prior to our evaluation, which had been managed conservatively. Since then, he had multiple episodes of *Pseudomonas aeruginosa* associated pneumonias, but no further hemoptysis.

He denied any shortness of breath, and his oxygen saturation had always been above 90% on room air. He had no other major comorbidities.

On examination, the relevant findings included raspy breathing with coarse conducted airway sounds, expiratory wheezes, and basilar crackles.

A computerized tomography (CT) scan of the chest showed extensive bronchiectasis in the lower lobes, lingula, and right middle lobe (Figure 34.1a–f). Interestingly, both upper lobes appeared relatively spared. A ventilation-perfusion scan (VQ scan) showed 70% of perfusion to the right lung with nearly equal distribution to the upper and lower lobes on both sides. Pulmonary function tests showed a forced expiratory volume in 1 second (FEV1) of 47% and a diffusion capacity (DLCO) of 72% of predicted.

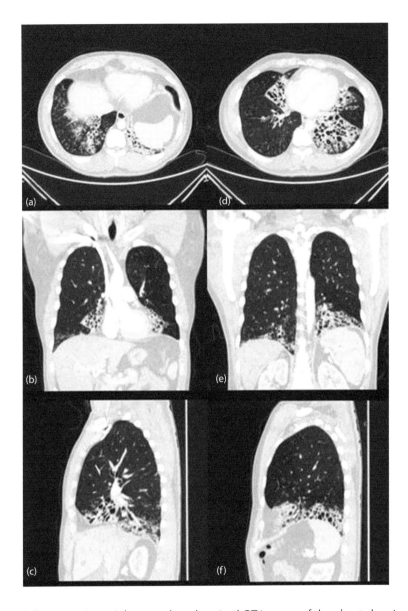

Figure 34.1 Preoperative axial, coronal, and sagittal CT images of the chest showing extensive right middle and lower lobe (a–c) and left lingula and lower lobe (d–f) bronchiectasis

Based on the CT findings and absence of shortness of breath with effort, we recommended bilateral sequential thoracoscopic resections (right middle and lower bilobectomy followed by left lower lobectomy and lingulectomy), instead of transplantation. He provided his consent.

We initially performed U-VATS right middle and lower bilobectomy through a 4 cm incision in the sixth intercostal space, between the anterior and midaxillary lines. A soft tissue wound protector (Alexis wound protector/retractor TM, Applied Medical Technology, USA) was used to prevent smudging of the camera. A 10-mm flexible 3D camera (Endoeye, Olympus, USA) was used for visualization, and the dissection was performed with Ligasure (Covidien, USA) bipolar vessel sealer device to take down adhesions. The adhesions were severe and quite vascular, which caused generalized bleeding. Due to the severe hilar adhesions and bulky consolidated lung, we decided to perform a standard lower lobectomy first, followed by the middle lobectomy. Once the lower lobe was removed, the bronchus intermedius (BI) could be dissected back to its takeoff from the right mainstem bronchus. The middle lobectomy was then completed by stapling off the BI at its origin from the right main bronchus. A bronchoscopy was performed to ensure that no stump was left behind. The chest was irrigated with 3 L of saline due to the abundant purulent secretions. The estimated blood loss was 150 mL. His postoperative recovery was rough, but he was discharged home after seven days without a chest tube. Two days later he was readmitted for noninfected pleural effusion that required a pigtail catheter drainage. He was discharged on daily intravenous cefepime infusion due to *Pseudomonas* in the sputum culture.

Six weeks after his first operation, he underwent a left U-VATS during which a lower lobectomy was performed first followed by an anatomical lingula segmentectomy. His recovery was less eventful than the first time, and he was discharged home eight days later with outpatient pulmonary rehabilitation. He was followed by our infectious disease and pulmonary teams: during his nine-month follow up, he had no residual symptoms and had gained 40 lbs from his preoperative weight. A repeat CT scan one year after surgery showed minimal residual disease in the remaining upper lobes (Figure 34.2).

Comments

Surgery for bronchiectasis has primarily included lobectomies, segmental resections, or wedge resections and most commonly performed on one side only. Bilateral lobectomies have been reported but much less frequently and have been staged at different times as in our patient [1]. Video-assisted thoracoscopic surgery (VATS) lobectomy and segmentectomies for bronchiectasis have been reported in some case series and individual case reports, but we have not identified any other report of bilateral thoracoscopic lobectomies in literature to date.

In a meta-analysis of 35 studies that included 4,788 patients with bronchiectasis who underwent surgical management, Fan et al. reported the following outcomes: mortality in 1.5%; morbidity in 17%; symptom resolution in 67%; symptoms improved in 28%; and no symptom improvement in 9% [2]. The low morbidity and mortality and high rates of symptom improvement after surgical treatment in localized bronchiectasis indicates that this should be considered when medical management is ineffective. In a retrospective analysis of 86 patients who underwent surgery for bronchiectasis, Balci et al. observed that, while complete resection independently

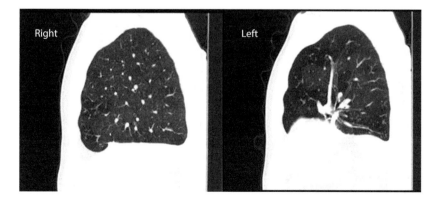

Figure 34.2 One year postoperative scans showing minimal bronchiectasis in both upper lobes

predicted symptom-free outcome (p < 0.05), an FEV1 of less than 60% of the predicted value, an incomplete resection, and preoperative antibiotic therapy independently predicted postoperative complications (p < 0.05) [1]. In an analysis of the United Network of Organs (UNOS) database by Hayes et al., the authors reported that the survival for non-CF bronchiectasis patients on the lung transplant wait list is much higher than those with CF bronchiectasis, suggesting that they are different pathophysiologies [3]. In non-CF patients, who are more likely to survive longer, surgical resection may be a better option than lung transplantation.

Patients being considered for bronchiectasis surgery should undergo thorough assessment to determine the extent of resection and medical candidacy. Preoperative workup should include a CT scan of the chest and a quantitative VQ scan in addition to pulmonary function tests. Patients with non-perfused, localized bronchiectasis appear to be the best candidates for resection. The role of antibiotics prior to surgery is not clear, but most patients with bronchiectasis have usually had multiple courses of antibiotics throughout their lifetime. It is advisable to wait for an acute exacerbation of infection to subside prior to operating.

Thoracoscopic management has been reported to be safe and feasible in retrospective studies of large series of patients with bronchiectasis [4,5]. In a retrospective comparison of 52 patients who had VATS resection with 52 who had thoracotomy for bronchiectasis at a single institution in China over 5 years, VATS was associated with shorter length of stay and fewer complications [5]. We believe that it is up to the individual surgeon to determine whether a minimally invasive resection can be performed or not since this is a much more difficult operation to perform by VATS.

In summary, unilateral or bilateral thoracoscopic lobectomy is feasible in patients with bronchiectasis although the operation can be challenging. The recovery of patients undergoing lung resection for bronchiectasis can be expected to be slower than most other diagnoses.

REFERENCES

1. Balci, A.E., Balci, T.A., Ozyurtan, M.O. Current surgical therapy for bronchiectasis: Surgical results and predictive factors in 86 patients. *Ann Thorac Surg.* 2014;97(1):211–217.
2. Fan, L.C., Liang, S., Lu, H.W., Fei, K., Xu, J.F. Efficiency and safety of surgical intervention to patients with non-cystic fibrosis bronchiectasis: A meta-analysis. *Sci Rep.* 2015;5:17382.
3. Hayes, D., Jr., Kopp, B.T., Tobias, J.D., Woodley, F.W., Mansour, H.M., Tumin, D., et al. Survival in patients with advanced non-cystic fibrosis bronchiectasis versus cystic fibrosis on the waitlist for lung transplantation. *Lung.* 2015;193(6):933–938.
4. Baysungur, V., Dogruyol, T., Ocakcioglu, I., Misirlioglu, A., Evman, S., Kanbur, S., et al. The feasibility of thoracoscopic resection in bronchiectasis. *Surg Laparosc Endosc Percutan Tech.* 2017;27(3):194–196.
5. Zhang, P., Zhang, F., Jiang, S., Jiang, G., Zhou, X., Ding, J., et al. Video-assisted thoracic surgery for bronchiectasis. *Ann Thorac Surg.* 2011;91(1):239–243.

CASE 35: ROBOTIC LOBECTOMY IN A PATIENT WITH BRONCHIECTASIS AND DIFFUSE PLEURAL ADHESIONS—ADVANTAGES OVER CHALLENGES

Adrian E. Rodrigues and Wickii T. Vigneswaran

 Key Words

- Bronchiectasis
- Robotic
- Minimally invasive
- Pleural adhesions
- Thoracic surgery

Introduction

The infancy of minimally invasive thoracic surgery (MITS) began in the 1990s, initially with the introduction of video-assisted thoracoscopic surgery (VATS) and ten years later with the advent of the da Vinci robot. When VATS emerged, it quickly became a common substitute for open thoracotomies, but when the da Vinci robot arrived, it offered even more advancements: increased dexterity, three-dimensional magnification, and enhanced precision and control of instrumentation. Although the robot offered better micromanagement of anatomical structures, it was criticized due to its cost and lack of showing greater effectiveness over its predecessor.

Today, both technologies are widely used to undertake various thoracic surgical procedures, and although they individually harbor different limitations, the da Vinci robot unavoidably inherited many of the contraindications attributed to VATS; including pleural adhesion.

No one doubts that pleural adhesions create a challenge in thoracic surgery, but robotic-assisted surgery offers a platform where in the hands of a skilled and well-experienced operator, adhesions can be taken down systematically and safely in selected cases. Proof of this took place at our institution in a case involving a male diagnosed with bronchiectasis; a disease well-known to produce extensive pleural adhesions. As the robotic surgery initiated, the peripheral density of adhesions was apparent, but as the procedure coursed, the true volume and location of adhesions became increasingly evident. Nevertheless, the surgical procedure concluded with a left lower lobe lobectomy that progressed wholly robotically, never requiring a thoracotomy. This case displays the technological capabilities the robot harbors, and with increased practice, surgeons can master its limits and use them in selective cases they would have otherwise done openly.

Case Report

We encountered a 29-year-old male with a history of bronchiectasis, chronic sinusitis, nasal polyps, persistent cough, and sinus fungal and pulmonary pseudomonas infections. The patient had a recent history of migrating to the United States from Mexico and reported chronic lung issues since childhood but affirmed his youth and current life incorporated an active lifestyle. Additionally, his sleep had consistently been associated with nasal congestion, while his pulmonary exacerbations had been accompanied with shortness of breath and blood-stained sputum. Nonetheless, he denied hemoptysis, fever, chills, chest pain, vomit, and diarrhea.

During general examination patient appeared well with no acute distress. Pulmonary auscultation exposed wheezing and crackles throughout the lung fields. Blood pressure measured 104/54 mmHg, pulse 81 bpm, respiratory rate was within normal limits, and he was afebrile with an SpO_2 of 95% and BMI of 27.8 kg/m^2.

A workup chest CT showed diffuse tree-in-bud opacities throughout the lungs, sparing the lung apices. There was focal severe bronchiectasis in the left lower lobe with associated volume loss (Figure 35.1). Scattered areas of bronchiectasis were also noted in the inferior portion of left upper lobe, right middle lobe, and inferior right lower lobe. There was mild air trapping on the expiratory views.

A pulmonary function test revealed a mildly reduced forced vital capacity (FVC), a moderate severely reduced forced expiratory volume in one second (FEV-1) and a reduced FEV-1/FVC with no response to albuterol. Total lung capacity (TLC) and residual volume (RV) were both mildly reduced, whereas diffusing lung capacity for carbon monoxide (DLCO) was normal. A sweat chloride test was negative for cystic fibrosis.

A fiber-optic video pharyngo-laryngoscopy showed right nasal polyps and left swollen and exudative nasal polys. Remaining pharynx and larynx were within normal limits. Prior to thoracic surgery, the patient underwent bilateral endoscopic sinus surgery with turbinate reduction and polyp removal. The procedure progressed without complications.

Approximately four months afterward, he underwent a robotic left lower lobe lobectomy. Although the left upper, right middle, and right lower lobe also showed evidence of bronchiectasis, the left lower lobe showed almost complete destruction and was very likely a nidus for microbes and respiratory symptom manifestation. It was therefore felt the patient would benefit from excising the destroyed lower lobe that was producing the respiratory concerns.

In the operating room, bronchoscopy revealed abundant bilateral purulent material that required suctioning, and a left video thoracoscopy exposed diffused lung adhesions with greater density between the left lower lobe and its adjacent diaphragm and pericardium. A da Vinci Si robotic system was used using one camera, two operating arms, and a utility port. The adhesions were taken down using bipolar cautery, and the lung mobilized from the chest wall, diaphragm, pericardium and mediastinum. The inferior pulmonary ligament was taken down using electrocautery, and systematic dissection was carried out in the lower part of the hilum, thereby facilitating left lower lobe pulmonary vein isolation. Once these were taken down with relative ease the hilum clearly visualized. Once in view, significant inflammation on both the hilum and mediastinum were observed.

Attention then focused on the fissure within the hilum, which after inspection showed a firm adherence throughout its oblique course. Electrocautery was therefore systematically used on the fissure, enabling successful separation of the upper and lower lobe. Hilum dissection then resumed, permitting neovascularized lymph node removal along with pulmonary arterial structure identification.

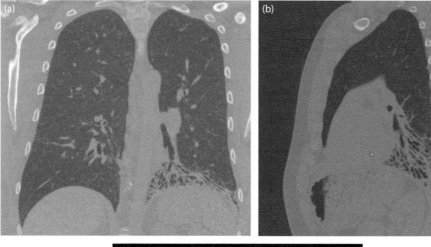

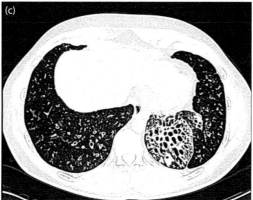

Figure 35.1 CT scan of the chest showing the involvement of the left lower lobe that is almost completely destroyed by chronic infection with relative sparing of the remaining lung. (a–c showing different views of the scan)

Then the lower lobe vein was transected using a linear endovascular stapler (Covidien). Vessel loops were then passed around the low basal segmental and superior segmental arterial branches of the lower lobe, and each were sequentially transected using an endovascular stapler. Hilum dissection ensued, allowing for lymph node removal near the bronchus along with adhesion take down along the lower lobe bronchus. Once the tissue surrounding the bronchus was dissected out, a thick Endo GIA stapler (Covidien, purple tri-staple) was introduced into the surgical field and used to transect the lower lobe bronchus. The left lower lobe specimen was then extracted through the utility port using a 12-mm Endo-bag. The thoraco-port closed with absorbable sutures.

The subsequent pathological report showed a left lower lobe consistent with bronchiectasis, follicular bronchitis, pneumocyte hyperplasia, bronchopneumonia, giant cell reaction, and dystrophic calcification; while its accompanying bronchus solely displayed chronic inflammation. Ultrastructural features of ciliary dyskinesia were also tested but failed to be observed via electron microscopy.

There were no complications during the surgical procedure or hospitalization. Follow-up revealed significant improvement and minimal sputum production and no other symptoms. Chest CT displayed stable minimal bronchiectasis in remaining lung tissue. He was able and eager to continue his active lifestyle at the six-month visit.

Comments

Although there are more than 16 known causes of bronchiectasis, most commonly cystic fibrosis, postinfectious, and COPD, the majority are categorized as idiopathic because most cases fail identifiable etiologies [1]. Yet regardless of cause, every case undergoes the same pathophysiology. Initially published in 1986, a process was identified and given the name "Cole's vicious cycle hypothesis" [2,3]; a model describing four phases that rotate cyclically: chronic bronchial infection, inflammation, impaired mucociliary clearance, and structural lung disease, with each independently being a starting point contingent on the etiology [3]. We now know this process generates repeated pulmonary exacerbations and is the culprit for the development of dense pleural adhesion formation; the main finding that causes some surgeons to avoid MITS in these patients.

Examining some history will allow us to recognize how this avoidance emerged. The incorporation of surgery in patients suffering from bronchiectasis is over a century old [3], and in the 1930s, the benefits of only removing the diseased pulmonary segment was becoming widely recognized [4]. As the 1950s approached, a decline in surgical intervention for bronchiectasis occurred due to the discovery and mass development of antibiotics [3]. Nevertheless, surgical treatment options for bronchiectasis never ceased due to the inability of antibiotics penetrating adequately in diseased areas. Four decades later, as VATS began to replace thoracotomies, many felt that pleural adhesions created a technical challenge for such approach [5]. As a result, VATS procedures in patients with adhesions was relatively contraindicated, and when the da Vinci robot was introduced, it unavoidably inherited the same relative contraindication without thoroughly testing its limits.

Regardless of surgical modality, pleural adhesions still create a challenge for surgeons today [6]. Adhesions can lead to hemorrhages, prolonged air leaks, longer surgeries, and increased surgical instrument alternation, and can influence a conversion to open [5,6]. They can also cause difficulty in recognizing anatomy, including interlobular fissure incompleteness and consequently create a hazardous surgical resection [3].

Some consider pleural adhesions as relative contraindication for the use of the da Vinci robot technique for lung resection [7] and some surgeons using adjunct techniques when using VATS [8]. In contrary to that belief, we feel the robotic technique is better for adhesionolysis, even when compared to open technique, and often when used in re-do operations [9]. In our experience, we observed this technology can decrease morbidity and shortens healing time and hospital length of stay as observed by others, even in the setting of complex and challenging scenarios [10,11].

REFERENCES

1. Lonni, S., Chalmers, J.D., Goeminne, P.C., et al. Etiology of non-cystic fibrosis bronchiectasis in adults and its correlation to disease severity. *Ann Am Thorac Soc.* 2015;12(12):1764–1770.
2. Cole, P.J. Inflammation: A two-edged sword: The model of bronchiectasis. *Eur J Respir Dis Suppl.* 1986;147:6–15.

3. Hiramatsu, M. and Shiraishi, Y. Surgical management of non-cystic fibrosis bronchiectasis. *J Thorac Dis*. 2018;10(Suppl 28):S3436–S3445.

4. Churchill, E.D., Belsey, R., London, F. Segmental pneumonectomy in bronchiectasis the lingula segment of the left upper lobe. *Ann Surg*. 1939;109(4):481.

5. Li, S.-J., Zhou K., Wu, Y.-M., et al. Presence of pleural adhesions can predict conversion to thoracotomy and postoperative surgical complications in patients undergoing video-assisted thoracoscopic lung cancer lobectomy. *J Thorac Dis*. 2018;10(1):416–431.

6. Qian, L., Chen, X., Huang, J., et al. A comparison of three approaches for the treatment of early-stage thymomas: Robot-assisted thoracic surgery, video-assisted thoracic surgery, and median sternotomy. *J Thorac Dis*. 2017;9(7):1997–2005.

7. Bonatti, J., Schachner, T., Bernecker, O., et al. Robotic totally endoscopic coronary artery bypass: Program development and learning curve issues. *J Thorac Cardiovasc Surg*. 2004;127(2):504–510.

8. Guerrero, W.G. and González-Rivas, D. Multiportal video-assisted thoracic surgery, uniportal video-assisted thoracic surgery and minimally invasive open chest surgery-selection criteria. *J Vis Surg*. 2017;3:56.

9. Latif, M.J and Park, B.J. Robotics in general thoracic surgery procedures. *J Vis Surg*. 2017;3:44.

10. Novellis, P., Bottoni, E., Voulaz, E., et al. Robotic surgery, video-assisted thoracic surgery, and open surgery for early stage lung cancer: Comparison of costs and outcomes at a single institute. *J Thorac Dis*. 2018;10(2):790–798.

11. Gallagher, S.P., Abolhoda, A., Kirkpatrick, V.E., Saffarzadeh, A.G., Thein, M.S., Wilson, S.E. Learning curve of robotic lobectomy for early-stage non-small cell lung cancer by a thoracic surgeon adept in open lobectomy. *Innov Technol Tech Cardiothorac Vasc Surg*. 2018;13(5):321–327.

Ashish Pulikal, Jason Long, and Benjamin Haithcock

Key Words
• Granulomatosis • Polyangiitis • ECMO

Introduction

Granulomatosis with polyangiitis (GPA), formerly known as Wegener's disease, is an auto-immune disease with features of medium-to-small vessel vasculitis and granulomatous inflammation most frequently affecting the pulmonary-renal axis. While the prevalence in the United States is only three cases per 100,000 people, there is a strong predominance to male individuals of northern European descent (>90% of cases in the US). The symptoms manifest with varying degrees of severity, and the development of pulmonary insufficiency necessitating extracorporeal oxygenation is exceedingly rare and infrequently reported in this patient population [1]. Our patient represents one of only thirteen reported cases of successful hospital discharge following severe pulmonary GPA treated with aggressive immunosuppressive therapies vvECMO. As well, our patient is the only reported case requiring adjunctive window thoracostomy for Stenotrophomonal/Pseudomonal cavitary superinfection and aspergillosis. All medical and surgical treatment was delivered at a major academic quaternary care hospital.

Case Report

A 53-years-old, Indian female with a height 157.5 cm, weight 61.3 kg, and body mass index (BMI) 24.7 kg/m² presented with progressive dyspnea and nonproductive cough to an outside institution. She presented to UNC Memorial hospital in Chapel Hill, North Carolina, as a transfer by ambulance from Alamance Hospital in Burlington, North Carolina, six months later.

The patient has a history of right breast invasive ductal adenocarcinoma (ER/PR+, Her2neu negative). This was treated with partial mastectomy and adjuvant targeted hormonal and radiation therapy. The patient was given steroids for presumed radiation pneumonitis at an outside facility prior to transfer. She does not have any other relevant past medical or surgical history. The patient is a lifelong non-smoker and non-drinker. The patient does not have a significant family history of medical illness or any relevant genetic history or genetic

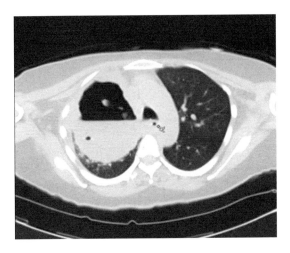

Figure 36.1 CT chest without contrast—cavitary destruction of the right upper lobe

predispositions. The patient was previously fully ambulatory and required no assistance for routine activities of daily living. She is a married, stay-at-home mother.

Numerous serologies and titers were sent during the patient's initial workup. Radiological imaging included a CT chest (Figure 36.1), as well as daily chest X-rays. Initial histopathologic data included the following:

1. Cytology, bronchoalveolar lavage on initial admission, no malignancy, abundant inflammation
2. Cytology, core biopsy—acid fast bacilli (AFB)/fungal stains negative. Atypical bronchial epithelium with squamous metaplasia, chronic inflammation, no malignancy
3. Right upper lobe biopsy—Reactive bronchial epithelium with squamous metaplasia and abundant necrosis with calcification, no malignancy

There were no barriers to access. There were no financial or cultural limitations to report. There were however diagnostic challenges in this case initially, while attempting to identify the root etiology for this patient's presentation with appropriate imaging and diagnostic modalities.

The initial differential diagnosis for this patient was quite broad with infectious etiologies felt to be most likely the etiology. Given the cavitary appearance of the lesions in the right upper lobe with evidence of extension to the contralateral lung as well as the indolent time course, mycobacterial and fungal etiologies were strongly considered by the infectious disease team. These include histoplasmosis, blastomycosis, and aspergillosis. As well, atypical pneumonia etiologies including *Pneumocystis*, *Legionella*, *Mucorales*, *Nocardia*, *Cryptococcus*, *Rhodococcus*, and *Actinomyces* were considered. Parasitic lung disease was considered with both *paragonamiasis* and *echinococcosis* in the differential, albeit lower on the list. Tuberculosis was initially a possibility but was ruled out given a nonreactive purified protein derivative(PPD) skin test as well as negative AFB sputum smears × 3. There certainly was concern for radiation-induced lung injury given the patient's recent adjuvant therapy for breast carcinoma. Vasculitis was highly suspected once the proteinase 3-anti-neutrophil cytoplasmic antibody (PR3-ANCA) titer was found to be strongly positive. The patient did have evidence of cavitary superinfection over the course of her hospitalization. Her *Aspergillus* Ag was elevated at the initial lavage. She also had *Pseudomonas aeruginosa* and *Stenotrophomonas maltophilia* from wound cultures obtained from her lung two months later.

The patient's prognosis was considered dynamic and in a state of constant flux. Day-to-day changes were reviewed with the family throughout the course of her hospitalization. We stratified our clinical outlook based on hemodynamic data, daily laboratory workup, end-organ perfusion metrics, and degree of support on the ECMO circuit (sweep, FiO$_2$).

Given the acuity of the patient's decline, no significant pre-interventional optimization or risk stratification was done. The patient was not on anticoagulation preoperatively.

On presentation, the patient's inciting etiologies were yet to be differentiated appropriately. Initial diagnostics included flexible bronchoscopy and endobronchial ultrasound with fine needle aspiration (EBUS-FNA). Once the diagnosis of PR3-ANCA positive granulomatosis with polyangiitis (GPA) was established, appropriate immunosuppressive therapies as directed by Rheumatology were administered. This included pulse-dosed intravenous Solumedrol (methylprednisolone) 1 g daily for three days, once monthly Cytoxan (cyclophosphamide) for three months, and therapeutic plasmapheresis every other day for approximately one week. Additional antibiotics used throughout the patient's hospital course were chosen based on culture and microbial sensitivity data.

The patient was brought for a diagnostic bronchoscopy and was found to have a large cavitary lesion in the right upper lobe with copious purulence. This drainage soiled the bilateral airways significantly such that the patient became difficult to oxygenate on maximal ventilator support. The decision was made to institute peripheral venovenous ECMO via the right internal jugular vein was established with an Avalon Elite® Bi-caval Dual Lumen Catheter under transesophageal echo (TEE) and fluoroscopic guidance. A percutaneous gastrostomy was placed for enteral feeding access. A tracheostomy with a Covidien 8-0 cuffed Shiley tube was placed for daily airway toileting. A right anterior window thoracostomy (Eloesser flap) was created for open-chest drainage due to right upper lobe cavitary superinfection (Figure 36.2). Daily dressing changes to this wound included Xeroform® (5″ × 9″) petrolatum gauze dressing for the base of the wound, followed by two Kerlix™ gauze bandage rolls packed tightly up to the level of the skin. Upon adequate rescue of pulmonary function after 32 days of ECMO support, the patient was decannulated. Areas of obvious bronchopleural fistulae at the base of the chest wound were closed primarily with permanent pledgeted Prolene suture. Aerosolized TISSEEL® (fibrin sealant) and Bioglue® were used to reinforce this closure. Finding of subdiagrammatic free air on routine chest X-ray gave concern for spontaneous viscus perforation in the setting of aggressive immunosuppression. A midline exploratory laparotomy was performed by general surgery service. No such perforation was found.

Several family members including the patient's husband were at the bedside every morning during rounds. As well, a stereo was brought into the room with Hindu prayers and spirituals playing throughout the day to uplift the patient's state of well-being. We feel each of these variables, albeit intangible, were of paramount importance in her positive outcome.

Upon discharge the patient spent approximately 11 days in acute in-patient rehabilitation and was followed subsequently in the UNC thoracic surgery outpatient clinic weekly. Multidisciplinary outpatient care was coordinated with the departments of infectious

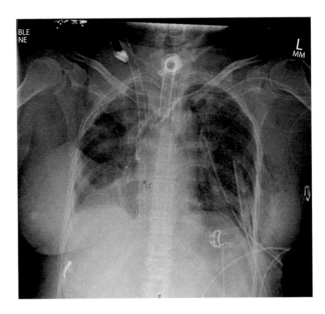

Figure 36.2 Chest X-ray—Two left-sided 28-Fr chest tubes, right internal jugular vein ECMO cannula, and silhouette of Eloesser flap overlying the right upper lobe anteriorly are all visible

disease, rheumatology, endocrinology, physical therapy, and occupational therapy. These visits included, but were not limited to, titration of immunosuppressive medications, antimicrobial therapies, as well as strength and endurance training. A referral to plastic surgery was also made for the consideration of Eloesser flap (Figure 36.3) closure with concurrent chest wall reconstruction. At three months post-discharge, maintains excellent functional status and is able to complete all activities of daily life independently. In order to close her BPF a bilobectomy was necessary through a right posterolateral thoracotomy - the eloesser was closed with a muscle flap. No overt technical, logistical, or treatment-related complications occurred over the course of this patient's hospital stay.

Comments

Eleven case reports of thirteen patients diagnosed with GPA and severe pulmonary insufficiency necessitating extracorporeal oxygenation exist in the literature. The average age of these patients was 34.6 +/− 13.2 years. The average duration of ECMO therapy was 12.4 +/− 4.9 days. All patients had evidence of alveolar hemorrhage, and seven of the thirteen patients required in-hospital renal replacement therapy. Immunosuppressive regimens were variable: however, all patients survived to decannulation and subsequent hospital discharge [2–12]. Interestingly, no patients underwent window thoracostomy. Our patient was statistically older (53 years, $p < 0.05$), remained on ECMO significantly longer (32 days, $p < 0.05$), and required open-chest drainage for cavitary superinfection.

We demonstrate that critically ill patients with severe, acute onset GPA requiring venovenous extracorporeal oxygenation can also undergo adjunctive window thoracostomy safely, with good long-term functional outcome at three months. Robust randomized studies on pulmonary autoimmune vasculitis and the available medical/surgical options for such disease are required to create a comprehensive treatment algorithm and further optimize patient outcomes.

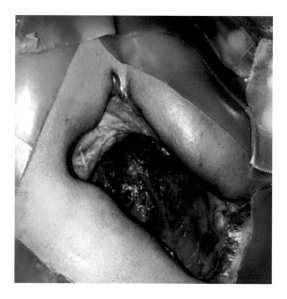

Figure 36.3 Right anterior window thoracostomy—Note, large cavitary lesion encompassing the right upper and right middle lobes

REFERENCES

1. Mukhtyar, C., Guillevin, L., Cid, M.C. EULAR recommendations for the management of primary small and medium vessel vasculitis. *Annals Rheumat Dis.* 2009; 68(3):310–317.
2. Hohenforst-Schmidt, W., Petermann, A., Visouli, A., et al. Successful application of extracorporeal membrane oxygenation due to pulmonary hemorrhage secondary to granulomatosis with polyangiitis. *Drug Design Develop Ther.* 2013;7:627–633.
3. Hartmann, A., Nordal, K.P., Svennevig, J., Noddeland, H., Pedersen, T., Skarbøvik, A.J., Fauchald, P. Successful use of artificial lung (ECMO) and kidney in the treatment of a 20-year-old female with Wegener's syndrome. *Nephrol Dial Transplant.* 1994;9:316–319.
4. Ahmed, S., Aziz, T., Cochran, J. Use of extracorporeal membrane oxygenation in a patient with diffuse alveolar hemorrhage. *Chest.* 2004;126:305–309.
5. Cerrati, E., Hartman, A., Gottlieb, M., Kohan, D. Sequential bilateral otitis media and bilateral facial nerve paralysis as presenting symptoms of Wegener's granulomatosis. *J Case Rep Med.* 2013;2:4.
6. Savran, Y., Gencpinar, T., Aydin, K., Eroz, E. Concurrent extracorporeal membrane oxygenation, plasmapheresis and continuous renal replacement therapy in a case of wegener's granulomatosis. *Annals Int Med Dental Res.* 2016;2(5):1–3.
7. Vanoli, J., Riva, M., Vergnano, B., et al. Granulomatosis with polyangiitis presenting with diffuse alveolar hemorrhage requiring extracorporeal membrane oxygenation with rapid multiorgan relapse: A case report. Dalar L, ed. *Medicine.* 2017;96(13):e6024.
8. Yusuff, H., Malagon, I., Robson, K., Parmar, J., Hamilton, P., Falter, F. Extracorporeal membrane oxygenation for life-threatening ANCA-positive pulmonary capillaritis. A review of UK experience. *Heart Lung Vessels.* 2015;7(2):159–167.

9. Rawal, G., Kumar, R., Yadav, S. ECMO rescue therapy in diffuse alveolar haemorrhage: A case report with review of literature. *J Clin Diag Res*. 2016;10(6):OD10–OD11.

10. Abrams, D., Agerstrand, C., Biscotti, M., Burkart, K., Bacchetta, M., Brodie, D. Extracorporeal membrane oxygenation in the management of diffuse alveolar hemorrhage. *ASAIO J*. 2015;61:216–218.

11. Guo, Z., Li, X., Jiang, L., Xu, L. Extracorporeal membrane oxygenation for the management of respiratory failure caused by diffuse alveolar hemorrhage. *J Extracorp Tech*. 2009;41(1):37–40.

12. Matsumoto, T., Ueki, K., Tamura, S., Ideura, H., Tsukada, Y., Maezawa, A., Nojima, Y., Naruse, T. Extracorporeal membrane oxygenation for the management of respiratory failure due to ANCA-associated vasculitis. *Scand J Rheumatol*. 2000;29(3):195–197.

Max Lacour and Isabelle Opitz

 Key Words

- Pulmonary artery
- Intimal sarcoma
- Pulmonary embolus

Introduction

Primary pulmonary artery sarcomas (PAS) are a very rare entity and usually associated with dismal outcomes. Since their first description by Moritz Mandelstamm in 1923, less than 300 cases have been reported [1]. As patients usually present with nonspecific symptoms such as dyspnea, chest pain, or cough, mimicking pulmonary embolism (PE), diagnosis can be difficult to establish. Misleading initial symptoms and pulmonary thromboembolism being the most common differential diagnosis, patients are often treated with therapeutic anticoagulation, leading to delay of diagnosis and therapy.

As reported by Bleisch and colleagues, pulmonary trunk is affected in 100% in patients presenting with PAS. Pulmonary valve is affected in around 57% of cases and right ventricle in 25% of the cases [2]. For this reason, to avoid dramatic hemodynamic consequences, early management of this aggressive tumor is mandatory, and whenever feasible, a surgical resection should be performed [3].

The establishment of a therapy plan for pulmonary artery sarcoma should always be discussed in a multidisciplinary tumor conference, and treatment allocation should preferably only be performed in high volume and experienced centers.

Median survival rates for patients with incomplete resection are reported as of 11 months [3]. For patients undergoing multimodality treatment, survival has been reported as of 24 months [3].

We present the case of an unusually favorable outcome after multimodality treatment for PAS.

Case Report

A 48-year-old female without comorbidities initially presented to the primary care physician with chest pain, shortness of breath, and fatigue. Transthoracic echocardiography was performed to rule out myocarditis and showed no signs of right ventricular failure. Apart from decrease in blood oxygen saturation, the performed bicycle stress testing was normal. Upon physical examination, the lungs were clear to auscultation with normal heart rate and rhythm. No murmurs were revealed. Clinical signs of right heart failure were also absent. The patient stated that there is no history of tobacco, alcohol, or illicit drug use.

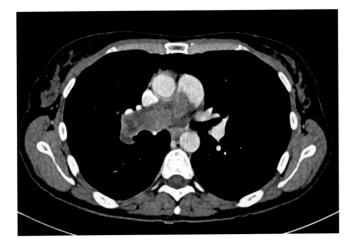

Figure 37.1 CT scan with contrast-enhancement showing the tumor mass in the right pulmonary artery

Due to persistent and aggravated shortness of breath, two weeks after initial presentation to the primary care physician, the patient was admitted to the hospital, and CT scan revealed an intravascular mass in the right pulmonary artery with suspicion of central embolism and consecutive infarction pneumonia on the right side (Figure 37.1).

Due to initial diagnosis of acute pulmonary embolism and infarction pneumonia, therapeutic anticoagulation and antibiotic therapy was initiated (Figure 37.2).

A follow-up CT-scan showed a persistent mass in the right pulmonary artery with suspicion of a malignant tumor. The subsequent PET-CT scan revealed an fludeoxyglucose (FDG)-positive mass in the right pulmonary artery (PA) with invasion of pulmonary trunk and no evidence of distant metastasis (Figure 37.3). In the transthoracic echocardiography, there were no signs of pulmonary hypertension, and the right ventricle to right atrial (RV-RA) gradient was 23 mm Hg.

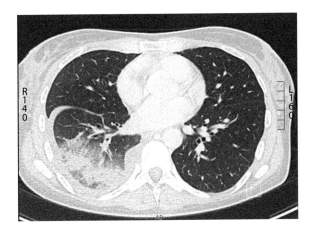

Figure 37.2 CT scan showing infarction pneumonia on the right side

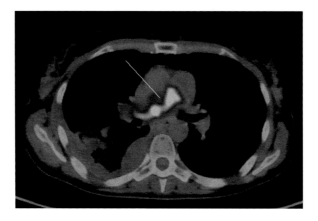

Figure 37.3 PET scan showing uptake of the tumor mass in the pulmonary artery

After discussion of the case in our multidisciplinary tumor conference, surgical resection with intraoperative frozen section was recommended.

The patient underwent a median sternotomy with extended right-sided pneumonectomy with resection of the pulmonary outflow tract and partial resection of left pulmonary artery with reconstruction and replacement of pulmonary valve under cardiopulmonary bypass in moderate hypothermia (Figure 37.4). Due to the extent of the tumor on the peripheral PA on the right side, right-sided pneumonectomy had to be performed. A preoperative perfusion-scan showed a significant decrease in perfusion on the right side, corresponding to only 2.3%. Furthermore, pulmonary function testing showed an FEV1 of 2.55 L. These preoperative findings showed no contraindication for performing a right-sided pneumonectomy in this situation.

Intraoperative frozen section and definitive histological examination showed intimal pulmonary sarcoma.

The postoperative course was uneventful, and the patient was discharged to rehabilitation two weeks after surgery.

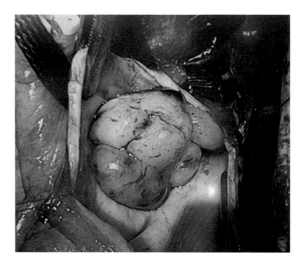

Figure 37.4 Intraoperative photo showing intimal sarcoma of the pulmonary artery

Due to positive surgical resection margins close to the pulmonary valve, adjuvant radiotherapy (50 Gy in total) and adjuvant chemotherapy were administered. A port-a-cath was inserted in preparation for chemotherapy. Four cycles of chemotherapy with doxorubicin and ifosfamid were administered. After the last cycle of chemotherapy with doxorubicin and ifosfamid, the patient needed to be hospitalized due to sepsis in neutropenia. Intravenous antibiotic therapy was initiated, and the patient's clinical status improved. Antibiotic therapy was continued orally for 10 days, and the patient was discharged home with a normalized blood count.

Postoperative anticoagulation was performed with a vitamin K antagonist. During chemotherapy, anticoagulation was temporarily stopped whenever platelets showed below 10 G/L.

After multimodality treatment including surgical resection, postoperative radiotherapy, and chemotherapy, the patient was enrolled to our regular follow-up program including CT scans.

More than two-years after resection (28.25 months), the patient is alive and in excellent condition, and follow-up CT scans are without evidence of local or distant recurrence.

Comments

Intimal sarcoma of the pulmonary artery is a very rare disease mimicking PE and often leads to initial inappropriate diagnosis and delay to the start of treatment. PAS is often initially mistaken for acute or chronic pulmonary thromboembolism (CTEPH). In PAS, however, there is usually a mismatch between the extent of intravascular obstruction and severity of pulmonary hypertension. This might be due to a more rapid progression of disease for PAS. Therefore, perioperative risks are increased in CTEPH patients compared to extended resections for PAS patients under cardiopulmonary bypass [4].

Surgical resection—whenever feasible in combination of neo- or adjuvant chemotherapy—is considered the mainstay of treatment for PAS [3]. However, due to the rarity of the disease, data for efficacy of treatment options have been limited up until today, and treatment allocation should always be discussed in multidisciplinary tumor conference.

Surgery for PAS includes pulmonary endarterectomy (PEA), tumor debulking with or without reconstruction of pulmonary artery, lobectomy, and even pneumonectomy. Depending on tumor localization and tumor extension, the extent of resection can often only be determined intraoperatively. Since PAS originates from vascular endothelium, it is often bilateral and complete resection is not achieved. However, in unilateral disease, surgical resection including pneumonectomy can be performed if the patient's functional reserve allows pneumonectomy. The surgical approach of choice is a median sternotomy, and PEA is performed using cardiopulmonary bypass and moderate hypothermia.

After surgical resection, regular follow-up with CT scans and physical examination is recommended in order to detect early recurrence [3].

Despite aggressive treatment of PAS, the prognosis remains dismal with median survival after incomplete resection reported as of 11 months and for patients undergoing multimodality treatment of 24 months [3].

The present case demonstrates that prolonged survival can be achieved with multimodality treatment approach.

REFERENCES

1. Kriz, J.P., Munfakh, N.A., King, G.S., Carden, J.O. Pulmonary artery intimal sarcoma: A case report. *Case Rep Oncol.* 2016;9(1):267–272.
2. Bleisch, V.R., Kraus, F.T. Polypoid sarcoma of the pulmonary trunk: Analysis of the literature and report of a case with leptomeric organelles and ultrastructural features of rhabdomyosarcoma. *Cancer.* 1980;46(2):314–324.
3. Blackmon, S.H., Rice, D.C., Correa, A.M., Mehran, R., Putnam, J.B., Smythe, W.R., et al. Management of primary pulmonary artery sarcomas. *Ann Thorac Surg.* 2009;87(3): 977–984.
4. Mussot, S., Ghigna, M.R., Mercier, O., Fabre, D., Fadel, E., Le Cesne, A., et al. Retrospective institutional study of 31 patients treated for pulmonary artery sarcoma. *Eur J Cardiothorac Surg.* 2013;43(4):787–793.

Reilly Hobbs and Rishindra M. Reddy

🔑	Key Words
	• Case report • Esophageal tumor • Fibroepithelial polyp • Esophagectomy

Introduction

Benign esophageal masses are commonly encountered during routine endoscopic and radiographic studies. Observation of asymptomatic lesions is reasonable depending on the size, malignant potential, and location of the lesion. The mainstay of treatment for symptomatic benign esophageal lesions is either surgical or endoscopic resection. When there is questionable malignant potential, oncologic principles should be considered when planning for resection and esophagectomy may be the best approach. When a benign diagnosis is suspected preoperatively, minimally invasive and alternative surgical strategies should be considered to decrease surgical morbidity.

Case Report

A 56-year-old Caucasian male in good overall health presented to his family practice physician with a two-year history of progressive chest discomfort, dysphagia to solids, nocturnal choking episodes, and orthopnea. His past medical history and physical exam were unremarkable. A barium esophagram was performed and demonstrated a large esophageal filling defect (Figure 38.1). He was referred to a thoracic surgeon in the local community who performed a subsequent esophago-gastro-duodenoscopy (EGD) with biopsy, which demonstrated a large submucosal mass occupying the entire lumen of the esophagus. The biopsy results were nondiagnostic. A follow-up chest CT scan with IV and oral contrast showed a large heterogeneous stalk-like mass arising in the cervical esophagus and extending 19.1 cm to the distal thoracic esophagus (Figure 38.2). At his original institution, it was recommended that he undergo an esophagectomy.

He sought a second opinion at a tertiary care center with a high volume of esophageal surgery. Upon review of his films and tests, it was felt that his lesion was consistent with a benign fibroepithelial polyp, and that resection of the polyp, with preservation of the esophagus was the preferred approach. He underwent a left-sided cervical neck incision with an esophagotomy in order to remove the polyp. An anterior myotomy was performed and the submucosal plane was explored. The mucosa was then entered to better delineate the anatomy of the polyp. The stalk was identified, arising from the submucosa.

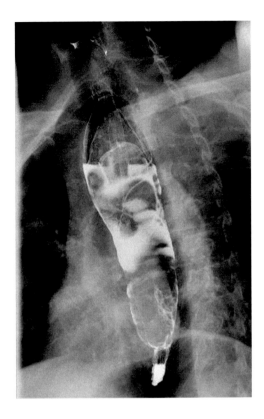

Figure 38.1 Preoperative barium esophagram showing a large esophageal filling defect

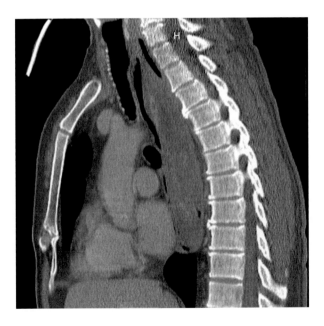

Figure 38.2 CT chest showing a large solid mass expanding into the esophageal lumen. White arrow shows a stalk arising in the cervical esophagus

The stalk was ligated and divided at the base with the esophageal mucosa repaired primarily. The mass was fully mobilized, but a manubrial split was necessary to remove the mass from the thoracic inlet due to its size. His manubrium was closed with wires, and a nasogastric tube was placed. The final pathology confirmed the diagnosis of a benign fibroepithelial polyp measuring 13 × 9 × 6 cm (Figure 38.3). No further surveillance imaging or testing was indicated. The nasogastric tube was removed on postoperative day 2, and an esophagram was performed that showed no signs of leak (Figure 38.4). He was discharged on postoperative day 4 tolerating a soft diet. He was able to transition to a regular diet shortly thereafter and had no symptoms of dysphagia on his postoperative follow-up.

Comments

Fibroepithelial polyps are benign slow-growing mesodermal lesions with low malignant potential. They typically manifest as cutaneous lesions (skin tags) and polyps along the urogenital tract, but they can manifest along the entirety of the gastrointestinal and respiratory tracts. Esophageal fibroepithelial polyps account for approximately 1% of all benign esophageal lesions and are the most common benign intraluminal tumor of the esophagus [1]. Identification of these lesions can be difficult endoscopically due to normal overlying mucosa.

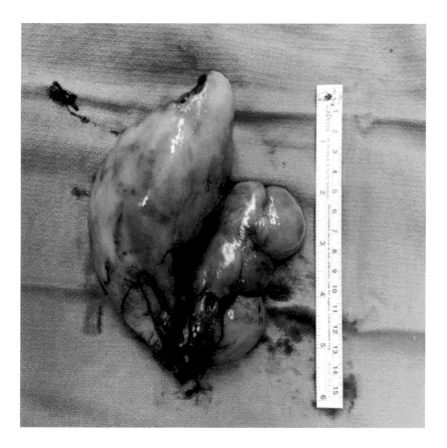

Figure 38.3 Gross pathologic image of the bilobed fibroepithelial polyp

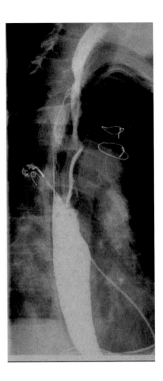

Figure 38.4 Barium esophagram performed on postoperative day 2 showing normal flow of contrast through the esophagus with resolution of the esophageal stasis and obstruction

Histologically, fibroepithelial polyps are pedunculated submucosal lesions composed of fibrovascular tissue and covered by squamous epithelium. Larger fibroepithelial polyps may have a lipomatous core. Malignant degeneration is rare, but transformation to squamous cell carcinoma and adenocarcinoma has been described. Fibroepithelial polyps typically arise from the upper third of the esophagus in the loose areolar tissue located near the pharyngoesophageal junction, also known as Laimer's triangle [2]. The polyps slowly enlarge and lengthen secondary to normal peristalsis before presenting as an elongated mass. Polyps that grow larger than 5 cm in any dimension are termed giant fibroepithelial polyps.

Esophageal fibroepithelial polyps predominately affect middle-aged and elderly males. Presenting symptoms are often nonspecific and include dysphagia, weight loss, bleeding due to ulceration, chest discomfort, orthopnea, breathing difficulties, and rarely asphyxia due to regurgitation into the airway [3]. Diagnosis can be challenging and relies on a thorough history and physical exam along with the thoughtful utilization of endoscopic and radiographic studies. Endoscopic findings are often nonspecific due to difficulty identifying a stalk in the proximal esophagus along with the epithelial covering of the polyp mimicking normal esophagus. Adjuncts such as endoscopic ultrasound and fine needle aspiration can increase the diagnostic utility of endoscopy. Barium swallow studies typically demonstrate a smooth luminal filling defect with varying degrees of lobulation and obstruction. Cross-sectional imaging such as CT and MRI typically demonstrates a well-defined homogenous mass that may contain adipose tissue [4]. Careful inspection for regional adenopathy is important to rule out potential malignancy. When there are questionable malignant characteristics, further attempts for tissue diagnosis or PET scan should be considered.

Treatment of giant fibroepithelial polyps is focused on either endoscopic or surgical resection. Endoscopic resection is an attractive option for those with favorable anatomy. Common challenges to endoscopic resection include the submucosal location, inability to control feeding vessels, and inability to dissect and extract the polyp from the submucosal plane [4]. Described techniques for surgical resection are varied and include esophagectomy, thoracotomy with esophagotomy and polypectomy, minimally invasive thoracoscopic polypectomy, and resection through a cervical esophagotomy [5]. Although not previously reported, a sternal split after exploration through the left neck is a reasonable approach for giant fibroepithelial polyps to avoid the morbidity of a thoracotomy incision. Esophagectomy should be avoided to reduce long-term comorbidity.

REFERENCES

1. Mufalli Behar, P., Arena, S., Marrangoni, A.G. Recurrent fibrovascular polyp of the esophagus. *Am J Otolaryngol Neck Med Surg.* 1995;16:209–212.
2. McLean, J.N., DelGaudio, J.M. Endoscopic resection of a giant esophageal polyp: Case report and review of the literature. *Am J Otolaryngol Head Neck Med Surg.* 2007;28:115–117.
3. Sargent, R.L., Hood, I.C. Asphyxiation caused by giant fibrovascular polyp of the esophagus. *Arch Pathol Lab Med.* 2006;130:725–727.
4. Ascenti, G., Racchiusa, S., Mazziotti, S., Bottari, M., Scribano, E. Giant fibrovascular polyp of the esophagus: CT and MR findings. *Abdom Imaging.* 1999;24:109–110.
5. Peltz, M., Estrera, A.S. Resection of a giant esophageal fibrovascular polyp. *Ann Thorac Surg.* 2010;90:1017–1019.

Grant Lewin, Samine Ravanbakhsh, Christopher W. Seder, and Ozuru Ukoha

 Key Words
- GIST
- Esophageal
- Case Report

Introduction

Gastrointestinal stromal tumors (GISTs) are the most common mesenchymal tumor of the gastrointestinal tract but account for only 0.1%–3% of all gastrointestinal malignancies. They occur most commonly in the stomach (60%–70%) and small intestine (20%–30%) [1,2]. Esophageal GISTs account for 1%–2% of all GIST cases, and their current management is generally extrapolated from their gastric and intestinal counterparts [3]. Historically, esophageal GISTs were most leiomyomas. With strides in immunohistochemistry, staining for CD117 (c-kit) and CD34 has helped to definitively distinguish these tumors as GISTs [1,4]. Nonetheless, the preoperative diagnostic workup remains difficult, given overlaps in radiographic and endoscopic appearance with other esophageal tumors or benign esophageal diseases. Furthermore, the question of optimal surgical management remains unanswered, with the options being enucleation or esophagectomy [5]. This case report outlines the diagnostic and therapeutic challenges of esophageal GISTs.

Case Report

A 50-year-old woman presented with a feeling of "food stuck" in her throat for eight days. She had experienced a progressive dysphagia to solids and liquids for the past four years. She noted a 5 kg weight loss during this time. Her medical history was otherwise unremarkable. Her physical exam was normal, and laboratory workup was within normal limits. Esophagram revealed right lateral displacement of the distal half of the esophagus without complete occlusion or significant delay of contrast (Figure 39.1). Upper endoscopy demonstrated extrinsic compression of the esophagus from 25 cm to 35 cm from the incisors with some luminal narrowing, preventing the endoscope from beyond the lesion (Figure 39.2). Computed tomography (CT) scan showed a large soft tissue mass with calcifications in the middle of the mediastinum, measuring 9.4 cm × 6.8 cm with moderate dilatation of the esophagus above the mass.

The patient was taken to the operating room in an elective manner, and her chest was explored through a right thoracotomy. A large mass was seen in the posterior mediastinum, extending from the level of the carina to the gastroesophageal junction. An intraoperative biopsy was

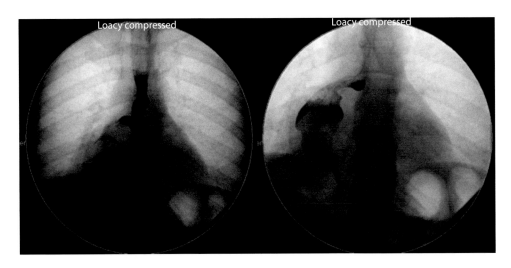

Figure 39.1 Preoperative esophagram showing displacement of the distal half of the esophagus without complete occlusion

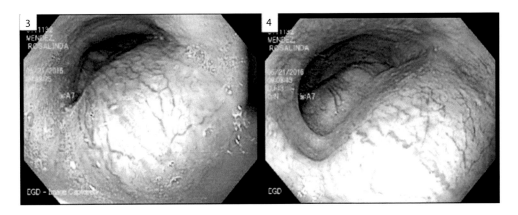

Figure 39.2 Preoperative upper endoscopy view demonstrated extrinsic compression of the esophagus

sent for frozen section, revealing spindle cells and smooth muscle. More dissection of the tumor showed that it was inseparably adherent to the esophageal mucosa, and the decision was made to proceed with an Ivor Lewis esophagectomy.

The patient tolerated the procedure well. Her postoperative course was uneventful. A swallow study on postoperative day 5 was normal. The patient was started on a clear liquid diet, which was advanced to soft diet in as tolerated. She had been on enteric feeding via a jejunostomy feeding tube placed during her operation. She was discharged home on postoperative day 8 without the need for more enteric feeding.

Pathologic analysis showed a GIST that measured 10.7 cm × 7.6 cm × 7.8 cm invading into the esophageal wall, extending to the overlying epithelium, and displaying areas of necrosis and fibrosis. There were no lymphovascular or perineural invasion, and all the regional lymph nodes were negative for metastatic disease. Two tumor nodules were found in the periesophageal adipose tissue. The margins of resection were negative for malignancy.

Immunohistochemical staining (IHC) was positive for CD117 (c-kit), CD34, DOG1, SMA, and Desmin; it was negative for AE1/AE3 and S-100. There were 5–6 mitoses per 50 high-power fields. Molecular genetic studies (e.g., KIT or platelet-derived growth factor receptor alpha (PDGFRA) mutational analysis) were not tested. It was determined she would be at high risk for progression of the disease based on the size of the tumor, the mitotic rate, and the metastatic tumor nodules in the periesophageal adipose tissue. She was started on Imatinib Mesylate at 300 mg/day but could not tolerate the dose, so it was decreased to 100 mg twice a day. She has been on that dose since her operation two years ago with out-patient clinic follow-up almost every two months. Surveillance chest CT scans and EGD (Esophagogastroduodenoscopy) have been negative for local or distant recurrent disease.

Comments

Esophageal GISTs present several notable diagnostic and therapeutic challenges, dysphagia, weight loss, and anemia [1,5]. The diagnostic workup for dysphagia consists of an esophagram, CT scan, and upper endoscopy. However, these clinical, radiographic, and endoscopic procedures are often quite similar in many disease entities, leaving a wide differential diagnosis, including GISTs, leiomyomas, leiomyoblastomas, and leiomyosarcomas [1,4]. In a series of 29 esophageal GISTs, authors observed no difference in clinical presentation, symptomatology, or endoscopic examination compared to leiomyomas [1]. This distinction is critical, however, as leiomyomas are significantly more common and truly benign, whereas esophageal GISTs have a greater potential for malignant behavior and often require more aggressive intervention [1,2].

Over time, there has been a relative increase in the diagnosis of GISTs and a decrease in diagnosis of leiomyosarcomas with a relatively stable total number of esophageal tumors, suggesting underdiagnosis of esophageal GISTs in the past [5]. This can be explained by the improved diagnostic accuracy of immunohistochemical staining for the common GIST markers, CD117 (c-kit) and CD34, which are not seen in leiomyomas. In addition, other mesenchymal tumors often stain for S-100 and Desmin, which typically represent neural- and muscle-derived tissues, respectively [4,5]. The identification of these specific markers has helped to differentiate GISTs from other tumors. However, this pathologic confirmation is often not obtained until after surgery, and biopsies are often not performed pre-operatively.

Many patients with dysphagia and the finding of a smooth, well-circumscribed, hypoechoic, submucosal esophageal mass on imaging do not require biopsy [5]. The high probability that such a finding is more consistent with a benign disease, such as leiomyoma, and a biopsy could induce scarring severe enough to complicate future enucleation. However, some authors have suggested that fine-needle aspiration at the time of endoscopy, as in Endoscopic Ultrasound (EUS), Fine Needle Aspiration (FNA), can be an effective tool to obtain a definitive diagnosis with low risk of complications and without compromising eventual resection [1–3].

The ultimate goal of surgery for GISTs is complete resection. The extent of resection must be guided by tumor size, characteristics, and location. GISTs of the esophagus must be approached differently than its gastric and intestinal counterparts based on anatomic considerations [5]. The stomach and intestine have a serosal layer that confines the tumor and a mesentery that allows for limited or "wedge" resections, whereas the options in esophageal resection are limited to enucleation or esophagectomy [1]. A local resection may be considered in cases of favorable histology (low mitotic count, no necrosis) and for small lesions (less than 2 cm) confined to the wall of the esophagus. However, in cases of larger tumors or those involving the gastroesophageal junction, most surgeons recommend esophagectomy [5]. Many authors identify a threshold of 6 cm to differentiate between the need for enucleation or esophagectomy [1–3]. Some studies used adjuvant therapy consisting of t Imatinib for tumors greater than 9 cm [1–3,5].

Long-term outcomes after esophageal GIST resection are largely unknown as most studies have very short follow-up [5]. In the limited reports to date, it appears that recurrence and mortality rates remain high. Mitotic index and size have been established as prognostic indicators for GISTs of the esophagus, similar to GIST of the stomach and small intestine. Imatinib Mesylate has been used with some success in such cases.

Esophageal GISTS are a rare entity, yet to be fully understood. Clinical presentation is typically that of dysphagia and differential diagnosis ranges from benign entities such as Gastroesophageal reflux disease, achalasia, and strictures to tumors of various benign and malignant potentials. Studies have shown that tumor size, mitotic activity, and surgical technique are critical in determining long-term outcome after esophageal GIST resection. Enucleation may be sufficient for small, well-encapsulated tumors with low mitotic index, whereas esophagectomy is ideal for larger tumors and those with more aggressive characteristics. The value of EUS-FNA should not be overlooked in esophageal tumors with the characteristic endoscopic appearance of extrinsic compression with intact mucosa. If the diagnosis of GIST is made in the larger tumors or those with aggressive potential, a neoadjuvant therapy followed by restaging and surgical resection could lead to improved survival. Although positron-emission tomography (PET) scan was not part of the diagnostic workup in this patient, GISTs are FDG-avid, so it is a recommended tool. Mutational analysis was not performed in this patient but should be considered in all these cases because it has an established value both in predicting response to tyrosine kinase inhibitors and improved prognosis in those with GIST tumor harboring PDGFRA mutation [6].

REFERENCES

1. Blum, M.G., Bilimoria, K.Y., Wayne, J.D., et al. Surgical considerations for the management and resection of esophageal gastrointestinal stromal tumors. *Ann Thorac Surg* 2007;84:1717.
2. Duffaud, F., Meeus, P., Bertucci, F., et al. French Sarcoma Group. Patterns of care and clinical outcomes in primary oesophageal gastrointestinal stromal tumours (GIST): A retrospective study of the French Sarcoma Group (FSG). *Eur J Surg Oncol.* 2017;43(6):1110–1116.
3. Maleddu, A., Pantaleo, M.A., Nannini, M., Biasco, G. The role of mutational analysis of KIT and PDGFRA in gastrointestinal stromal tumors in a clinical setting. *J Transl Med.* 2011. 9:75. PMC 3224648

4. Miettinen, M., Sarlomo-Rikala, M., Sobin, L.H., Lasota, J. Esophageal stromal tumors: A clinicopathologic, immunohistochemical, and molecular genetic study of 17 cases and comparison with esophageal leiomyomas and leiomyosarcomas. *Am J Surg Pathol* 2000;24:211–222.
5. Robb, W.B., Bruyere, E., Amielh, D., et al. Esophageal gastrointestinal Stromal Tumor: Is tumoral enucleation a viable therapeutic option? *Ann Surg* 2015;261(1):117–124.
6. Shinigare AB, Zukotynski, K.A., Krajewski, K.M., et al. Esophageal gastrointestinal stromal tumor: Report of 7 patients. *Cancer Imaging* 2012;12:100–108.

Danuel V. Laan, Betty Allen, John Agzarian, Phillip G. Rowse, and Shanda H. Blackmon

---

 Key Words

- Acute esophageal necrosis
- Black esophagus
- Prader–Willi syndrome

Introduction

"Black esophagus" is an extremely rare endoscopic finding, with an incidence only approaching 0.001%. Approximately 100 case reports are in the English literature. The disease most commonly affects men (4:1) in their sixties, although it has been diagnosed in every age group. Diffuse esophageal necrosis, while most common in older patients, can be seen in younger patients with risk factors for thrombosis. Awareness of this rare condition aids in identification and successful treatment.

Case Report

A 46-year-old male with Prader–Willi Syndrome was admitted to a medicine service for treatment of a presumed right lower lobe pneumonia having symptoms of breathlessness. A chest roentgenogram showed a right lower lobe consolidation associated with leukocytosis. On hospital day (HD) two, he had unprovoked hematemesis associated with an acute 2 g/dL drop in hemoglobin. An esophagogastroduodenoscopy (EGD) was performed showing circumferential black discoloration with areas of whitish exudates within the lower two-thirds of the esophagus (Figure 40.1). Biopsy was avoided because of concern for necrosis and risk of perforation. Computed tomographic angiography (CTA) of the chest was obtained revealing diffuse dilatation and mural thickening of the esophagus (Figure 40.2). Arterial supply to the esophagus was not well visualized on the chest CTA. The patient was otherwise hemodynamically stable, and serial labs revealed no further drop in hemoglobin. Proton Pump inhibitor therapy was initiated (pantoprazole 80 mg intravenous, twice daily), and the patient was made *nil per os*. On HD four, a barium esophagram was obtained showing no contrast extravasation (Figure 40.3). A clear liquid diet was initiated. The patient was discharged on HD five on oral pantoprazole with plans to advance to a soft diet within one week. Follow-up at two weeks revealed uncomplicated progression of diet with no signs of dysphagia. At six months, the patient was tolerating a general diet and was taken off all acid reducing medications. At one-year follow-up, the patient had no difficulties with swallowing and continued on a general diet. No repeat esophagram or endoscopy has been attempted given lack of symptoms.

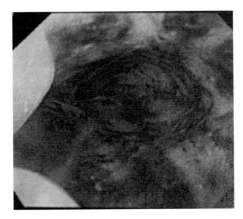

Figure 40.1 EGD showing circumferential black discoloration with areas of whitish exudates within the lower two-thirds of the esophagus

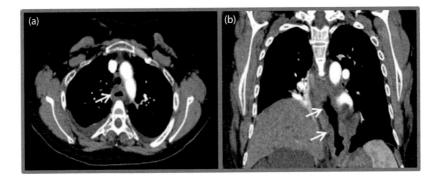

Figure 40.2 CTA of the chest showing diffuse dilatation and mural thickening of the esophagus. (a) Cross-sectional view, (b) coronal view, white arrows indicate esophagus

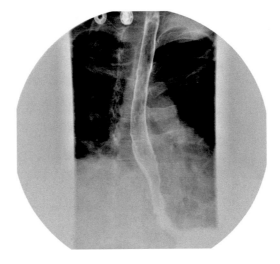

Figure 40.3 Esophagram showing no leak present on hospital day 4

Comments

AEN, or "black esophagus," is an extremely rare endoscopic finding, with an incidence only approaching 0.001% [1]. With only approximately 100 case reports in the English literature, it is an orphan diagnosis, and the most widely cited review is by Gurvits [2]. The disease most commonly affects men (4:1) in their sixties, although it has been diagnosed in every age group. Identifiable risk factors for development of AEN include diabetes mellitus (24%), malignancy (20%), hypertension (20%), alcohol abuse (10%), and coronary artery disease (9%). The most common clinical presentation of AEN is evidence of a gastrointestinal bleed characterized by hematemesis, coffee ground emesis, and melena [2].

Development of AEN is most likely multifactorial resulting from tissue hypoperfusion (low flow state), impaired mucosal barrier, and backflow injury from gastric secretions. While biopsy was not performed in this case, reported histologic findings include circumferential inflammation and necrosis of the mucosa and submucosa [2].

We believe the etiology of AEN in our patient is most likely associated with his underlying diagnosis of Prader–Willi syndrome given no other vasculopathic risk factors, cancer, or diabetes. The patient had syndromic features of Prader–Willi including infantile hypotonia, feeding difficulties at birth, poor growth, and delayed development. He also had characteristic features including a narrow forehead, almond-shaped eyes, short stature, and small hands and feet. Previous genetic testing in this patient revealed a paternal deletion involving chromosome 15, securing the diagnosis. The association of Prader–Willi and spontaneous thrombosis is well documented in the literature [3]. To our knowledge, esophageal ischemia resulting from Prader–Willi Syndrome has not previously been reported.

Pillars of nonoperative management of AEN include prompt resuscitation to correct hypoperfusion or low flow state, *nil per os* to avoid esophageal perforation, intravenous proton pump inhibitor or histamine receptor blocker to neutralize mucosal barrier injury, and correction of any underlying critical illness [2]. Nasogastric tube insertion should be avoided due to the risk of perforation. Empiric broad-spectrum antibiotics are appropriate in the setting of underlying sepsis, immunocompromise, rapid deterioration, or suspected perforation. A review of AEN by Gurvits et al. estimated that one-third of patients with AEN expire; however, the majority of deaths are related to an underlying critical illness. The rate of esophageal perforation in AEN approaches 7% and is the primary reason for AEN-specific mortality [4].

Surgical intervention is indicated when an uncontained esophageal perforation has been confirmed. AEN typically involves the lower two-thirds of the esophagus, and primary closure in the setting of a perforation in most cases should not be attempted due to grossly devitalized tissues. Esophageal diversion is likely the best approach [5]. However, given the complexity and the spectrum of presentation, endoscopic, minimally invasive, and hybrid therapies may be considered when clinically appropriate. Operative management of AEN-related esophageal stricture refractory to dilation should follow the principals of esophageal reconstruction with either esophagogastrostomy or alternative conduit reconstruction where applicable.

REFERENCES

1. Moretó, M., Ojembarrena, E., Zaballa, M., Tánago, J.G., Ibánez, S. Idiopathic acute esophageal necrosis: Not necessarily a terminal event. *Endoscopy*. 1993;25(8):534–538. http://www.ncbi.nlm.nih.gov/pubmed/8287816. Accessed September 24, 2017.
2. Gurvits, G.E. Black esophagus: Acute esophageal necrosis syndrome. *World J Gastroenterol*. 2010;16(26):3219–3225. doi:10.3748/WJG.V16.I26.3219.
3. Page, S.R., Nussey, S.S., Haywood, G.A., Jenkins, J.S. Premature coronary artery disease and the Prader–Willi syndrome. *Postgrad Med J*. 1990;66(773):232–234. http://www.ncbi.nlm.nih.gov/pubmed/2362894. Accessed September 24, 2017.
4. Gurvits, G.E., Shapsis, A., Lau, N., Gualtieri, N., Robilotti, J.G. Acute esophageal necrosis: A rare syndrome. *J Gastroenterol*. 2007;42(1):29–38. doi:10.1007/s00535-006-1974-z.
5. Sancheti, M.S. and Fernandez, F.G. Surgical management of esophageal perforation. *Oper Tech Thorac Cardiovasc Surg*. 2015;20(3):234–250. doi:10.1053/J.OPTECHSTCVS.2016.02.002.

Tessa Watt and Rishindra M. Reddy

 Key Words
- Case report
- Esophageal repair
- Giant esophageal leiomyoma

Introduction

Benign esophageal tumors are rare, with esophageal leiomyomas making up two-thirds of benign primary tumors of the esophagus [1]. Most patients are asymptomatic, and lesions are found incidentally, with approximately half of the tumors smaller than 5 cm in diameter [2]. Smaller lesions in asymptomatic patients (<5 cm) may be amenable to conservative management and surveillance with regular endoscopic or CT follow-up [3]. For midsize tumors (5–8 cm), transthoracic extramucosal blunt enucleation is the standard of care. However, giant leiomyomas (>8–10 cm) may require esophagectomy due to extensive mucosal involvement and damage [4,5]. This case report details a case in which a giant leiomyoma was resected and the esophagus spared with primary repair.

Case Report

A 41-year-old obese Caucasian female presented to her primary care physician with back pain and progressive shortness of breath over a nine month timespan. CT scan revealed a lower esophageal mass (Figure 41.1). A barium swallow revealed compression of her esophagus with distal narrowing (Figure 41.2). A repeat CT chest one month later showed no change in the size of the mass. A PET scan the following month revealed a large, hypermetabolic distal esophageal mass. Biopsy revealed a low-grade smooth muscle neoplasm consistent with leiomyoma. She was referred to thoracic surgery clinic for surgical evaluation.

On re-review of her original imaging, we measured a 12-cm esophageal mass. The tissue biopsy was re-reviewed as well and revealed normal stomach tissue rather than definitive leiomyoma. An esophageal ultrasound (EUS) and biopsy were repeated, and pathology was consistent with aleiomyoma. The patient elected to proceed with transthoracic enucleation of the tumor with esophageal repair, possible Belsey fundoplication, and possible esophagectomy, if the esophagus could not be primarily repaired or intraoperative frozen pathology revealed esophageal cancer.

The patient was taken to the operating room and a standard left posterolateral thoracotomy was performed entering the sixth intercostal space. The esophagus was mobilized above the level of the inferior pulmonary vein. The mass was identified and found to be firm and

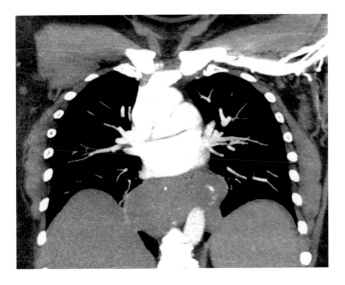

Figure 41.1 CT scan demonstrating large esophageal mass

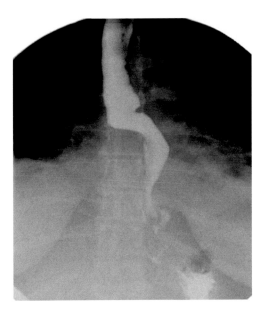

Figure 41.2 Barium esophagogram showing the mass distorting the distal esophageal passage of contrast

pushing into right pleural space without obvious hernia. During the dissection, we were noted to have transected the thoracic duct, which was ligated. The mass and esophagus were mobilized en-bloc off the aorta and pericardium and freed from the right chest without entering the right pleural space. The entire mass was confirmed to be above the gastroesophageal junction. The mass formed a dumbbell shape, encompassing the anterior and lateral sides of the esophageal mucosa approximately 270° around the circumference. The mass was then enucleated. A 5-cm injury to the esophageal mucosa was noted and repaired primarily using a running

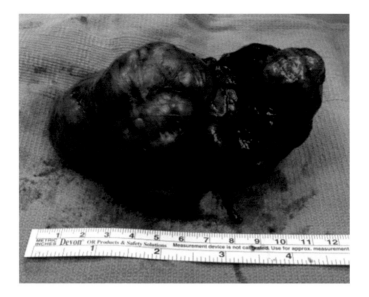

Figure 41.3 Bilobed esophageal leiomyoma, removed intact

4-0 vicryl. Clips were used to mark the top and bottom of the mucosal defects. The nasogastric tube, placed by Anesthesia, was advanced into the stomach under direct vision and feel. We then placed saline into the chest and performed an air test of the repair by clamping the esophagus at the gastroesophageal junction and asking Anesthesia to insufflate air through the nasogastric tube. There was no evidence of any leak in the mucosa. The attenuated esophageal muscle was then laid over the area of repair and secured with absorbable suture.

The mass was sent to pathology (Figure 41.3). The tumor measured $12 \times 8 \times 6$ cm in size and was consistent with leiomyoma on gross examination and frozen pathology. Final pathology revealed esophageal leiomyomatosis.

The patient immediately noted improvement in her shortness of breath after surgery. She had an unremarkable postoperative course and was discharged home without complication. At her three-month clinic follow-up, she was tolerating a regular diet without dysphagia. She also noted mild bloating with belching and occasional reflux, but no heartburn or regurgitation. Her chest pain and difficulty breathing had completely resolved.

Comments

Among benign esophageal tumors, leiomyomas are the most common. Larger leiomyomas often require esophagectomy due to mucosal damage and transformation to malignant leiomyosarcoma. We present a case where we successfully enucleated a giant leiomyosarcoma with primary esophageal repair and spared esophagectomy. Postoperatively the patient had no major complications and noted immediate resolution in her shortness of breath. Given the significant morbidity associated with esophagectomy, our experience demonstrates the importance of carefully considering resection and primary repair for leiomyomas of all sizes. Even though successful enucleation and avoiding esophagectomy may not always be possible for large leiomyomas, it is worthwhile to at least attempt an esophageal-sparing approach whenever possible.

REFERENCES

1. Seremetis, M.G., Lyons, W.S., deGuzman ,V.C., et al. Leiomyomata of the esophagus: An analysis of 838 cases. *Cancer.* 1976;38:2166–2177.
2. Lee, L.S., Singhal, S., Brinster, C.J., et al. Current management of esophageal leiomyoma. *J Am Coll Surg.* 2004;198:136–146.
3. Xu, G.Q., Qian, J.J., Chen, M.H., et al. Endoscopic ultrasonography for the diagnosis and selecting treatment of esophageal leiomyoma. *J Gastroenterol Hepatol.* 2012;27:521–525.
4. Rijcken, E., Kersting, C.M., Sinninger, N., et al. Esophageal resection for giant leiomyoma: Report of two cases and a review of the literature. *Langenbecks Arch Surg.* 2009;394:623–629.
5. Qi-Xin, S., Yu-Shang, Y., Wen-Ping, W., et al. Missed diagnosis of esophageal leiomyoma leading to esophagectomy: A case report and review of literatures. *J Thorac Dis.* 2018;10(1):E65–E69.

Alexander A. Brescia, Mark B. Orringer, and Rishindra M. Reddy

 Key Words

- Transhiatal esophagectomy
- Colon interposition
- Esophageal cancer
- Colon cancer
- Case report

Introduction

In current practice, many surgical centers perform transhiatal esophagectomy (THE) through abdominal and neck incisions with a cervical esophagogastric anastomosis (CEGA) for benign and malignant esophageal pathology. The largest THE series published reported neo-esophageal conduits formed from the stomach in 97% of patients and with colon interposition conduits in 3% [1], while separate reports have described using a "supercharged" jejunum as an alternative to the stomach [2]. While THE using a gastric conduit is performed with variable results across the country, utilization of a colon interposition or pedicled jejunal conduit is typically performed at a tertiary high-volume esophageal center. Postsurgical surveillance is of critical importance in cancer patients to evaluate for recurrence, but new primary cancers in the conduit can also occur [3].

Case Report

A 58-year-old Caucasian male was evaluated at his local community hospital for reflux and was found to have long segment Barrett's esophagitis. He received a THE with final pathology showing Barrett's esophagus with high-grade dysplasia. His postoperative course was complicated by acute respiratory distress syndrome, left vocal cord paralysis, anastomotic leak, and anastomotic breakdown with mediastinitis, requiring a reoperation eight days later with takedown of esophagogastric anastomosis, cervical esophagostomy, laparotomy with takedown of stomach, and placement of a feeding tube. After seven months, he had recovered his strength and received a substernal left colonic interposition graft to re-establish alimentary continuity (Figure 42.1). Postoperatively, he did well, eating without dysphagia or regurgitation.

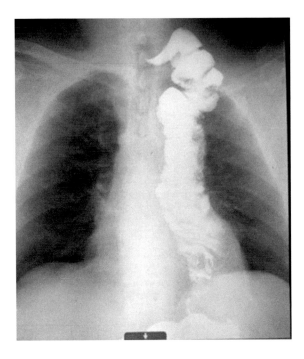

Figure 42.1 Barium esophagogram after initial colon interposition

On surveillance using upper endoscopy six years after his operation, the patient was found to have a very small polyp at the cervical esophagocolic anastomosis, with a biopsy revealing benign tissue. He underwent follow-up endoscopy intermittently over the next 6 years, until 12 years after his colon interposition operation, when a 3.5–4 cm mass was found at 20 cm from the incisors just beyond the cervical esophagocolic anastomosis, while the remainder of the colon graft and anastomosis were normal with redundant colon. A biopsy showed invasive adenocarcinoma, consistent with a colon primary cancer. A barium esophagogram and CT scan of the neck, chest, and abdomen revealed subtle colon wall thickening (Figure 42.2), but no evidence of further disease. Thus, he was taken to the operating room for a partial colectomy of 8 cm of proximal left substernal colon via a partial sternal split, and a redo of the cervical esophagocolonic anastomosis. There was some redundant length of colon allowing for a resection of 8 cm of colon length with primary anastomosis (Figure 42.3). Final pathology showed a 3.5-cm segment of adenocarcinoma invading into the muscularis propria with negative margins and two negative lymph nodes, pathologic T2N0M0, stage I colon adenocarcinoma. The patient had a brief episode of atrial fibrillation postoperatively and was discharged on postoperative day 10.

Postoperatively the patient experienced increased drainage from his wound, which was reopened and packed. Approximately two months after his operation, he underwent sternal debridement. He was last seen 14 years after his partial colectomy for colon cancer, 26 years after his initial THE, and he reported no complaints about his health, eating well orally with regular bowel movements.

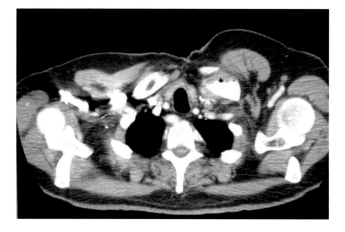

Figure 42.2 CT chest with white arrow showing mucosal thickening at site of new colon cancer

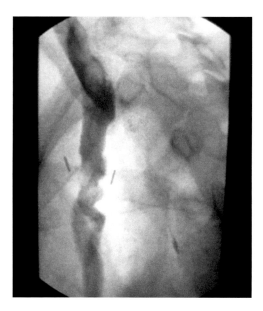

Figure 42.3 Barium esophagogram after colon resection showing elimination of redundant colon

Comments

This case is an unusual account of a patient undergoing THE for high-grade Barrett's dysplasia complicated by anastomotic breakdown requiring esophagostomy and subsequent substernal colon interposition grafting, then found to contain a primary colonic invasive adenocarcinoma 12 years later, which was successfully resected. Despite a series of postoperative complications after each procedure, the patient is doing well 26 years later.

This patient's clinical course highlights effective surgical reconstruction of the alimentary tract, and the importance of oncological surveillance. After the initial THE, anastomotic leak incidence has been cited between 9% and 14% [1]. Despite undergoing CEGA, the patient unfortunately had a leak into his chest causing mediastinitis. The patient was a smoker with 35-pack-years, quitting the month prior to surgery. In total, he had a 57-day hospitalization associated with this initial operation. Risk factors for CEGA leaks include a number of pre-operative comorbidities, active smoking history, postoperative arrhythmia, higher pathologic stage disease, and anastomotic technique (e.g., side-to-side stapled versus manually sewn) [4].

On initial evaluation at our center, the patient was deconditioned and still recovering from his index hospitalization and associated complications. As with first-time esophagectomy patients, we have found a rigorous preoperative regimen including abstinence of cigarette smoking, the use of an incentive spirometer, and a walk of 1–3 miles per day to improve fitness for esophagectomy, all of which helps to improve outcomes [1]. For cancer patients undergo-ing neoadjuvant chemoradiation, we would ideally obtain restaging imaging and perform esophagectomy within 4–6 weeks following completion of therapy. In this case, pathology showed Barrett's with high-grade dysplasia, and the patient recovered for seven months prior to performing a substernal colon interposition conduit reconstruction.

Following colon interposition, focus shifted to recovery and surveillance. In this case of high-grade dysplasia and colon interposition, surveillance consisted of postoperative visits 1 month, 2 months, 6 months, 18 months, and 42 months after the operation, as well as sur-veillance endoscopies of the colon interposition conduit as clinically indicated. At surveil-lance endoscopy 12 years after colon interposition, the suspicious mass was found.

At that point, workup for suspected colon cancer ensued. Importantly, imaging and endos-copy should be performed to rule out metastatic and locally invasive disease. Upon discovery of a suspicious polyp or mass in a colon interposition, multidisciplinary collaboration with the gastroenterologists should prioritize diagnosing the suspicious lesion as an esophageal recurrence versus primary colon cancer versus metastasis from elsewhere. In this case, a recurrent esophageal mass was unlikely with high-grade Barrett's pathology in the original resected specimen and no other distant primary was found, making primary colon malig-nancy the most likely etiology. After the colon resection, surveillance was performed for stage I colon cancer, including history and physical, CEA monitoring, and colonoscopy at regular intervals as indicated by NCCN guidelines [5].

This case presented a unique constellation of postoperative complications and strategies for management and surveillance of two primary diseases, Barrett's esophagus with high-grade dysplasia followed by invasive colon adenocarcinoma discovered within a colon interposition conduit.

REFERENCES

1. Orringer, M.B., Marshall, B., Chang, A.C., Lee, J., Pickens, A., Lau, C.L. Two thou-sand transhiatal esophagectomies: Changing trends, lessons learned. *Ann Surg.* 2007;246(3):363–372; discussion 372–374.
2. Blackmon, S.H., Correa, A.M., Skoracki, R., et al. Supercharged pedicled jejunal interposition for esophageal replacement: A 10-year experience. *Ann Thorac Surg.* 2012;94(4):1104–1111.

3. Shersher, D.D., Hong, E., Warren, W., Penfield Faber, L., Liptay, M.J. Adenocarcinoma in a 40-year-old colonic interposition treated with Ivor Lewis esophagectomy and esophagogastric anastomosis. *Ann Thorac Surg.* 2011;92(6):e113–e114.
4. Cooke, D.T., Lin, G.C., Lau, C.L., Zhang, L., Si, M.S., Lee, J., Chang, A.C., Pickens, A., Orringer, M.B. Analysis of cervical esophagogastric anastomotic leaks after transhiatal esophagectomy: Risk factors, presentation, and detection. *Ann Thorac Surg.* 2009;88(1):177–184; discussion 184–185.
5. Engstrom, P.F., Arnoletti, J.P., Benson, A.B., III, et al., National comprehensive cancer network. NCCN Clinical Practice Guidelines in Oncology: Colon cancer. *J Natl Compr Canc Netw.* 2009;7(8):778–831.

Kimberly Song, Christopher W. Seder, and Ozuru Ukoha

🔨 Key Words

- Esophageal hemangioma-lymphangioma
- Esophageal neoplasms
- Benign esophageal tumors
- Vascular anomalies
- Esophagectomy

Introduction

Esophageal hemangiomas are tumors of vascular origin arising from the submucosal layer of the esophagus. They are rare, comprising only 3% of benign esophageal tumors, and often asymptomatic [1]. Symptoms most commonly include dysphagia and hematemesis, the latter being potentially lethal. Mixed hemangioma-lymphangiomas (or hemangiolymphangiomas) are proliferations of vessels of varied nature lined by endothelium and forming a tumor [2]. Hemangiolymphangiomas are exceedingly rare, with only a few pediatric esophageal cases documented in the literature. We report an adult patient with a symptomatic mixed cavernous hemangioma-lymphangioma of the gastroesophageal junction who was treated with esophagectomy.

Case Report

A 61-year-old Hispanic man with a history of gastroesophageal reflux disease and hypertension presented with increasing fatigue. He denied any history of unintentional weight loss, hematochezia, or hematemesis. He did not drink alcohol or use tobacco and had a maternal history of esophageal cancer. Physical exam revealed a well-nourished man with mild epigastric tenderness. Routine bloodwork revealed anemia with a hemoglobin of 12 g/dL. He was referred to gastroenterology for an endoscopy. His colonoscopy was normal, but upper endoscopy demonstrated a soft, bluish polypoid lesion 25 cm from the incisors extending submucosally to the gastroesophageal junction (Figure 43.1). The stomach and duodenal bulb appeared normal. Biopsy was not performed due to its hypervascular appearance. Positron-emission tomography-computed tomography (PET-CT) demonstrated esophageal thickening with a low-attenuating $12 \times 11 \times 8$ cm mass extending from the carina to gastroesophageal junction with areas of increased metabolic activity ranging from SUV 2.5 to 7.6 (Figure 43.2). No axillary, mediastinal, or hilar lymphadenopathy was identified. Endoscopic ultrasound further characterized the mass as being nearly circumferential and heterogeneous in composition with cystic and hypervascular areas (Figure 43.3).

The patient was lost to follow-up and returned to clinic six months later with dysphagia and a hemoglobin of 10.6 g/dL. Due to his persistent symptoms, the decision was made to treat the

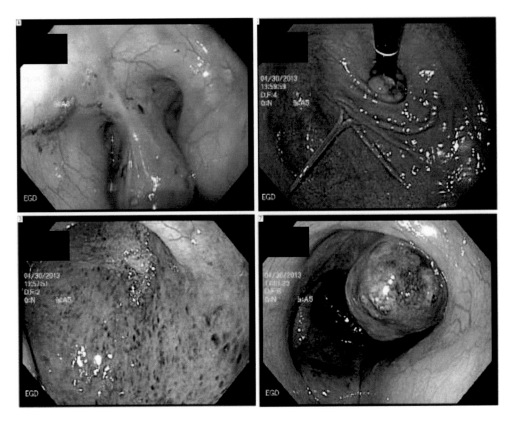

Figure 43.1 Endoscopic images of a large, bluish polypoid esophageal mass

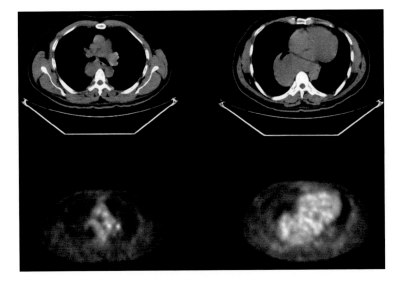

Figure 43.2 PET-avid 12 × 11 × 8 cm mass extending from the carina to gastroesophageal junction

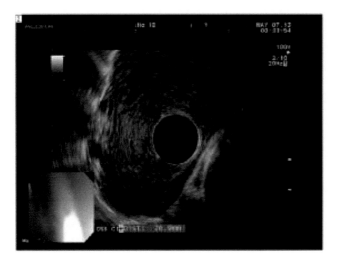

Figure 43.3 Endoscopic ultrasound demonstrating a heterogeneous, hypervascular mass encircling the esophagus

patient with an Ivor Lewis esophagectomy. Upon right posterolateral thoracotomy, a vascular mass was externally visible in the distal one-third of the esophagus. The distal esophagus and proximal stomach were removed with intraoperative confirmation of negative margins, in the standard fashion. The patient recovered well from surgery and was discharged on post-operative day 7, without complication, on a liquid diet. Final pathology revealed a mixed cavernous hemangioma-lymphangioma.

Comments

Hemangiomas and hemangiolymphangiomas of the esophagus are very rare. Observation of asymptomatic hemangiomas is an accepted management strategy [1], but treatment is indicated for those that produce symptoms of dysphagia or bleeding. However, due to the rarity of hemangiolymphangiomas, treatment guidelines are not well established. In the current case, it was felt that a hypermetabolic esophageal tumor causing ongoing dysphagia should not be observed.

One of the few published series examining such tumors is a histopathological review of 27 gastrointestinal tract vascular malformations, in which 12 were hemangiomas, lymphangiomas, or mixed hemangiolymphomas [2]. None were located in the esophagus. The most common location was the small bowel and 27% of patients presented with gastrointestinal bleeding. Associations with esophageal carcinoma [3] and malignant degeneration have been rarely reported in esophageal hemangiomas, generally in tumors greater than 3 cm [4]. Due to their similar appearance and symptomatology, these lesions must be distinguished from esophageal varices. A proximal lesion may suggest vascular malformation since isolated cervical varices are extremely rare in cirrhotic patients [5]. CT, MRI, physical exam, and blood work can be utilized to assess for signs of cirrhosis. Biopsy of hypervascular esophageal tumors is not typically recommended due to the potential for bleeding [6].

We chose to treat this patient with transthoracic esophagectomy, given the good functional status of the patient, unknown pathology, and hypermetabolism on PET-CT scan. However, there have been isolated reports of endoscopic management of patients with esophageal hemangiomas [7,8]. Though typically solitary, multiple esophageal hemangiomas can be seen in conditions such as congenital blue rubber bleb nevus syndrome (BRBNS) [7]. A report by Takasumi et al [7]. demonstrated successful endoscopic management of a patient with BRBNS found to have a large esophageal hemangioma upon hospital admission for hematemesis. Injection of 1% polidocanol sclerosant to inflow vessels followed by incision, decompression, and argon coagulation resulted in a hemostatic lesion that resolved and remained absent at the two-month follow-up. Shigemitsu et al [8]. used potassium titanyl phosphate/yttrium aluminum garnet (KTP/YAG) laser to fulgurate an 11-cm esophageal hemangioma, repeating the process every week for one month, with good results. Treatment by endoscopic resection, sclerotherapy, and laser fulguration have not been specifically described for hemangiolymphangiomas.

In conclusion, we report the surgical management of a mixed cavernous hemangioma-lymphangioma of the gastroesophageal junction. Although there are reports of these rare lesions being treated endoscopically, malignancy could not be excluded, prompting us to proceed with transthoracic esophagectomy for diagnostic and therapeutic purposes.

REFERENCES

1. Ha, C., Regan, J., Cetindag, I.B., Ali, A., Mellinger, J.D. Benign esophageal tumors. *Surg Clin North Am*. 2015;95(3):491–514.
2. Handra-Luca, A. and Montgomery, E. Vascular malformations and hemangiolymph-angiomas of the gastrointestinal tract: morphological features and clinical impact. *Int J Clin Experiment Pathol*. 2011;4(5):430–443.
3. Kusumi, F., Takakuwa, H., Hajiro, K. A case of esophageal cancer with cavernous hemangioma: Endoscopic and endosonographic assessment. *Endoscopy*. 1999;31(5):S36.
4. Bandoh, T., Isoyama, T., Toyoshima, H. Submucosal tumors of the stomach: A study of 100 operative cases. *Surgery*. 1993;113(5):498–506.
5. Won, J.W., Lee, H.W., Yoon, K.H., Yang, S.Y., Moon, I.S., Lee, T.J. Extended hemangioma from pharynx to esophagus that could be misdiagnosed as an esophageal varix on endoscopy. *Digest Endosc*. 2013;25(6):626–629.
6. Yoo, S. GI-associated hemangiomas and vascular malformations. *Clin Colon Rect Surg*. 2011;24(3):193–200.
7. Takasumi, M., Hikichi, T., Takagi, T., et al. Endoscopic therapy for esophageal hematoma with blue rubber bleb nevus syndrome. *World J of Gastrointest Endosc*. 2014;6(12):630–634.
8. Shigemitsu, K., Naomoto, Y., Yamatsuji, T., et al. Esophageal hemangioma successfully treated by fulguration using potassium titanyl phosphate/yttrium aluminum garnet (KTP/YAG) laser: A case report. *Dis Esophagus*. 2000;13(2):161–164.

Adrian E. Rodrigues, James L. Lubawski Jr.,
and Wickii T. Vigneswaran

🔑	Key Words
	• Aortoesophageal
	• Esophagealpleural
	• Fistula
	• Stricture
	• Stent

Introduction

Esophageal strictures have numerous etiologies and can occur at any age. To name a few, they can develop from neuromuscular complications (achalasia, esophageal rings), inflammatory processes (infectious, Crohn's, Behcet's, reflux), and iatrogenic causes (chemoradiation, endoscopic submucosal dissection, prolonged intubation), and they can be congenital such as an esophageal atresia.[1] The most effective treatment modality always involves treating the cause of the stricture, although this isn't always possible [1].

Treatment options vary, from simple dilation to resection. A refractory stricture can be treated by placing one or more self-expanding stents into the esophageal lumen. The concept behind this approach is that the esophageal wall will remodel itself after prolonged radial force and prevent restenosis [2]. However, this approach comes with numerous complications, including perforation and stent migration [3]. In a study with 444 patients, 40% showed an effective response to stenting and 28.6% showed stent migration [4]. Stents classically migrate distally, and if not repositioned, they can enter the stomach. To hinder their movement, clips or endoscopic suturing to the esophageal wall has shown success [5]. Although stent fixation by suturing addresses the movement concern, the procedure can unintentionally injure the adjacent structures.

Case Report

A 72-year-old Caucasian female complained of dysphagia at an outside hospital. Her past medical history involved a lumpectomy for breast cancer and a hysterectomy for uterine cancer; both of which exceeded 10 years from the time we first encountered her. The dysphagia was induced by an esophageal stricture, and she underwent esophageal dilation that became complicated by an esophageal perforation with subsequent empyema development. She was admitted to the operating room where the right empyema was evacuated, the esophagus was repaired, and a decortication was performed. Throughout the hospital course she continued to have high output chest tube drainage, and a chest CT showed the development of an esophageal-pleural fistula. At this stage, the decision was made to transfer the patient to our hospital.

At our facility, the patient rejected surgical management and was therefore treated with an esophageal stent and endoscopic clip closure. Her stay was complicated by respiratory failure and was subsequently intubated, and subsequently a tracheotomy was performed due to failed attempts to wean her off the ventilator. A gastrostomy tube was also placed, and after a 10-day hospital course, the patient was discharged.

The patient followed medical management for a course of several months. Eight months after her initial treatment at our facility, she underwent a thoracentesis for loculated air and fluid collection of the right hemithorax, and the old esophageal stents was replaced with a new stent and included fixation by endoscopic suturing. Four months later the patient returned complaining of a one-day history of "bloody stools, difficulty swallowing, and red saliva."

Upon arrival the patient was in distress and tachycardic at 104/min. She complained of a one-day history of bloody stools, dysphagia, red sputum, and light headedness. Hemoccult test was positive, and stools were indicative of melena. A complete blood count was remarkable for red blood cells of 3.37 mil/ul, Hemoglobin 9.3 g/dl and Hematocrit of 30%. An upper endoscopy showed fresh blood clots throughout the esophagus, and an aortic angiogram (Figure 44.1) confirmed the presence of an aortoesophageal fistula.

The patient was transfused four units of packed red blood cells and one unit of fresh frozen plasma. An emergent percutaneous thoracic aortic stent graft was placed and successfully provided fistula control. Six days later she underwent a partial gastrectomy using left thoracoabdominal approach. During this procedure, we observed the endoscopic esophageal suture traversing the aortic wall, we therefore followed with a fistula take down and gastroesophagectomy, then placed a feeding jejunostomy. Examination of the esophagus showed a suture that was placed for a stent and travelled outside of the esophagus, thereby causing an aortoesophageal fistula with acute inflammation and ulceration.

Her second hospitalization coursed for 12 days, and aside from the surgery, she was treated for anxiety, sepsis, multiple self-extubations, and another tracheostomy. She was discharged in stable condition to a skilled nursing facility. Four months later, the patient returned complaining of difficulty with swallowing. A barium swallow study was ordered, but the patient failed to follow through with both the study and her future appointments. Months later, our hospital was informed the patient had expired with no further details.

Comments

The most common etiologies for the formation of aortoesophageal fistulas are from aortic aneurysms, foreign bodies, esophageal malignancy, esophagitis, stent-graft repair of the aorta, esophageal surgery, and metallic esophageal stent placement soon after chemotherapy and radiation [6–8]. As a rule, if the esophagus becomes perforated, a subsequent fistula may develop [9]. And although aortoesophageal fistulas are not common, when they do occur, their most devastating complication is a fatal hemorrhage [3].

In this case, however, we found that the fistula was induced by fixating the esophageal stent to the wall by suturing it in place. Although stents have shown that they are safe—with and without suture fixation—this case demonstrates the need for careful techniques and spatial awareness of the proximity of the surrounding viscera. The sentinel hemorrhage and early surgical intervention helped to avoid the fatal outcome that is often seen in these patients.

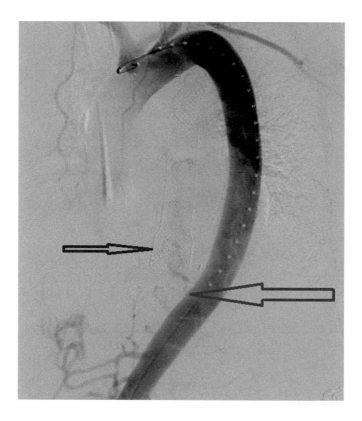

Figure 44.1 Aortogram—Intraarterial contrast is visible inside the esophageal stent

REFERENCES

1. Ravich, W.J. Endoscopic management of benign esophageal strictures. *Curr Gastroenterol Rep.* 2017;19:50. doi:10.1007/s11894-017-0591-8.
2. Hindy, P., Hong, J., Lam-Tsai, Y., Gress, F. A comprehensive review of esophageal stents. *Gastroenterol Hepatol (N Y).* 2012;8(8):526–534.
3. Qiang, W.M., Sze, D.Y., Pu, W.Z., Qiang, W.Z., Ao, G.Y., Dake, M.D. Delayed complications after esophageal stent placement for treatment of malignant esophageal obstructions and esophagorespiratory fistulas. *J Vasc Interv Radiol.* 2001;12:465–474. doi:10.1016/S1051-0443(07)61886-7.
4. Fuccio, L., Hassan, C., Frazzoni, L., Miglio, R., Repici, A. Clinical outcomes following stent placement in refractory benign esophageal stricture: A systematic review and meta-analysis. *Endoscopy.* 2015;48(2):141–148. doi:10.1055/s-0034-1393331.
5. Sharaiha, R.Z., Kumta, N.A., Doukides, T.P., et al. Esophageal stenting with sutures time to redefine our standards. *J Clin Gastroenterol.* 2015;49:e57–e50. doi:10.1097/MCG.0000000000000198.
6. Chiesa, R., Melissano, G., Marone, E.M., Marrocco-Trischitta, M.M., Kahlberg, A. Aorto-oesophageal and aortobronchial fistulae following thoracic endovascular aortic repair: A national survey. *Eur J Vasc Endovasc Surg.* 2010;39(3):273–279. doi:10.1016/J.EJVS.2009.12.007.

7. Um. S.-J., Park. B.H., Son. C. An aortoesophageal fistula in patient with lung cancer after chemo-irradiation and subsequent esophageal stent implantation. *J Thorac Oncol.* 2009;4:263–265. doi:10.1097/JTO.0b013e318194fc68.

8. Unosawa, S., Hata, M., Sezai, A., et al. Surgical treatment of an aortoesophageal fistula caused by stent implantation for esophageal stenosis: Report of a case. *Surg Today.* 2008;38(1):62–64. doi:10.1007/s00595-007-3569-6.

9. Dash, M., Mohanty, T., Patnaik, J., Mishra, N., Subhankar, S., Parida, P. An unusual case of spontaneous esophagopleural fistula. *Lung India.* 2017;34(3):287–289. doi:10.4103/0970-2113.205327.

Wickii T. Vigneswaran and James L. Lubawski Jr.

 Key Words

- Benign esophageal stricture
- Esophageal stent
- Esophagectomy

Introduction

Benign esophageal strictures are caused by a variety of esophageal disorders, including peptic, caustic, and radiotherapy induced injuries, Schatzki ring, eosinophilic esophagitis, granulomatous infection such as mycobacterial and histoplasma infections, strictures after surgical or endoscopic mucosal or submucosal resections, and other ablative therapies. Benign esophageal strictures are subdivided into simple and complex strictures. Simple strictures are short (<2 cm), focal, straight, and frequently allow passage of a normal diameter endoscope, whereas complex strictures are longer (>2 cm), angulated, irregular, and are severely narrowed. Treatment for simple strictures may consist of 3–5 dilations, which is usually sufficient to relieve symptoms. On the contrary, treatment for complex strictures are more difficult and they have a higher tendency to become refractory or recurrent [1].

Endoscopic stent placement is a well-accepted and effective alternative treatment modality for complex and refractory esophageal strictures. Currently, partially or fully covered self-expanding metal stents, plastic stents, and biodegradable stents have been used with varying success. Hyperplastic tissue ingrowth, stent migration, and erosion of the esophageal wall with fistula formation are some long-term sequelae, and therefore, the outcome is disappointing in patients with benign strictures. Surgical resection and reconstruction may be the ultimate solution for refractory stricture. We describe a young man with a long segment benign esophageal stricture of unknown etiology that was treated with repeated dilations and stent placements, ultimately developing complications and recurrence requiring subtotal esophagectomy.

Case Report

A 32-year-old male presented with dysphagia and chest tightness. The dysphagia was first to solids. This progressed to needing to "wash" foods down with liquids when they would get stuck—either at the base of the neck or mid-chest. This then progressed to not being able to get liquids down either. The chest tightness was severe at times, and he couldn't catch his breath during these episodes. The pain radiated around the sides of his chest. He also had some coughing that was associated with a small amount of blood. He lost a lot of weight during this time. He was initially treated in an outside institution, where he underwent esophageal dilation that was followed by multiple self-expanding metal stents. As his dysphagia became intractable, a Percutaneous endoscopic gastrostomy (PEG) tube was placed to combat his poor nutritional status. He was treated with dilations and repeated stent placements for almost five years and subsequently presented with worsening dysphagia to our institution. Initially, he underwent multiple endoscopic interventions where the stents were refashioned in the interventional Gastro Intestinal (GI) service. This was performed five times over the course of one year, then was referred to thoracic surgery for definitive treatment. He was a non-smoker, did not drink any alcohol, or use any recreational drugs. He was an immigrant from Liberia and, on direct questioning, did not reveal any history of caustic ingestion or chronic infection.

On presentation, the patient was significantly stressed and was depressed. Clinical examination revealed that he weighed 63.7 kg with a height of 1.651, a calculated body mass index (BMI) of 23.40 kg/m^2, blood pressure (BP) 110/70 mm Hg, pulse 94/min in sinus rhythm of SpO$_2$ 98%. Clinical examination was unremarkable. His imaging studies showed stents in the esophagus just below the cricopharygeous to the gastro esophageal (GE) junction (Figure 45.1a). An esophagram performed showed a contained trachea-esophageal fistula in the mid-esophagus and a long segment stricture of esophagus and stents from thoracic inlet to the stomach (Figure 45.1b). This was confirmed on CT scan examination of his neck and chest (Figure 45.2). Plans were made for subtotal resection of the esophagus, repair of the trachea-esophageal fistula, and cervical esophagogastric anastomosis.

During the operation, a bronchoscopy examination confirmed a trachea-esophageal fistulous track at 3 cm above the carina. The operative procedure included a right thoracotomy followed by laparotomy and left cervical incision. First, a right posterolateral thoracotomy was performed with the plans of resection of esophagus and repair of the trachea-esophageal

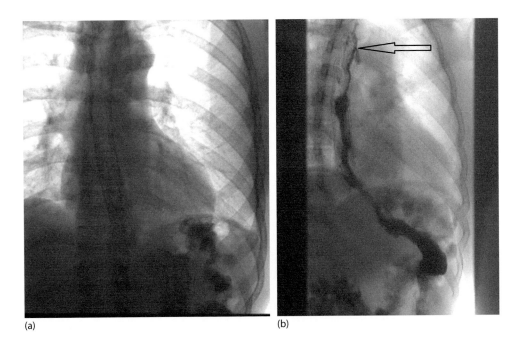

(a) (b)

Figure 45.1 Preoperative oral contrast study. (a) Demonstrate multiple stents in the esophagus from thoracic inlet to GE junction. (b) Demonstrate a contained fistulous track into the airway

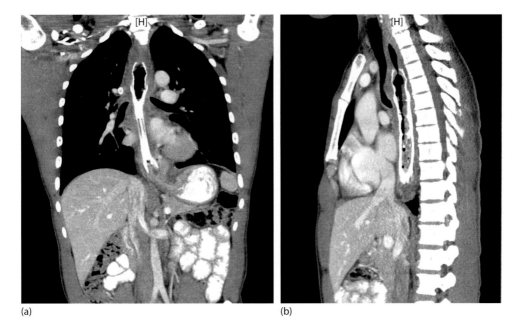

(a)   (b)

Figure 45.2 (a and b) CT scan of chest showing multiple, straddling stents almost the full length of the esophagus

fistula. After the entry into the chest, first an incision was made in the esophagus at the level of the azygos vein and the metal stents within the esophagus were extracted through the esophagotomy. The esophagus was mobilized and encircled in the upper end close to the thoracic outlet. Then the esophagus below the carina was mobilized and encircled and then the remaining inferior esophageal mobilization was completed. Once this was completed, the esophagus was transected just below the thoracic inlet and at the carinal level. Then segment of esophagus that was attached to the trachea was filleted open along the right border, and the trachea-esophageal fistulous tract was identified. The mucosal layer of this segment of the esophagus was almost completely destroyed by the previously placed stents, but the muscular layer appeared healthy. Any residual mucosa was removed leaving the muscle attached to the posterior tracheal wall. The posterior wall of the esophagus was then turned over on itself and sutured to the opposite side of the trachea closing the trachea-esophageal fistula with the esophageal muscle patch and reinforcing the posterior tracheal wall, in a "top-hat" fashion suturing the edges together (Figure 45.3). Thickened mediastinal pleura was then mobilized and was used to cover this repair. Then, the chest was closed in the standard fashion with the chest tube in the posterior mediastinum.

Then, the patient was placed supine, and an upper abdominal laparoscopy was performed. Upon entrance into the abdomen, it was noted that the loop of jejunum pexied to the anterior abdominal wall consistent with a previous feeding jejunostomy. The stomach was mobilized on the gastroepiploic artery. It appeared healthy and distensible and would be a viable source for conduit. The duodenum was then Kocherized completely. After dividing the left gastric artery and vein, the gastric conduit was created with six fires of the

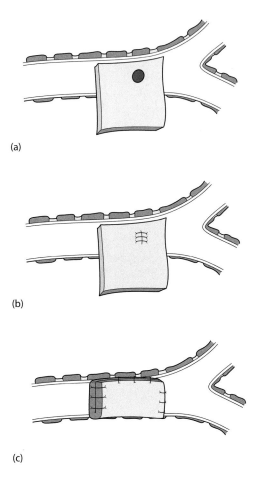

(a)

(b)

(c)

Figure 45.3 Cartoon diagram of an esophageal muscle patch to close the trachea-esophageal fistula. (a) Segment of posterior esophageal wall opened longitudinally showing fistulos connection to trachea. (b) Fistula closed directly with simple sutures. (c) The esophageal muscle is turned back on itself to reinforce the repair with vascularized esophageal muscle patch

Endo GIA. Then two additional tacking sutures were placed to the portion of small bowel that was attached to the anterior abdominal wall. After verifying proximal and distal orientation of the bowel, an enterotomy was then made, the 16-French Malecot tube was introduced into the lumen, and the feeding tube was established. Simultaneously, a left cervical incision was made, and the proximal esophagus was delivered into the neck. The distal esophagus was then attached to the Foley catheter and then delivered through the mediastinum into the neck. A near total esophagectomy was completed. Then the gastric conduit was brought into the neck. Esophagogastrostomy was then fashioned and the liner stapled posterior anastomosis completing anterior anastomosis with interrupted (4-0 polydioxanone PDS) sutures [2,3]. The neck wound was then closed in layers as well as the abdominal port sites.

Patient recovered well, and a postoperative swallow on postoperative day 7 showed good anastomosis and prompt outflow of the contrast into the small bowel. He was discharged home on the tenth day. At follow-up at six months, he had gained weight and was running ten miles two to three times a week, regularly with no limitations.

Comments

The most common cause of benign esophageal stricture in African countries is ingestion of corrosives. The ingestion of these corrosives are accidental, suicidal, or for medicinal purposes. This stricture is long, narrow, and irregular. Most extend from the cervical esophagus to the GE junction [4]. Our patient was born in Nigeria and spent his early childhood there before emigrating to the US. We could not elicit a history of ingestion of any corrosive intentionally or accidentally on direct questioning. Additionally, it appears that his stricture initially affected the lower esophagus rather than the cricopharyngeus as generally would be in cases of ingestion of corrosive agents or thermal injury.

Many novel techniques have been suggested for the treatment of refractory benign esophageal strictures, at present, including incisional therapy, stenting, or the injection of steroids and antifibrotic agents, all with limited success. In a multicenter series, Repici et al. showed a disappointing long-term outcome for endoscopic therapy for refractory benign esophageal strictures, with only one of three achieving clinical a resolution. The dysphagia-free period was relatively short following these interventions, therefore affecting the quality of life like in our patient. In a meta-analysis, endoprosthetics did not appear to affect the natural history of benign esophageal strictures. Stent placement was effective in about 40% of the patients. Additionally, stents that have been in place for a long period can erode into surrounding structures and cause other complications. As observed in our patient, a self-expanding metal stent eroded into the membranous posterior tracheal wall, thereby leading to fistula formation often untreated fatal. Resection and reconstruction of the esophagus is the ultimate solution for refractory benign strictures or those associated with complications. A careful appraisal of the situation and planning of the operative procedure is mandatory for a successful outcome. We were able to use the patient's own esophageal tissue to close the tracheal esophageal fistula. This was available to us because we were dealing with a benign esophageal pathology. In a malignant fistula, a pedicle muscle flap for reinforcement would be appropriate. Because we used in situ muscle reinforcement, we were able to use the gastric conduit in the orthotopic position for reconstruction. In a relatively short follow-up period, our patient appeared to have recovered well and have a good quality of life without limitations.

REFERENCES

1. Repici, A, Small, A.J., Mendelson, A., Jovani, M., Correale, L., Hassan, C., Ridola, L., Anderloni, A., Ferrara, E.C., Kochman, M.L. Natural history and management of refractory benign esophageal strictures. *Gastrointest Endosc.* 2016;84(2):222–228. doi:10.1016/j.gie.2016.01.053.
2. Orringer, M.B., Marshall, B., Iannettoni, M.D. Transhiatal esophagectomy for treatment of benign and malignant esophageal disease. *World J Surg.* 2001;25(2):196–203.
3. Steven, J.M. Esophageal anastomosis. *Oper Tech Thorac Cardiovasc Surg.* 2000;5(4):231–241.
4. Ajao, O.G. and Solanke T.F. Benign esophageal stricture in a tropical African population. *J Natl Med Assoc.* 1978;70(7):497–499.

Curtis S. Bergquist and Rishindra M. Reddy

🔑	Key Words
	• Transhiatal esophagectomy • Stroke • Diaphragm • Colon hernia • Case report

Introduction

Esophagectomy can be performed safely with low mortality in experienced hands. All esophageal resections though carry the risk of postoperative complications, such as anastomotic leak, chylothorax, and stricture. Nonspecific complications like heart attack, stroke, and respiratory failure are also possible. Intraoperative or postoperative stroke is a relatively uncommon complication, with none reported in a series of 2,000 transhiatal esophagectomies [1]. Delayed herniation of the colon or other abdominal organs can be seen in the acute setting or delayed, even decades after surgery [2]. Management of hernias, when found, should be performed quickly to reduce the risk of strangulation of the herniated contents.

Case Report

The patient was a 74-year-old Caucasian female with history of brain aneurysms and diabetes who was diagnosed with a distal esophageal adenocarcinoma during a workup of lower gastrointestinal bleeding by her local primary care physician and a gastroenterologist. She experienced a 30-lb weight loss, which she attributed to a weight loss program, and denied symptoms of heartburn, dysphagia, or regurgitation. She was able to walk one mile and up two flights of stairs, had only smoked for four years, and quit nearly thirty years ago. Her medical history was notable for diabetes mellitus and brain aneurysms, which were treated with coiling or were being observed.

Her physical exam at her initial preoperative consultation was normal; she was a well-nourished woman with a soft abdomen with no gross neurological deficits. An esophagogastroduodenoscopy revealed semi-circumferential thickening with central ulceration at the esophagogastric junction, a hiatal hernia, and antral erosions. A biopsy of the suspicious lesion was positive for adenocarcinoma. Other testing included an endoscopic ultrasound, which showed a T1N0 lesion, and a PET scan, which demonstrated only local disease. It was felt that she was a surgical candidate, but she was referred to Neurosurgery for evaluation of her untreated brain aneurysms. The neurosurgeon noted that her two brain aneurysms were small and asymptomatic and therefore recommended she follow-up in one year with imaging.

She underwent initially robot-assisted approach that was, converted to open transhiatal esophagectomy. The operation was converted to open due to dense adhesions around the liver and duodenum. Both pleural spaces were entered requiring the placement of thoracostomy tubes. No hypotensive episodes were recorded in the anesthetic record. After the gastric conduit was delivered into the neck, the diaphragmatic hiatus was narrowed to allow the tips of two fingerbreadths with simple interrupted #1 Silk suture on the crura. In the post-anesthesia unit, she was not speaking or moving her right side. Neurology was emergently consulted. A non-contrast CT scan of the head showed changes consistent with an ischemic stroke, and a CT-angiogram did not show any proximal occlusion. The neurology team recommended medical treatment for her stroke, and she continued to recovery in the surgical ICU. Her recovery from her operation was otherwise uneventful, and she was discharged to a subacute rehabilitation facility on postoperative day 8. She was discharged on tube feeds but ultimately recovered most of her function and resumed eating by mouth. She remained in skilled nursing due to limitations from her stroke but was happy with her quality of life.

Eleven months after her esophagectomy, she presented to a community hospital with shortness of breath and chest pain. A chest X-ray showed an effusion in her left chest, but a CT of the chest showed a large left-sided diaphragmatic hernia with her colon and omentum in her left chest, compressing her left lung with a dilated conduit (Figure 46.1). The decision to repair this was delayed due to the patient's perceived frailty, and she was discharged with a new jejunostomy feeding tube and strict *nil per os* (NPO) instructions because of a possible herniated colon compressing her gastric conduit and resulting obstruction. In a follow-up with her initial surgeon, her quality of life was related to her ability to share meals with her friends. Despite her frailty, which was improving per the patient and her family, she wished to have the hernia repaired so that she could eat.

She was brought to the operating room for an endoscopy, and a robot-assisted laparoscopy and attempted hiatal hernia repair. The hiatus was found to be widely open, and there was little scar tissue. The transverse colon and omentum were easily reduced back into the abdomen through the hiatus, the lung re-expanded, a left thoracostomy tube was placed, and the gastric conduit inspected and not damaged. The diaphragmatic hiatus was then narrowed and

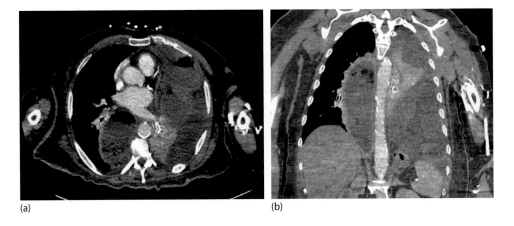

(a)   (b)

Figure 46.1 (a and b) CT chest 11 months post-THE showing colon and omentum in left chest

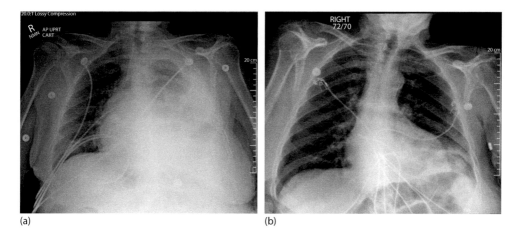

Figure 46.2 (a and b) Postoperative films showing hemothorax after hernia reduction and subsequent resolution of the hemothorax

was tacked to the gastric conduit in multiple places, obliterating all potential space. Three days later, a routine blood count showed an acute decrease in hemoglobin, and a follow-up chest radiograph demonstrated a new left effusion (Figure 46.2). She was thus brought to the operating room for thoracoscopic hemothorax evacuation. Approximately one liter of old blood was removed from the left chest, but no source of bleeding was identified. The remainder of her hospitalization was unremarkable, and she was discharged several days later eating by mouth. In a follow-up, her jejunostomy feeding tube was removed, and she was back to her initial postoperative "baseline" eating with her friends.

Comments

The patient had a difficult postoperative recovery period after her transhiatal esophagectomy. The esophagectomy is a major operation for which patient selection is a crucial component. However, rigorous preoperative workup does not eliminate all complications. Failure to rescue has emerged as an area of interest and describes what happens to patients who suffer complications. Her stroke was recognized as early as was feasible, and appropriate consultants were involved immediately. No obvious event is found in the operative record to suggest why or when she had a stroke, but in retrospect, she was at baseline hypertensive. Systolic blood pressures of 100 and mean arterial pressures of greater than 60 were maintained during surgery and during the mediastinal dissection, but in retrospect, these may not have been high enough for this patient. Hypotension can occur with a tension pneumothorax, during displacement of the heart during posterior mediastinal dissection or in episodes of hemorrhage. Care was paid to the arterial line tracing while the surgeon's hand is behind the heart to monitor for hypotension, but despite this, an ischemic event happened during her operation.

Hiatal hernia after esophagectomy is a recognized complication. Routine closure of the crura as a part of the esophagectomy is practiced by most if not all experienced esophageal surgeons [1–3] and was performed in this patient. Regardless of setting (e.g., post-esophagectomy or in case of isolated hiatal hernia with no prior operation), surgery is the recommended treatment for large, symptomatic hiatal hernias [4]. Torsion of the superiorly displaced abdominal organs is a feared sequalae. Bleeding after surgery is an unfortunate complication, made even more frustrating when no source is identified when the patient is brought to the operation for exploration. The surgical team must be aware of signs of bleeding and not delay a return trip to the operating room. Here, a drop in the blood count followed by an opaque radiograph was sufficient evidence; further studies would have only delayed the care of the patient unnecessarily.

REFERENCES

1. Orringer, M.B., Marshall, B., Chang, A.C., Lee, J., Pickens, A., Lau, C.L. Two thousand transhiatal esophagectomies: Changing trends, lessons learned. *Ann Surg.* 2007;246(3):363–372; discussion 372–374.
2. Gooszen, J.A.H., Slaman, A.E., van Dieren, S., Gisbertz, S.S., van Berge Henegouwen, M.I. The incidence and treatment of a symptomatic diaphragmatic hernia following esophagectomy for cancer. *Ann Thorac Surg.* 2018;106(1):199–206. doi:10.1016/j.athoracsur.2018.02.034.
3. Orringer, M.B. Transhiatal esophagectomy: How I teach it. *Ann Thorac Surg.* 2016;102(5):1432–1437. doi:10.1016/j.athoracsur.2016.09.044.
4. Skinner, D.B. and Belsey, R.H. Surgical management of esophageal reflux and hiatus hernia: Long-term results with 1,030 patients. *J Thorac Cardiovasc Surg* 1967;53:33–54.

Claudio Caviezel, Didier Schneiter, and Walter Weder

 Key Words

- Lung volume reduction surgery
- Hypercapnia
- COPD
- Emphysema

Introduction

Lung volume reduction surgery (LVRS) improves lung function, decreases dyspnea, and increases survival in selected emphysema patients [1]. Chronic hypercapnia is considered as a contraindication for LVRS [2]. Several single center studies from the late 1990s showed no higher perioperative risk for this group of patients, although there is no randomized evidence. The multicenter randomized controlled National Emphysema Treatment Trial (NETT) excluded patients with hypercapnia [1]. However, in heterogeneous disease with obvious volume reduction target zones, patients with chronic hypercapnia can still be considered for LVRS as long as they are severely overinflated. We present a successful LVRS in an emphysema patient with severe hyperinflation and chronic hypercapnia.

Case Report

A 64-year-old female patient was admitted to our department to be evaluated for a lung volume reduction procedure. Because of her chronic pulmonary obstructive disease (COPD), she suffered from severe dyspnea on exertion and needed oxygen therapy. First expiratory volume in one second (FEV1) was 0.4 liter (L) and 20% predicted. Total lung capacity (TLC) was 9.38 L (205% predicted), and her residual volume (RV) was 7.28 L (390% predicted). The RV-TLC-ratio, the so-called hyperinflation, was 78. Carbon monoxide diffusion capacity for (DLCO) was 27% predicted. The computer tomography (CT) of the chest showed a bilateral heterogeneous emphysema, predominant on the right side. There was a bullous part in the right lower lobe and an additional upper lobe predominant target zone (Figure 47.1). Perfusion scintigraphy confirmed these findings. Her body mass index was 20.7. She had a treated systemic arterial hypertension and a slight pulmonary hypertension. The latter was only observed by transthoracic echocardiography (TTE) and showed a systolic pulmonary arterial pressure (sPAP) of 34 mmHg. We only perform right-sided heart catheter when the screening by TTE showed sPAP values above 35 mmHg.

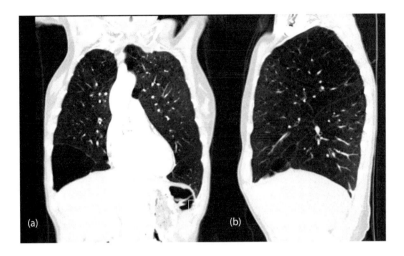

Figure 47.1 Heterogeneous emphysema with bullous emphysema in the right lower lobe (a) and target zone in the right upper lobe (b)

The left ventricle had a normal function. Blood gas analysis showed a global insufficiency with a carbon dioxide partial pressure ($PaCO_2$) of 60 mmHg (8 kPa) and an oxygen partial pressure (pO_2) of 55 mmHg (7.34 kPa).

Unilateral LVRS on the right side was performed. The patient was operated in a left-sided lateral decubitus position, and general anesthesia was conducted with a left-sided double-lumen tube. We performed the video-assisted thoracic surgery (VATS) with three ports. Figure 47.2a shows the massive bulla on the lower lobe. After penetrating the bulla for deflation, volume reduction was performed with stapling devices. Only a small verge of normal parenchyma was resected (Figure 47.2b). The volume reduction was continued on the upper lobe. The resection line followed a hockey-stick like shape from anterior to posterior above the azygos vein (Figure 47.2c). Both specimens were harvested through one port. One chest tube was placed, and the surgery terminated. The postoperative course was uneventful. The chest tube was removed on the third day, and the patient dismissed to an in-patient rehabilitation center on the sixth day after the operation. The postoperative chest X-ray already showed the elevated diaphragm on the right side compared to the preoperative situation (Figure 47.3).

After the operation, $paCO_2$ dropped to 36 mmHg (4.8 kPa) and PaO_2 rose to 68.3 mmHg (9.1 kPa) without oxygen. Table 47.1 shows the course of the blood gas analysis. The patient reported a significant benefit from the operation, and long-term oxygen therapy was omitted. The improvement was also shown in pulmonary function tests (PFTs): FEV1% predicted increased by 150%. PFT values are listed in Table 47.1. Both blood gases and PFT values remained stable for at least six months.

Comments

Hypercapnia as exclusion criteria for LVRS was possibly established from the Massachusetts General Hospital cohort between 1994 and 1995 [2]. Forty-seven consecutive patients underwent bilateral LVRS by median sternotomy. Patients with resting hypercapnia (11 of

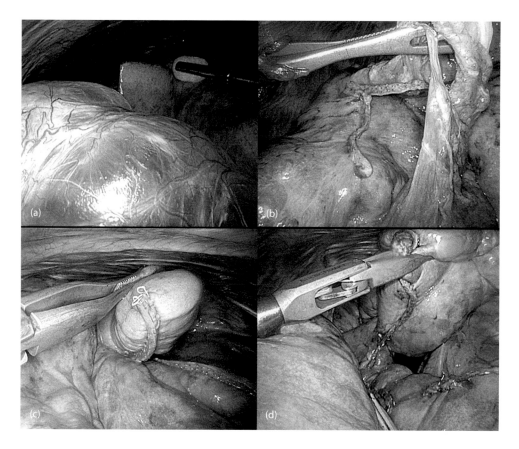

Figure 47.2 Intraoperative situs. (a) Bullous destruction in the lower lobe. (b) Resection of opened bulla. (c and d) Apical LVRS by hockey-stick shaped resection from anterior to posterior

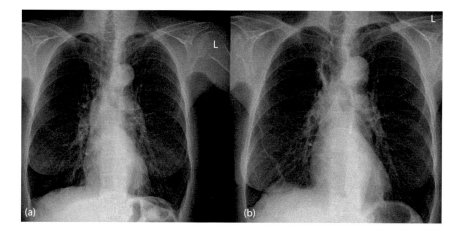

Figure 47.3 Pre- (a) and postoperative (b) chest X-ray: re-shaped diaphragm on the right side

Table 47.1 Lung function values and blood gases preoperative, 3 months and 6 months after LVRS

	Preoperative	Day Six	4 Weeks	3 Months	6 Months
FEV1 mL	400	—	—	1010	990
FEV1%p	20	—	—	50	49
TLC mL	9380	—	—	7050	6310
TLC%p	205	—	—	154	138
RV mL	7280	—	—	4970	4430
RV%p	390	—	—	269	238
RV/TLC	78	—	—	70	70
PaCO$_2$ (mmHg/kPa)	60/8	36/4.8	34/4.5	—	34/4.5
PaO$_2$ (mmHg/kPa)	55/7.34	68.3/9.1	70/9.3	—	68/9

Abbreviations: FEV1: forced expiratory volume in 1 second, TLC: total lung capacity, RV: residual volume, RV/TLC: hyperinflation, PaO$_2$: oxygen partial pressure, PaCO$_2$: carbon dioxide partial pressure, mL: milliliters, %p: percent predicted, mmHg: millimeters mercury, kPA: kilopascal.

47 patients with PaCO$_2$ ≥ 45 mm Hg) had an unacceptable outcome, defined as hospital courses >21 days and/or death within 6 months postoperative. Only one of the 11 hypercapnic patients had hospital stays ≤21 days, and five of the 11 hypercapnic patients died. Total mortality in all patients was relatively high at 19.1%. Considering the learning curve, all deaths occurred in the first 32 patients. Nevertheless, these outcomes of patients with hypercapnia were not confirmed in several following single center studies. In a recent review by Ariyaratnam and colleagues, 14 papers, predominantly from the late 1990s, were found to address this topic [3]. Whereas six to seven studies show improvements in FEV1 and PaCO$_2$, only two papers showed increased mortality in the hypercapnic group compared to the normocapnic group. Nine studies showed no difference in perioperative mortality, five papers did not compare the two groups regarding mortality. The NETT group reported their high-risk patients already in 2001 and showed increased mortality for patients with a FEV1 < 20 predicted and homogeneous emphysema or FEV1 < 20% predicted and DLCO < 20% predicted [4]. Patients with hypercapnia were excluded, and there was no mention about the blood gases in the high-risk and low-risk groups. Therefore, these lung function parameters in combination shall still guide the clinician accepting patients for LVRS. Our group showed that patients with DLCO < 20% predicted as sole high-risk factor can still be considered for LVRS as long as severe hyperinflation and obvious heterogeneous target zones exist [5]. The same might be true for patients with hypercapnia if no other exclusion criteria like homogeneous emphysema morphology or low FEV1 and low DLCO are met at the same time.

REFERENCES

1. Fishman, A., Martinez, F., Naunheim, K., Piantadosi, S., Wise, R., Ries, A., et al. A randomized trial comparing lung-volume-reduction surgery with medical therapy for severe emphysema. *N Engl J Med.* 2003;348(21):2059–2073.
2. Szekely, L.A., Oelberg, D.A., Wright, C., Johnson, D.C., Wain, J., Trotman-Dickenson, B., et al. Preoperative predictors of operative morbidity and mortality in COPD patients undergoing bilateral lung volume reduction surgery. *Chest.* 1997;111(3):550–558.

3. Ariyaratnam, P., Tcherveniakov, P., Milton, R., Chaudhuri, N. Is preoperative hypercapnia a justified exclusion criterion for lung volume reduction surgery? *Interact Cardiovasc Thorac Surg.* 2017;24(2):273–279.
4. National Emphysema Treatment Trial Research, Fishman, A., Fessler, H., Martinez, F., McKenna, R.J., Jr., Naunheim, K., et al. Patients at high risk of death after lung-volume-reduction surgery. *N Engl J Med.* 2001;345(15):1075–1083.
5. Caviezel, C., Schaffter, N., Schneiter, D., Franzen, D., Inci, I., Opitz, I., et al. Outcome after lung volume reduction surgery in patients with severely impaired diffusion capacity. *Ann Thorac Surg.* 2018;105(2):379–385.

CASE 48: BILATERAL LOBAR LUNG TRANSPLANTATION WITH EXTRA-CORPORAL LIFE SUPPORT (ECLS) IN A JEHOVAH'S WITNESS

Bastian Grande, Isabelle Opitz, and Ilhan Inci

Key Words
• Lung transplantation • Jehovah's witness • ECLS • Anemia management

Introduction

The refusal of blood transfusion represents a relative contraindication in solid organ transplantation because of anticipated high blood loss in the context of organ scarcity. The expected outcome of the candidates becomes even poorer with extra-corporal life support (ECLS) due to the associated heparin-related thrombin inactivation. Recent publications suggest a similar outcome on patients who refuse transfusion after cardiac surgery [1]. Referring to our knowledge, lung transplantation on ECLS with size reduction has never been performed so far in a patient refusing blood transfusions.

Case Report

The 42-year-old woman suffering from a progressive interstitial lung disease presented to the University Hospital Zürich for lung transplantation listing process. Overall, she was a suitable candidate with a single organ failure. The lung function, the right heart function, and the preoperative blood and coagulation assessments met all criteria for lung transplantation. The aspect of the blood refusal had been discussed within the interdisciplinary lung transplantation team. Based on recent literature and our team experience, we accepted listing in this special case. The patient did not accept red blood cells, white blood cells, platelets, and plasma. She agreed to the use of normovolemic hemodilution, cardiopulmonary bypass (CPB), ECSL, intraoperative blood salvage with re-transfusion, and hemostatic agents including purified coagulation factor concentrates.

To minimize intraoperative blood loss, she was listed for single-lung transplantation without CPB. The first organ to be offered was a size mismatch (body height +10.6 cm). Also, based on the fact that she was a candidate with the rare blood type AB, we decided to accept and perform the transplantation with size reduction (lobar transplantation) on ECLS, because the patient had secondary pulmonary arterial hypertension and most important to protect the transplanted lobe from reperfusion injury during implantation of the second graft.

The patient was informed about these modifications in the procedure and the inherent increased risk of blood loss and mortality. Written consent had been obtained.

Two months after listing, the patient was admitted to our institution a few hours before transplantation. Because of the rapid progression of the disease, she was now suffering from exercise dyspnea, although she has been in good condition (70 kg, 157 cm height, BMI 28.5) without oxygen. Her actual two years survival rate was estimated at 20%.

The preoperative hemoglobin level was 123 g/L, platelet count was 488,000 per cubic millimeter, INR was 1.1, and the fibrinogen level was at 4.7 g/L. Before the operation started, 40,000 IU synthetic erythropoietin (epoetin alfa) subcutaneous, 1,000 mg of ferric carboxymaltose intravenous, and 1,000 mcg cyanocobalamin (vitamin B12) subcutaneous had been administered to optimize the production of red blood cells.

The AB donor organ (male, 187 cm, 90 kg) was offered. The organ was considered for lobar transplant because of the significant size mismatch. We decided to perform the lung transplantation on ECLS to protect the allograft (lobes) from reperfusion injury due to secondary pulmonary arterial hypertension.

Therefore, careful interdisciplinary teamwork aiming at minimal blood loss was mandatory. Before the induction of general anesthesia, an arterial catheter was placed. Anesthesia was induced using fentanyl, and propofol as target-controlled infusion and rocuronium. Propofol and remifentanil were used to maintain anesthesia, rocuronium was administered for neuromuscular blockade, and bispectral index (BIS) was used to control the depth of anesthesia. After a four-luminal central venous catheter and a pulmonal arterial catheter were placed, autologous harvest was performed through a 14 G peripheral venous cannula by removing two bags of whole blood (a total of 380 cc, each). The blood remained in a closed-circuit connected to the patient, and this blood withdrawal was primarily not replaced because the patient remained hemodynamically totally stable throughout the scavenging process. The patient underwent a clamshell access and central cannulation for venoarterial ECLS, which was performed under standardized heparin protocol. For arterial cannulation, we used the ascending aorta, and for venous cannulation, the right atrium. After administering heparin, an application error was detected; 15,000 IU heparin had been given instead of 1,500 IU. The activated clotting time (ACT) increased from 141 to 270 seconds and decreased thereafter to 200 seconds throughout the procedure. During the transplantation, 1,500 cc crystalloid and 500 cc gelatin solutions were infused. Perioperative blood loss was 660 cc estimated with the hemoglobin dilution method. Cell saver blood as well as patient's own scavenged blood was reinfused at the end of the bilateral left lower lobe lung transplantation (Figures 48.1 and 48.2). The patient could be weaned from ECLS in the OR. Total ECLS time was 198 minutes. Subsequently, she was transferred to ICU in a stable hemodynamic condition, without bleeding complications.

In the ICU, pulmonary weaning from the respirator failed, and the patient developed primary organ dysfunction grade 3 within 72 hours. Attempts to improve oxygenation and the treatment of the increasing pulmonary vascular resistance with inhalative Nitric Oxide (NO) and illoprost were ineffective. Venoarterial ECLS had to be installed and immunosuppressive medication was augmented. The empiric antibiotic and antifungal therapy was expanded broadly because of escalating signs of inflammation in face of negative cultures. Despite bone marrow stimulation with erythropoietin, discontinuation of hematotoxic medication and minimal diagnostic blood sampling, a steady decrease of the Hb level over three weeks to a minimal value of 27 g/L (two weeks after transplantation) was documented. Blood transfusion was not permitted following the patient's and her family's will. In the context of pronounced anemia, hypoxic organ damage evolved causing multiorgan failure. The patient died in the presence of her relatives.

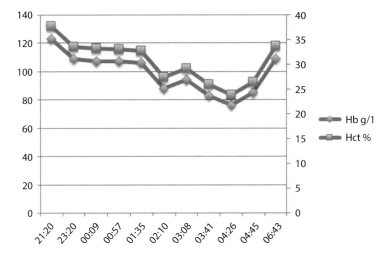

Figure 48.1 Intraoperative hemoglobin and hematocrit level

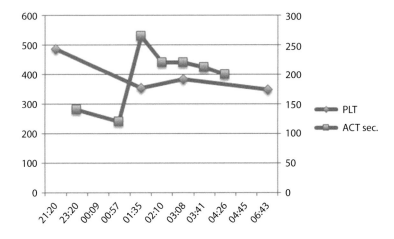

Figure 48.2 Intraoperative ACT and platelets

Comments

This is the first description of bilateral sequential lobar lung transplantation on ECLS in a Jehovah's Witness. The belief of a Jehovah's Witness prohibits blood transfusions, and storage and donation of blood, but some Jehovah's Witnesses accept solid organs for transplantation [2,3].

Patients refusing blood transfusions should be evaluated at least four weeks before surgery and should be treated with supplements like erythropoietin alpha, iron, vitamin B12, and folic acid to avoid perioperative anemia [4]. Intraoperative blood loss should be minimized with all available techniques including cell salvage, hemodilution, careful operation technique, meticulous hemostasis, minimized blood samples, coagulation monitoring, and pharmacotherapy [5].

Intraoperative complications regarding the blood loss may occur suddenly and unexpectedly. In our case, a heparin dose error led to a prolonged ACT without any signs of exaggerated clinical bleeding. The ACT level to be aimed at during ECLS is controversial because the test is not reliable. It varies 10% on repeated testing. Also, it varies depending on the ATIII level of the patient, specific activant, prewarming of the test, and stand-alone ACT values cannot always be interpreted in the same way. We believe that an experienced multidisciplinary team has to interpret laboratory or point of care data together with clinical findings in order to decide on therapeutic consequences.

The present case demonstrates that intraoperative management of bilateral sequential lobar lung transplantation in a Jehovah's Witness is feasible, even in the challenging context of CPB, with careful intraoperative planning and interdisciplinary teamwork.

However, postoperative complications such as graft failure, pulmonary edema, or the necessity of prolonged ECLS therapy cannot be avoided in all cases, which results in fatal outcome despite best available treatment, was applied.

REFERENCES

1. Pattakos, G., Koch, C.G., Brizzio, M.E., Batizy, L.H., Sabik, J.F., III, Blackstone, E.H., Lauer, M.S. Outcome of patients who refuse transfusion after cardiac surgery: A natural experiment with severe blood conservation. *Arch Intern Med.* 2012;172:1154–1160.
2. Lin, E.S., Kaye, A.D., Baluch, A.R. Preanesthetic assessment of the Jehovah's Witness patient. *Ochsner J.* 2012;12:61–69.
3. Chand, N.K., Subramanya, H.B., Rao, G.V. Management of patients who refuse blood transfusion. *Indian J Anaesth.* 2014;58:658–664.
4. Conte, J.V. and Orens, J.B. Lung transplantation in a Jehovah's Witness. *J Heart Lung Transplant.* 1999;18:796–800.
5. Spahn, D.R. and Goodnough, L.T. Alternatives to blood transfusion. *Lancet.* 2013;381:1855–1865.

Adrian E. Rodrigues and Wickii T. Vigneswaran

🔑 Key Words
• Lung • Transplant • Cancer • Metastasis • Donor

Introduction

Lung transplantation is the final medical option for many people with end-state pulmonary disease, and since its introduction in 1983 [1], survival has progressively improved throughout the years [2]. Although lung transplantation is contraindicated in patients diagnosed with pulmonary cancer, pulmonary malignancies are occasionally found after a transplant. Data shows that 13% of 5-year survivors and 28% of 10-year survivors will develop some type of malignancy after their transplant [2]. Moreover, patients who undergo a single-lung transplant (SLTx) are more likely to develop pulmonary cancer than their double-lung transplant (DLTx) counterparts [3]. In these patients, the origin of primary cancer can be in either the native lung or the donor lung. And during workup, the recipient or the donor may have an undiagnosed malignancy outside of the respiratory system that metastasizes to a lung that is not detected by conventional imaging. Conventionally, it is taught that carcinomas spread through the lymphatic system first. In a transplanted lung recipient, the lymphatic connections do not exist early after transplantation. A sparse network may develop later, but it's uncommon. We report a native lung primary malignancy metastasizing to the donor lung relatively early following in a SLTx recipient.

Case Report

We report on a 68-year-old male retired clerical worker who presented to our institution with increased dyspnea on exertion. His past medical history was remarkable for depression, dyslipidemia, pneumonia, and type 2 diabetes mellitus. He had a social history of 30-pack-years cigarette use and extensive ethanol abuse.

A few days prior to his initial visit with us, the patient contracted pneumonia and sought medical attention at a neighboring hospital. He was treated with antibiotics and was discharged on oxygen at 2 LPM at rest and 5 LPM with activities. The day following his discharge he presented to our institution. Upon evaluation, the patient looked chronically sick but was nevertheless robust and had a body mass index (BMI) of 31.59 kg/m^2. His cognition and orientation were intact, and he denied all constitutional symptoms except for dyspnea on exertion and bilateral lower extremity edema.

After workup, a diagnosis of idiopathic pulmonary fibrosis and pulmonary hypertension was attributed. Five months afterward, he underwent a left SLTx at our institution. The procedure was remarkable for a pulmonary pressure of 70 systolic after pulmonary artery clamping but was quickly controlled with inhaled nitric oxide. The mediastinum had significant adipose tissue along with calcified and fibrotic lymph nodes, which were successfully removed. The chest cavity was somewhat small for the donor lung, but it was accommodated into the recipient's pleural space with minimal difficulty. The hospital stay was uneventful, and at postoperative day eight, the patient was discharged to home health care. Pathological report of native lung was notable for end-stage lung fibrosis, bronchiolar metaplasia with honeycombing, and fibroblastic foci consistent with interstitial pneumonia.

During follow-up of the left single-lung transplant, a chest CT at four months showed a soft tissue density measuring 2.2 × 1.4 cm in the right lung base, suspected as scar, pleural thickening, or atelectasis. Examination at another four months later reported the finding as stable chronic appearing interstitial opacity of right lung base. However, a CT scan at an additional six months later showed growth of the right lower lung mass and an additional new lung nodule in the middle lobe (1.6 × 1.2 cm) and in the left (donor, 0.7 cm) upper lobe. In retrospect, the mass that was favored as fibrotic or infective change was a missed growth in the right lower lobe that was masked by the pre-existing fibrotic changes in the bases due to pulmonary fibrosis. The right lower lobe showed a mass that was now 7.7 × 6.7 cm (Figures 49.1 through 49.3). A 7-mm nodule was also noted in the left upper lobe. A PET-CT showed abnormal fluoro-deoxyglucose (FDG) accumulation along the periphery with a central area of necrosis and a Standardized Uptake Value (SUV) max of 18.9 in the right base. A right middle lobe nodule showed an SUV max of 12.6, and the left upper lobe also showed a mass of 7 mm with a SUV max of 5.8 and a subcarinal lymph node (1.1 cm) with an SUV of 9.5. A brain MRI showed an enhancing left frontal lobe mass (1.6 × 1.0 cm) extending to the dura with moderate local edema and sulcal effacement. Pulmonary fine-needle biopsies were subsequently obtained and reported metastatic carcinoma consistent with metastatic squamous cell carcinoma from the lung.

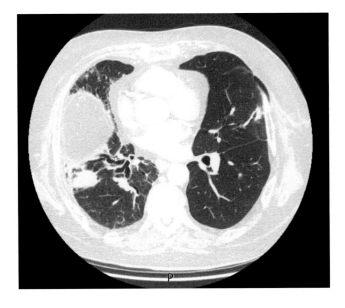

Figure 49.1 Five months post-transplant

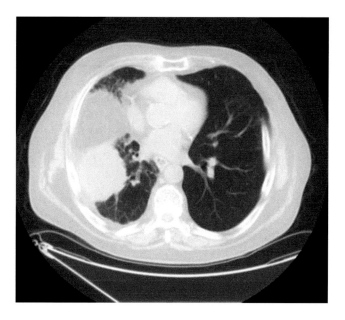

Figure 49.2 One year post-transplant

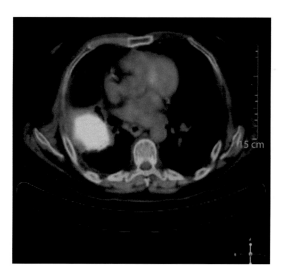

Figure 49.3 PET scan

With a diagnosis of stage IV non-small cell lung cancer, the patient was treated with carboplatin and paclitaxel chemotherapy. He was also seen by Neurosurgery and underwent stereotactic radiosurgery of the frontal lobe, of which he tolerated well. Five months after we diagnosed his pulmonary cancer, the patient died under hospice care.

Comments

Pulmonary cancer following lung transplantation is not common, but this can occur in the native or the transplanted lung. The risks of this morbidity can increase under certain circumstances and has a reported incidence of 0.46%–6.9% in some studies [4]. In patients who undergo single-lung transplants, the risk for native lung cancer is increased in advanced age, a history of smoking, and immunosuppression [2,3,5,6]. And in this patient, all of these risks were present. Risks for developing cancer in the donated lung include receiving one from a person who smoked or was advanced in age [2]. The donor in this case was a non-smoker and died at the age of 40.

In a retrospective chart review study by Grewal et al. [3], 9 out of 462 lung transplant patients were found to have pulmonary cancer, and out of those 9, only one had a tumor in the donor allograft lung, which they state was potentially of donor origin but could not confirm due to inclusive cytogenetic studies. In another retrospective review by Belli et al. [4], 13 out of 335 lung transplant recipients were found to subsequently develop lung cancer with one confirmed to be from donor origin, confirming native lung cancer is more common than a donor lung cancer.

Although developing pulmonary cancer after a lung transplant is significant, what is remarkable about this case is having a primary pulmonary malignancy metastasize from the patient's native lung to his donor lung early. The pathway on which this can happen is via blood stream, as the lymphatic connection to the transplanted lung is severed. The origin of our patient's native lung primary malignancy is highly suspected to have developed after his transplant. Although the possibility that it was unrecognized before the transplant does exist given that lung cancers arising under the cover of interstitial lung changes such as honeycombing are difficult to diagnose [7]. Although this patient's primary tumor could have developed before or after the transplant, what is most noteworthy is the mode of metastasis to the donor lung allograft. This malignancy very likely metastasized early via the blood to the donor lung.

REFERENCES

1. Toronto Lung Transplant Group. Unilateral Lung Transplantation for Pulmonary Fibrosis. *N Engl J Med.* 1986;314(18):1140–1145. doi:10.1056/NEJM198605013141802.
2. Olland, A.B.M., Falcoz, P.-E., Santelmo, N., Kessler, R., Massard, G. Primary lung cancer in lung transplant recipients. *Ann Thorac Surg.* 2014;98:362–371. doi:10.1016/j.athoracsur.2014.04.014.
3. Grewal, A.S., Padera, R.F., Boukedes, S., et al. Prevalence and outcome of lung cancer in lung transplant recipients. *Respir Med.* 2015;109:427–433. doi:10.1016/j.rmed.2014.12.013.
4. Belli, E.V., Landolfo, K., Keller, C., Thomas, M., Odell, J. Lung cancer following lung transplant: Single institution 10 year experience. *Lung Cancer.* 2013;81:451–454. doi:10.1016/j.lungcan.2013.05.018.
5. Raviv, Y., Shitrit, D., Amital, A., et al. Lung cancer in lung transplant recipients: Experience of a tertiary hospital and literature review. *Lung Cancer.* 2011;74:280–283. doi:10.1016/j.lungcan.2011.02.012.
6. Nakajima, T., Cypel, M., De Perrot, M., et al. Retrospective analysis of lung transplant recipients found to have unexpected lung cancer in explanted lungs. *Semin Thorac Cardiovasc Surg.* 2015;27:9–14. doi:10.1053/j.semtcvs.2015.02.006.
7. Yoshida, R., Arakawa H., Kaji Y. Lung cancer in chronic interstitial pneumonia: Early manifestation from serial CT Observations. *Am J Roentgenol.* 2012;199(1):85–90. doi:10.2214/AJR.11.7516.

Mathew Thomas

Key Words
• Cystic fibrosis • Lung transplantation • Aortic homograft • Superior vena cava

Introduction

Patients requiring lung transplantation may have complex intrathoracic anatomy, either due to congenital anomalies, prior surgery, or from progression of their primary disease. In some cases, these anatomic abnormalities can be severe enough to contraindicate lung transplantation. One such challenging problem is superior vena cava (SVC) obstruction, which can occur due to mediastinal pathology such as fibrosing mediastinitis, chronic non-fibrosing inflammation, tumors, or intravascular obstruction from chronic indwelling venous catheters. Approximately 9% of cystic fibrosis patients may have SVC stenosis or obstruction [1]. Percutaneous recanalization of the SVC can be successful in most cases of stenosis [2] but can be extremely difficult when complete occlusion is present. SVC reconstruction using spiral saphenous vein graft or synthetic grafts have been also been described before as a way to bypass SVC obstruction [3,4] but not in cystic fibrosis patients prior to lung transplantation.

We describe an innovative, staged approach where we performed successful bilateral lung transplantation in a patient with SVC occlusion and patent foramen ovale.

Case Report

A 21-year-old male with hypoxia secondary to cystic fibrosis was evaluated for lung transplantation at our institution. He had a significant history of multiple lung infections and left pneumothorax treated with a chest tube. Upon further evaluation, he was found to have complete occlusion of the SVC between the insertion of the azygous vein and right atrium with exuberant collateral drainage of the left innominate vein through the azygous, hemiazygous, and left superior intercostal veins (Figure 50.1). In addition, a patent foramen ovale (PFO) with moderate right-to-left shunt and giant, hypervascular, mediastinal lymph nodes were also present. Multiple attempts at recanalization of the occluded SVC by interventional vascular radiologists were unsuccessful. The risks of interrupting the collateral blood flow

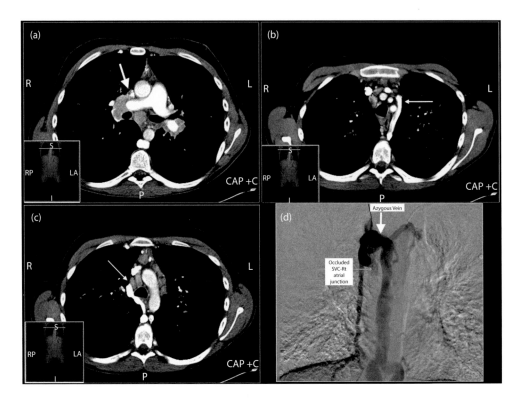

Figure 50.1 (a–c) CT-angiogram images showing (a) occluded SVC-right atrial junction (arrow) with collateral drainage through (b) hemiazygous (arrow) and (c) azygous (arrow) venous systems, and (d) venogram by fluoroscopy prior to SVC bypass

during bilateral transplantation and causing an immediate SVC syndrome were considered to be too high, and he was considered to be a poor candidate for lung transplantation without first addressing the SVC occlusion and PFO.

The following options were discussed:

1. Concurrent SVC reconstruction or bypass and PFO closure during bilateral lung transplantation. This option was considered to be contraindicated due to the following reasons:
    a. The median sternotomy approach required for SVC bypass and PFO closure was different from the clamshell or bilateral thoracotomy that would be preferred for bilateral lung transplantation.
    b. Extensive pleural adhesions from prior infections were anticipated to lead to severe bleeding and consequently prolong the operative time if all procedures were performed at the same time.
    c. Concerns of severe bleeding from the highly pressurized mediastinal and pleural venous collaterals were raised.
2. Closure of the PFO through percutaneous approach followed by bypass of the SVC occlusion and then bilateral lung transplantation later. We did not feel that there was any significant advantage to this approach over surgical repair of the PFO at the same time as SVC bypass.

3. Multistage approach to relieve the SVC obstruction and repair the PFO first followed by listing for bilateral lung transplantation, if the initial operation was successful.

The third option was chosen as the most appropriate, with the understanding that ultimate success was dependent on timely availability of a donor and that a bridge to transplantation such as extracorporeal membrane oxygenation (ECMO) would be required if he could not be extubated.

Stage 1: A midline sternotomy was made; large collateral veins were observed on the anterior chest wall as well as on the anterior pericardium. Cardiopulmonary bypass was initiated through the aorta and right atrium. The PFO was repaired primarily through a right atriotomy. Due to large hypervascular lymph nodes on the right lateral surface of the SVC near the entry of the azygous vein and concerns of injuring the right phrenic nerve, we decided to bypass the SVC obstruction from the innominate vein to the right atriotomy using a 19-mm aortic homograft in an end-to-side fashion. He was successfully weaned off cardiopulmonary bypass.

Stage 2: The patient remained intubated and, four days later, underwent venoarterial ECMO via femoral vessels in anticipation of lung transplantation. A CT-angiogram showed the innominate-to-right atrial graft to be patent with significantly decreased intrathoracic collaterals (Figure 50.2).

Stage 3: A donor became available a week later, and the patient underwent bilateral lung transplantation via bilateral sequential thoracotomies. As a result of decompression of the intrathoracic collaterals, no excessive bleeding was encountered.

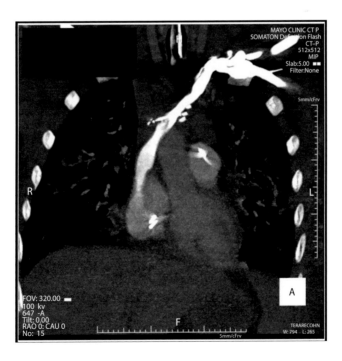

Figure 50.2 CT-angiogram before transplantation showing patent left innominate-to-right atrial bypass

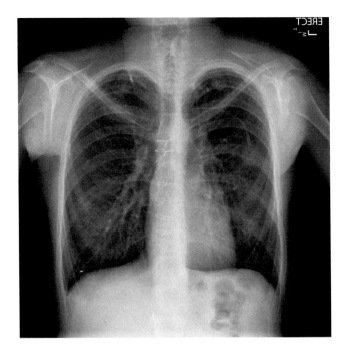

Figure 50.3 Chest X-ray at four years after bilateral lung transplantation

Following recovery from his surgery, he was eventually discharged from the hospital and was maintained on anticoagulation with Warfarin. He returned to a normal life and graduated successfully from college. Four years later, he remains healthy with no signs of rejection (Figure 50.3) and continues to have a patent bypass graft.

Comments

Severe SVC stenosis or obstruction can be usually managed with stents or a balloon and should not be considered an absolute contraindication to lung transplantation. However, when SVC obstruction cannot be relieved by percutaneous intervention, surgical reconstruction or bypass of the SVC should be considered prior to lung transplantation. Such patients should be referred to more experienced centers for consideration of surgery. It is also important to discuss with the patient and the patient's family that multiple surgeries might be required in a staged approach until lung transplantation can be safely performed. As in our patient, success of the multi-staged approach depends not only on the re-establishment of adequate drainage from the head and upper extremities, but also on the timely availability of donor lungs.

Risks of SVC reconstruction with any graft include bleeding, possible thrombosis of the graft, or obstruction due to kinking. Although there is no data to guide the use of anticoagulation in patients with aortic homograft central venous reconstruction, we recommended lifelong anticoagulation because of the low pressure and flow in the venous system.

We are unaware of any other reports in literature that describe a similar staged approach that included surgical bypass of the SVC using an aortic homograft prior to lung transplantation in a cystic fibrosis patient.

REFERENCES

1. Otani, S., et al. Managing central venous obstruction in cystic fibrosis recipients: Lung transplant considerations. *J Cyst Fibros.* 2015;14(2):255–261.
2. Rizvi, A.Z., et al. Benign superior vena cava syndrome: Stenting is now the first line of treatment. *J Vasc Surg.* 2008;47(2):372–380.
3. Doty, J.R., et al. Superior vena cava obstruction: Bypass using spiral vein graft. *Ann Thorac Surg.* 1999;67(4):1111–1116.
4. Magnan, P.E., et al. Surgical reconstruction of the superior vena cava. *Cardiovasc Surg.* 1994;2(5):598–604.

INDEX

Note: Page numbers in italic and bold refer to figures and tables, respectively.

Index

Fundamental Mass Transfer Concepts in Engineering Applications

İsmail Tosun

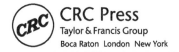

CRC Press

Taylor & Francis Group
Boca Raton   London   New York

CRC Press is an imprint of the
Taylor & Francis Group, an **informa** business

CRC Press
Taylor & Francis Group
6000 Broken Sound Parkway NW, Suite 300
Boca Raton, FL 33487-2742

© 2019 by Taylor & Francis Group, LLC
CRC Press is an imprint of Taylor & Francis Group, an Informa business

International Standard Book Number-13: 978-1-138-55227-2 (Hardback)

Library of Congress Cataloging-in-Publication Data

Names: Tosun, Ismail, author.
Title: Fundamental mass transfer concepts in engineering applications / Ismail Tosun.
Description: Boca Raton : Taylor & Francis, a CRC title, part of the Taylor & Francis imprint, a member of the Taylor & Francis Group, the academic division of T&F Informa, plc, 2019. | Includes bibliographical references.
Identifiers: LCCN 2019007036 | ISBN 9781138552272 (hardback : acid-free paper)
Subjects: LCSH: Mass transfer–Mathematical models. | MathCAD.
Classification: LCC TP156.M3 T67 2019 | DDC 660/.28423–dc23
LC record available at https://lccn.loc.gov/2019007036

Visit the Taylor & Francis Web site at
http://www.taylorandfrancis.com

and the CRC Press Web site at
http://www.crcpress.com

Dedication

To Nurten and Derviş Şamlı

Contents

Preface

This book is intended as a text for upper undergraduate and graduate courses on mass transfer. The focus is to teach the foundations of mass transfer and to equip students with sufficient mathematical skills to tackle problems with confidence. An overview of this book is shown schematically in Figure P.1. The presented material is for a one-semester course, and it provides sufficient background for students interested in pursuing further research on the topics not covered in this book.

Since mathematics is an integral part of mass transfer, readers should go over Appendices A, C, D, and E before they start reading Chapter 1. Students usually struggle with the elimination of terms in the governing equations because they do not know the order of magnitude values or the physical significance of these terms. The purpose of Appendix B is to introduce the order of magnitude (or scale) analysis to students in order to enable them to make reasonable estimations.

Chapter 1 covers the basic concepts and their characteristics. The terms appearing in the conservation equations for mass, momentum, and energy are discussed qualitatively, and the similarities between mass, momentum, and energy transport are pointed out. Chapter 2 provides the foundations for the formulation of mass transfer problems. Those who do not want to cover multicomponent mass transfer may skip Chapter 3. Mass transfer in binary systems without bulk flow is covered in Chapters 4–6. Steady-state, pseudosteady-state, and unsteady-state examples are given in Chapters 4, 5, and 6, respectively. Chapter 7 deals with the mass transfer in binary systems in the case of bulk flow. Chapter 9 is optional; it shows how the area averaging technique together with two-point Hermite expansion is used to obtain an approximate solution.

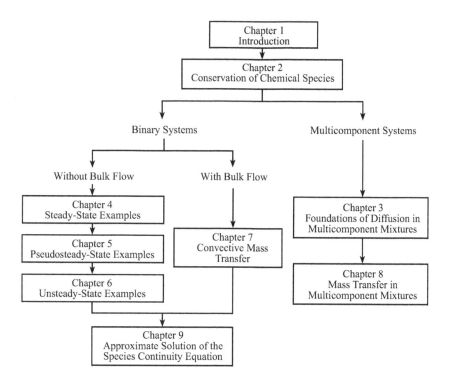

Figure P.1 Arrangement of the chapters.

Nowadays engineering calculations are carried out by mathematical software packages, such as Mathcad, Matlab, and Polymath. It is extremely important for engineering students to learn and practice the use of these modern computational tools. Mathcad worksheets provided in this book show the steps to be followed in the calculations.

Chapters 3 and 8 talk about mass transfer in multicomponent mixtures. Maxwell–Stefan multicomponent mass transfer calculations are lengthy and time-consuming. Students usually become bogged down in the details of the calculations and lose the big picture. The Mathcad subroutine given in Chapter 8 for the "shooting method" carries out the complex calculations in a straightforward manner and enables students to conduct a parametric study.

Not only are answers to all the problems in this book provided, but also step-by-step solution procedures are given in most problem statements, facilitating its use as a self-study reference book.

My colleagues Harun Koku, Canan Özgen, Turgut Tokdemir, and Hayrettin Yücel made many helpful suggestions during the preparation of this book. Their efforts are greatly appreciated. Above all, I am grateful to my wife, Ayşe, for her unwavering support and understanding ever since we got married.

Suggestions and criticisms from instructors and students using this book would be appreciated.

İsmail Tosun
Ankara, Turkey
January 2019
(itosun@metu.edu.tr)

Author

Professor İsmail Tosun received his BS and MS degrees from the Middle East Technical University (METU) in 1972 and 1974, respectively, and a PhD degree from the University of Akron, Ohio in 1977, all in Chemical Engineering.

After spending a year as a post-doctoral fellow at the University of Akron and completing his military service in Ankara, he started his academic career as an assistant professor at the METU Chemical Engineering Department in 1981. He was promoted to Associate Professorship in 1984 and to full Professorship in 1989. As a Fulbright Scholar and a Visiting Professor, Prof. Tosun was in the United States from 1987 to 1989.

From 1990 to 1993, Prof. Tosun was the Assistant-Dean of the Graduate School at METU. Then he acted as the Dean of Graduate School until 1997. In January of 1997, Prof. Tosun was appointed to the Council of Higher Education (YÖK), which, in a way, acts as the National Board of Trustees. After completing his term of 4 years as the Vice-President, he returned to his academic career at METU in January of 2001.

His research and teaching interests are mathematical modeling, solid–liquid separation processes, transport phenomena, and thermodynamics. He is the author or co-author of more than 60 publications. Prof. Tosun is also the author of the following books:

1. *Modeling in Transport Phenomena – A Conceptual Approach*, 2nd Ed., Elsevier, 2007.
2. *The Thermodynamics of Phase and Reaction Equilibria*, Elsevier, 2012.
3. *Thermodynamics – Principles and Applications*, World Scientific, 2015.

Notation

Dimensions are given in terms of mass (M), length (L), time (t), temperature (T), and dimensionless (—). Boldface symbols are vectors or tensors.

A	area, L^2
a_v	surface area per unit volume, L^{-1}
$\widehat{C}_P$	heat capacity at constant pressure, ML^2/t^2
c	total concentration, mol/L^3
c_i	concentration of species i, mol/L^3
D	diameter of a cylinder or a sphere, L
D_h	hydraulic equivalent diameter, L
$\mathcal{D}_{AB}$	diffusion coefficient for system $A-B$, L^2/t
$\mathcal{D}_{eff}$	effective diffusion coefficient, L^2/t
$\mathcal{D}_{im}$	effective diffusion coefficient of species i in a mixture, Eq. (3.153), L^2/t
$\mathcal{D}_{ik}^*$	Fick diffusion coefficients with reference to molar-average velocity, L^2/t
$\mathcal{D}_{ik}^m$	Fick diffusion coefficients with reference to mass-average velocity, L^2/t
$\mathcal{D}_{ik}^{\blacksquare}$	Fick diffusion coefficients with reference to volume-average velocity, L^2/t
$\mathcal{D}_{i,self}$	self-diffusion coefficient of species i, L^2/t
$Đ_{ik}$	Maxwell–Stefan diffusion coefficient, L^2/t
$\mathbf{d}_i$	diffusional driving force for species i, L^{-1}
$\mathbf{e}_i$	unit vector in the i-direction, —
F	force, ML/t^2
$\widehat{F}_i$	body force per unit mass acting on species i, L/t^2
$\mathbf{F}$	Faraday's constant
f	friction factor, —
$\widehat{f}_i$	fugacity of species i in a mixture, M/Lt^2
G	Gibbs energy, ML^2/t^2
g	acceleration of gravity, L/t^2
h	heat transfer coefficient, M/t^3T
$\mathcal{H}$	Henry's law constant, —
I	unit matrix, Eq. (C.19)
$\mathbf{J}_i$	diffusive molar flux of species i relative to mass-average velocity, mol/L^2t
$\mathbf{J}_i^*$	diffusive molar flux of species i relative to molar-average velocity, mol/L^2t
$\mathbf{J}_i^{\blacksquare}$	diffusive molar flux of species i relative to volume-average velocity, mol/L^2t
$\mathbf{j}_i$	diffusive mass flux of species i relative to mass-average velocity, M/L^2t
$\mathbf{j}_i^*$	diffusive mass flux of species i relative to molar-average velocity, M/L^2t
$\mathbf{j}_i^{\blacksquare}$	diffusive mass flux of species i relative to volume-average velocity, M/L^2t

K_i	partition coefficient of species i, —
K_i^{ow}	octanol–water partition coefficient, Eq. (2.237), —
K_T	overall mass transfer coefficient, Eq. (5.24), L/t
k	thermal conductivity, $ML/t^3 T$
k_c	mass transfer coefficient, L/t
k_n''	heterogeneous chemical reaction rate coefficient, $\text{mol}^{1-n}/L^{2-3n}t$
k_n'''	homogeneous chemical reaction rate coefficient, $\text{mol}^{1-n}/L^{3-3n}t$
L	length, L
M	molecular weight of the mixture, M/mol
M_i	molecular weight of species i, M/mol
m	mass, M
$\mathbf{N}_i$	total molar flux of species i, $\text{mol}/L^2 t$
$\mathbb{N}$	number of moles, mol
$\mathcal{N}$	number of species in a multicomponent mixture, —
$\mathbf{n}_i$	total mass flux of species i, $M/L^2 t$
P	pressure, M/Lt^2
P_M	permeability (Ex. 4.1), $\text{mol} t/M$
P_M^*	permeability (Ex. 4.1), L^3/tM
P_i^{vap}	vapor (saturation) pressure of species i, M/Lt^2
$\overline{P}_i$	partial pressure of species i, M/Lt^2
$\mathcal{P}$	modified pressure, M/Lt^2
$\dot{Q}$	volumetric flow rate, L^3/t
q	heat flux, M/t^3
R	gas constant (in $P\widetilde{V} = RT$), $ML^2/t^2 T\text{mol}$
R	radius of a cylinder or a sphere, L
$\mathcal{R}_i$	molar rate of production of species i per unit volume by homogeneous chemical reaction, mol/tL^3
r	$\sqrt{x^2 + y^2}$, radial coordinate in cylindrical coordinates, L
r	$\sqrt{x^2 + y^2 + z^2}$, radial coordinate in spherical coordinates, L
$\mathfrak{r}$	rate of a chemical reaction, $\text{mol}/L^3 t$
S	entropy, $ML^2/t^2 T$
S_i	solubility coefficient of species i, Eq. (2.235)
T	absolute temperature, T
t	time, t
V	volume, L^3
v	speed, L/t
$\mathbf{v}$	mass-average velocity, L/t
$\mathbf{v}^*$	molar-average velocity, L/t
$\mathbf{v}^{\blacksquare}$	volume-average velocity, L/t

W	width, L
$\mathcal{W}_i$	molar flow rate of species i, mol/t
$\mathbf{w}$	velocity of the dividing surface, L/t
w_i	mass flow rate of species i, M/t
X	fractional conversion, —
x, y, z	rectangular coordinates, L
x_i	mole fraction of species i, —
y_i	mole fraction of species i in the gas phase, —
Z	compressibility factor, —
z_i	ionic charge, equiv/mol

Greek symbols

α	$k/\rho \widehat{C}_P$, thermal diffusivity, L^2/t
α_i	stoichiometric coefficient of species i
γ_i	activity coefficient of species i, —
Δ	difference
δ	Film thickness, L
δ_{ij}	Kronecker delta, Eq. (A.17), —
ε	molar extent of reaction, mol
ε_{ijk}	alternating unit tensor, Eq. (A.19), —
ε	Lennard-Jones energy parameter, ML^2/t^2
ε	porosity (void volume fraction), —
η	effectiveness factor, —
θ	arctan(y/x), angle in cylindrical coordinates, —
θ	arctan($\sqrt{x^2+y^2}/z$), angle in spherical coordinates, —
κ	Boltzmann constant
λ	unit normal vector, —
λ_i	molar Gibbs energy of pure species i at unit fugacity, ML^2/t^2mol
μ	viscosity, M/Lt
ν	kinematic viscosity, L^2/t
π	3.14159...
ρ	total density of a mixture, M/L^3
ρ_i	density of species i, M/L^3
σ, σ_{AB}	collision diameter, L
σ	standard deviation
τ_{ij}	shear stress (flux of j-momentum in the i-direction), M/Lt^2
$\widehat{\phi}_i$	fugacity coefficient of species i in a mixture, —
Ω_D	collision integral, —

Γ_{ik}	thermodynamic factor, —
ψ	electrostatic potential, volts
ω_i	mass fraction of species i, —
ω_i	acentric factor of species i, —

Overlines

$\tilde{}$	per mole
$\hat{}$	per unit mass
$\overline{}$	partial molar

Bracket

$\langle a \rangle$	average value of a

Superscripts

eq	equilibrium
f	fluid
G	gas
L	liquid
o	standard state
V	vapor
∞	at infinite dilution

Subscripts

A, B	species in binary systems
b	bulk
c	critical point property
ch	characteristic
exp	exposure
GM	geometric mean
i	species in multicomponent systems
in	inlet
int	interface
LM	log-mean
max	maximum
mix	mixture
out	out
r	reduced property
ref	reference
sys	system
w	wall or surface
∞	free-stream

Dimensionless Numbers

Bi_M	Biot number for mass transfer, Eq. (2.232)
Gz	Graetz number, Eq. (5.62)
Le	Lewis number, Eq. (1.20)
Pe_H	Peclet number for heat transfer, Eq. (1.26)
Pe_M	Peclet number for mass transfer, Eq. (1.26)
Pr	Prandtl number, Eq. (1.18)
Re	Reynolds number, Eq. (5.27)
Sc	Schmidt number, Eq. (1.19)
Sh	Sherwood number, Eq. (5.26)
St_H	Stanton number for heat transfer, Eq. (1.34)
St_M	Stanton number for mass transfer, Eq. (1.35)
τ	Fourier number, Eq. (6.14)

Mathematical Operations

D/Dt	substantial (material) derivative, t^{-1}
∇	del operator, L^{-1}
$\ln x$	the logarithm of x to the base e
$\log x$	the logarithm of x to the base 10
$\exp x$	e^x, the exponential function of x
$\mathrm{erf}\, x$	error function of x
erfc	complementary error function of x
$\Gamma(x)$	the gamma function, Eq. (7.37)
$\Gamma(x, u)$	the incomplete gamma function
δ	Dirac delta function
$O(\ )$	"of the order of"

1 Introduction

1.1 BASIC CONCEPTS

Chemical species, total mass, momentum, and energy are the *conserved* quantities encountered in engineering analysis. That is, once these quantities are transformed from one form to another, their total amount does not change. Inventory of the conserved quantity is based on a specified unit of time, which is reflected in the term *rate*. In other words, rate is a conserved quantity per unit time.

Any region that occupies a volume and has a boundary is called a *system*. The volume outside the boundary is called the *surroundings* of the system. Once the system is specified, the inventory rate equation for any conserved quantity φ is expressed as

$$\left(\begin{array}{c} \text{Rate of} \\ \text{input of } \varphi \end{array} \right) - \left(\begin{array}{c} \text{Rate of} \\ \text{output of } \varphi \end{array} \right) + \left(\begin{array}{c} \text{Rate of} \\ \text{generation of } \varphi \end{array} \right) = \left(\begin{array}{c} \text{Rate of} \\ \text{accumulation of } \varphi \end{array} \right) \quad (1.1)$$

The rate of input of φ is the amount of φ entering the system in unit time, while the rate of output of φ is the amount of φ leaving the system in unit time. The quantity φ may be generated (or depleted) within the volume of the system in unit time. The rate of accumulation of φ is the time rate of change of φ within the volume of the system.

Conservation equations for chemical species, total mass, momentum, and energy are also called *basic concepts*. The basic concepts are applied at all levels, i.e., subatomic, atomic, molecular (or nano), microscopic, and macroscopic. Application of the basic concepts at the microscopic and macroscopic levels is shown in Table 1.1.

Conservation equations at the microscopic level are called *equations of change*, and they are written in tensor notation. When these equations are applied to a specific geometry, they become partial differential equations in three independent space variables and time. The number of unknowns in the equations of change exceeds the number of independent equations unless the material properties are identified. The additional equations describing material behavior are called *constitutive* (or phenomenological) *equations*, and the parameters in the constitutive equations are called *material properties*. Once the equations of change and the constitutive equations are solved using the initial and/or boundary conditions describing the system of interest, the results are the *theoretical solutions* leading to velocity, temperature, pressure, and concentration profiles.

Integration of the equations of change over the volume of a system gives the basic concepts at the macroscopic level. Integration eliminates position dependence, and the resulting equations are ordinary differential equations, with time as the only independent variable. These equations are

Table 1.1

Levels of Application of the Basic Concepts

Level	Theory	Experiment
Microscopic	Equations of change	Constitutive equations
Macroscopic	Design equations	Process correlations

called *design equations* or *macroscopic balances*. When the mathematical description at the microscopic level is not possible, theoretical solutions are replaced by experimental information called *process correlations*. Process correlations, however, are limited to a specific geometry, equipment configuration, boundary conditions, and material.

1.2 DEFINITIONS

The functional notation

$$\varphi = \varphi(x, y, z, t) \tag{1.2}$$

indicates that there are three *independent space variables* (x, y, z) and one *independent time variable* (t). The φ on the right side of Eq. (1.2) represents the functional form, and the φ on the left side represents the value of the dependent variable, φ.

1.2.1 STEADY-STATE

The term *steady-state* means that at a particular location in space, the dependent variable does not change as a function of time. If the dependent variable is φ, then

$$\left(\frac{\partial \varphi}{\partial t}\right)_{x,y,z} = 0 \tag{1.3}$$

The partial derivative notation indicates that the dependent variable is a function of more than one independent variable. In this particular case, the independent variables are x, y, z, and t. The specified location in space is indicated by the subscripts (x, y, z), and Eq. (1.3) implies that φ is not a function of time. When an ordinary derivative is used, i.e., $d\varphi/dt = 0$, this implies that φ is a constant. It is important to distinguish between partial and ordinary derivatives because the conclusions are very different.

Each process experiences an unsteady-state period before reaching steady-state conditions. The time it takes for the process to reach steady-state is dependent on the characteristics of the process. While for some processes this period is of the order of seconds, it may be of the order of hours (or days) for other processes. Mathematically speaking, processes reach steady-state conditions as time approaches infinity, i.e., $t \to \infty$.

1.2.2 UNIFORM

The term *uniform* means that at a particular instant in time, the dependent variable is not a function of position. This requires that all three of the partial derivatives with respect to position be zero. In other words, the gradient of a quantity must be zero, i.e.,

$$\nabla \varphi = 0 \tag{1.4}$$

for a uniform condition to exist with respect to that quantity.

1.2.3 EQUILIBRIUM

A system is in *equilibrium* if both steady-state and uniform conditions are met simultaneously. An equilibrium system does not exhibit any variations with respect to position or time. *Property correlation* is the name given to the response of a material under equilibrium conditions. The ideal gas law is an example of a thermodynamic property correlation that is called an *equation of state*.

1.2.4 FLUX

The flux of a certain quantity is defined by

$$\text{Flux of a quantity} = \frac{\text{Flow of a quantity/Time}}{\text{Area}} = \frac{\text{Flow rate of a quantity}}{\text{Area}}, \tag{1.5}$$

where area is normal to the direction of flow. The units of momentum, energy, mass, and molar fluxes are Pa (N/m^2 or $kg/m.s^2$), W/m^2 ($J/m^2.s$), $kg/m^2.s$, and $kmol/m^2.s$, respectively. The flux of a quantity may be either constant or dependent on position. Thus, the rate of a quantity can be determined as

$$\text{Rate} = \begin{cases} (\text{Flux})(\text{Area}) & \text{If flux is constant} \\[2ex] \displaystyle\iint_A \text{Flux } dA & \text{If flux is position dependent} \end{cases} \tag{1.6}$$

The total flux of any quantity is the sum of the molecular and convective fluxes. The fluxes arising from potential gradients or driving forces are called *molecular fluxes*. Molecular fluxes are expressed in the form of *constitutive equations* for momentum, energy, and mass transport. Momentum, energy, and mass can also be transported by bulk fluid motion or bulk flow, and the resulting flux is called *convective flux*.

1.3 MOLECULAR FLUX

Materials behave differently when subjected to the same gradients. Constitutive equations identify the characteristics of a particular material. For example, if the gradient is momentum, then the viscosity is defined by the constitutive equation called *Newton's law of viscosity*. If the gradient is energy, then the thermal conductivity is defined by *Fourier's law of heat conduction*. If the gradient is concentration, then the diffusion coefficient is defined by *Fick's first law of diffusion*. Viscosity, thermal conductivity, and diffusion coefficient are called *transport properties*.

1.3.1 NEWTON'S LAW OF VISCOSITY

Consider a fluid contained between two large parallel plates of area A, separated by a very small distance H. The system is initially at rest, but at time $t = 0$ the lower plate is set in motion in the z-direction at a constant velocity V by applying a force F in the z-direction, while the upper plate is kept stationary. The resulting velocity profiles are shown in Figure 1.1 for various times. At $t = 0$, the velocity is zero everywhere except at the lower plate, which has a velocity V. Then, the velocity distribution starts to develop as a function of time. As $t \to \infty$, i.e., under steady-state conditions, a linear velocity distribution is obtained.

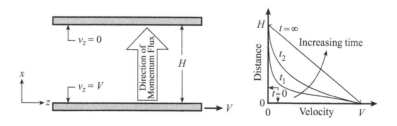

Figure 1.1 Velocity profile development in flow between parallel plates.

Experimental results show that the force, F, required to maintain the motion of the lower plate per unit area (or momentum flux) is proportional to the velocity gradient, i.e.,

$$\underbrace{\frac{F}{A}}_{\substack{\text{Momentum}\\\text{flux}}} = \underbrace{\mu}_{\substack{\text{Transport}\\\text{property}}} \underbrace{\frac{V}{H}}_{\substack{\text{Velocity}\\\text{gradient}}} \tag{1.7}$$

and the proportionality constant, μ, is the *viscosity*. Equation (1.7) is a macroscopic equation. The microscopic form of this equation is given by

$$\tau_{xz} = -\mu \frac{dv_z}{dx} = -\mu \dot{\gamma}_{xz} \tag{1.8}$$

which is known as *Newton's law of viscosity*, and any fluid obeying Eq. (1.8) is called a *Newtonian fluid*. The term $\dot{\gamma}_{xz}$ is called the *rate of strain*,[1] *rate of deformation*, or *shear rate*. The term τ_{xz} is called *shear stress*. It contains two subscripts: z, which represents the direction of force, and x, which represents the direction of the normal to the surface on which the force is acting. Therefore, it is possible to interpret τ_{xz} as the flux of z-momentum in the x-direction. Since the velocity gradient is negative, i.e., v_z decreases with increasing x, a negative sign is placed on the right side of Eq. (1.8) so that the stress in tension is positive.

In SI units, τ_{xz} is in N/m^2 (Pa), dv_z/dx in $1/s$, and μ in Pa.s or kg/m.s.

1.3.2 FOURIER'S LAW OF HEAT CONDUCTION

Consider a slab of solid material of area A between two large parallel plates of a distance H apart. Initially, the solid material is at a temperature T_o throughout. Then, the lower plate is suddenly brought to a slightly higher temperature T_w and maintained at that temperature. The second law of thermodynamics states that heat flows spontaneously from the higher temperature T_w to the lower temperature T_o. As time proceeds, the temperature profile in the slab changes, and ultimately a linear steady-state temperature is attained as shown in Figure 1.2.

Experimental measurements made at steady-state indicate that the rate of heat flow, $\dot{Q}$, per unit area is proportional to the temperature gradient, i.e.,

$$\underbrace{\frac{\dot{Q}}{A}}_{\substack{\text{Energy}\\\text{flux}}} = \underbrace{k}_{\substack{\text{Transport}\\\text{property}}} \underbrace{\frac{T_w - T_o}{H}}_{\substack{\text{Temperature}\\\text{gradient}}} \tag{1.9}$$

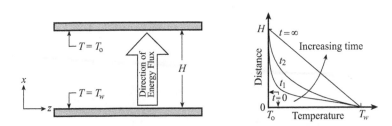

Figure 1.2 Temperature profile development in a solid slab between two plates.

---

[1] Strain is defined as deformation per unit length. For example, if a spring of original length L_o is stretched to a length L, then the strain is $(L - L_o)/L_o$.

and the proportionality constant, k, is the *thermal conductivity*. The microscopic form of Eq. (1.9) is known as *Fourier's law of heat conduction* and is given by

$$q_x = -k\frac{dT}{dx},\tag{1.10}$$

where q_x represents the conductive energy flux in the x-direction. The negative sign in Eq. (1.10) indicates that heat flows in the direction of decreasing temperature.

In SI units, q_x is in W/m^2, dT/dx in K/m, and k in W/m.K.

1.3.3 FICK'S FIRST LAW OF DIFFUSION

Consider two large parallel plates separated by a small distance H. The lower one is coated with a material A that has a very low solubility in the stagnant fluid B filling the space between the plates. Suppose that the saturation concentration of A is ρ_{A_o} and A undergoes a rapid chemical reaction at the upper plate surface so that its concentration is zero at that surface. At $t = 0$ the lower plate is exposed to the fluid B, and as time proceeds, the concentration profile develops as shown in Figure 1.3. Since the solubility of A is low, an almost linear distribution is obtained under steady conditions.

Experimental measurements indicate that the mass flow rate of A, w_A, per unit area is proportional to the concentration gradient, i.e.,

$$\underbrace{\frac{w_A}{A}}_{\substack{\text{Mass} \\ \text{flux of } A}} = \underbrace{\mathcal{D}_{AB}}_{\substack{\text{Transport} \\ \text{property}}} \underbrace{\frac{\rho_{A_o}}{H}}_{\substack{\text{Concentration} \\ \text{gradient}}}\tag{1.11}$$

and the proportionality constant, $\mathcal{D}_{AB}$, is the *diffusion coefficient* (*or diffusivity*) of species A through B. The microscopic form of Eq. (1.11) is known as *Fick's first law of diffusion* and is given by

$$j_{A_x} = -\mathcal{D}_{AB}\,\rho\,\frac{d\omega_A}{dx},\tag{1.12}$$

where j_{A_x} and ω_A represent the molecular mass flux of species A in the x-direction and mass fraction of species A, respectively. The term ρ is the total density of the mixture, i.e., $\rho_A + \rho_B$.

In SI units, j_{A_x} is in $\text{kg/m}^2\text{.s}$, ρ in kg/m^3, $d\omega_A/dx$ in m^{-1}, and $\mathcal{D}_{AB}$ in m^2/s.

1.3.4 DIMENSIONLESS NUMBERS

In reality, Newton's "law" of viscosity, Fourier's "law" of heat conduction, and Fick's first "law" of diffusion are not laws[2] but defining equations for viscosity, μ, thermal conductivity, k, and diffusion coefficient, $\mathcal{D}_{AB}$. These equations can be generalized as

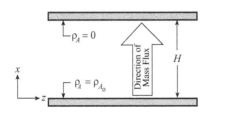
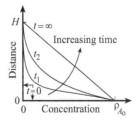

Figure 1.3 Concentration profile development between parallel plates.

---

[2]These constitutive equations are postulated and cannot be derived from the fundamental principles. The mathematical form of a constitutive equation is constrained by the second law of thermodynamics so as to yield positive entropy generation.

$$
\left(\begin{array}{c} \text{Molecular flux of} \\ \text{Quantity} \end{array} \right) = \left(\begin{array}{c} \text{Transport} \\ \text{property} \end{array} \right) \left(\begin{array}{c} \text{Gradient of} \\ \text{driving force} \end{array} \right) \quad (1.13)
$$

However, they are not completely analogous since the transport properties $(\mu, k, \mathcal{D}_{AB})$ have different units. Equations (1.8), (1.10), and (1.12) can be rearranged in the following forms:

$$
\tau_{xz} = -\frac{\mu}{\rho} \frac{d(\rho v_z)}{dx} \qquad \rho = \text{constant} \qquad \rho v_z = \text{momentum/volume} \quad (1.14)
$$

$$
q_x = -\frac{k}{\rho \widehat{C}_P} \frac{d(\rho \widehat{C}_P T)}{dx} \qquad \rho \widehat{C}_P = \text{constant} \qquad \rho \widehat{C}_P T = \text{energy/volume} \quad (1.15)
$$

$$
j_{A_x} = -\mathcal{D}_{AB} \frac{d\rho_A}{dx} \qquad \rho = \text{constant} \qquad \rho_A = \text{mass of } A/\text{volume} \quad (1.16)
$$

The term μ/ρ in Eq. (1.14) is called *momentum diffusivity* or *kinematic viscosity*, and the term $k/\rho\widehat{C}_P$ in Eq. (1.15) is called *thermal diffusivity*. Momentum and thermal diffusivities are designated by ν and α, respectively. Note that the terms ν, α, and $\mathcal{D}_{AB}$ all have the same unit, m^2/s, and Eqs. (1.14)–(1.16) are expressed in the general form as

$$
\left(\begin{array}{c} \text{Molecular flux of} \\ \text{Quantity} \end{array} \right) = (\text{Diffusivity}) \left(\begin{array}{c} \text{Gradient of} \\ \text{Quantity/Volume} \end{array} \right) \quad (1.17)
$$

Since the terms ν, α, and $\mathcal{D}_{AB}$ all have the same unit, the ratio of any two of these diffusivities results in a dimensionless number. For example, the ratio of the momentum diffusivity to thermal diffusivity gives the *Prandtl number*, Pr:

$$
\text{Pr} = \frac{\nu}{\alpha} = \frac{\widehat{C}_P \mu}{k} \quad (1.18)
$$

The *Schmidt number*, Sc, is defined as the ratio of the momentum to mass diffusivities:

$$
\text{Sc} = \frac{\nu}{\mathcal{D}_{AB}} = \frac{\mu}{\rho \mathcal{D}_{AB}} \quad (1.19)
$$

For gases and liquids, the order of magnitude estimates of the Prandtl and Schmidt numbers are given by

$$
O(\text{Pr}) \sim \left\{ \begin{array}{ll} 1 & \text{Gases} \\ 10 & \text{Liquids} \end{array} \right. \qquad \text{and} \qquad O(\text{Sc}) \sim \left\{ \begin{array}{ll} 1 & \text{Gases} \\ 1,000 & \text{Liquids} \end{array} \right.
$$

Finally, the ratio of the thermal to mass diffusivities gives the *Lewis number*, Le:

$$
\text{Le} = \frac{\alpha}{\mathcal{D}_{AB}} = \frac{k}{\rho \widehat{C}_P \mathcal{D}_{AB}} = \frac{\text{Sc}}{\text{Pr}} \quad (1.20)
$$

1.4 CONVECTIVE FLUX

The convective flux or bulk flux of a quantity is expressed as

$$
\left(\begin{array}{c} \text{Convective flux of} \\ \text{Quantity} \end{array} \right) = (\text{Quantity/Volume}) \left(\begin{array}{c} \text{Characteristic} \\ \text{velocity} \end{array} \right) \quad (1.21)
$$

For a single phase and a single component system, there is no ambiguity in defining the characteristic velocity. In the case of a single phase but multicomponent system, however, characteristic velocity can be defined in different forms. These will be covered in Section 2.1.2.

1.5 TOTAL FLUX

Since the total flux of any quantity is the sum of its molecular and convective fluxes, then from Eqs. (1.17) and (1.21)

$$
\begin{pmatrix} \text{Total flux of} \\ \text{Quantity} \end{pmatrix} = \underbrace{(\text{Diffusivity}) \begin{pmatrix} \text{Gradient of} \\ \text{Quantity/Volume} \end{pmatrix}}_{\text{Molecular flux}} + \underbrace{\begin{pmatrix} \dfrac{\text{Quantity}}{\text{Volume}} \end{pmatrix} \begin{pmatrix} \text{Characteristic} \\ \text{velocity} \end{pmatrix}}_{\text{Convective flux}}
$$

(1.22)

The ratio of the convective flux to the molecular flux is given by

$$
\frac{\text{Convective flux}}{\text{Molecular flux}} = \frac{(\text{Quantity/Volume})(\text{Characteristic velocity})}{(\text{Diffusivity})(\text{Gradient of Quantity/Volume})}
$$

(1.23)

Since the gradient of a quantity represents the variation of that particular quantity over a characteristic length, the gradient of "Quantity/Volume" can be expressed as

$$
\text{Gradient of "Quantity/Volume"} = \frac{\text{Quantity/Volume}}{\text{Characteristic length}}
$$

(1.24)

The use of Eq. (1.24) in Eq. (1.23) gives

$$
\frac{\text{Convective flux}}{\text{Molecular flux}} = \frac{(\text{Characteristic length})(\text{Characteristic velocity})}{\text{Diffusivity}}
$$

(1.25)

The ratio of the convective flux to the molecular flux is known as the *Peclet number*, Pe. Therefore, Peclet numbers for heat and mass transfers are

$$
\text{Pe}_H = \frac{L_{ch} v_{ch}}{\alpha} \quad \text{and} \quad \text{Pe}_M = \frac{L_{ch} v_{ch}}{\mathcal{D}_{AB}}
$$

(1.26)

Hence, the total flux of any quantity is given by

$$
\text{Total flux} = \begin{cases} \text{Molecular flux} & \text{Pe} \ll 1 \\ \text{Molecular flux} + \text{Convective flux} & \text{Pe} \simeq 1 \\ \text{Convective flux} & \text{Pe} \gg 1 \end{cases}
$$

(1.27)

1.6 TRANSFER COEFFICIENTS

In engineering calculations, we are interested in the determination of the rate of momentum, heat, and mass transfer from one phase to another across the phase interface. This can be accomplished by first evaluating the total flux of a quantity using Eq. (1.22) and then integrating it over the interfacial area. For this purpose, equations of change and constitutive equations must be solved to obtain the distribution of "quantity/volume" as a function of position and time. In most cases, however, analytical solutions cannot be obtained. In that case, we resort to experimental data and correlate the results by the transfer coefficients, namely the friction factor, the heat transfer coefficient, and the mass transfer coefficient.

The shear stress (or momentum flux) at the interface, τ_{int}, is expressed in terms of a dimensionless term called the *friction factor*, f, in the form

$$
\boxed{\tau_{int} = \frac{1}{2} \rho v_{ch}^2 f,}
$$

(1.28)

where v_{ch} is the characteristic velocity.

The heat flux at the interface, q_{int}, is expressed in terms of the *heat transfer coefficient*, h, as

$$\boxed{q_{int} = h\,\Delta T_{ch},}\tag{1.29}$$

where ΔT_{ch} is the characteristic temperature difference. In the literature, Eq. (1.29) is known as *Newton's law of cooling*.[3] The unit of the heat transfer coefficient is $W/m^2.K$. It depends on the fluid flow mechanism, fluid properties (density, viscosity, thermal conductivity, and heat capacity), and flow geometry.

The molar flux of species A at the interface, $N_{A_{int}}$, is expressed in terms of the *mass transfer coefficient*, k_c, as

$$\boxed{N_{A_{int}} = k_c\,(\Delta c_A)_{ch},}\tag{1.30}$$

where $(\Delta c_A)_{ch}$ is the characteristic molar concentration difference of species A. Equation (1.30) may be called *Newton's law of mass transfer* as suggested by Slattery (1999). The unit of the mass transfer coefficient is m/s. It depends on the fluid flow mechanism, fluid properties (density, viscosity, and diffusion coefficient), and flow geometry.

1.6.1 DIMENSIONLESS NUMBERS

Rearrangement of Eqs. (1.28)–(1.30) gives

$$\tau_{int} = \frac{1}{2}f v_{ch}\,\Delta(\rho\,v_{ch})\tag{1.31}$$

$$q_{int} = \frac{h}{\rho\,\widehat{C}_P}\Delta(\rho\,\widehat{C}_P T_{ch})\tag{1.32}$$

$$N_{A_{int}} = k_c\,\Delta c_{A_{ch}}\tag{1.33}$$

Note that the terms $f v_{ch}/2$, $h/\rho\widehat{C}_P$, and k_c all have the same unit, m/s. Thus, the ratio of these quantities yields dimensionless Stanton numbers as follows:

$$\text{Heat transfer Stanton number} \; = \; \text{St}_H = \frac{h}{\rho\,\widehat{C}_P v_{ch}}\tag{1.34}$$

$$\text{Mass transfer Stanton number} \; = \; \text{St}_M = \frac{k_c}{v_{ch}}\tag{1.35}$$

Since the term $f/2$ is dimensionless itself, it is omitted in Eqs. (1.34) and (1.35).

REFERENCE

Slattery, J. C. 1999. *Advanced Transport Phenomena*. Cambridge: Cambridge University Press.

---

[3]Newton's law of cooling is not a law but a defining equation for the heat transfer coefficient. In addition, the use of the word "cooling" is misleading and confusing since Eq. (1.29) is used whether the system of interest is heated or cooled.

2 Conservation of Chemical Species

The *conservation of species equation*, also referred to as the *species continuity equation*, is the governing equation for mass transfer. The transport property appearing in this equation is the diffusion coefficient. The solution of the species continuity equation requires the initial and/or boundary conditions to be specified. This chapter provides the foundations for the formulation of mass transfer problems.

Since more than one species is involved in the transport process, one has to be precise in defining concentrations, velocities, and mass/molar fluxes. Velocity of the mixture as a whole is different from individual species velocities. As a result, mass and molar fluxes are defined with respect to various reference velocity frames. These definitions are succinctly given in Section 2.1, and the equations relating different types of mass and molar fluxes are developed.

In Section 2.2, the derivation of the species continuity equation is given in terms of the total flux. Formulation of the rate of generation by a homogeneous reaction, which appears as a source term in the continuity equation, is also presented.

The total flux is the summation of diffusive and convective fluxes. Depending on the choice of the diffusive flux (mass and molar) and the characteristic velocity used in the convective flux (mass-average, molar-average, and volume-average), different forms of the species continuity equation are given in Section 2.3.

Section 2.4 is devoted to the governing equations for mass transfer in binary systems. In that respect, Fick's first and second laws are introduced.

Contrary to the common belief, it is the gradient of partial molar Gibbs energy and not the concentration gradient that is responsible for mass transfer taking place. Mass transfer is also facilitated by the existence of other driving forces. The thermodynamics preliminaries covered in Section 2.5 explain these concepts.

In Section 2.6, various equations available to estimate the diffusion coefficients in gases and liquids are presented.

Formulation of a mass transport problem is not complete unless the initial and/or boundary conditions are specified. Various boundary conditions encountered in mass transfer are explained in Section 2.7.

2.1 DEFINITIONS

2.1.1 CONCENTRATIONS

The mass density of species i, ρ_i, is the mass of species i, m_i, per unit volume of the mixture, V_{mix}

$$\rho_i = \frac{m_i}{V_{mix}} \tag{2.1}$$

In a multicomponent mixture consisting of $\mathcal{N}$ species, the total mass density, ρ, is the sum of all species' densities present in the mixture and is defined by

$$\rho = \sum_{k=1}^{\mathcal{N}} \rho_k \tag{2.2}$$

The mass fraction of species i, ω_i, is defined as the mass of species i per unit mass of the mixture, i.e.,

$$\omega_i = \frac{\rho_i}{\rho} = \frac{\rho_i}{\displaystyle\sum_{k=1}^{\mathcal{N}} \rho_k} \tag{2.3}$$

The molar concentration of species i, c_i, is the moles of species i per unit volume of the mixture and is defined by

$$c_i = \frac{\rho_i}{M_i}, \tag{2.4}$$

where M_i represents the molecular weight of species i. The total molar concentration, c, is the sum of all species' molar concentrations present in the mixture and is defined by

$$c = \sum_{k=1}^{\mathcal{N}} c_k \tag{2.5}$$

The mole fraction of species i is defined as the moles of species i per unit mole of the mixture, i.e.,[1]

$$x_i \text{ (or } y_i) = \frac{c_i}{c} = \frac{c_i}{\displaystyle\sum_{k=1}^{\mathcal{N}} c_k} \tag{2.6}$$

Mole fractions are converted to mass fractions or *vice versa* by the following formulas:

$$\omega_i = \frac{x_i M_i}{\displaystyle\sum_{k=1}^{\mathcal{N}} x_k M_k} = x_i \frac{M_i}{M} \quad \text{and} \quad x_i = \frac{\dfrac{\omega_i}{M_i}}{\displaystyle\sum_{k=1}^{\mathcal{N}} \frac{\omega_k}{M_k}} = \omega_i \frac{M}{M_i} \tag{2.7}$$

Note that the molecular weight of the mixture, M, is defined by

$$M = \sum_{k=1}^{\mathcal{N}} x_k M_k = \left(\sum_{k=1}^{\mathcal{N}} \frac{\omega_k}{M_k} \right)^{-1} \tag{2.8}$$

In expressing mass and/or molar concentrations, one has to be careful when defining volumetric units. For example, if the molar concentration is given as mol/cm^3, does cm^3 represent the volume of the mixture or the volume of the pure component? The following example clarifies this point.

Example 2.1 When two liquids, A and B, are mixed to form a homogeneous mixture (for example, water and ethyl alcohol), the molar volume of the resulting mixture, $\widetilde{V}_{mix}$, is given by

$$\widetilde{V}_{mix} = x_A \widetilde{V}_A + x_B \widetilde{V}_B + \Delta \widetilde{V}_{mix}, \tag{1}$$

where $\widetilde{V}_A$ and $\widetilde{V}_B$ represent molar volumes of pure A and pure B, respectively, and $\Delta \widetilde{V}_{mix}$ is the molar volume change on mixing. For an ideal mixture, $\Delta \widetilde{V}_{mix} = 0$, and the molar concentration of the mixture, c, is expressed as

$$c = \frac{1}{x_A \widetilde{V}_A + x_B \widetilde{V}_B} \tag{2}$$

---

[1] In the literature, mole fractions in liquid and vapor mixtures are represented by x_i and y_i, respectively. In the derivation of the general equations, x will be used throughout the text to represent the mole fraction. In example problems involving a gas phase, x will be replaced by y.

Molar volumes of pure A and B are represented by

$$\widetilde{V}_A = \frac{M_A}{\rho_A} = \frac{1}{\dfrac{\rho_A}{M_A}} \quad \text{and} \quad \widetilde{V}_B = \frac{M_B}{\rho_B} = \frac{1}{\dfrac{\rho_B}{M_B}} \tag{3}$$

The use of Eq. (2.4) reduces Eq. (3) to

$$\widetilde{V}_A = \frac{1}{c_A} \quad \text{and} \quad \widetilde{V}_B = \frac{1}{c_B} \tag{4}$$

Substitution of Eq. (4) into Eq. (2) yields

$$c = \frac{1}{\dfrac{x_A}{c_A} + \dfrac{x_B}{c_B}} \tag{5}$$

Since $c_i = cx_i$, Eq. (5) becomes

$$c = \frac{1}{\dfrac{1}{c} + \dfrac{1}{c}} = \frac{c}{2} \quad \Rightarrow \quad 1 \overset{?}{=} \frac{1}{2} \tag{6}$$

What went wrong in the derivation?

Solution

The conflict arises as a result of using two different types of volumetric units. $\widetilde{V}_A$ is the molar volume of pure A expressed as m^3 of pure A/mol of A. On the other hand, c_A is the molar concentration of A in the mixture expressed as mol of A/m^3 of mixture. Therefore, Eq. (4) is not correct.

2.1.2 VELOCITIES

The species present in a multicomponent mixture move with different velocities. Let $\mathbf{v}_i$ be the velocity of species i relative to fixed coordinates. The characteristic (or reference) velocity of the mixture is calculated by averaging the species velocities as

$$\mathbf{v}_{ch} = \sum_{k=1}^{\mathcal{N}} \beta_k \mathbf{v}_k, \tag{2.9}$$

where β_k is the weighting factor with the following constraint:

$$\sum_{k=1}^{\mathcal{N}} \beta_k = 1 \tag{2.10}$$

The three most common characteristic velocities are given in Table 2.1. The term $\overline{V}_k$ in the definition of volume-average velocity is the *partial molar volume of species k*, defined by

$$\overline{V}_k = \left(\frac{\partial V_{mix}}{\partial n_k} \right)_{T,P,n_j \neq k} \tag{2.11}$$

The subscripts on the partial derivative mean that temperature, pressure, and number of moles of all components other than k are kept constant. It should be kept in mind that, besides temperature and pressure, $\overline{V}_k$ is dependent on the composition of the mixture. Partial molar volumes are determined

Table 2.1
Common Characteristic Velocities

Characteristic Velocity	Weighting Factor	Formulation	
Mass-average	Mass fraction (ω_k)	$\mathbf{v} = \displaystyle\sum_{k=1}^{N} \omega_k \mathbf{v}_k = \frac{1}{\rho} \sum_{k=1}^{N} \rho_k \mathbf{v}_k$	(A)
Molar-average	Mole fraction (x_k)	$\mathbf{v}^* = \displaystyle\sum_{k=1}^{N} x_k \mathbf{v}_k = \frac{1}{c} \sum_{k=1}^{N} c_k \mathbf{v}_k$	(B)
Volume-average	Volume fraction $(c_k \overline{V}_k)$	$\mathbf{v}^\blacksquare = \displaystyle\sum_{k=1}^{N} c_k \overline{V}_k \mathbf{v}_k$	(C)

experimentally. In the absence of experimental data, partial molar volumes can be approximated by pure component molar volumes, i.e., $\overline{V}_k = \widetilde{V}_k$.

Characteristic velocities have found use in problems related to the transport of species. In general, both magnitudes and directions of these three average velocities are different from each other.

Example 2.2 Calculate the molar-average velocity for a binary mixture of A and B if the following quantities are provided:

$$x_A = \frac{1}{4} \qquad 4M_A = M_B \qquad \mathbf{v} = 10\,\text{mm/min} \qquad \mathbf{v}_A - \mathbf{v}^* = 6\,\text{mm/min}$$

Solution

Note that
$$\mathbf{v}_A - \mathbf{v}^* = \mathbf{v}_A - (x_A \mathbf{v}_A + x_B \mathbf{v}_B) = 6 \qquad \Rightarrow \qquad x_B(\mathbf{v}_A - \mathbf{v}_B) = 6$$

or
$$\frac{3}{4}(\mathbf{v}_A - \mathbf{v}_B) = 6 \qquad \Rightarrow \qquad \mathbf{v}_A - \mathbf{v}_B = 8 \tag{1}$$

The use of Eq. (2.7) gives the mass fraction of species A as

$$\omega_A = \frac{\dfrac{1}{4} M_A}{\dfrac{1}{4} M_A + \dfrac{3}{4}(4M_A)} = \frac{1}{13}$$

Using the definition of mass-average velocity, one can write

$$\frac{1}{13}\mathbf{v}_A + \frac{12}{13}\mathbf{v}_B = 10 \qquad \Rightarrow \qquad \mathbf{v}_A + 12\mathbf{v}_B = 130 \tag{2}$$

Simultaneous solution of Eqs. (1) and (2) gives

$$\mathbf{v}_A = \frac{226}{13}\,\text{mm/min} \qquad \text{and} \qquad \mathbf{v}_B = \frac{122}{13}\,\text{mm/min}$$

Thus, the molar-average velocity is

$$\mathbf{v}^* = \mathbf{v}_A - 6 = \frac{226}{13} - 6 = \frac{148}{13}\,\text{mm/min}$$

2.1.3 MASS AND MOLAR FLUXES

As stated in Section 1.2.4, the flux of a certain quantity is defined by

$$\text{Flux} = \frac{\text{Flow of a quantity/Time}}{\text{Area}} = \frac{\text{Flow rate}}{\text{Area}}, \tag{2.12}$$

where area is normal to the direction of flow. The units of mass and molar fluxes are $kg/m^2.s$ and $kmol/m^2.s$, respectively.

In a multicomponent mixture consisting of $\mathcal{N}$ species, total mass flux of species i, i.e., mass of i per unit area per unit time, is the sum of the diffusive (or molecular) and convective (or advective) fluxes

$$\begin{pmatrix} \text{Total mass flux} \\ \text{of species } i \end{pmatrix} = \begin{pmatrix} \text{Diffusive mass flux} \\ \text{of species } i \end{pmatrix} + \begin{pmatrix} \text{Convective mass flux} \\ \text{of species } i \end{pmatrix} \tag{2.13}$$

The total mass flux of species i is given by

$$\boxed{\begin{pmatrix} \text{Total mass flux} \\ \text{of species } i \end{pmatrix} = \begin{pmatrix} \dfrac{\text{Mass of } i}{\text{Volume}} \end{pmatrix} \begin{pmatrix} \text{Velocity} \\ \text{of species } i \end{pmatrix}} \tag{2.14}$$

On the other hand, convective mass flux is expressed as

$$\boxed{\begin{pmatrix} \text{Convective mass flux} \\ \text{of species } i \end{pmatrix} = \begin{pmatrix} \dfrac{\text{Mass of } i}{\text{Volume}} \end{pmatrix} \begin{pmatrix} \text{Characteristic} \\ \text{velocity} \end{pmatrix}} \tag{2.15}$$

Substitution of Eqs. (2.14) and (2.15) into Eq. (2.13) gives the diffusive mass flux of species i in the form

$$\boxed{\begin{aligned} \begin{pmatrix} \text{Diffusive mass flux} \\ \text{of species } i \end{pmatrix} &= \begin{pmatrix} \text{Total mass flux} \\ \text{of species } i \end{pmatrix} - \begin{pmatrix} \text{Convective mass flux} \\ \text{of species } i \end{pmatrix} \\ &= \begin{pmatrix} \dfrac{\text{Mass of } i}{\text{Volume}} \end{pmatrix} \left[\begin{pmatrix} \text{Velocity} \\ \text{of species } i \end{pmatrix} - \begin{pmatrix} \text{Characteristic} \\ \text{velocity} \end{pmatrix} \right] \end{aligned}} \tag{2.16}$$

Similarly, the diffusive molar flux of species i is defined by

$$\boxed{\begin{pmatrix} \text{Diffusive molar flux} \\ \text{of species } i \end{pmatrix} = \begin{pmatrix} \dfrac{\text{Mole of } i}{\text{Volume}} \end{pmatrix} \left[\begin{pmatrix} \text{Velocity} \\ \text{of species } i \end{pmatrix} - \begin{pmatrix} \text{Characteristic} \\ \text{velocity} \end{pmatrix} \right]} \tag{2.17}$$

In the literature, it is customary to use lowercase and capital letters for representing mass and molar fluxes, respectively. Note that dividing the mass flux by the molecular weight gives the molar flux.

Let $\mathbf{v}_i$ be the velocity of species i passing through a fixed differential surface area dA as shown in Figure 2.1. According to Eq. (2.14), the total mass flux vector of species i relative to fixed coordinates, $\mathbf{n}_i$, is expressed as

$$\boxed{\mathbf{n}_i = \rho_i \mathbf{v}_i} \tag{2.18}$$

Figure 2.1 Schematic of a mass flux $\mathbf{n}_i$ passing through a stationary differential surface area dA.

Let λ be the unit normal vector[2] perpendicular to dA and $\mathbf{n}_i$ be the total mass flux vector of species i passing through dA. The dot product of the vectors λ and $\mathbf{n}_i$, i.e., $\lambda \cdot \mathbf{n}_i$, gives the component of the mass flux vector in the direction of λ, which is perpendicular to dA. Thus, mass flow rate of species i passing through the total surface area A is given by

$$\text{Mass flow rate of species } i = w_i = \iint_A \lambda \cdot \mathbf{n}_i \, dA \tag{2.19}$$

Dividing Eq. (2.18) by the molecular weight of species i gives the total molar flux vector of species i relative to fixed coordinates, $\mathbf{N}_i$, as

$$\boxed{\mathbf{N}_i = c_i \mathbf{v}_i} \tag{2.20}$$

so that

$$\text{Molar flow rate of species } i = \mathcal{W}_i = \iint_A \lambda \cdot \mathbf{N}_i \, dA \tag{2.21}$$

Example 2.3 The total mass flux vector for species i is given by

$$\mathbf{n}_i(\text{g/cm}^2.\text{s}) = 3.5 \times 10^{-8} xy \mathbf{e}_x + 7.6 \times 10^{-7} x^2 z \mathbf{e}_y - 1 \times 10^{-8} yz \mathbf{e}_z,$$

where $\mathbf{e}_x$, $\mathbf{e}_y$, and $\mathbf{e}_z$ are the unit vectors in the direction of the x, y, and z axes, respectively. Calculate the mass flow rate of species i in the y-direction through the rectangular surface perpendicular to the xz-plane as shown in the figure below.

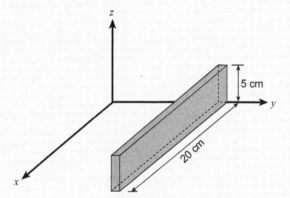

Solution

Since $\lambda = \mathbf{e}_y$, the component of the total mass flux vector in the y-direction is

$$\mathbf{e}_y \cdot \mathbf{n}_i = 7.6 \times 10^{-7} x^2 z$$

The mass flow rate is

$$w_i = \int_0^{0.05} \int_0^{0.2} 7.6 \times 10^{-7} x^2 z \, dx dz = 2.533 \times 10^{-12} \text{g/s}$$

---

[2]In the literature, unit normal vector to the surface is usually designated by $\mathbf{n}$. Since $\mathbf{n}$ expresses mass flux, λ is used for unit normal vector to avoid confusion.

The characteristic velocities defined in Table 2.1 can also be expressed in terms of mass and molar fluxes as follows:

$$\mathbf{v} = \frac{1}{\rho} \sum_{k=1}^{N} \rho_k \mathbf{v}_k = \frac{1}{\rho} \sum_{k=1}^{N} \mathbf{n}_k \tag{2.22}$$

$$\mathbf{v}^* = \frac{1}{c} \sum_{k=1}^{N} c_k \mathbf{v}_k = \frac{1}{c} \sum_{k=1}^{N} \mathbf{N}_k \tag{2.23}$$

$$\mathbf{v}^\blacksquare = \sum_{k=1}^{N} c_k \overline{V}_k \mathbf{v}_k = \sum_{k=1}^{N} \overline{V}_k \mathbf{N}_k \tag{2.24}$$

Depending on the choice of characteristic velocity, three different types of diffusive (or molecular) mass fluxes can be defined according to Eq. (2.16):

$$\mathbf{j}_i = \rho_i(\mathbf{v}_i - \mathbf{v}) \quad \text{Diffusive mass flux of } i \text{ relative to mass-average velocity} \tag{2.25}$$

$$\mathbf{j}_i^* = \rho_i(\mathbf{v}_i - \mathbf{v}^*) \quad \text{Diffusive mass flux of } i \text{ relative to molar-average velocity} \tag{2.26}$$

$$\mathbf{j}_i^\blacksquare = \rho_i(\mathbf{v}_i - \mathbf{v}^\blacksquare) \quad \text{Diffusive mass flux of } i \text{ relative to volume-average velocity} \tag{2.27}$$

These three fluxes are shown in Figure 2.2. On the other hand, the following diffusive molar flux expressions can be written according to Eq. (2.17):

$$\mathbf{J}_i = c_i(\mathbf{v}_i - \mathbf{v}) \quad \text{Diffusive molar flux of } i \text{ relative to mass-average velocity} \tag{2.28}$$

$$\mathbf{J}_i^* = c_i(\mathbf{v}_i - \mathbf{v}^*) \quad \text{Diffusive molar flux of } i \text{ relative to molar-average velocity} \tag{2.29}$$

$$\mathbf{J}_i^\blacksquare = c_i(\mathbf{v}_i - \mathbf{v}^\blacksquare) \quad \text{Diffusive molar flux of } i \text{ relative to volume-average velocity} \tag{2.30}$$

Thus, total mass and molar fluxes of species i are expressed in the forms

$$\mathbf{n}_i = \rho_i \mathbf{v}_i = \begin{cases} \mathbf{j}_i + \rho_i \mathbf{v} & = \mathbf{j}_i + \omega_i \sum_{k=1}^{N} \mathbf{n}_k \\[2mm] \mathbf{j}_i^* + \rho_i \mathbf{v}^* & = \mathbf{j}_i^* + M_i x_i \sum_{k=1}^{N} \mathbf{N}_k \\[2mm] \mathbf{j}_i^\blacksquare + \rho_i \mathbf{v}^\blacksquare & = \mathbf{j}_i^\blacksquare + \rho_i \sum_{k=1}^{N} \overline{V}_k \mathbf{N}_k \end{cases} \tag{2.31}$$

and

$$\mathbf{N}_i = c_i \mathbf{v}_i = \begin{cases} \mathbf{J}_i + c_i \mathbf{v} & = \mathbf{J}_i + \frac{\omega_i}{M_i} \sum_{k=1}^{N} \mathbf{n}_k \\[2mm] \mathbf{J}_i^* + c_i \mathbf{v}^* & = \mathbf{J}_i^* + x_i \sum_{k=1}^{N} \mathbf{N}_k \\[2mm] \mathbf{J}_i^\blacksquare + c_i \mathbf{v}^\blacksquare & = \mathbf{J}_i^\blacksquare + c_i \sum_{k=1}^{N} \overline{V}_k \mathbf{N}_k \end{cases} \tag{2.32}$$

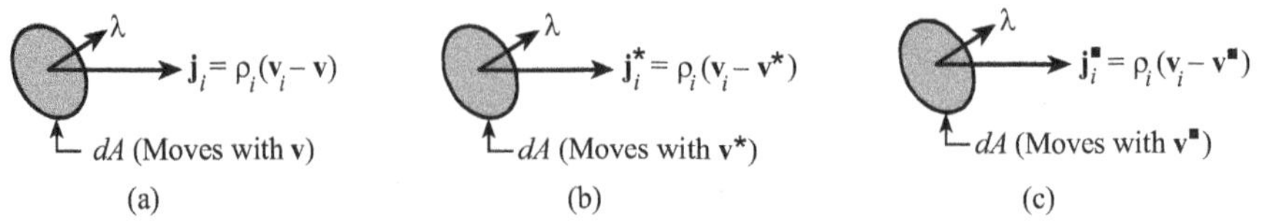

$$j_i = \rho_i(v_i - v) \qquad j_i^* = \rho_i(v_i - v^*) \qquad j_i^\bullet = \rho_i(v_i - v^\bullet)$$

(a) dA (Moves with **v**)   (b) dA (Moves with **v***)   (c) dA (Moves with **v**$^\bullet$)

Figure 2.2 Schematic of diffusive mass fluxes passing through a differential surface area dA moving with a) mass-average velocity, b) molar-average velocity, c) volume-average velocity.

Example 2.4 A binary gas mixture containing 70 mol % helium (A) and 30% argon (B) at 1 atm and 298 K is flowing in a tube. The mass- and molar-average velocities of the mixture in the axial direction are 10 and 2 mm/s, respectively.

a) Calculate the diffusive mass fluxes of species with reference to mass-average velocity.
b) Calculate the diffusive molar fluxes of species with reference to molar-average velocity.
c) Calculate the diffusive molar fluxes of species with reference to volume-average velocity.

Solution

a) From Appendix F

$$M_A = 4.003 \, \text{kg/kmol} \qquad \text{and} \qquad M_B = 39.948 \, \text{kg/kmol}$$

The molecular weight of the mixture is

$$M = y_A M_A + y_B M_B = (0.7)(4.003) + (0.3)(39.948) = 14.7865 \, \text{kg/kmol}$$

The mass fractions are

$$\omega_A = \frac{y_A M_A}{M} = \frac{(0.7)(4.003)}{14.7865} = 0.1895 \qquad \text{and} \qquad \omega_B = \frac{y_B M_B}{M} = \frac{(0.3)(39.948)}{14.7865} = 0.8105$$

Using the definitions of mass- and molar-average velocities, one can write

$$v_z = \omega_A v_{A_z} + \omega_B v_{B_z} \qquad \Rightarrow \qquad 10 = 0.1895 \, v_{A_z} + 0.8105 \, v_{B_z} \qquad (1)$$

$$v_z^* = x_A v_{A_z} + x_B v_{B_z} \qquad \Rightarrow \qquad 2 = 0.7 \, v_{A_z} + 0.3 \, v_{B_z} \qquad (2)$$

Simultaneous solution of Eqs. (1) and (2) yields

$$v_{A_z} = -2.7013 \, \text{mm/s} \qquad \text{and} \qquad v_{B_z} = 12.9696 \, \text{mm/s}$$

Assuming ideal gas behavior, the density of the mixture is

$$\rho = \frac{PM}{RT} = \frac{(1)(14.7865)}{(0.08205)(298)} = 0.6047 \, \text{kg/m}^3$$

Therefore, diffusive mass fluxes of helium and argon with reference to mass-average velocity are

$$j_{A_z} = \rho_A \left(v_{A_z} - v_z \right) = (0.6047)(0.1895)(-2.7013 - 10) \times 10^{-3} = -1.455 \times 10^{-3} \text{kg/m}^2.\text{s}$$

$$j_{B_z} = \rho_B \left(v_{B_z} - v_z \right) = (0.6047)(0.8105)(12.9696 - 10) \times 10^{-3} = 1.455 \times 10^{-3} \text{kg/m}^2.\text{s}$$

Note that $j_{A_z} + j_{B_z} = 0$, which is a consequence of the conservation of mass.

b) The molar concentration of the mixture is

$$c = \frac{\rho}{M} = \frac{0.6047}{14.7865} = 0.0409 \, \text{kmol/m}^3$$

Diffusive molar fluxes of helium and argon with reference to molar-average velocity are

$$J_{A_z}^* = c_A \left(v_{A_z} - v_z^*\right) = (0.0409)(0.7)(-2.7013 - 2) \times 10^{-3} = -1.346 \times 10^{-4} \, \text{kmol/m}^2.\text{s}$$

$$J_{B_z}^* = c_B \left(v_{B_z} - v_z^*\right) = (0.0409)(0.3)(12.9696 - 2) \times 10^{-3} = 1.346 \times 10^{-4} \, \text{kmol/m}^2.\text{s}$$

Again note that $J_{A_z}^* + J_{B_z}^* = 0$.

c) Diffusive molar fluxes of helium and argon with reference to volume-average velocity are

$$J_{A_z}^\blacksquare = c_A(v_{A_z} - v_z^\blacksquare) \qquad \text{and} \qquad J_{B_z}^\blacksquare = c_B(v_{B_z} - v_z^\blacksquare)$$

The definition of the partial molar volume is

$$\overline{V}_k = \left(\frac{\partial V_{mix}}{\partial n_k}\right)_{T,P,n_j \neq k} = \left[\frac{\partial (n\widetilde{V}_{mix})}{\partial n_k}\right]_{T,P,n_j \neq k} = \left[\frac{\partial (n/c)}{\partial n_k}\right]_{T,P,n_j \neq k} \tag{3}$$

Since the total molar concentration, c, is constant, Eq. (3) simplifies to

$$\overline{V}_k = \frac{1}{c}\left(\frac{\partial n}{\partial n_k}\right)_{T,P,n_j \neq k} = \frac{1}{c} \quad \Rightarrow \quad c_k \overline{V}_k = \frac{c_k}{c} \quad \Rightarrow \quad c_k \overline{V}_k = x_k$$

Equality of volume and mole fractions leads to $v_z^\blacksquare = v_z^*$. Thus

$$J_{A_z}^\blacksquare = J_{A_z}^* = -1.346 \times 10^{-4} \, \text{kmol/m}^2.\text{s}$$

$$J_{B_z}^\blacksquare = J_{B_z}^* = 1.346 \times 10^{-4} \, \text{kmol/m}^2.\text{s}$$

Example 2.5 Using the following data provided for a quaternary gas mixture of carbon dioxide (1), oxygen (2), nitrogen (3), and water (4) at 1 atm and 298 K, calculate the following:

a) The diffusive mass fluxes of species with reference to mass-average velocity,
b) The diffusive mass fluxes of species with reference to molar-average velocity.

Species	ω_i	$n_i \, (\text{g/cm}^2.\text{s})$
CO_2	0.05	-0.5×10^{-4}
O_2	0.20	7.5×10^{-4}
N_2	0.70	1.8×10^{-3}
H_2O	0.05	-1.1×10^{-4}

Solution

a) From Appendix F

$$M_1 = 44.010 \, \text{g/mol} \qquad M_2 = 31.999 \, \text{g/mol} \qquad M_3 = 28.013 \, \text{g/mol} \qquad M_4 = 18.016 \, \text{g/mol}$$

The molecular weight of the mixture is calculated from Eq. (2.8) as

$$M = \left(\frac{0.05}{44.010} + \frac{0.20}{31.999} + \frac{0.70}{28.013} + \frac{0.05}{18.016}\right)^{-1} = 28.449 \, \text{g/mol}$$

Assuming ideal gas behavior, the density of the mixture is given by

$$\rho = \frac{PM}{RT} = \frac{(1)(28.449)}{(82.05)(298)} = 1.164 \times 10^{-3} \text{g/cm}^3$$

From Eq. (2.31)

$$\mathbf{j}_i = \mathbf{n}_i - \omega_i \sum_{k=1}^{4} \mathbf{n}_k \tag{1}$$

The summation of the total mass fluxes is

$$\sum_{k=1}^{4} \mathbf{n}_k = -0.5 \times 10^{-4} + 7.5 \times 10^{-4} + 1.8 \times 10^{-3} - 1.1 \times 10^{-4} = 2.39 \times 10^{-3} \, \mathrm{g/cm^2.s}$$

Therefore, diffusive mass fluxes with reference to mass average velocity are calculated from Eq. (1) as

$$\mathbf{j}_1 = -0.5 \times 10^{-4} - (0.05)(2.39 \times 10^{-3}) = -1.695 \times 10^{-4} \mathrm{g/cm^2.s}$$
$$\mathbf{j}_2 = 7.5 \times 10^{-4} - (0.20)(2.39 \times 10^{-3}) = 2.720 \times 10^{-4} \mathrm{g/cm^2.s}$$
$$\mathbf{j}_3 = 1.8 \times 10^{-3} - (0.70)(2.39 \times 10^{-3}) = 1.270 \times 10^{-4} \mathrm{g/cm^2.s}$$
$$\mathbf{j}_4 = -1.1 \times 10^{-4} - (0.05)(2.39 \times 10^{-3}) = -2.295 \times 10^{-4} \mathrm{g/cm^2.s}$$

b) From Eq. (2.31)

$$\mathbf{j}_i^* = \mathbf{n}_i - M_i y_i \sum_{k=1}^{\mathcal{N}} \mathbf{N}_k \tag{2}$$

The mole fractions and the total molar fluxes of each species are as follows:

Species	$y_i = \omega_i M/M_i$	$\mathbf{N}_i = \mathbf{n}_i/M_i \, (\mathrm{mol/cm^2.s})$
CO_2	0.032	-1.136×10^{-6}
O_2	0.178	2.344×10^{-5}
N_2	0.711	6.426×10^{-5}
H_2O	0.079	-6.111×10^{-6}

The summation of the total molar fluxes is

$$\sum_{k=1}^{4} \mathbf{N}_k = -1.136 \times 10^{-6} + 2.344 \times 10^{-5} + 6.426 \times 10^{-5} - 6.111 \times 10^{-6} = 8.045 \times 10^{-5} \mathrm{mol/cm^2.s}$$

Therefore, diffusive mass fluxes with reference to molar average velocity are calculated from Eq. (2) as

$$\mathbf{j}_1^* = -0.5 \times 10^{-4} - (44.010)(0.032)(8.045 \times 10^{-5}) = -1.633 \times 10^{-4} \mathrm{g/cm^2.s}$$
$$\mathbf{j}_2^* = 7.5 \times 10^{-4} - (31.999)(0.178)(8.045 \times 10^{-5}) = 2.918 \times 10^{-4} \mathrm{g/cm^2.s}$$
$$\mathbf{j}_3^* = 1.8 \times 10^{-3} - (28.013)(0.711)(8.045 \times 10^{-5}) = 1.977 \times 10^{-4} \mathrm{g/cm^2.s}$$
$$\mathbf{j}_4^* = -1.1 \times 10^{-4} - (18.016)(0.079)(8.045 \times 10^{-5}) = -2.245 \times 10^{-4} \mathrm{g/cm^2.s}$$

2.1.4 DIFFUSIVE MASS/MOLAR FLUXES IN DIFFERENT REFERENCE VELOCITY FRAMES

In a mixture consisting of $\mathcal{N}$ species, the sum of all mole fractions is unity,

$$\sum_{k=1}^{\mathcal{N}} x_k = 1, \tag{2.33}$$

indicating that mole fractions are **not** all independent. In other words, if x_k values are known for $(\mathcal{N}-1)$ species, the value of the remaining one, $x_{\mathcal{N}}$, is automatically fixed as

$$x_{\mathcal{N}} = 1 - \sum_{k=1}^{\mathcal{N}-1} x_k \tag{2.34}$$

The same argument is also true for mass fractions.

Total mass and molar fluxes of species i, $\mathbf{n}_i$ and $\mathbf{N}_i$, are all independent. However, like mole/mass fractions, diffusive mass and molar fluxes are **not** all independent. The reason for this is the fact that appropriately weighted diffusive mass/molar fluxes sum to zero, i.e.,

$$\sum_{k=1}^{\mathcal{N}} \beta_k \, (\text{Diffusive mass/molar flux})_k = 0, \tag{2.35}$$

where β_k is the weighting factor. Equation (2.35) leads to

$$(\text{Diffusive mass/molar flux})_{\mathcal{N}} = -\frac{1}{\beta_{\mathcal{N}}} \sum_{k=1}^{\mathcal{N}-1} \beta_k \, (\text{Diffusive mass/molar flux})_k \tag{2.36}$$

The determination of β_k depending on different reference velocity frames is explained below.

● **Mass fluxes**

Summation of diffusive mass fluxes defined by Eqs. (2.25)–(2.27) over all species present in the mixture and replacing the "dummy variable" i by k give

$$\sum_{k=1}^{\mathcal{N}} \mathbf{j}_k = \sum_{k=1}^{\mathcal{N}} \rho_k (\mathbf{v}_k - \mathbf{v}) = \underbrace{\sum_{k=1}^{\mathcal{N}} \rho_k \mathbf{v}_k}_{\rho\mathbf{v}} - \mathbf{v} \underbrace{\sum_{k=1}^{\mathcal{N}} \rho_k}_{\rho} = 0 \tag{2.37}$$

$$\sum_{k=1}^{\mathcal{N}} \mathbf{j}_k^* = \sum_{k=1}^{\mathcal{N}} \rho_k (\mathbf{v}_k - \mathbf{v}^*) = \underbrace{\sum_{k=1}^{\mathcal{N}} \rho_k \mathbf{v}_k}_{\rho\mathbf{v}} - \mathbf{v}^* \underbrace{\sum_{k=1}^{\mathcal{N}} \rho_k}_{\rho} = \rho\,(\mathbf{v} - \mathbf{v}^*) \tag{2.38}$$

$$\sum_{k=1}^{\mathcal{N}} \mathbf{j}_k^{\blacksquare} = \sum_{k=1}^{\mathcal{N}} \rho_k (\mathbf{v}_k - \mathbf{v}^{\blacksquare}) = \underbrace{\sum_{k=1}^{\mathcal{N}} \rho_k \mathbf{v}_k}_{\rho\mathbf{v}} - \mathbf{v}^{\blacksquare} \underbrace{\sum_{k=1}^{\mathcal{N}} \rho_k}_{\rho} = \rho\,(\mathbf{v} - \mathbf{v}^{\blacksquare}) \tag{2.39}$$

Equation (2.37) indicates that diffusive mass fluxes relative to mass-average velocity are not all independent ($\beta_k = 1$); when $\mathbf{j}_k$ values are known for $(\mathcal{N}-1)$ species, the value of $\mathbf{j}_{\mathcal{N}}$ is automatically fixed as

$$\boxed{\mathbf{j}_{\mathcal{N}} = -\sum_{k=1}^{\mathcal{N}-1} \mathbf{j}_k} \tag{2.40}$$

If the diffusive mass flux relative to molar-average velocity, $\mathbf{j}_i^*$ in Eq. (2.26), is multiplied by x_i/ω_i, the result is

$$\frac{x_i}{\omega_i} \mathbf{j}_i^* = \frac{\rho_i}{\omega_i} x_i (\mathbf{v}_i - \mathbf{v}^*) \qquad \Rightarrow \qquad \frac{x_i}{\omega_i} \mathbf{j}_i^* = \rho x_i (\mathbf{v}_i - \mathbf{v}^*) \tag{2.41}$$

Summation of Eq. (2.41) over all species present in the mixture and replacing the "dummy variable" i by k yield

$$\sum_{k=1}^{\mathcal{N}} \frac{x_k}{\omega_k} \mathbf{j}_k^* = \rho \underbrace{\sum_{k=1}^{\mathcal{N}} x_k \mathbf{v}_k}_{\mathbf{v}^*} - \rho \mathbf{v}^* \underbrace{\sum_{k=1}^{\mathcal{N}} x_k}_{1} = 0, \tag{2.42}$$

indicating that $\beta_k = x_k/\omega_k$. Thus

$$\sum_{k=1}^{\mathcal{N}-1} \frac{x_k}{\omega_k} \mathbf{j}_k^* + \frac{x_{\mathcal{N}}}{\omega_{\mathcal{N}}} \mathbf{j}_{\mathcal{N}}^* = 0 \qquad \Rightarrow \qquad \boxed{\mathbf{j}_{\mathcal{N}}^* = -\frac{\omega_{\mathcal{N}}}{x_{\mathcal{N}}} \sum_{k=1}^{\mathcal{N}-1} \frac{x_k}{\omega_k} \mathbf{j}_k^*} \tag{2.43}$$

If the diffusive mass flux relative to volume-average velocity, $\mathbf{j}_i^{\blacksquare}$ in Eq. (2.27), is multiplied by $c_i \overline{V}_i / \omega_i$, the result is

$$\frac{c_i \overline{V}_i}{\omega_i} \mathbf{j}_i^{\blacksquare} = \frac{\rho_i}{\omega_i} c_i \overline{V}_i \left(\mathbf{v}_i - \mathbf{v}^{\blacksquare} \right) \qquad \Rightarrow \qquad \frac{\overline{V}_i}{M_i} \mathbf{j}_i^{\blacksquare} = c_i \overline{V}_i \left(\mathbf{v}_i - \mathbf{v}^{\blacksquare} \right) \tag{2.44}$$

Summation of Eq. (2.44) over all species present in the mixture and replacing the "dummy variable" i by k yield

$$\sum_{k=1}^{\mathcal{N}} \frac{\overline{V}_k}{M_k} \mathbf{j}_k^{\blacksquare} = \underbrace{\sum_{k=1}^{\mathcal{N}} c_k \overline{V}_k \mathbf{v}_k}_{\mathbf{v}^{\blacksquare}} - \mathbf{v}^{\blacksquare} \underbrace{\sum_{k=1}^{\mathcal{N}} c_k \overline{V}_k}_{1} = 0, \tag{2.45}$$

indicating that $\beta_k = \overline{V}_k/M_k$. Thus,

$$\sum_{k=1}^{\mathcal{N}-1} \frac{\overline{V}_k}{M_k} \mathbf{j}_k^{\blacksquare} + \frac{\overline{V}_{\mathcal{N}}}{M_{\mathcal{N}}} \mathbf{j}_{\mathcal{N}}^{\blacksquare} = 0 \qquad \Rightarrow \qquad \boxed{\mathbf{j}_{\mathcal{N}}^{\blacksquare} = -\frac{M_{\mathcal{N}}}{\overline{V}_{\mathcal{N}}} \sum_{k=1}^{\mathcal{N}-1} \frac{\overline{V}_k}{M_k} \mathbf{j}_k^{\blacksquare}} \tag{2.46}$$

• Molar fluxes

Summation of diffusive molar fluxes defined by Eqs. (2.28)–(2.30) over all species present in the mixture and replacing the "dummy variable" i by k give

$$\sum_{k=1}^{\mathcal{N}} \mathbf{J}_k = \sum_{k=1}^{\mathcal{N}} c_k \left(\mathbf{v}_k - \mathbf{v} \right) = \underbrace{\sum_{k=1}^{\mathcal{N}} c_k \mathbf{v}_k}_{c\mathbf{v}^*} - \mathbf{v} \underbrace{\sum_{k=1}^{\mathcal{N}} c_k}_{c} = c \left(\mathbf{v}^* - \mathbf{v} \right) \tag{2.47}$$

$$\sum_{k=1}^{\mathcal{N}} \mathbf{J}_k^* = \sum_{k=1}^{\mathcal{N}} c_k \left(\mathbf{v}_k - \mathbf{v}^* \right) = \underbrace{\sum_{k=1}^{\mathcal{N}} c_k \mathbf{v}_k}_{c\mathbf{v}^*} - \mathbf{v}^* \underbrace{\sum_{k=1}^{\mathcal{N}} c_k}_{c} = 0 \tag{2.48}$$

$$\sum_{k=1}^{\mathcal{N}} \mathbf{J}_k^{\blacksquare} = \sum_{k=1}^{\mathcal{N}} c_k \left(\mathbf{v}_k - \mathbf{v}^{\blacksquare} \right) = \underbrace{\sum_{k=1}^{\mathcal{N}} c_k \mathbf{v}_k}_{c\mathbf{v}^*} - \mathbf{v}^{\blacksquare} \underbrace{\sum_{k=1}^{\mathcal{N}} c_k}_{c} = c \left(\mathbf{v}^* - \mathbf{v}^{\blacksquare} \right) \tag{2.49}$$

Equation (2.48) indicates that diffusive molar fluxes relative to molar-average velocity are not all independent ($\beta_k = 1$); when $\mathbf{J}_k^*$ values are known for $(\mathcal{N} - 1)$ species, the value of $\mathbf{J}_{\mathcal{N}}^*$ is automatically fixed, i.e.,

$$\boxed{\mathbf{J}_{\mathcal{N}}^* = -\sum_{k=1}^{\mathcal{N}-1} \mathbf{J}_k^*} \tag{2.50}$$

Table 2.2

Weighting Factor, β_k, Values Satisfying Eq. (2.35)

Diffusive Mass Flux	β_k	Diffusive Molar Flux	β_k
$\mathbf{j}_k$	1	$\mathbf{J}_k$	ω_k/x_k
$\mathbf{j}_k^*$	x_k/ω_k	$\mathbf{J}_k^*$	1
$\mathbf{j}_k^{\blacksquare}$	$\overline{V}_k/M_k$	$\mathbf{J}_k^{\blacksquare}$	$\overline{V}_k$

If the diffusive molar flux relative to mass-average velocity, $\mathbf{J}_i$ in Eq. (2.28), is multiplied by ω_i/x_i, the result is

$$\frac{\omega_i}{x_i}\mathbf{J}_i = \frac{c_i}{x_i}\omega_i(\mathbf{v}_i - \mathbf{v}) \quad \Rightarrow \quad \frac{\omega_i}{x_i}\mathbf{J}_i = c\,\omega_i(\mathbf{v}_i - \mathbf{v}) \tag{2.51}$$

Summation of Eq. (2.51) over all species present in the mixture and replacing the "dummy variable" i by k yield

$$\sum_{k=1}^{\mathcal{N}} \frac{\omega_k}{x_k}\mathbf{J}_k = c\underbrace{\sum_{k=1}^{\mathcal{N}} \omega_k \mathbf{v}_k}_{\mathbf{v}} - c\mathbf{v}\underbrace{\sum_{k=1}^{\mathcal{N}} \omega_k}_{1} = 0, \tag{2.52}$$

indicating that $\beta_k = \omega_k/x_k$. Thus,

$$\sum_{k=1}^{\mathcal{N}-1} \frac{\omega_k}{x_k}\mathbf{J}_k + \frac{\omega_{\mathcal{N}}}{x_{\mathcal{N}}}\mathbf{J}_{\mathcal{N}} = 0 \quad \Rightarrow \quad \boxed{\mathbf{J}_{\mathcal{N}} = -\frac{x_{\mathcal{N}}}{\omega_{\mathcal{N}}}\sum_{k=1}^{\mathcal{N}-1} \frac{\omega_k}{x_k}\mathbf{J}_k} \tag{2.53}$$

Noting that $\mathbf{J}_i^{\blacksquare} = \mathbf{j}_i^{\blacksquare}/M_i$, Eq. (2.45) takes the form

$$\sum_{k=1}^{\mathcal{N}} \overline{V}_k \mathbf{J}_k^{\blacksquare} = 0, \tag{2.54}$$

indicating that $\beta_k = \overline{V}_k$. Thus

$$\sum_{k=1}^{\mathcal{N}-1} \overline{V}_k \mathbf{J}_k^{\blacksquare} + \overline{V}_{\mathcal{N}} \mathbf{J}_{\mathcal{N}}^{\blacksquare} = 0 \quad \Rightarrow \quad \boxed{\mathbf{J}_{\mathcal{N}}^{\blacksquare} = -\frac{1}{\overline{V}_{\mathcal{N}}}\sum_{k=1}^{\mathcal{N}-1} \overline{V}_k \mathbf{J}_k^{\blacksquare}} \tag{2.55}$$

Table 2.2 summarizes the weighting factors for different types of mass/molar diffusive fluxes.

Example 2.6   For a binary system of species A and B, show that

$$\mathbf{J}_A^* = \frac{M}{M_A M_B}\mathbf{j}_A$$

Solution

By definition, the diffusive mass flux of species A with respect to mass-average velocity is written as

$$\mathbf{j}_A = \rho_A(\mathbf{v}_A - \mathbf{v}) \quad \Rightarrow \quad \frac{\mathbf{j}_A}{\rho_A} = \mathbf{v}_A - \mathbf{v} \tag{1}$$

Similarly, for species B,

$$\mathbf{j}_B = \rho_B(\mathbf{v}_B - \mathbf{v}) \quad \Rightarrow \quad \frac{\mathbf{j}_B}{\rho_B} = \mathbf{v}_B - \mathbf{v} \tag{2}$$

Subtraction of Eq. (2) from Eq. (1) gives

$$\frac{\mathbf{j}_A}{\rho_A} - \frac{\mathbf{j}_B}{\rho_B} = \mathbf{v}_A - \mathbf{v}_B \tag{3}$$

Since $\mathbf{j}_A + \mathbf{j}_B = 0$, Eq. (3) simplifies to

$$\frac{\rho}{\rho_A \rho_B} \mathbf{j}_A = \mathbf{v}_A - \mathbf{v}_B \tag{4}$$

By definition, the diffusive molar flux of species A with respect to molar-average velocity is written as

$$\mathbf{J}_A^* = c_A(\mathbf{v}_A - \mathbf{v}^*) \quad\Rightarrow\quad \frac{\mathbf{J}_A^*}{c_A} = \mathbf{v}_A - \mathbf{v}^* \tag{5}$$

Similarly, for species B

$$\mathbf{J}_B^* = c_B(\mathbf{v}_B - \mathbf{v}^*) \quad\Rightarrow\quad \frac{\mathbf{J}_B^*}{c_B} = \mathbf{v}_B - \mathbf{v}^* \tag{6}$$

Subtraction of Eq. (6) from Eq. (5) gives

$$\frac{\mathbf{J}_A^*}{c_A} - \frac{\mathbf{J}_B^*}{c_B} = \mathbf{v}_A - \mathbf{v}_B \tag{7}$$

Since $\mathbf{J}_A^* + \mathbf{J}_B^* = 0$, Eq. (7) simplifies to

$$\frac{c}{c_A c_B} \mathbf{J}_A^* = \mathbf{v}_A - \mathbf{v}_B \tag{8}$$

From Eqs. (4) and (8)

$$\frac{\rho}{\rho_A \rho_B} \mathbf{j}_A = \frac{c}{c_A c_B} \mathbf{J}_A^* \tag{9}$$

Since $\rho = cM$, $\rho_A = c_A M_A$, and $\rho_B = c_B M_B$, Eq. (9) simplifies to

$$\mathbf{J}_A^* = \frac{M}{M_A M_B} \mathbf{j}_A \tag{10}$$

2.1.5   DIFFUSIVE FLUX TRANSFORMATIONS

After encountering various mass/molar diffusive flux expressions, the obvious question that comes to mind is how to transform diffusive fluxes from one reference velocity frame to another.

• Transformation of j* to j

Once the diffusive mass fluxes relative to molar-average velocity, $\mathbf{j}_i^*$, are known, how can we obtain the diffusive mass fluxes relative to mass-average velocity, $\mathbf{j}_i$? Using Eqs. (2.25) and (2.26), these two fluxes are related by

$$\mathbf{j}_i = \mathbf{j}_i^* - \rho_i(\mathbf{v} - \mathbf{v}^*) \tag{2.56}$$

Elimination of the term $(\mathbf{v} - \mathbf{v}^*)$ in Eq. (2.56) with the help of Eq. (2.38) gives

$$\mathbf{j}_i = \mathbf{j}_i^* - \omega_i \sum_{k=1}^{\mathcal{N}} \mathbf{j}_k^* = \mathbf{j}_i^* - \omega_i \left(\sum_{k=1}^{\mathcal{N}-1} \mathbf{j}_k^* + \mathbf{j}_{\mathcal{N}}^* \right) \tag{2.57}$$

The use of Eq. (2.43) in Eq. (2.57) yields

$$\mathbf{j}_i = \mathbf{j}_i^* - \omega_i \sum_{k=1}^{\mathcal{N}-1} \left(1 - \frac{\omega_{\mathcal{N}}}{x_{\mathcal{N}}} \frac{x_k}{\omega_k} \right) \mathbf{j}_k^* \tag{2.58}$$

Note that

$$\mathbf{j}_i^* = \sum_{k=1}^{\mathcal{N}-1} \delta_{ik} \mathbf{j}_k^*, \tag{2.59}$$

where δ_{ik} is the *Kronecker delta*, defined by

$$\delta_{ik} = \begin{cases} 1 & \text{if} \quad i = k \\ 0 & \text{if} \quad i \neq k \end{cases} \tag{2.60}$$

Substitution of Eq. (2.59) into Eq. (2.58) and rearrangement result in

$$\boxed{\mathbf{j}_i = \sum_{k=1}^{\mathcal{N}-1} \left[\delta_{ik} - \omega_i \left(1 - \frac{\omega_{\mathcal{N}}}{x_{\mathcal{N}}} \frac{x_k}{\omega_k} \right) \right] \mathbf{j}_k^*} \tag{2.61}$$

In matrix notation, Eq. (2.61) is written as

$$\boxed{[\mathbf{j}] = [\mathbf{B}^{m*}] [\mathbf{j}^*],} \tag{2.62}$$

where $[\mathbf{B}^{m*}]$ is a square matrix of order $(\mathcal{N} - 1)$ and $[\mathbf{j}]$ and $[\mathbf{j}^*]$ are $(\mathcal{N} - 1)$ column vectors. The transformation matrix $[\mathbf{B}^{m*}]$ is given by

$$[\mathbf{B}^{m*}] = \begin{pmatrix} 1 & 0 & \cdots & 0 \\ 0 & 1 & \cdots & 0 \\ \vdots & \vdots & \vdots & \vdots \\ 0 & 0 & \cdots & 1 \end{pmatrix} - \begin{pmatrix} \omega_1 \\ \omega_2 \\ \vdots \\ \omega_{\mathcal{N}-1} \end{pmatrix} \cdot \begin{pmatrix} 1 - \dfrac{\omega_{\mathcal{N}}}{x_{\mathcal{N}}} \dfrac{x_1}{\omega_1} \\ 1 - \dfrac{\omega_{\mathcal{N}}}{x_{\mathcal{N}}} \dfrac{x_2}{\omega_2} \\ \vdots \\ 1 - \dfrac{\omega_{\mathcal{N}}}{x_{\mathcal{N}}} \dfrac{x_{\mathcal{N}-1}}{\omega_{\mathcal{N}-1}} \end{pmatrix}^{\mathrm{T}}, \tag{2.63}$$

where the superscript ^{m*} indicates the transformation from mass-average to molar-average reference frame.

• Transformation of j to j*

To obtain the diffusive mass fluxes relative to molar-average velocity, $\mathbf{j}_i^*$, once the diffusive mass fluxes relative to mass-average velocity, $\mathbf{j}_i$, are known, Eq. (2.62) must be multiplied by the inverse of the matrix $[\mathbf{B}^{m*}]$. The result is

$$[\mathbf{j}^*] = [\mathbf{B}^{m*}]^{-1} [\mathbf{j}] \tag{2.64}$$

or

$$\boxed{[\mathbf{j}^*] = [\mathbf{B}^{*m}][\mathbf{j}]} \tag{2.65}$$

Equation (2.63) can be expressed in the form of

$$[\mathbf{B}^{m*}] = [\mathbf{I}] - [\mathbf{u}][\mathbf{v}]^T, \tag{2.66}$$

where

$$[\mathbf{u}] = \begin{pmatrix} \omega_1 \\ \omega_2 \\ \vdots \\ \omega_{\mathcal{N}-1} \end{pmatrix} \quad \text{and} \quad [\mathbf{v}] = \begin{pmatrix} 1 - \dfrac{\omega_{\mathcal{N}}}{x_{\mathcal{N}}} \dfrac{x_1}{\omega_1} \\ 1 - \dfrac{\omega_{\mathcal{N}}}{x_{\mathcal{N}}} \dfrac{x_2}{\omega_2} \\ \vdots \\ 1 - \dfrac{\omega_{\mathcal{N}}}{x_{\mathcal{N}}} \dfrac{x_{\mathcal{N}-1}}{\omega_{\mathcal{N}-1}} \end{pmatrix} \tag{2.67}$$

According to the Sherman–Morrison formula given in Appendix C, i.e., Eq. (C.33), the inverse of the matrix $[\mathbf{B}^{m*}]$ is

$$[\mathbf{B}^{m*}]^{-1} = [\mathbf{I}] + \frac{[\mathbf{u}][\mathbf{v}]^T}{1 - [\mathbf{v}]^T[\mathbf{u}]} \tag{2.68}$$

Noting that

$$1 - [\mathbf{v}]^T[\mathbf{u}] = \frac{\omega_{\mathcal{N}}}{x_{\mathcal{N}}} \tag{2.69}$$

Eq. (2.68) leads to

$$[\mathbf{B}^{m*}]^{-1} = [\mathbf{B}^{*m}] = \begin{pmatrix} 1 & 0 & \cdots & 0 \\ 0 & 1 & \cdots & 0 \\ \vdots & \vdots & \vdots & \vdots \\ 0 & 0 & \cdots & 1 \end{pmatrix} - \begin{pmatrix} \omega_1 \\ \omega_2 \\ \vdots \\ \omega_{\mathcal{N}-1} \end{pmatrix} \cdot \begin{pmatrix} \dfrac{x_1}{\omega_1} - \dfrac{x_{\mathcal{N}}}{\omega_{\mathcal{N}}} \\ \dfrac{x_2}{\omega_2} - \dfrac{x_{\mathcal{N}}}{\omega_{\mathcal{N}}} \\ \vdots \\ \dfrac{x_{\mathcal{N}-1}}{\omega_{\mathcal{N}-1}} - \dfrac{x_{\mathcal{N}}}{\omega_{\mathcal{N}}} \end{pmatrix}^T \tag{2.70}$$

and Eq. (2.65) is expressed as

$$\boxed{\mathbf{j}_i^* = \sum_{k=1}^{\mathcal{N}-1} \left[\delta_{ik} - \omega_i \left(\frac{x_k}{\omega_k} - \frac{x_{\mathcal{N}}}{\omega_{\mathcal{N}}} \right) \right] \mathbf{j}_k} \tag{2.71}$$

Example 2.7   Let us calculate $\mathbf{j}_i^*$ using the following data given in Example 2.5:

Species	ω_i	y_i	$\mathbf{j}_i \times 10^4$ (g/cm^2.s)
CO_2	0.05	0.032	-1.695
O_2	0.20	0.178	2.720
N_2	0.70	0.711	1.270
H_2O	0.05	0.079	-2.295

The Mathcad worksheet is given below. The slight differences in the calculated $\mathbf{j}_i^*$ values from those calculated in Example 2.5 come from the round-off errors.

ORIGIN:= 1

$$\omega := \begin{pmatrix} 0.05 \\ 0.20 \\ 0.70 \\ 0.05 \end{pmatrix} \qquad y := \begin{pmatrix} 0.032 \\ 0.178 \\ 0.711 \\ 0.079 \end{pmatrix} \qquad j := \begin{pmatrix} -1.695 \\ 2.720 \\ 1.270 \\ -2.295 \end{pmatrix} \cdot 10^{-4}$$

$$jstar := \left[\begin{pmatrix} 1 & 0 & 0 \\ 0 & 1 & 0 \\ 0 & 0 & 1 \end{pmatrix} - \begin{pmatrix} \omega_1 \\ \omega_2 \\ \omega_3 \end{pmatrix} \cdot \begin{pmatrix} \dfrac{y_1}{\omega_1} - \dfrac{y_4}{\omega_4} \\[2mm] \dfrac{y_2}{\omega_2} - \dfrac{y_4}{\omega_4} \\[2mm] \dfrac{y_3}{\omega_3} - \dfrac{y_4}{\omega_4} \end{pmatrix}^{T} \right] \cdot \begin{pmatrix} j_1 \\ j_2 \\ j_3 \end{pmatrix} = \begin{pmatrix} -1.645 \times 10^{-4} \\ 2.92 \times 10^{-4} \\ 1.97 \times 10^{-4} \end{pmatrix}$$ Equation (2.71)

$$jstar_4 := \dfrac{-\omega_4}{y_4} \cdot \sum_{k=1}^{3} \left(\dfrac{y_k}{\omega_k} \cdot jstar_k \right) = -2.245 \times 10^{-4}$$ Equation (2.43)

Mathcad worksheet of Example 2.7.

• Transformation of $\mathbf{J}_i^{\blacksquare}$ to $\mathbf{J}^*$

Once the diffusive molar fluxes relative to volume-average velocity, $\mathbf{J}_i^{\blacksquare}$, are known, how can we obtain the diffusive molar fluxes relative to molar-average velocity, $\mathbf{J}_i^*$? Using Eqs. (2.29) and (2.30), these two fluxes are related by

$$\mathbf{J}_i^* = \mathbf{J}_i^{\blacksquare} - c_i \left(\mathbf{v}^* - \mathbf{v}^{\blacksquare} \right) \tag{2.72}$$

Elimination of the term $(\mathbf{v}^* - \mathbf{v}^{\blacksquare})$ in Eq. (2.73) with the help of Eq. (2.49) gives

$$\mathbf{J}_i^* = \mathbf{J}_i^{\blacksquare} - x_i \sum_{k=1}^{\mathcal{N}} \mathbf{J}_k^{\blacksquare} = \mathbf{J}_i^{\blacksquare} - x_i \left(\sum_{k=1}^{\mathcal{N}-1} \mathbf{J}_k^{\blacksquare} + \mathbf{J}_{\mathcal{N}}^{\blacksquare} \right) \tag{2.73}$$

The use of Eq. (2.55) in Eq. (2.73) yields

$$\mathbf{J}_i^* = \mathbf{J}_i^{\blacksquare} - x_i \sum_{k=1}^{\mathcal{N}-1} \left(1 - \frac{\overline{V}_k}{\overline{V}_{\mathcal{N}}} \right) \mathbf{J}_k^{\blacksquare} \tag{2.74}$$

Expressing

$$\mathbf{J}_i^{\blacksquare} = \sum_{k=1}^{\mathcal{N}-1} \delta_{ik} \mathbf{J}_k^{\blacksquare} \tag{2.75}$$

Eq. (2.74) becomes

$$\mathbf{J}_i^* = \sum_{k=1}^{\mathcal{N}-1} \left[\delta_{ik} - x_i \left(1 - \frac{\overline{V}_k}{\overline{V}_{\mathcal{N}}} \right) \right] \mathbf{J}_k^{\blacksquare} \tag{2.76}$$

In matrix notation, Eq. (2.76) is written as

$$[\mathbf{J}^*] = [\mathbf{G}^{*\blacksquare}][\mathbf{J}^{\blacksquare}], \tag{2.77}$$

where the superscript $^{*\blacksquare}$ indicates the transformation from molar-average to volume-average reference frame. Note that $[\mathbf{G}^{*\blacksquare}]$ is a square matrix of order $(\mathcal{N}-1)$ and $[\mathbf{J}^*]$ and $[\mathbf{J}^{\blacksquare}]$ are $(\mathcal{N}-1)$ column vectors. The transformation matrix $[\mathbf{G}^{*\blacksquare}]$ is given by

$$[\mathbf{G}^{*\blacksquare}] = \begin{pmatrix} 1 & 0 & \cdots & 0 \\ 0 & 1 & \cdots & 0 \\ \vdots & \vdots & \vdots & \vdots \\ 0 & 0 & \cdots & 1 \end{pmatrix} - \begin{pmatrix} x_1 \\ x_2 \\ \vdots \\ x_{\mathcal{N}-1} \end{pmatrix} \cdot \begin{pmatrix} 1 - \dfrac{\overline{V}_1}{\overline{V}_{\mathcal{N}}} \\ 1 - \dfrac{\overline{V}_2}{\overline{V}_{\mathcal{N}}} \\ \vdots \\ 1 - \dfrac{\overline{V}_{\mathcal{N}-1}}{\overline{V}_{\mathcal{N}}} \end{pmatrix}^{\mathrm{T}} \tag{2.78}$$

• Transformation of J* to J■

To obtain the diffusive molar fluxes relative to volume-average velocity, $\mathbf{J}_i^{\blacksquare}$, once the diffusive molar fluxes relative to molar-average velocity, $\mathbf{J}_i^*$, are known, Eq. (2.68) must be multiplied by the inverse of the matrix $[\mathbf{G}^{*\blacksquare}]$. The result is

$$[\mathbf{J}^{\blacksquare}] = [\mathbf{G}^{*\blacksquare}]^{-1}[\mathbf{J}^*] \tag{2.79}$$

or

$$[\mathbf{J}^{\blacksquare}] = [\mathbf{G}^{\blacksquare*}][\mathbf{J}^*], \tag{2.80}$$

where the superscript $^{\blacksquare*}$ indicates the transformation from volume-average to molar-average reference frame. The inverse of $[\mathbf{G}^{*\blacksquare}]$ can be calculated by application of the Sherman–Morrison formula, Eq. (C.33) in Appendix C. Noting that

$$1 - \mathbf{v}^{\mathrm{T}}\mathbf{u} = \frac{\widetilde{V}_{mix}}{\overline{V}_{\mathcal{N}}} \tag{2.81}$$

the inverse of the matrix $[\mathbf{G}^{*\blacksquare}]$ becomes

$$[\mathbf{G}^{*\blacksquare}]^{-1} = [\mathbf{G}^{\blacksquare*}] = \begin{pmatrix} 1 & 0 & \cdots & 0 \\ 0 & 1 & \cdots & 0 \\ \vdots & \vdots & \vdots & \vdots \\ 0 & 0 & \cdots & 1 \end{pmatrix} - \begin{pmatrix} x_1 \\ x_2 \\ \vdots \\ x_{\mathcal{N}-1} \end{pmatrix} \cdot \begin{pmatrix} \dfrac{\overline{V}_1 - \overline{V}_{\mathcal{N}}}{\widetilde{V}_{mix}} \\ \dfrac{\overline{V}_2 - \overline{V}_{\mathcal{N}}}{\widetilde{V}_{mix}} \\ \vdots \\ \dfrac{\overline{V}_{\mathcal{N}-1} - \overline{V}_{\mathcal{N}}}{\widetilde{V}_{mix}} \end{pmatrix}^{\mathrm{T}}, \tag{2.82}$$

where $\widetilde{V}_{mix}$ is the molar volume of the mixture, defined by

$$\widetilde{V}_{mix} = \sum_{k=1}^{\mathcal{N}} x_k \overline{V}_k = \frac{1}{c} \tag{2.83}$$

Thus, Eq. (2.80) is expressed as

$$\mathbf{J}_i^{\blacksquare} = \sum_{k=1}^{\mathcal{N}-1} \left[\delta_{ik} - x_i \left(\frac{\overline{V}_k - \overline{V}_{\mathcal{N}}}{\widetilde{V}_{mix}} \right) \right] \mathbf{J}_k^* \tag{2.84}$$

2.2 THE SPECIES CONTINUITY EQUATION

Let us consider any arbitrary Eulerian volume element[3] V at the macroscopic level as shown in Figure 2.3. The surface area enclosing volume V is represented by A. The conservation statement for mass of species i is expressed as

$$\left(\begin{array}{c} \text{Net rate of input} \\ \text{of species } i \end{array} \right) + \left(\begin{array}{c} \text{Rate of generation of species } i \\ \text{by homogeneous chem. rxn.} \end{array} \right)$$

$$= \left(\begin{array}{c} \text{Rate of accumulation} \\ \text{of species } i \end{array} \right) \tag{2.85}$$

Net rate of outflow, i.e., out – in, of species i through surface A of volume V is given by

$$\text{Net rate of outflow of species } i = \int_A \lambda \cdot \mathbf{n}_i \, dA \tag{2.86}$$

Note that $\lambda \cdot \mathbf{n}_i$ is the component of $\mathbf{n}_i$ in the direction of the outwardly directed unit normal vector λ. Thus,

$$\text{Net rate of input of species } i = - \int_A \lambda \cdot \mathbf{n}_i \, dA \tag{2.87}$$

Application of the divergence theorem transforms the surface integral into a volume integral as

$$\text{Net rate of input of species } i = - \int_V \nabla \cdot \mathbf{n}_i \, dV \tag{2.88}$$

Let r_i be the mass rate of production of species i by homogeneous chemical reaction[4] per unit volume. Then

$$\text{Rate of generation of species } i \text{ by homogeneous chem. rxn.} = \int_V r_i \, dV \tag{2.89}$$

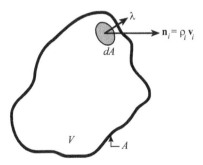

Figure 2.3 Eulerian volume element of volume V and surface area A.

---

[3] A volume element that is fixed in space.

[4] A chemical reaction that takes place in a single phase.

The rate of accumulation of species i is the time rate of change of total mass of i in volume V and is given by

$$\text{Rate of accumulation of species } i = \frac{d}{dt} \int_V \rho_i \, dV \tag{2.90}$$

Since V is independent of time, application of Leibniz's rule gives

$$\text{Rate of accumulation of species } i = \int_V \frac{\partial \rho_i}{\partial t} \, dV \tag{2.91}$$

Substitution of Eqs. (2.88), (2.89), and (2.91) into Eq. (2.85) and rearrangement yield

$$\int_V \left(\frac{\partial \rho_i}{\partial t} + \nabla \cdot \mathbf{n}_i - r_i \right) dV = 0 \tag{2.92}$$

Since V is arbitrary, the only way of satisfying Eq. (2.92) is to set the integrand to be equal to zero. Thus

$$\boxed{\frac{\partial \rho_i}{\partial t} + \nabla \cdot \mathbf{n}_i = r_i} \quad i = 1, 2, \dots, \mathcal{N}, \tag{2.93}$$

which is usually called the *equation of continuity for species i*.

Summation of Eq. (2.93) over all species present in the mixture and replacing the "dummy variable" i by k result in

$$\frac{\partial}{\partial t} \sum_{k=1}^{\mathcal{N}} \rho_k + \nabla \cdot \sum_{k=1}^{\mathcal{N}} \mathbf{n}_k = \sum_{k=1}^{\mathcal{N}} r_k \tag{2.94}$$

The total mass density of a multicomponent mixture, ρ, is

$$\rho = \sum_{k=1}^{\mathcal{N}} \rho_k \tag{2.95}$$

The use of Eq. (2.21) gives

$$\sum_{k=1}^{\mathcal{N}} \mathbf{n}_k = \rho \mathbf{v} \tag{2.96}$$

Since mass is neither created nor destroyed by homogeneous chemical reactions,

$$\sum_{k=1}^{\mathcal{N}} r_k = 0 \tag{2.97}$$

The use of Eqs. (2.95)–(2.97) in Eq. (2.94) leads to

$$\boxed{\frac{\partial \rho}{\partial t} + \nabla \cdot \rho \mathbf{v} = 0,} \tag{2.98}$$

which is the *equation of continuity for the mixture*.

Reaction rates and phase equilibrium relationships are generally expressed in terms of molar quantities. Therefore, sometimes it is more convenient to work in terms of molar concentration $c_i = \rho_i / M_i$, where M_i is the molecular weight of species i. Dividing each term of Eq. (2.98) by M_i results in

$$\boxed{\frac{\partial c_i}{\partial t} + \nabla \cdot \mathbf{N}_i = \mathcal{R}_i,} \tag{2.99}$$

Table 2.3

The Equation of Continuity for Species i in Various Coordinate Systems

Cartesian Coordinates

$$\frac{\partial c_i}{\partial t} + \left(\frac{\partial N_{i_x}}{\partial x} + \frac{\partial N_{i_y}}{\partial y} + \frac{\partial N_{i_z}}{\partial z} \right) = \mathcal{R}_i \qquad\qquad (A)$$

Cylindrical Coordinates

$$\frac{\partial c_i}{\partial t} + \left[\frac{1}{r} \frac{\partial}{\partial r} (r N_{i_r}) + \frac{1}{r} \frac{\partial N_{i_\theta}}{\partial \theta} + \frac{\partial N_{i_z}}{\partial z} \right] = \mathcal{R}_i \qquad\qquad (B)$$

Spherical Coordinates

$$\frac{\partial c_i}{\partial t} + \left[\frac{1}{r^2} \frac{\partial}{\partial r} (r^2 N_{i_r}) + \frac{1}{r \sin\theta} \frac{\partial}{\partial \theta} (N_{i_\theta} \sin\theta) + \frac{1}{r \sin\theta} \frac{\partial N_{i_\phi}}{\partial \phi} \right] = \mathcal{R}_i \qquad (C)$$

where $\mathcal{R}_i$ is the molar rate of production of species i per unit volume by homogeneous chemical reactions. Equation (2.99) is presented in the Cartesian, cylindrical, and spherical coordinate systems in Table 2.3.

Summation of Eq. (2.99) over all species present in the mixture and replacing the "dummy variable" i by k result in

$$\frac{\partial}{\partial t} \sum_{k=1}^{\mathcal{N}} c_k + \nabla \cdot \sum_{k=1}^{\mathcal{N}} \mathbf{N}_k = \sum_{k=1}^{\mathcal{N}} \mathcal{R}_k \qquad\qquad (2.100)$$

The total molar concentration of a multicomponent mixture, c, is

$$c = \sum_{k=1}^{\mathcal{N}} c_k \qquad\qquad (2.101)$$

The use of Eq. (2.22) gives

$$\sum_{k=1}^{\mathcal{N}} \mathbf{N}_k = c\mathbf{v}^* \qquad\qquad (2.102)$$

The use of Eqs. (2.101) and (2.102) in Eq. (2.100) gives the *equation of continuity for the mixture in terms of molar quantities* as

$$\boxed{\frac{\partial c}{\partial t} + \nabla \cdot c\mathbf{v}^* = \sum_{k=1}^{\mathcal{N}} \mathcal{R}_k} \qquad\qquad (2.103)$$

Note that $\sum\limits_{k=1}^{\mathcal{N}} \mathcal{R}_k \neq 0$ since, in general, moles are not conserved.

To determine the rate of generation by homogeneous reaction per unit volume (r_i or $\mathcal{R}_i$), one must know the stoichiometry and kinetics of chemical reaction(s). It is the homogeneous reaction rate expression that appears in the conservation equation, i.e., in either Eq. (2.93) or (2.99). The heterogeneous reaction rate expression, on the other hand, appears in the boundary conditions.

2.2.1 HOMOGENEOUS REACTION RATE EXPRESSION

A chemical reaction is expressed in the form of

$$\sum_{i=1}^{s} \alpha_i A_i = 0, \qquad\qquad (2.104)$$

where α_i is the stoichiometric coefficient of the ith chemical species (positive if the species is a product, negative if the species is a reactant), s is the total number of species in the reaction, and A_i is the chemical symbol for the ith chemical species (it represents the molecular weight of the species). Stoichiometric coefficients have the units of moles of i per mole of the basis species, where the basis species is arbitrarily chosen. The *law of combining proportions* states that

$$\frac{\text{Moles of } i \text{ reacted}}{(\text{Moles of } i/\text{Mole of basis species})} = \text{Moles of basis species} \tag{2.105}$$

or

$$\frac{n_i - n_{i_o}}{\alpha_i} = \varepsilon, \tag{2.106}$$

where ε is called the *molar extent* of the reaction.[5] Rearrangement of Eq. (2.106) gives

$$\boxed{n_i = n_{i_o} + \alpha_i \varepsilon} \tag{2.107}$$

Note that once ε has been determined, the number of moles of any chemical species participating in the reaction can be determined by using Eq. (2.107).

The molar extent of the reaction should not be confused with the *fractional conversion variable*, which can only take values between 0 and 1. The molar extent of the reaction is an extensive property measured in Moles, and its value can be greater than unity.

The *rate of a chemical reaction*, $\mathfrak{r}$, is defined by

$$\boxed{\mathfrak{r} = \frac{1}{V}\frac{d\varepsilon}{dt},} \tag{2.108}$$

where V is the volume physically occupied by the reacting fluid. Since both V and $d\varepsilon/dt$ are positive, then the reaction rate is intrinsically positive. Note that the reaction rate has the units of moles reacted per unit time per unit volume of the reaction mixture and has the following characteristics: (1) it is an intensive property, (2) it is independent of the reactor type, and (3) it is independent of a process.

Changes in the molar extent of the reaction can be related to the changes in the number of moles of species i by differentiating Eq. (2.107). The result is

$$d\varepsilon = \frac{1}{\alpha_i}dn_i \tag{2.109}$$

Substitution of Eq. (2.109) into Eq. (2.108) gives

$$\mathfrak{r} = \frac{1}{\alpha_i}\frac{1}{V}\frac{dn_i}{dt} \tag{2.110}$$

Since the rate of generation of species i per unit volume, $\mathcal{R}_i$, is defined by

$$\mathcal{R}_i = \frac{1}{V}\frac{dn_i}{dt} \tag{2.111}$$

---

[5]The term ε has been given various names in the literature, such as degree of advancement, reaction of coordinate, degree of reaction, and progress variable.

and then,

$$\boxed{\mathcal{R}_i = \alpha_i \mathfrak{r}} \tag{2.112}$$

Therefore, $\mathcal{R}_i$ is negative if i appears as a reactant; $\mathcal{R}_i$ is positive if i is a product.

In the case of several reactions, $\mathcal{R}_i$ is defined by

$$\boxed{\mathcal{R}_i = \sum_j \alpha_{ij} \mathfrak{r}_j,} \tag{2.113}$$

where α_{ij} is the stoichiometric coefficient of the ith species in the jth reaction and $\mathfrak{r}_j$ is the rate of the jth reaction.

2.2.2 HETEROGENEOUS REACTION RATE EXPRESSION

Heterogeneous chemical reactions take place at phase interfaces, such as catalytic surfaces. As a result, they appear in the boundary conditions. For heterogeneous reactions, the rate of reaction is empirically specified as

$$\mathbf{N}_i \cdot \lambda \big|_{\text{surface}} = k_n'' \, c_i^n \big|_{\text{surface}}, \tag{2.114}$$

where λ is the unit normal to the surface in the direction of diffusing species i and k_n'' is the surface reaction rate constant (n indicates the order of the reaction). In the case of an instantaneous reaction, i.e., $k_n'' \to \infty$, the concentration of reacting species on the surface of the catalyst can be considered zero.

For a heterogeneous chemical reaction represented by Eq. (2.104), molar fluxes are related by

$$\frac{\mathbf{N}_{A_1}}{\alpha_1} = \frac{\mathbf{N}_{A_2}}{\alpha_2} = \cdots = \frac{\mathbf{N}_{A_s}}{\alpha_s} \tag{2.115}$$

2.3   THE SPECIES CONTINUITY EQUATION IN TERMS OF FLUXES

2.3.1 MASS BASIS

The total mass flux, $\mathbf{n}_i$, is the summation of diffusive and convective mass fluxes, i.e.,

$$\mathbf{n}_i = \mathbf{j}_i + \rho_i \mathbf{v} \tag{2.116}$$

Substitution of Eq. (2.116) into Eq. (2.93) gives

$$\boxed{\underbrace{\frac{\partial \rho_i}{\partial t}}_{\text{Accumulation}} + \underbrace{\nabla \cdot \rho_i \mathbf{v}}_{\text{Convection}} = \underbrace{-\nabla \cdot \mathbf{j}_i}_{\text{Diffusion}} + \underbrace{r_i}_{\text{Reaction}}} \tag{2.117}$$

Substituting $\rho_i = \omega_i \rho$ into the left side of Eq. (2.117) and expanding the terms lead to

$$\rho \left(\frac{\partial \omega_i}{\partial t} + \mathbf{v} \cdot \nabla \omega_i \right) + \omega_i \underbrace{\left(\frac{\partial \rho}{\partial t} + \nabla \cdot \rho \mathbf{v} \right)}_{0} = -\nabla \cdot \mathbf{j}_i + r_i \tag{2.118}$$

or

$$\boxed{\rho \left(\frac{\partial \omega_i}{\partial t} + \mathbf{v} \cdot \nabla \omega_i \right) = -\nabla \cdot \mathbf{j}_i + r_i} \tag{2.119}$$

2.3.2 MOLAR BASIS

Since convective molar flux can be expressed in terms of either molar-average or volume-average velocity, we can express the species continuity equation in two different forms.

• **In terms of molar-average velocity**

The total molar flux, $\mathbf{N}_i$, is the summation of diffusive and convective molar fluxes, i.e.,

$$\mathbf{N}_i = \mathbf{J}_i^* + c_i \mathbf{v}^* \tag{2.120}$$

Substitution of Eq. (2.120) into Eq. (2.99) gives

$$\underbrace{\frac{\partial c_i}{\partial t}}_{\text{Accumulation}} + \underbrace{\nabla \cdot c_i \mathbf{v}^*}_{\text{Convection}} = \underbrace{-\nabla \cdot \mathbf{J}_i^*}_{\text{Diffusion}} + \underbrace{\mathcal{R}_i}_{\text{Reaction}} \tag{2.121}$$

Substituting $c_i = cx_i$ into the left side of Eq. (2.121) and expanding the terms lead to

$$c\left(\frac{\partial x_i}{\partial t} + \mathbf{v}^* \cdot \nabla x_i\right) + x_i \underbrace{\left(\frac{\partial c}{\partial t} + \nabla \cdot c\mathbf{v}^*\right)}_{\Sigma_{k=1}^{\mathcal{N}} \mathcal{R}_k} = -\nabla \cdot \mathbf{J}_i^* + \mathcal{R}_i \tag{2.122}$$

or

$$c\left(\frac{\partial x_i}{\partial t} + \mathbf{v}^* \cdot \nabla x_i\right) = -\nabla \cdot \mathbf{J}_i^* + \mathcal{R}_i - x_i \sum_{k=1}^{\mathcal{N}} \mathcal{R}_k \tag{2.123}$$

The main disadvantage of Eqs. (2.121) and (2.123) is the appearance of molar-average velocity in the convective term. Note that the solutions of the equations of continuity and motion yield the mass-average velocity and not the molar-average velocity.

The molar-average velocity in the convective term can be eliminated in favor of the mass-average velocity with the help of Eq. (2.37) as

$$\mathbf{v}^* = \mathbf{v} - \frac{1}{\rho} \sum_{k=1}^{\mathcal{N}} \mathbf{j}_k^* \tag{2.124}$$

Substitution of $\rho = cM$ and $\mathbf{j}_k^* = M_k \mathbf{J}_k^*$ into Eq. (2.124) yields

$$\mathbf{v}^* = \mathbf{v} - \frac{1}{c} \sum_{k=1}^{\mathcal{N}} \frac{M_k}{M} \mathbf{J}_k^* \tag{2.125}$$

Substitution of Eq. (2.125) into Eq. (2.121) gives

$$\frac{\partial c_i}{\partial t} + \nabla \cdot c_i \mathbf{v} = -\nabla \cdot \left(\mathbf{J}_i^* - x_i \sum_{k=1}^{\mathcal{N}} \frac{M_k}{M} \mathbf{J}_k^*\right) + \mathcal{R}_i \tag{2.126}$$

The first term on the right side of Eq. (2.126) is expressed as

$$\nabla \cdot \left(\mathbf{J}_i^* - x_i \sum_{k=1}^{\mathcal{N}} \frac{M_k}{M} \mathbf{J}_k^*\right) = \nabla \cdot \left[\mathbf{J}_i^* - x_i \left(\sum_{k=1}^{\mathcal{N}-1} \frac{M_k}{M} \mathbf{J}_k^* + \frac{M_{\mathcal{N}}}{M} \mathbf{J}_{\mathcal{N}}^*\right)\right] \tag{2.127}$$

The use of Eq. (2.49) in Eq. (2.127) leads to

$$\nabla \cdot \left(\mathbf{J}_i^* - x_i \sum_{k=1}^{\mathcal{N}} \frac{M_k}{M} \mathbf{J}_k^* \right) = \nabla \cdot \left\{ \mathbf{J}_i^* - x_i \left[\sum_{k=1}^{\mathcal{N}-1} \left(\frac{M_k - M_{\mathcal{N}}}{M} \right) \mathbf{J}_k^* \right] \right\} \qquad (2.128)$$

Noting that

$$\mathbf{J}_i^* = \sum_{k=1}^{\mathcal{N}-1} \delta_{ik} \mathbf{J}_k^* \qquad (2.129)$$

Eq. (2.126) finally takes the form

$$\boxed{ \frac{\partial c_i}{\partial t} + \nabla \cdot c_i \mathbf{v} = -\nabla \cdot \left\{ \sum_{k=1}^{\mathcal{N}-1} \left[\delta_{ik} - x_i \left(\frac{M_k - M_{\mathcal{N}}}{M} \right) \right] \mathbf{J}_k^* \right\} + \mathcal{R}_i } \qquad (2.130)$$

If we consider the diffusion of a trace amount of species i through a mixture, i.e., $x_i \ll 1$, Eq. (2.130) simplifies to

$$\boxed{ \frac{\partial c_i}{\partial t} + \nabla \cdot c_i \mathbf{v} = -\nabla \cdot \mathbf{J}_k^* + \mathcal{R}_i } \quad x_i \ll 1 \qquad (2.131)$$

• In terms of volume-average velocity

The total molar flux, $\mathbf{N}_i$, is the summation of molecular and convective molar fluxes, i.e.,

$$\mathbf{N}_i = \mathbf{J}_i^{\blacksquare} + c_i \mathbf{v}^{\blacksquare} \qquad (2.132)$$

Substitution of Eq. (2.132) into Eq. (2.99) gives

$$\boxed{ \underbrace{\frac{\partial c_i}{\partial t}}_{\text{Accumulation}} + \underbrace{\nabla \cdot c_i \mathbf{v}^{\blacksquare}}_{\text{Convection}} = \underbrace{-\nabla \cdot \mathbf{J}_i^{\blacksquare}}_{\text{Diffusion}} + \underbrace{\mathcal{R}_i}_{\text{Reaction}} } \qquad (2.133)$$

The volume-average velocity in the convective term can be eliminated in favor of the mass-average velocity with the help of Eq. (2.38) as follows:

$$\mathbf{v}^{\blacksquare} = \mathbf{v} - \frac{1}{\rho} \sum_{k=1}^{\mathcal{N}} \mathbf{j}_k^{\blacksquare} \qquad (2.134)$$

Substitution of $\rho = cM$ and $\mathbf{j}_k^{\blacksquare} = M_k \mathbf{J}_k^{\blacksquare}$ into Eq. (2.134) yields

$$\mathbf{v}^{\blacksquare} = \mathbf{v} - \frac{1}{c} \sum_{k=1}^{\mathcal{N}} \frac{M_k}{M} \mathbf{J}_k^{\blacksquare} \qquad (2.135)$$

Substitution of Eq. (2.135) into Eq. (2.133) gives

$$\frac{\partial c_i}{\partial t} + \nabla \cdot c_i \mathbf{v} = -\nabla \cdot \left(\mathbf{J}_i^{\blacksquare} - x_i \sum_{k=1}^{\mathcal{N}} \frac{M_k}{M} \mathbf{J}_k^{\blacksquare} \right) + \mathcal{R}_i \qquad (2.136)$$

The first term on the right side of Eq. (2.136) is expressed as

$$\nabla \cdot \left(\mathbf{J}_i^{\blacksquare} - x_i \sum_{k=1}^{\mathcal{N}} \frac{M_k}{M} \mathbf{J}_k^{\blacksquare} \right) = \nabla \cdot \left[\mathbf{J}_i^{\blacksquare} - x_i \left(\sum_{k=1}^{\mathcal{N}-1} \frac{M_k}{M} \mathbf{J}_k^{\blacksquare} + \frac{M_{\mathcal{N}}}{M} \mathbf{J}_{\mathcal{N}}^{\blacksquare} \right) \right] \qquad (2.137)$$

The use of Eq. (2.54) in Eq. (2.137) leads to

$$\nabla \cdot \left(\mathbf{J}_i^\blacksquare - x_i \sum_{k=1}^{\mathcal{N}} \frac{M_k}{M} \mathbf{J}_k^\blacksquare \right) = \nabla \cdot \left\{ \mathbf{J}_i^\blacksquare - x_i \left[\sum_{k=1}^{\mathcal{N}-1} \frac{1}{M} \left(M_k - \frac{\overline{V}_k}{\overline{V}_{\mathcal{N}}} M_{\mathcal{N}} \right) \mathbf{J}_k^\blacksquare \right] \right\} \tag{2.138}$$

Noting that

$$\mathbf{J}_i^\blacksquare = \sum_{k=1}^{\mathcal{N}-1} \delta_{ik} \mathbf{J}_k^\blacksquare \tag{2.139}$$

Eq. (2.136) finally takes the form

$$\boxed{\frac{\partial c_i}{\partial t} + \nabla \cdot c_i \mathbf{v} = -\nabla \cdot \left\{ \sum_{k=1}^{\mathcal{N}-1} \left[\delta_{ik} - x_i \left(\frac{M_k}{M} - \frac{\overline{V}_k}{\overline{V}_{\mathcal{N}}} \frac{M_{\mathcal{N}}}{M} \right) \right] \mathbf{J}_k^\blacksquare \right\} + \mathcal{R}_i} \tag{2.140}$$

If we consider the diffusion of a trace amount of species i through a mixture, i.e., $x_i \ll 1$, Eq. (2.140) simplifies to

$$\boxed{\frac{\partial c_i}{\partial t} + \nabla \cdot c_i \mathbf{v} = -\nabla \cdot \mathbf{J}_k^\blacksquare + \mathcal{R}_i} \quad x_i \ll 1 \tag{2.141}$$

2.4 GOVERNING EQUATIONS FOR A BINARY SYSTEM

For a binary system consisting of species A and B, Eqs. (2.93) and (2.99) become

$$\frac{\partial \rho_A}{\partial t} + \nabla \cdot \mathbf{n}_A = r_A \tag{2.142}$$

$$\frac{\partial c_A}{\partial t} + \nabla \cdot \mathbf{N}_A = \mathcal{R}_A \tag{2.143}$$

The total mass and molar fluxes are expressed from Eqs. (2.31) and (2.32), respectively, as

$$\boxed{\underbrace{\mathbf{n}_A}_{\text{Total mass flux}} = \underbrace{\mathbf{j}_A}_{\text{Diffusive mass flux}} + \underbrace{\rho_A \mathbf{v}}_{\text{Convective mass flux}} = \mathbf{j}_A + \omega_A \left(\mathbf{n}_A + \mathbf{n}_B \right)} \tag{2.144}$$

$$\boxed{\underbrace{\mathbf{N}_A}_{\text{Total molar flux}} = \underbrace{\mathbf{J}_A^*}_{\text{Diffusive molar flux}} + \underbrace{c_A \mathbf{v}^*}_{\text{Convective molar flux}} = \mathbf{J}_A^* + x_A \left(\mathbf{N}_A + \mathbf{N}_B \right)} \tag{2.145}$$

$$\boxed{\underbrace{\mathbf{N}_A}_{\text{Total molar flux}} = \underbrace{\mathbf{J}_A^\blacksquare}_{\text{Diffusive molar flux}} + \underbrace{c_A \mathbf{v}^\blacksquare}_{\text{Convective molar flux}} = \mathbf{J}_A^\blacksquare + c_A \left(\overline{V}_A \mathbf{N}_A + \overline{V}_B \mathbf{N}_B \right)} \tag{2.146}$$

Examination of Eqs. (2.144)–(2.146) indicates that there is no need to have a bulk motion of the mixture as a result of external forces, such as pressure gradient, in order to have a nonzero convective flux term. For example, the convective flux term in Eq. (2.144) is nonzero unless either $\mathbf{n}_A = -\mathbf{n}_B$ or $\omega_A \ll 1$. Similar arguments hold for Eqs. (2.145) and (2.146). Thus, when mass transfer occurs only as a result of driving forces, the convective flux may be nonzero. In other words, diffusion creates its own convection. This phenomenon is called *diffusion-induced convection*.

Substitution of total mass flux, Eq. (2.144), into Eq. (2.142) gives the species continuity equation on a mass basis. On the other hand, substitution of total molar flux, either Eq. (2.145) or (2.146), into Eq. (2.143) gives the species continuity equation on a molar basis. To proceed further, one needs a constitutive equation for diffusive flux. *Fick's first law of diffusion* provides relationships for diffusive fluxes relative to characteristic velocities.

2.4.1 FICK'S FIRST LAW OF DIFFUSION

In 1995, to celebrate the 100th volume of the *Journal of Membrane Science*, the journal editors decided to publish 12 classic contributions to membrane science, one of which was the paper by Fick.[6] Fick's original paper in German was published in 1855 and abstracted in English by "The London, Edinburgh, and Dublin Philosophical Magazine and Journal of Science" in the same year[7]. Fick (1995) describes his purpose as follows:

> "A few years ago Graham published an extensive investigation on the diffusion of salts in water, in which he more especially compared the diffusivity of different salts. It appears to me a matter of regret, however, that in such an exceedingly valuable and extensive investigation, the development of a fundamental, for the operation of diffusion in a single element of space, was neglected, and I have therefore endeavored to supply this omission."

Using the analogy with Fourier's law for heat conduction and Ohm's law for electricity, he proposed that "the transfer of salt and water occurring in a unit of time, between two elements of space filled with differently concentrated solutions of the same salt, must be directly proportional to the difference of concentration, and inversely proportional to the distance of the elements from one another." Mathematically, this statement is generalized as

$$\boxed{\mathbf{j}_A = -\rho \mathcal{D}_{AB} \nabla \omega_A,}$$

(2.147)

where $\mathcal{D}_{AB}$ is the binary diffusion coefficient with $\mathcal{D}_{AB} = \mathcal{D}_{BA}$. The minus sign comes from the fact that diffusion takes place in the direction of decreasing ω_A. Since $\nabla \omega_A < 0$, the minus sign assures that the flux is a positive quantity.

- **Fick's first law in terms of mole fraction gradient**

The gradient of mass fraction is

$$\nabla \omega_A = \nabla \left(\frac{M_A}{M} x_A \right) = \frac{M_A}{M} \nabla x_A - \frac{x_A M_A}{M^2} \nabla M = \frac{M_A}{M^2} (M \nabla x_A - x_A \nabla M)$$

(2.148)

The term ∇M can be calculated as

$$\nabla M = \nabla (x_A M_A + x_B M_B) = M_A \nabla x_A + M_B \nabla x_B$$

(2.149)

Note that

$$x_A + x_B = 1 \quad \Rightarrow \quad \nabla x_A + \nabla x_B = 0 \quad \Rightarrow \quad \nabla x_B = -\nabla x_A$$

(2.150)

Substitution of Eq. (2.150) into Eq. (2.149) yields

$$\nabla M = (M_A - M_B) \nabla x_A$$

(2.151)

The use of Eq. (2.151) in Eq. (2.148) yields

$$\nabla \omega_A = \frac{M_A M_B}{M^2} \nabla x_A$$

(2.152)

---

[6] Adolf Eugen Fick (1829–1901), German mathematician, physicist, and physiologist.

[7] Readers interested in the history of diffusion may refer to Philibert (2006).

Substitution of Eq. (2.152) into Eq. (2.147) gives

$$\mathbf{j}_A = -\rho \mathcal{D}_{AB} \frac{M_A M_B}{M^2} \nabla x_A \tag{2.153}$$

Note that $\rho = cM$ and from Example 2.6

$$\mathbf{J}_A^* = \frac{M}{M_A M_B} \mathbf{j}_A \tag{2.154}$$

Thus, Eq. (2.153) takes the form

$$\boxed{\mathbf{J}_A^* = -c\mathcal{D}_{AB} \nabla x_A} \tag{2.155}$$

• Fick's first law in terms of molar concentration gradient

From Problem 2.1

$$\mathbf{J}_A^{\blacksquare} = c\overline{V}_B \frac{M}{M_A M_B} \mathbf{j}_A \tag{2.156}$$

Substitution of Eqs. (2.152) and (2.156) into Eq. (2.147) gives

$$\mathbf{J}_A^{\blacksquare} = -c^2 \overline{V}_B \mathcal{D}_{AB} \nabla x_A \tag{2.157}$$

Note that

$$\nabla x_A = \nabla \left(\frac{c_A}{c} \right) = \frac{1}{c} \nabla c_A - \frac{c_A}{c^2} \left(\nabla c_A + \nabla c_B \right) = \frac{1}{c^2} \left(c_B \nabla c_A - c_A \nabla c_B \right) \tag{2.158}$$

Substitution of Eq. (2.158) into Eq. (2.157) results in

$$\mathbf{J}_A^{\blacksquare} = -\mathcal{D}_{AB} \left(c_B \overline{V}_B \nabla c_A - c_A \overline{V}_B \nabla c_B \right) \tag{2.159}$$

Since volume fractions sum to unity, the volume fraction of species B is

$$c_B \overline{V}_B = 1 - c_A \overline{V}_A \tag{2.160}$$

Substitution of Eq. (2.160) into Eq. (2.159) yields

$$\mathbf{J}_A^{\blacksquare} = -\mathcal{D}_{AB} \left[\nabla c_A - c_A \left(\overline{V}_A \nabla c_A + \overline{V}_B \nabla c_B \right) \right] \tag{2.161}$$

From Problem 2.7

$$\overline{V}_A \nabla c_A + \overline{V}_B \nabla c_B = 0 \tag{2.162}$$

Thus, Eq. (2.161) becomes

$$\boxed{\mathbf{J}_A^{\blacksquare} = - \mathcal{D}_{AB} \nabla c_A}$$ (2.163)

2.4.2 TOTAL MASS/MOLAR FLUX EXPRESSIONS

Substitution of Eqs. (2.147), (2.155), and (2.163) into Eqs. (2.144), (2.145), and (2.146), respectively, gives the following expressions for the total mass and molar fluxes:

$$\boxed{\mathbf{n}_A = - \rho \mathcal{D}_{AB} \nabla \omega_A + \omega_A \left(\mathbf{n}_A + \mathbf{n}_B \right)}$$ (2.164)

$$\boxed{\mathbf{N}_A = - c \mathcal{D}_{AB} \nabla x_A + x_A \left(\mathbf{N}_A + \mathbf{N}_B \right)}$$ (2.165)

$$\boxed{\mathbf{N}_A = - \mathcal{D}_{AB} \nabla c_A + c_A \left(\overline{V}_A \mathbf{N}_A + \overline{V}_B \mathbf{N}_B \right)}$$ (2.166)

2.4.3 VARIOUS FORMS OF THE SPECIES CONTINUITY EQUATION

• **Simplification of Eq. (2.119)**

Substitution of Eq. (2.147) into Eq. (2.119) results in

$$\boxed{\rho \left(\frac{\partial \omega_A}{\partial t} + \mathbf{v} \cdot \nabla \omega_A \right) = \nabla \cdot (\rho \mathcal{D}_{AB} \nabla \omega_A) + r_A}$$ (2.167)

For diffusion in dilute liquid solutions at constant temperature and pressure, total density and diffusion coefficient are considered constant. Under these circumstances, Eq. (2.167) simplifies to

$$\frac{\partial \rho_A}{\partial t} + \mathbf{v} \cdot \nabla \rho_A = \mathcal{D}_{AB} \nabla^2 \rho_A + r_A$$ (2.168)

Division of Eq. (2.168) by the molecular weight of species A leads to

$$\boxed{\frac{\partial c_A}{\partial t} + \mathbf{v} \cdot \nabla c_A = \mathcal{D}_{AB} \nabla^2 c_A + \mathcal{R}_A} \quad \rho, \mathcal{D}_{AB} = \text{const.}$$ (2.169)

Equation (2.169) is presented in the Cartesian, cylindrical, and spherical coordinate systems in Table 2.4.

• **Simplification of Eq. (2.123)**

Substitution of Eq. (2.155) into Eq. (2.123) results in

$$\boxed{c \left(\frac{\partial x_A}{\partial t} + \mathbf{v}^* \cdot \nabla x_A \right) = \nabla \cdot (c \mathcal{D}_{AB} \nabla x_A) + \mathcal{R}_A - x_A (\mathcal{R}_A + \mathcal{R}_B)}$$ (2.170)

Table 2.4

The Equation of Continuity for Species A for Constant ρ and $\mathcal{D}_{AB}$ (Dilute Liquid Solutions)

Cartesian Coordinates

$$\frac{\partial c_A}{\partial t} + \left(v_x \frac{\partial c_A}{\partial x} + v_y \frac{\partial c_A}{\partial y} + v_z \frac{\partial c_A}{\partial z} \right) = \mathcal{D}_{AB} \left(\frac{\partial^2 c_A}{\partial x^2} + \frac{\partial^2 c_A}{\partial y^2} + \frac{\partial^2 c_A}{\partial z^2} \right) + \mathcal{R}_A \qquad (A)$$

Cylindrical Coordinates

$$\frac{\partial c_A}{\partial t} + \left(v_r \frac{\partial c_A}{\partial r} + v_\theta \frac{1}{r} \frac{\partial c_A}{\partial \theta} + v_z \frac{\partial c_A}{\partial z} \right)$$

$$= \mathcal{D}_{AB} \left[\frac{1}{r} \frac{\partial}{\partial r} \left(r \frac{\partial c_A}{\partial r} \right) + \frac{1}{r^2} \frac{\partial^2 c_A}{\partial \theta^2} + \frac{\partial^2 c_A}{\partial z^2} \right] + \mathcal{R}_A \qquad (B)$$

Spherical Coordinates

$$\frac{\partial c_A}{\partial t} + \left(v_r \frac{\partial c_A}{\partial r} + v_\theta \frac{1}{r} \frac{\partial c_A}{\partial \theta} + v_\phi \frac{1}{r \sin \theta} \frac{\partial c_A}{\partial \phi} \right)$$

$$= \mathcal{D}_{AB} \left[\frac{1}{r^2} \frac{\partial}{\partial r} \left(r^2 \frac{\partial c_A}{\partial r} \right) + \frac{1}{r^2 \sin \theta} \frac{\partial}{\partial \theta} \left(\sin \theta \frac{\partial c_A}{\partial \theta} \right) + \frac{1}{r^2 \sin^2 \theta} \frac{\partial^2 c_A}{\partial \phi^2} \right] + \mathcal{R}_A \qquad (C)$$

For low-density gases at constant temperature and pressure, total molar concentration[8] and the diffusion coefficient are considered constant. Under these circumstances, Eq. (2.170) simplifies to

$$\boxed{\frac{\partial c_A}{\partial t} + \mathbf{v}^* \cdot \nabla c_A = \mathcal{D}_{AB} \nabla^2 c_A + \mathcal{R}_A - x_A \left(\mathcal{R}_A + \mathcal{R}_B \right)} \quad c, \mathcal{D}_{AB} = \text{const.} \qquad (2.171)$$

- **Simplification of Eq. (2.130)**

For a binary system, Eq. (2.130) reduces to

$$\frac{\partial c_A}{\partial t} + \nabla \cdot c_A \mathbf{v} = -\nabla \cdot \left(\frac{M_B}{M} \right) \mathbf{J}_A^* + \mathcal{R}_A \qquad (2.172)$$

When $x_A \ll 1$, then $M \simeq M_B$ and Eq. (2.172) becomes

$$\boxed{\frac{\partial c_A}{\partial t} + \nabla \cdot c_A \mathbf{v} = \mathcal{D}_{AB} \nabla^2 c_A + \mathcal{R}_A} \quad \mathcal{D}_{AB} = \text{const.} \ \& \ x_A \ll 1 \qquad (2.173)$$

- **Simplification of Eq. (2.140)**

For a binary system, Eq. (2.140) reduces to

$$\frac{\partial c_A}{\partial t} + \nabla \cdot c_A \mathbf{v} = -\nabla \cdot \left[1 - x_A \left(\frac{M_A}{M} - \frac{\overline{V}_A}{\overline{V}_B} \frac{M_B}{M} \right) \right] \mathbf{J}_A^* + \mathcal{R}_A \qquad (2.174)$$

When $x_A \ll 1$,

$$1 - x_A \left(\frac{M_A}{M} - \frac{\overline{V}_A}{\overline{V}_B} \frac{M_B}{M} \right) \simeq 1 \qquad (2.175)$$

---

[8]For an ideal gas, $c = P/RT$, where R represents the gas constant.

Thus, substitution of Eq. (2.175) into Eq. (2.174) yields

$$\boxed{\frac{\partial c_A}{\partial t} + \nabla \cdot c_A \mathbf{v} = \mathcal{D}_{AB} \nabla^2 c_A + \mathcal{R}_A} \quad \mathcal{D}_{AB} = \text{const. } \& \; x_A \ll 1, \tag{2.176}$$

which is identical with Eq. (2.173).

Example 2.8   Consider the case in which species A diffuses through a stagnant gas film B.

a) Show that the molar-average velocity is given by

$$\mathbf{v}^* = -\frac{c\mathcal{D}_{AB}}{1 - y_A} \nabla y_A$$

b) Consider steady-state diffusion with no homogeneous chemical reaction. If c and $\mathcal{D}_{AB}$ are constants, show that the continuity equation for species A reduces to

$$\nabla y_B \cdot \nabla y_B = y_B \nabla^2 y_B$$

Solution

a) Since $\mathbf{N}_B = 0$, Eq. (2.165) simplifies to

$$\mathbf{N}_A = -\frac{c\mathcal{D}_{AB}}{1 - y_A} \nabla y_A \tag{1}$$

The molar-average velocity is defined as

$$\mathbf{v}^* = \frac{\mathbf{N}_A + \mathbf{N}_B}{c} = \frac{\mathbf{N}_A}{c} \tag{2}$$

Substitution of Eq. (1) into Eq. (2) gives

$$\mathbf{v}^* = -\frac{c\mathcal{D}_{AB}}{1 - y_A} \nabla y_A \tag{3}$$

b) For steady-state diffusion with no homogeneous chemical reaction, Eq. (2.143) reduces to

$$\nabla \cdot \mathbf{N}_A = 0 \tag{4}$$

The use of Eq. (1) in Eq. (4) yields

$$\nabla \cdot \left(-\frac{c\mathcal{D}_{AB}}{1 - y_A} \nabla y_A \right) = 0 \tag{5}$$

Since c and $\mathcal{D}_{AB}$ are constants and $\nabla y_A = -\nabla y_B$, Eq. (6) simplifies to

$$\nabla \cdot \left(\frac{1}{y_B} \nabla y_B \right) = 0 \tag{6}$$

Expanding Eq. (6),

$$-\frac{1}{y_B^2} \nabla y_B \cdot \nabla y_B + \frac{1}{y_B} \nabla \cdot \nabla y_B = 0 \tag{7}$$

or

$$\nabla y_B \cdot \nabla y_B = y_B \nabla^2 y_B \tag{8}$$

2.4.4 FICK'S SECOND LAW OF DIFFUSION

Fick's second law of diffusion expressed in terms of mass and molar concentrations is given by

$$\boxed{\frac{\partial \rho_A}{\partial t} = \mathcal{D}_{AB} \nabla^2 \rho_A} \tag{2.177}$$

and

$$\boxed{\frac{\partial c_A}{\partial t} = \mathcal{D}_{AB} \nabla^2 c_A} \tag{2.178}$$

What are the assumptions involved in simplifying Eqs. (2.167) and (2.170) to Eqs. (2.177) and (2.178), respectively? The first requirement is obviously the absence of a homogeneous chemical reaction. Since Fick's second law does not contain a convection term, either $\mathbf{v}$ must be zero in Eq. (2.167) or $\mathbf{v}^*$ must be zero in Eq. (2.170). Furthermore, total density (ρ), total molar concentration (c), and the diffusion coefficient must be all constant.

In the literature, Fick's second law of diffusion is used for diffusion in solids and stationary liquids. In these cases, the mass-average velocity is practically zero. The molar average velocity, on the other hand, is zero for diffusion in gases with $\mathbf{N}_A = -\mathbf{N}_B$. This condition is referred to as *equimolar counterdiffusion*.

The absence of a homogeneous chemical reaction is a prerequisite to use Fick's second law of diffusion. In some cases, however, it is possible to end up with either Eq. (2.177) or (2.178) without making the other simplifying assumptions mentioned above. Consider, for example, one-dimensional unsteady-state diffusion of species A through a solid matrix B. From Eq. (2.164), the total mass flux of species A in the z-direction is given by

$$n_{A_z} = -\rho \mathcal{D}_{AB} \frac{\partial \omega_A}{\partial z} + \omega_A (n_{A_z} + n_{B_z}) \tag{2.179}$$

Since $n_{B_z} = 0$, Eq. (2.179) simplifies to

$$n_{A_z} = -\frac{\rho \mathcal{D}_{AB}}{1 - \omega_A} \frac{\partial \omega_A}{\partial z} \tag{2.180}$$

Noting that ρ_B is a constant, the gradient of species A mass fraction, ω_A, is expressed as

$$\frac{\partial \omega_A}{\partial z} = \frac{\partial}{\partial z} \left(\frac{\rho_A}{\rho_A + \rho_B} \right) = \frac{\rho_B}{\rho^2} \frac{\partial \rho_A}{\partial z} \tag{2.181}$$

The use of Eq. (2.181) in Eq. (2.180) gives

$$n_{A_z} = \mathcal{D}_{AB} \frac{\partial \rho_A}{\partial z} \tag{2.182}$$

Finally, substitution of Eq. (2.182) into Eq. (2.142) under the condition of constant $\mathcal{D}_{AB}$ gives

$$\frac{\partial \rho_A}{\partial t} = \mathcal{D}_{AB} \frac{\partial^2 \rho_A}{\partial z^2} \tag{2.183}$$

Note that Eq. (2.183) is obtained without assuming $\mathbf{v} = 0$ and ρ is a constant.

2.5 DRIVING FORCES FOR DIFFUSION

The expressions representing Fick's first law of diffusion, Eqs. (2.147), (2.155), and (2.163), indicate that the driving force for diffusive flux is the concentration gradient. In other words, species diffuse in the direction of decreasing concentration. It is interesting to note that while the motion of molecules is due to imbalance of forces, concentration gradient does not have the dimensions of force.

In general, however, thermodynamics of irreversible processes indicates that the driving force for diffusion is not the concentration gradient but the gradient of partial molar Gibbs energy. In the literature, partial molar Gibbs energy, $\overline{G}_i$, is also referred to as the *chemical potential*, μ_i. To clarify this point, let us consider a pure component and note that pressure is defined as the force per unit area. Thus, pressure gradient (pressure/distance) is equal to force per unit volume. In other words, $F/V = \nabla P$. Remember that this equation is widely used in fluid mechanics. For a pure substance, Gibbs energy is defined in differential form as

$$dG = V\,dP - S\,dT, \tag{2.184}$$

where S indicates the entropy. Under isothermal conditions, Eq. (2.184) reduces to

$$dG = V\,dP \tag{2.185}$$

or

$$\nabla G = V\,\nabla P, \tag{2.186}$$

indicating that the gradient of Gibbs energy is equal to force.

2.5.1 THERMODYNAMICS PRELIMINARIES[9]

• **Criteria for equilibrium**

The following conditions should be met when α- and β-phases of a multicomponent system are in equilibrium with each other:

$$
\begin{aligned}
T^\alpha &= T^\beta & &\text{Thermal equilibrium (Equality of temperatures)} \\
P^\alpha &= P^\beta & &\text{Mechanical equilibrium (Equality of pressures)} \\
\overline{G}_i^\alpha &= \overline{G}_i^\beta & &\text{Chemical equilibrium (Equality of partial molar Gibbs energies)}
\end{aligned}
\tag{2.187}
$$

Equality of partial molar Gibbs energies implies there are no chemical driving forces to move species from one phase to another. Partial molar Gibbs energy is expressed in terms of fugacity, $\widehat{f}$, as

$$\overline{G}_i(T, P, x_i) = \lambda_i(T) + RT \ln \widehat{f}_i(T, P, x_i), \tag{2.188}$$

where λ_i is the molar Gibbs energy of pure species i at unit fugacity.

Letting $T^\alpha = T^\beta = T$ and $P^\alpha = P^\beta = P$, equality of partial molar Gibbs energies leads to

$$\lambda_i(T) + RT \ln \widehat{f}_i^\alpha(T, P, x_i^\alpha) = \lambda_i(T) + RT \ln \widehat{f}_i^\beta(T, P, x_i^\beta) \tag{2.189}$$

or

$$\boxed{\widehat{f}_i^\alpha(T, P, x_i^\alpha) = \widehat{f}_i^\beta(T, P, x_i^\beta)} \tag{2.190}$$

Thus, at equilibrium, fugacities of each component are equal in all phases.

---

[9]For details, see Tosun (2013).

• **Partial molar property**

When nonidentical liquids are mixed, the total property of the mixture, φ_{mix}, is different from the sum of the properties of the pure liquids, i.e.,

$$\varphi_{mix} \neq \sum_{k=1}^{\mathcal{N}} n_k \widetilde{\varphi}_k, \tag{2.191}$$

where $\widetilde{\varphi}_k$ is the molar property of pure species k. The inequality sign in Eq. (2.191) can be removed by the introduction of a *partial molar property*, $\overline{\varphi}_k$, so that

$$\varphi_{mix} = \sum_{k=1}^{\mathcal{N}} n_k \overline{\varphi}_k \tag{2.192}$$

A partial molar property is the rate at which an extensive property of the entire mixture, φ_{mix}, changes with the number of moles of component k in the mixture when temperature, pressure, and number of moles of all components other than k are kept constant. Mathematically, it is expressed as

$$\overline{\varphi}_k = \left(\frac{\partial \varphi_{mix}}{\partial n_k} \right)_{T,P,n_j \neq k} \tag{2.193}$$

Note that $\overline{\varphi}_k$ is a property of the mixture and not simply a property of component k. The partial molar property is an intensive property that is generally dependent on the composition of the mixture besides temperature and pressure.

A mixture is said to be an *ideal mixture* when (1) it is homogeneous, (2) the sizes of the molecules are equal, and (3) the forces between unlike molecules of the mixture are the same as the forces between like molecules. For an ideal mixture, the partial molar volume of species k is equal to the molar volume of pure species k, i.e.,

$$\overline{V}_k(T,P,x_i) = \widetilde{V}_k(T,P) \tag{2.194}$$

Partial molar properties are determined experimentally. For a binary mixture, one of the methods used to calculate partial molar properties is the *method of tangent intercepts*. In this method, once the molar property of the mixture, $\widetilde{\varphi}_{mix}$, is experimentally determined as a function of composition, $\widetilde{\varphi}_{mix}$ is plotted versus mole fraction (either x_1 or x_2). Then the intercepts of the tangent drawn to this curve at a given composition give partial molar properties as shown in Figure 2.4.

2.5.2 TWO-BULB DIFFUSION EXPERIMENT

Consider two bulbs, A and B, each containing a binary mixture of species 1 and 2 at different compositions as shown in Figure 2.5. The two bulbs are connected by a capillary tube, and the

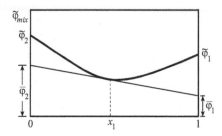

Figure 2.4 Graphical determination of partial molar properties for a binary mixture.

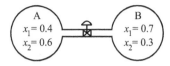

Figure 2.5 A two-bulb diffusion cell.

stopcock is initially closed. The whole system is kept at constant pressure and temperature. When the stopcock is opened, species 1 diffuses from bulb B to bulb A and species 2 diffuses from bulb A to bulb B until equilibrium is reached. In this specific case, diffusion is indeed in the direction of decreasing concentration. This phenomenon is explained in terms of partial molar Gibbs energy as follows.

A typical $\widetilde{G}_{mix}$ versus composition (say x_1) curve is shown in Figure 2.6. Since $\overline{G}_1^B > \overline{G}_1^A$, species 1 diffuses from bulb B to bulb A. On the other hand, $\overline{G}_2^A > \overline{G}_2^B$ and species 2 diffuses from bulb A to bulb B.

An interesting case arises when $\widetilde{G}_{mix}$ versus x_1 exhibits more than one minimum[9] as shown in Figure 2.7. In this case, $\overline{G}_1^A > \overline{G}_1^B$ and $\overline{G}_2^B > \overline{G}_2^A$. Therefore, while species 1 diffuses from bulb A to bulb B, species 2 diffuses from bulb B to bulb A. In other words, diffusion takes place from a region of low concentration to a region of high concentration! This is called *reverse* (or uphill) *diffusion*.

Movement of species from a region of low concentration to one of higher concentration may be conceptually difficult to grasp for some readers. An experiment described by Job and Herrmann (2006) clarifies this point. Consider a beaker containing pure water. If some iodine is added, it dissolves in the water and the solution turns brown. Now let us add a chemical to the solution that does not mix with water, such as ether. Even if the solution is mixed, the water and ether will form two distinct and separate layers, with the ether on top since it is less dense. As time progresses, while the ether turns brown, the color of the water fades and it becomes almost colorless. This is an indication of transfer of iodine from the water into the ether. Obviously, the initial concentration of iodine in the water is higher. As the mass transfer takes place, the concentration of iodine in the water decreases and the concentration of iodine in the ether increases. Does the mass transfer stop when the concentrations of iodine equalize in the water and the ether phases? The answer is no; mass transfer stops only when the partial molar Gibbs energies of iodine in the water and in the ether are equal to each other. At that point, the concentration of iodine in the ether phase is much higher than the iodine concentration in the water. In other words, iodine has moved against a concentration difference.

In addition to reverse diffusion, Duncan and Toor (1962) mentioned two other types of diffusion. When diffusion takes place even though there is no concentration gradient, this is called *osmotic*

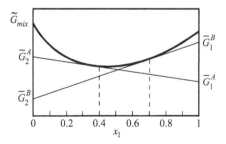

Figure 2.6 Determination of partial molar Gibbs energy from the $\widetilde{G}_{mix}$ versus x_1 plot.

---

[9]This type of phenomenon leads to phase splitting of liquid mixtures.

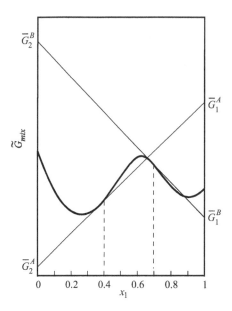

Figure 2.7 $\tilde{G}_{mix}$ versus x_1 plot with two minima.

diffusion. In the case of a *diffusion barrier*, no diffusion takes place even though there is a concentration gradient! These will be covered in detail in Chapter 8.

2.5.3 OTHER DRIVING FORCES OF MASS TRANSFER

It should be kept in mind that the gradient of partial molar Gibbs energy is not the sole driving force for diffusion. Gradient of temperature, gradient of pressure, gradient of electrical potential, and external forces, such as centrifugal force, are also responsible for the transfer of species.

Mass transfer of species as a result of temperature gradient is called *thermal diffusion*. This phenomenon is also known as the *Soret effect*. Since the separation as a result of temperature gradient is quite small, it is combined with free convection in a thermal diffusion column. A thermal diffusion column has an electrically heated wire located in the center of a vertical, water-cooled tube. It is usually used to separate isotopes, i.e., separation of the isotopes of neon. While the large radial temperature gradient causes radial separation of isotopes, the free convection current moving upward near the hot wire sweeps the lighter isotope to the top of the column and the free convection current moving downward near the cold wall drags the heavier isotope to the bottom of the column.

Separation of the isotopes of uranium is a typical example of mass transfer by a pressure gradient. Natural uranium constitutes approximately 0.71 wt % U^{235}, while the rest is U^{238}. Being a fissionable material, U^{235} is used as a fuel in nuclear reactors for producing steam at high temperature and pressure. The fuel for the reactor, however, must be enriched with a higher fraction of U^{235}, typically 4.4% in today's light water (ordinary water) reactors. Separation of U^{235} from U^{238} is accomplished by gas centrifuges. The rotor spinning at very high speed provides the pressure gradient for separation. The fission of 1g of U^{235} produces 1MW-day worth of nuclear energy.

When a gradient of electrical potential is applied to ionic solutions, each ion experiences a force that is the product of the ionic charge and the field strength of the electric field. Separation is accomplished by the movement of the positive and the negative ions toward the cathode and the anode, respectively.

2.6   ESTIMATION OF DIFFUSION COEFFICIENTS

Problems related to mass transfer require diffusion coefficients to be known. Diffusion coefficients can be estimated from experiments, correlations, and existing tabulated values. Diffusion coefficients for gases are of the order of $10^{-5} m^2/s$ $(0.1 cm^2/s)$ under atmospheric conditions. Diffusion coefficients for liquids are usually of the order of $10^{-9} m^2/s$ $(10^{-5} cm^2/s)$. Diffusion coefficients for solids vary from $10^{-10} m^2/s$ to $10^{-14} m^2/s$ $(10^{-6}$ to $10^{-10} cm^2/s)$.

Table 2.5
Diffusion Coefficients for Some Binary Systems as a Function of Temperature and Pressure

System	$\dfrac{\mathcal{D}_{AB}P}{(\mathbf{cm^2/s}).\mathbf{atm}}$	T Range (K)
Air–CO_2	$\dfrac{2.70 \times 10^{-5} T^{1.590}}{\exp\left(\dfrac{102.1}{T}\right)}$	280–1,800
CO–N_2	$\dfrac{4.40 \times 10^{-3} T^{1.576}}{\left[\ln\left(\dfrac{T}{1.57 \times 10^8}\right)\right]^2 \exp\left(\dfrac{-36.2}{T}\right) \exp\left(\dfrac{3,825}{T^2}\right)}$	78–10,000
H_2–Ar	$\dfrac{2.35 \times 10^{-2} T^{1.519}}{\left[\ln\left(\dfrac{T}{4.88 \times 10^7}\right)\right]^2 \exp\left(\dfrac{39.8}{T}\right)}$	14–10,000
H_2–CO_2	$\dfrac{3.14 \times 10^{-5} T^{1.750}}{\exp\left(\dfrac{11.7}{T}\right)}$	200–550
H_2–CO	$\dfrac{1.539 \times 10^{-2} T^{1.548}}{\left[\ln\left(\dfrac{T}{3.16 \times 10^7}\right)\right]^2 \exp\left(\dfrac{-2.80}{T}\right) \exp\left(\dfrac{1,067}{T^2}\right)}$	65–10,000
N_2–CO_2	$\dfrac{3.15 \times 10^{-5} T^{1.570}}{\exp\left(\dfrac{113.6}{T}\right)}$	288–1,800
N_2–O_2	$1.13 \times 10^{-5} T^{1.724}$	285–10,000
H_2O–Air	$1.87 \times 10^{-6} T^{2.072}$ $2.75 \times 10^{-5} T^{1.632}$	$282 - 450$ $450 - 1,070$
H_2O–CO_2	$\dfrac{9.24 \times 10^{-5} T^{1.500}}{\exp\left(\dfrac{307.9}{T}\right)}$	$296 - 1,640$
H_2O–N_2	$1.87 \times 10^{-6} T^{2.072}$ $1.89 \times 10^{-6} T^{2.072}$	$282 - 373$ $282 - 450$
H_2O–O_2	$2.78 \times 10^{-5} T^{1.632}$	$450 - 1,070$

Source: (Marrero and Mason, 1972)

2.6.1 DIFFUSION COEFFICIENTS FOR GASES

Marrero and Mason (1972) summarized the experimental methods used to measure binary diffusion coefficients. They also fitted the published experimental data to an equation, some of which are given in Table 2.5. Poling et al. (2001) summarized the theoretical and empirical correlations to predict diffusion coefficients for binary gas systems at low pressures. Some of these correlations are given below.

2.6.1.1 Chapman–Enskog theory

Based on the Chapman–Enskog kinetic theory, the binary diffusion coefficients for nonpolar gases at low density are given by[10]

$$
\mathcal{D}_{AB} = 1.8583 \times 10^{-3} \frac{T^{3/2} \sqrt{\dfrac{1}{M_A} + \dfrac{1}{M_B}}}{P \sigma_{AB}^2 \Omega_{\mathcal{D}}} \ (\text{cm}^2/\text{s}),
\tag{2.195}
$$

where T is the absolute temperature in K, P is the pressure in atm, and M_A and M_B represent the molecular weights (g/mol or kg/kmol) of species A and B, respectively. The Lennard-Jones collision diameter, σ_{AB}, in angstroms[11] is calculated from

$$
\sigma_{AB} = \frac{\sigma_A + \sigma_B}{2}
\tag{2.196}
$$

The diffusion collision integral, $\Omega_{\mathcal{D}}$, in Eq. (2.195) is expressed as (Neufeld et al., 1972)

$$
\Omega_{\mathcal{D}} = \frac{1.06036}{(T^*)^{0.15610}} + \frac{0.19300}{\exp(0.47635\,T^*)} + \frac{1.03587}{\exp(1.52996\,T^*)} + \frac{1.76474}{\exp(3.89411\,T^*)} \quad 0.3 \leq T^* \leq 100,
\tag{2.197}
$$

where the dimensionless temperature, T^*, is defined by

$$
T^* = \frac{T}{\sqrt{\left(\dfrac{\varepsilon_A}{\kappa}\right)\left(\dfrac{\varepsilon_B}{\kappa}\right)}},
\tag{2.198}
$$

in which κ is the Boltzmann constant; ε_A and ε_B are Lennard-Jones energy parameters for species A and B, respectively. Table 2.6 lists the values of σ and ε/κ for several substances. It should be pointed out that the values of σ and ε/κ may differ from one reference to another. For example, the values given by Bird et al. (2007) are very different from those given by Poling et al. (2001) for some substances.

A log-log plot of $\Omega_{\mathcal{D}}$ versus T^*, shown in Figure 2.8, indicates that at low values of dimensionless temperature ($0.3 \leq T^* \leq 2$), $\Omega_{\mathcal{D}}$ is approximately proportional to $T^{-0.5}$. On the other hand, when $T^* \geq 5$, $\Omega_{\mathcal{D}}$ is proportional to $T^{-0.16}$. Therefore, temperature dependence of the diffusion coefficient is expressed as

$$
\mathcal{D}_{AB} \propto
\begin{cases}
T^2 & 0.3 \leq T^* \leq 2 \\[2mm]
T^{1.66} & 5 \leq T^* \leq 100
\end{cases}
\tag{2.199}
$$

---

[10] The derivation of this equation is given by Bird et al. (2007).

[11] One angstrom (Å) $= 0.1$ nanometer (nm) $= 10^{-10}$ m.

Table 2.6
Lennard-Jones Potential Parameters[a]

Name	Molecular Weight	σ (Å)	ε/κ (K)
Light Gases			
Helium	4.003	2.551	10.22
Hydrogen	2.016	2.827	59.7
Noble Gases			
Argon	39.948	3.542	93.3
Neon	20.180	2.820	32.8
Simple Polyatomic Gases			
Air	28.964	3.617	97.0
Chlorine	70.906	4.217	316.0
Carbon dioxide	44.010	3.941	195.2
Carbon monoxide	28.010	3.690	91.7
Iodine	253.809	5.160	474.2
Nitric oxide	30.006	3.492	116.7
Nitrogen	28.013	3.798	71.4
Nitrous oxide	44.013	3.828	232.4
Oxygen	31.999	3.467	106.7
Sulfur dioxide	64.064	4.112	335.4
Hydrocarbons			
Acetylene	26.037	4.033	231.8
Benzene	78.112	5.349	412.3
n-Butane	58.122	4.687	531.4
Cyclohexane	84.160	6.182	297.1
Ethane	30.069	4.443	215.7
Ethylene	28.053	4.163	224.7
Isobutane	58.122	5.278	330.1
Methane	16.043	3.758	148.6
n-Pentane	72.149	5.784	341.1
Propane	44.096	5.118	237.1
Propylene	42.080	4.678	298.9
Organic Compounds			
Carbon disulfide	76.141	4.483	467
Carbon tetrachloride	153.823	5.947	322.7
Chloroform	119.378	5.389	340.2
Methyl acetate	74.079	4.936	469.8

[a]Molecular weights are compiled from NIST Chemistry WebBook; Lennard-Jones potential parameters are taken from Poling et al. (2001).

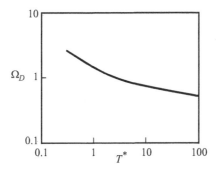

Figure 2.8 Variation in the diffusion collision integral, $\Omega_{\mathcal{D}}$, with dimensionless temperature, T^*.

Example 2.9   Estimate the diffusion coefficient for a binary mixture of helium (A) and nitrogen (B) at 850 K and 1 atm.

Solution

From Table 2.6

$$M_A = 4.003 \, \text{g/mol} \qquad \sigma_A = 2.551 \, \text{Å} \qquad \varepsilon_A/\kappa = 10.22 \, \text{K}$$

$$M_B = 28.013 \, \text{g/mol} \qquad \sigma_B = 3.798 \text{Å} \qquad \varepsilon_B/\kappa = 71.4 \, \text{K}$$

As can be seen from the Mathcad worksheet shown below, the diffusion coefficient is predicted as $3.945 \, \text{cm}^2/\text{s}$.

ORIGIN:= 1

$$M := \begin{pmatrix} 4.003 \\ 28.013 \end{pmatrix} \qquad \sigma := \begin{pmatrix} 2.551 \\ 3.798 \end{pmatrix} \qquad \varepsilon := \begin{pmatrix} 10.22 \\ 71.4 \end{pmatrix} \qquad T := 850 \qquad P := 1$$

$$D := \quad \sigma m \leftarrow \frac{\sigma_1 + \sigma_2}{2}$$

$$Tr \leftarrow \frac{T}{\sqrt{\varepsilon_1 \cdot \varepsilon_2}}$$

$$\Omega \leftarrow \frac{1.06036}{Tr^{0.1561}} + \frac{0.193}{\exp(0.47635Tr)} + \frac{1.03587}{\exp(1.52996Tr)} + \frac{1.76474}{\exp(3.89411Tr)}$$

$$D \leftarrow \frac{1.85831\,0^{-3} \cdot T^{\frac{3}{2}} \cdot \sqrt{\dfrac{1}{M_1} + \dfrac{1}{M_2}}}{P \cdot \sigma m^2 \cdot \Omega}$$

$$D$$

$$D = 3.945$$

Mathcad worksheet of Example 2.9.

Comment: Marrero and Mason (1972) proposed the following equation for a helium–nitrogen system:

$$\mathcal{D}_{AB} P = \frac{1.58 \times 10^{-2} \, T^{1.524}}{\left[\ln \left(\dfrac{T}{2.65 \times 10^7} \right) \right]^2} \; (\text{cm}^2/\text{s}) \,.\text{atm}$$

Thus

$$\mathcal{D}_{AB} = \frac{1.58 \times 10^{-2} \, (850)^{1.524}}{\left[\ln \left(\dfrac{850}{2.65 \times 10^7} \right) \right]^2} = 4.3 \, \text{cm}^2/\text{s}$$

Table 2.7

Special Atomic Diffusion Volumes

Atomic and Structural Diffusion Volume Increments, v_i's (cm^3)			
C	15.9	Cl	21.0
H	2.31	Br	21.9
O	6.11	I	29.8
N	4.54	Aromatic ring	−18.3
S	22.9	Heterocyclic ring	−18.3
F	14.7		

Diffusion Volumes of Atom and Simple Molecules, $\sum v_i$'s (cm^3)			
He	2.67	CO	18.0
Ne	5.98	CO_2	26.7
Ar	16.2	N_2O	35.9
Kr	24.5	NH_3	20.7
Xe	32.7	H_2O	13.1
H_2	6.12	SF_6	71.3
D_2	6.84	Cl_2	38.4
N_2	18.5	Br_2	69.0
O_2	16.3	SO_2	41.8
Air	19.7		

Source: (Fuller et al., 1969)

2.6.1.2   Fuller–Schettler–Giddings correlation

Fuller et al. (1966) developed a correlation equation based on special atomic diffusion volumes as

$$\mathcal{D}_{AB} = 1.01 \times 10^{-3} \frac{T^{1.75} \sqrt{\frac{1}{M_A} + \frac{1}{M_B}}}{P\left[(\Sigma v_i)_A^{1/3} + (\Sigma v_i)_B^{1/3}\right]^2} \ (cm^2/s), \tag{2.200}$$

where T is the absolute temperature in K, P is the pressure in atm, M_A and M_B are the molecular weights (g/mol or kg/kmol) of species A and B, respectively, and v_i's are the atomic diffusion volume increments (cm^3) to be summed over the atoms, groups, and structural features of each diffusing species. Numerous v_i's and the 1.75 exponent of T were determined from a nonlinear least-squares analysis of over 300 experimental points. Later, Fuller et al. (1969) expanded the data collection to 512 points. The revised v_i values are listed in Table 2.7. Although the temperature exponent was found to be 1.776, it was retained as 1.75 for simplicity.

For chemicals in air, Eq. (2.200) simplifies to

$$\mathcal{D}_{A(air)} = 1.01 \times 10^{-3} \frac{T^{1.75} \sqrt{\frac{1}{M_A} + 0.0345}}{P\left[(\Sigma v_i)_A^{1/3} + 2.7\right]^2} \ (cm^2/s) \tag{2.201}$$

Example 2.10   Estimate the diffusion coefficient of hydrogen (A) in methane (B) at 425 K and 1 atm.

Solution

From Table 2.6

$$M_A = 2.016 \, g/mol \qquad M_B = 16.043 \, g/mol$$

From Table 2.7

$$(\Sigma v_i)_A = 6.12\,\text{cm}^3 \qquad (\Sigma v_i)_B = 15.9 + (4)(2.31) = 25.14\,\text{cm}^3$$

Substitution of the values into Eq. (2.200) gives

$$\mathcal{D}_{AB} = 1.01 \times 10^{-3}\, \frac{(425)^{1.75}\sqrt{\dfrac{1}{2.016} + \dfrac{1}{16.043}}}{(1)\left[(6.12)^{1/3} + (25.14)^{1/3}\right]^2} = 1.326\,\text{cm}^2/\text{s}$$

Comment: Marrero and Mason (1972) proposed the following equation for a hydrogen–methane system:

$$\mathcal{D}_{AB}P = 3.13 \times 10^{-5}\,T^{1.765}\ \left(\text{cm}^2/\text{s}\right).\text{atm}$$

Thus

$$\mathcal{D}_{AB} = 3.13 \times 10^{-5}\,(425)^{1.765} = 1.364\,\text{cm}^2/\text{s}$$

2.6.2 DIFFUSION COEFFICIENTS FOR LIQUIDS

Correlations as well as the experimental techniques for the determination of liquid diffusion coefficients are summarized by Johnson and Babb (1956), Himmelblau (1964), and Poling et al. (2001). Besides temperature and pressure, liquid diffusion coefficients are strong functions of concentration. For example, for a binary system of acetone (A) and water (B) at 298K, variation in diffusion coefficients as a function of mole fraction of acetone is shown in Figure 2.9.

The terms $\mathcal{D}_{AB}^{\infty}$ and $\mathcal{D}_{BA}^{\infty}$ represent diffusion coefficients at infinite dilution. $\mathcal{D}_{AB}^{\infty}$ is the value of the diffusion coefficient as $x_A \to 0$, i.e., a small amount of A in a very large amount of B. On the other hand, $\mathcal{D}_{BA}^{\infty}$ is the value of the diffusion coefficient as $x_B \to 0$, i.e., a small amount of B in a very large amount of A. Some of the existing correlations to estimate liquid diffusion coefficients at infinite dilution are given below.

2.6.2.1 Stokes–Einstein equation

Einstein (1905) assumed diffusion of large rigid spheres (solute A) through a medium of small particles (solvent B), such as diffusion of colloidal particles through a liquid. To predict the diffusion coefficient of a dilute solute A in a solvent B, he proposed the following equation:

$$\mathcal{D}_{AB}^{\infty} = \frac{\kappa T}{6\pi \mu_B R_A}, \qquad (2.202)$$

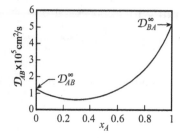

Figure 2.9 Diffusion coefficients for an acetone (A)–water (B) system (Tyn and Calus, 1975b).

Table 2.8

Molecular and van der Waals Volumes of Some Liquids

Substance	v_M (Å³)	v_W (Å³)
Benzene	148.6	80.4
Cyclohexane	179.4	102.0
Ethylene glycol	92.4	60.8
Glycerol	121.3	88.5
Methanol	67.0	36.1
n-Pentane	192	96.4

Source: (Edward, 1970)

---

where κ is the Boltzmann constant (1.3806×10^{-23} J/K), T is the absolute temperature, μ_B is the viscosity of solvent, and R_A is the spherical solute radius. Equation (2.202) indicates that the diffusion coefficient is dependent on the radius (or diameter) of the diffusing molecules and the viscosity of the solvent.

One of the assumptions used in the derivation of Eq. (2.202) is that there is no slip at the surface of the solute sphere. If the solvent does not stick to the diffusing species,[12] then it is recommended to replace the numerical factor 6 in the denominator of Eq. (2.202) with 4.

The use of Eq. (2.202) requires the radius (or diameter) of the solute molecule to be known. As a rough estimate, R_A can be taken as $\sigma_A/2$, where σ_A is the collision diameter[13] of solute given in Table 2.6. If the molecular volume, v, is known, then R_A can be determined from

$$R_A = \left(\frac{3v}{4\pi} \right)^{1/3} \tag{2.203}$$

However, there is no unique method for the determination of molecular volume. The van der Waals volume, v_w, is the total volume occupied by its atoms. Bondi (1964) calculated v_w as the sum of volumes of mutually intersecting spheres centered on single atoms based on the bond distances, bond angles, and intermolecular van der Waals radii. On the other hand, the molecular volume, v_M, is obtained by dividing the molar volume of a solid or liquid by Avogadro's number (6.02×10^{23} molecules/mol). Furthermore, there are other methods used for the determination of molecular volume (Edward, 1970). Molecular and van der Waals volumes of some liquids at room temperature (293–298 K) are listed in Table 2.8. While the use of v_w in the calculation of R_A is more suitable for small molecules of 2–6 Å radius, it is recommended to use v_M for large molecules (Edward, 1970).

In the literature, the Stokes–Einstein equation is generally used to estimate R_A (also named the *hydrodynamic radius*) once the diffusion coefficient is experimentally measured.

Example 2.11 Diffusion coefficients of lactalbumin, ovalbumin, and bovine serum albumin (BSA) in 0.1 M phosphate buffered saline (PBS) solution at 298 K are reported by Pluen et al. (1999) as 1.14×10^{-6}, 7.8×10^{-7}, and 6.4×10^{-7} cm²/s, respectively. If the viscosity of the solvent is 0.8705 cP, calculate the radii of these macromolecules.

Solution

Rearrangement of Eq. (2.202) gives

$$R_A = \frac{\kappa T}{6\pi \mu_B \mathcal{D}_{AB}^{\infty}} \tag{1}$$

---

[12] Slip takes place at the surface of the solute sphere when $R_A < 5$ Å.

[13] The collision diameter, σ, is the center-to-center distance between two molecules of the same species.

Substitution of the numerical values into Eq. (1) gives

Lactalbumin $\qquad R_A = \dfrac{(1.3806 \times 10^{-23})(298)}{6\pi(0.8705 \times 10^{-3})(1.14 \times 10^{-10})} = 2.199 \times 10^{-9}\,\mathrm{m} = 2.199\,\mathrm{nm}$

Ovalbumin $\qquad R_A = \dfrac{(1.3806 \times 10^{-23})(298)}{6\pi(0.8705 \times 10^{-3})(7.8 \times 10^{-11})} = 3.215 \times 10^{-9}\,\mathrm{m} = 3.215\,\mathrm{nm}$

BSA $\qquad R_A = \dfrac{(1.3806 \times 10^{-23})(298)}{6\pi(0.8705 \times 10^{-3})(6.4 \times 10^{-11})} = 3.918 \times 10^{-9}\,\mathrm{m} = 3.918\,\mathrm{nm}$

2.6.2.2 Wilke–Chang equation

The equation proposed by Wilke and Chang (1955) was evolved from the Stokes–Einstein equation. Noting that the group $\mathcal{D}_{AB}\mu_B/T$, designated as the diffusion factor, is essentially independent of temperature, they proposed the following equation for calculating the diffusion coefficient of solute A at very low concentrations in solvent B:

$$\mathcal{D}_{AB}^{\infty} = 7.4 \times 10^{-8} \frac{T \sqrt{\phi_B M_B}}{\mu_B \widetilde{V}_A^{0.6}} \; (\mathrm{cm}^2/\mathrm{s}),\tag{2.204}$$

where T is the absolute temperature in K, ϕ_B is an "association parameter"[14] for the solvent, M_B is the molecular weight of the solvent in g/mol, μ_B is the viscosity of the solvent in centipoises, and $\widetilde{V}_A$ is the molar volume of the solute at its normal boiling point in $\mathrm{cm}^3/\mathrm{mol}$. Recommended values of the association parameter for common solvents are given as follows:

$$\phi_B = \begin{cases} 2.6 & \text{Water} \\ 1.9 & \text{Methanol} \\ 1.5 & \text{Ethanol} \\ 1 & \text{Unassociated solvents (benzene, ether, heptane)} \end{cases}\tag{2.205}$$

2.6.2.3 Modified Tyn–Calus equation

This equation was also evolved from the Stokes–Einstein equation. Since the sizes of the solute and solvent molecules are of the same order of magnitude, Tyn and Calus (1975a) introduced the size of the solvent molecule as an additional variable. The modified form of this equation is presented by Poling et al. (2001) as

$$\mathcal{D}_{AB}^{\infty} = 8.93 \times 10^{-8} \frac{\widetilde{V}_B^{0.267}}{\widetilde{V}_A^{0.433}} \frac{T}{\mu_B} \; (\mathrm{cm}^2/\mathrm{s}),\tag{2.206}$$

where T is the absolute temperature in K, μ_B is the viscosity of the solvent in centipoises, and $\widetilde{V}_A$ and $\widetilde{V}_B$ are the molar volumes of the solute and solvent, respectively, at their respective normal boiling points in $\mathrm{cm}^3/\mathrm{mol}$. The molar volumes are obtained from

$$\widetilde{V}_i = 0.285 \left(\widetilde{V}_c\right)_i^{1.048} \qquad i = A, B,\tag{2.207}$$

---

[14] *Association parameter* defines the effective molecular weight of the solvent with respect to the diffusion process. It has to be estimated from experimental data.

where $\widetilde{V}_c$ is the critical molar volume in cm^3/mol. Note that Eq. (2.207) can also be used to calculate $\widetilde{V}_A$ in the Wilke–Chang equation, Eq. (2.204).

Example 2.12 Estimate the infinitely dilute diffusion coefficient of acetone (A) in chloroform (B) at 313 K and 1 atm using

a) The Wilke–Chang equation,
b) The modified Tyn–Calus equation.

Solution

From Appendix F

$$M_A = 58.079\,kg/kmol \qquad (\widetilde{V}_c)_A = 215.98\,cm^3/mol \qquad M_B = 119.378\,kg/kmol$$

From the Dortmund Data Bank,[15] the viscosity of chloroform at 313 K is

$$\mu_B = 0.473\,cP$$

From the Dortmund Data Bank,[16] the density of chloroform at its normal boiling point (334.3 K) is

$$\rho_B = 1410.73\,kg/m^3$$

Thus

$$\widetilde{V}_B = \frac{119.378 \times 10^3}{1410.73} = 84.621\,cm^3/mol$$

The use of Eq. (2.206) gives

$$\widetilde{V}_A = 0.285(215.98)^{1.048} = 79.673\,cm^3/mol$$

a) Substitution of the numerical values into Eq. (2.204) gives

$$\mathcal{D}_{AB}^{\infty} = 7.4 \times 10^{-8}\frac{(313)\sqrt{(1)(119.378)}}{(0.473)(79.673)^{0.6}} = 3.869 \times 10^{-5}\,cm^2/s$$

b) Substitution of the numerical values into Eq. (2.206) gives

$$\mathcal{D}_{AB}^{\infty} = 8.93 \times 10^{-8}\frac{(84.621)^{0.267}}{(79.673)^{0.433}}\frac{(313)}{(0.473)} = 2.903 \times 10^{-5}\,cm^2/s$$

Comment: Poling et al. (2001) reported the experimental value as $2.9 \times 10^{-5}\,cm^2/s$. While the modified Tyn–Calus equation predicts the diffusion coefficient accurately, the error introduced by using the Wilke–Chang equation is

$$Error = \left(\frac{3.689 - 2.9}{2.9}\right) \times 100 = 27\%$$

---

[15]http://ddbonline.ddbst.de/VogelCalculation/VogelCalculationCGI.exe

[16]http://ddbonline.ddbst.de/DIPPR105DensityCalculation/DIPPR105CalculationCGI.exe

Example 2.13 Use the Wilke–Chang equation to calculate

a) The infinitely dilute diffusion coefficient of chlorobenzene in bromobenzene at 303 K and 1 atm,

b) The infinitely dilute diffusion coefficient of bromobenzene in chlorobenzene at 303 K and 1 atm.

DATA:

Component	μ (cP)	$\widetilde{V}$ (cm^3/mol)
Bromobenzene	1.016	107.07
Chlorobenzene	0.714	103.76

Solution

Let A and B designate chlorobenzene and bromobenzene, respectively. From Appendix F

$$M_A = 112.557 \, \text{kg/kmol} \quad \text{and} \quad M_B = 157.008 \, \text{kg/kmol}$$

a) From Eq. (2.204)

$$\mathcal{D}_{AB}^{\infty} = 7.4 \times 10^{-8} \frac{(303) \sqrt{(1)(157.008)}}{(1.016)(103.76)^{0.6}} = 1.71 \times 10^{-5} \, \text{cm}^2/\text{s}$$

b) From Eq. (2.204)

$$\mathcal{D}_{BA}^{\infty} = 7.4 \times 10^{-8} \frac{(303) \sqrt{(1)(112.557)}}{(0.714)(107.07)^{0.6}} = 2.02 \times 10^{-5} \, \text{cm}^2/\text{s}$$

Comment: Unlike binary diffusion coefficients in gases, $\mathcal{D}_{AB}^{\infty} \neq \mathcal{D}_{BA}^{\infty}$. The experimental diffusion coefficients reported by Burchard and Toor (1962) are

$$\mathcal{D}_{AB}^{\infty} = 1.36 \times 10^{-5} \text{cm}^2/\text{s} \quad \text{and} \quad \mathcal{D}_{BA}^{\infty} = 1.76 \times 10^{-5} \text{cm}^2/\text{s}$$

2.7 BOUNDARY CONDITIONS AT PHASE INTERFACES

As stated in Section 2.5.1, when α- and β-phases of a multicomponent system are in equilibrium, the fugacities of each component are equal in both phases, i.e.,

$$\widehat{f}_i^{\alpha}(T,P,x_i^{\alpha}) = \widehat{f}_i^{\beta}(T,P,x_i^{\beta}) \tag{2.208}$$

The starting point for obtaining boundary conditions at phase interfaces is Eq. (2.208).

2.7.1 VAPOR–LIQUID INTERFACE

Let α and β be the vapor and liquid phases, respectively. Therefore, Eq. (2.208) becomes

$$\widehat{f}_i^{V}(T,P,y_i) = \widehat{f}_i^{L}(T,P,x_i) \tag{2.209}$$

The fugacity of component i in the vapor phase is expressed in terms of the fugacity coefficient, $\widehat{\phi}_i^{V}$, and the fugacity of component i in the liquid phase is expressed in terms of the activity coefficient, γ_i. Thus, Eq. (2.209) takes the following form[17]:

$$y_i P \widehat{\phi}_i^{V}(T,P,y_i) = x_i f_i^{L}(T,P) \gamma_i(T,P,x_i) \tag{2.210}$$

---

[17]For details, see Tosun (2013).

The fugacity of pure liquid is given by

$$f_i^L(T,P) = P_i^{vap} \phi_i^V(T,P_i^{vap}) \exp\left[\frac{\widetilde{V}_i^L(P - P_i^{vap})}{RT}\right], \tag{2.211}$$

where the exponential term is known as the *Poynting correction factor* (PCF). It accounts for the compression of the liquid to a pressure P greater than its vapor pressure, P_i^{vap}, and its value is practically unity at low and moderate pressures.

Substitution of Eq. (2.211) into Eq. (2.210) gives the general equation representing the equilibrium condition at the vapor–liquid interface as

$$y_i P \widehat{\phi}_i^V(T,P,y_i) = x_i P_i^{vap} \phi_i^V(T,P_i^{vap}) \exp\left[\frac{\widetilde{V}_i^L(P - P_i^{vap})}{RT}\right] \gamma_i(T,P,x_i) \tag{2.212}$$

The fugacity coefficient of component i, $\widehat{\phi}_i^V$, and the fugacity coefficient of pure i, ϕ_i^V, are calculated from the equation of state. Boundary conditions at the vapor–liquid interface can be obtained by simplifying Eq. (2.212) depending on the assumptions made in the solution of the problem.

• Pure liquid is in contact with a gas mixture

Consider pure liquid A in contact with a gas mixture containing A as shown in Figure 2.10. Note that the concentration distribution is not continuous at the gas–liquid interface. For a pure liquid, x_A and γ_A are unity, and Eq. (2.212) reduces to

$$y_A P \widehat{\phi}_A^V(T,P,y_A) = P_A^{vap} \phi_A^V(T,P_A^{vap}) \exp\left[\frac{\widetilde{V}_A^L(P - P_A^{vap})}{RT}\right] \tag{2.213}$$

At low pressures, PCF = 1, and it is plausible to consider the gas phase as an ideal gas mixture, i.e.,

$$\widehat{\phi}_A^V(T,P,y_A) = \widehat{\phi}_A^{IGM}(T,P,y_A) = 1, \tag{2.214}$$

where the superscript ^{IGM} stands for "ideal gas mixture." Moreover, $\phi_A^V(T,P_A^{vap}) \simeq 1$ when the vapor pressure is not very high. Under these circumstances, Eq. (2.213) simplifies to

$$y_A = \frac{P_A^{vap}}{P} \tag{2.215}$$

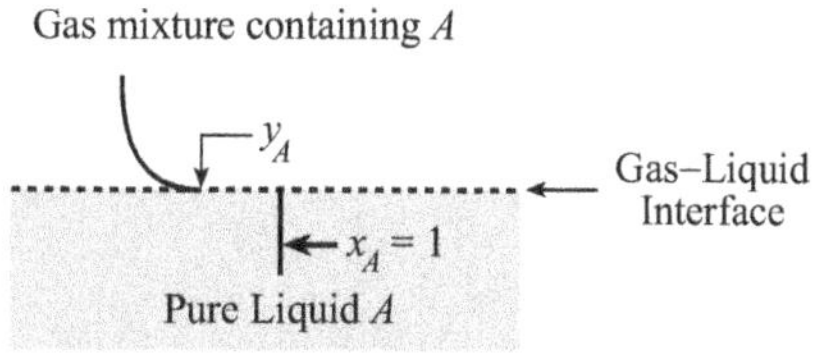

Figure 2.10   Gas–liquid interface.

• One of the species in a gas mixture is dissolving in a liquid

This is the case encountered in gas absorption. Let us consider absorption of species A in a gas mixture by a liquid solvent B. The equilibrium condition at the gas–liquid interface is given by

$$y_A P \widehat{\phi}_A^V(T,P,y_A) = \widehat{f}_A^L(T,P,x_A)$$
$$= x_A f_A^L(T,P) \gamma_A(T,P,x_A) \tag{2.216}$$

When the temperature of the system is greater than the critical temperature of species A, then the pure species A exists only as a gas and it is impossible to calculate $f_A^L(T,P)$. To circumvent this problem, Henry's law is defined as

$$\widehat{f}_A^L(T,P,x_A) = \mathcal{H}_A(T,P) x_A \qquad \text{when } x_A \to 0, \tag{2.217}$$

where $\mathcal{H}_A$ is called *Henry's law constant* and has the units of pressure.[18] While $\mathcal{H}_A$ is a strong function of temperature, its dependence on pressure is generally weak. Substitution of Eq. (2.217) into Eq. (2.216) leads to

$$y_A P \widehat{\phi}_A^V(T,P,y_A) = \mathcal{H}_A x_A \tag{2.218}$$

At low pressures, the gas phase may be considered an ideal gas mixture, i.e., $\widehat{\phi}_A^V(T,P,y_A) = \widehat{\phi}_A^{IGM}(T,P,y_A) = 1$, and Eq. (2.218) becomes

$$y_A P = \mathcal{H}_A x_A \qquad \Rightarrow \qquad \overline{P}_A = \mathcal{H}_A x_A, \tag{2.219}$$

where $\overline{P}_A$ represents the partial pressure of species A. It should be kept in mind that Eq. (2.219) holds when pressure is low and $x_A \ll 1$.

Rearrangement of Eq. (2.219) gives

$$\boxed{\mathcal{H}_A = \frac{\overline{P}_A}{x_A}} \tag{2.220}$$

Thus, Henry's law constant can be interpreted as the ratio of compositions in the gas and liquid phases. Partial pressure represents the composition in the gas phase, and mole fraction represents the composition in the liquid phase. Unfortunately, depending on the discipline, the various forms of Henry's law constant used in the literature create a great deal of confusion.

Sander (2015) classifies Henry's law constants used in the literature into two fundamental types as either

$$\text{Henry's law constant} = \frac{\text{Gas phase composition}}{\text{Liquid phase composition}} \tag{2.221}$$

or

$$\text{Henry's law constant} = \frac{\text{Liquid phase composition}}{\text{Gas phase composition}} \tag{2.222}$$

Typical choices for the gas phase composition are partial pressure ($\overline{P}$) and molar concentration (c). For the liquid phase, mole fraction (x), molar concentration (c), and molality are often used. Depending on the different choices of compositions, one can also express Eq. (2.221) as

$$\mathcal{H}_A^* = \frac{\overline{P}_A}{c_A^L} \tag{2.223}$$

and

$$K_A = \frac{c_A^V}{c_A^L} \tag{2.224}$$

---

[18]The SI unit for $\mathcal{H}_A$ is Pa. However, atm is still frequently used.

The SI unit for $\mathcal{H}_A^*$ is Pa.m^3/mol. The dimensionless term K_A is generally called the *partition coefficient*. Sander (2015) provided tables for conversion between the different units of so-called "Henry's law constants" used in the literature.

2.7.2 SOLID–FLUID INTERFACE

• Physical significance of the Biot number

Let us consider the transport of species A from the solid phase (species B) to the fluid phase through a solid–fluid interface. Since the molar flux of A is continuous at the interface

$$\mathbf{N}_A\big|_{\text{solid}\to\text{interface}} = \mathbf{N}_A\big|_{\text{interface}\to\text{fluid}} \tag{2.225}$$

Within the solid phase, the total molar flux of species A is

$$\mathbf{N}_A = -c\mathcal{D}_{AB}\nabla x_A + x_A\left(\mathbf{N}_A + \mathbf{N}_B\right) \tag{2.226}$$

Note that

$$O\left(-c\mathcal{D}_{AB}\nabla x_A\right) \gg O\left[x_A\left(\mathbf{N}_A + \mathbf{N}_B\right)\right] \tag{2.227}$$

In other words, the order of magnitude of the diffusive flux is much greater than that of the convective flux. Therefore, the left side of Eq. (2.225) is expressed as

$$\mathbf{N}_A\big|_{\text{solid}\to\text{interface}} = -c\mathcal{D}_{AB}\nabla x_A\big|_{\text{interface}} \tag{2.228}$$

The right side of Eq. (2.225) is expressed with the help of Eq. (1.30) in the form

$$\mathbf{N}_A\big|_{\text{interface}\to\text{fluid}} = k_c\left(\Delta c_A\right)_{\text{fluid}} \tag{2.229}$$

Substitution of Eqs. (2.228) and (2.229) into Eq. (2.227) yields

$$-c\mathcal{D}_{AB}\nabla x_A\big|_{\text{interface}} = k_c\left(\Delta c_A\right)_{\text{fluid}} \tag{2.230}$$

The gradient of a quantity represents the variation in that particular quantity over a characteristic length, L_{ch}. Thus, the orders of magnitude of the terms in Eq. (2.230) are more or less equal to each other, i.e.,

$$0\left[\frac{\mathcal{D}_{AB}\left(\Delta c_A\right)_{\text{solid}}}{L_{ch}}\right] \sim 0\left[k_c\left(\Delta c_A\right)_{\text{fluid}}\right] \tag{2.231}$$

or

$$\boxed{\text{Bi}_\text{M} = \frac{\left(\Delta c_A\right)_{\text{solid}}}{\left(\Delta c_A\right)_{\text{fluid}}} = \frac{k_c L_{ch}}{\mathcal{D}_{AB}},} \tag{2.232}$$

where Bi_M is the *Biot number for mass transfer*.[19] When $\text{Bi}_\text{M} \ll 1$, the concentration distribution in the fluid is much larger than that in the solid. In other words, the resistance to mass transfer lies within the fluid phase, and the concentration distribution is considered uniform within the solid phase. When $\text{Bi}_\text{M} \gg 1$, on the other hand, the resistance to mass transfer in the fluid phase is considered negligible. Thus, the concentration distribution is considered uniform within the fluid phase. Representative concentration profiles within the solid and fluid phases depending on the value of the

---

[19]The Biot number for mass transfer is sometimes confused with the Sherwood number (see, for example, Siepmann et al., 1999). Although the Sherwood number has a form similar to Eq. (2.232), $\mathcal{D}_{AB}$ terms are different from each other. Diffusion coefficients in the Biot and Sherwood numbers are in the solid and fluid phases, respectively.

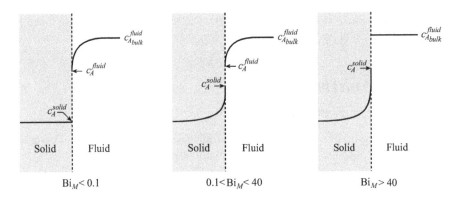

Figure 2.11   Effect of Bi_M on the concentration distribution.

Biot number are shown in Figure 2.11. When $Bi_M > 40$, the boundary condition at the solid–fluid interface is given by

$$K_A = \frac{c_A^{solid}}{c_{A_{bulk}}^{fluid}}, \tag{2.233}$$

where K_A is a partition coefficient. When $0.1 < Bi_M < 40$, Eq. (2.230) gives the boundary condition at the interface as

$$-c\mathcal{D}_{AB}\nabla x_A \cdot \lambda = k_c \left(c_A^{fluid} - c_{A_{bulk}}^{fluid} \right), \tag{2.234}$$

where λ is the unit normal vector to the phase interface that is directed into the fluid.

- **Liquid–pure solid interface**

Adding a small amount of sugar to a cup filled with tea and stirring result in disappearance of the sugar. This means the tea is *unsaturated* with sugar. If we continue adding sugar to the tea at constant temperature, a point comes where the liquid is *saturated* with sugar. This corresponds to a thermodynamic equilibrium, i.e., equality of fugacities, between solid and liquid phases. After this point, any additional sugar does not dissolve and appears as a solid phase. In other words, *saturation concentration* represents the maximum amount of solute that the solvent can hold. Thus, $c_A = c_A^{sat}$ at a pure solid–liquid phase interface as shown in Figure 2.12.

- **Gas–polymer membrane interface**

The equilibrium molar concentration of a penetrant gas, c_A, dissolved in a polymer membrane is called *solubility* and is given by

$$c_A = S_A \overline{P}_A, \tag{2.235}$$

where S_A is the *solubility coefficient* for the gas/membrane system and $\overline{P}_A$ is the partial pressure. Comparison of Eq. (2.235) with Eq. (2.223) indicates that $S_A = 1/\mathcal{H}_A^*$.

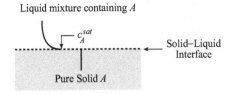

Figure 2.12   Solid–liquid interface.

In the literature, solubility, c_A, is expressed either in mol of A/m^3 of polymer or m^3 of A at STP/m^3 of polymer. STP stands for standard temperature and pressure, i.e., 273.15 K and 1 atm. At STP, the volume of 1 mol of an ideal gas is 22.4 L.

2.7.3 LIQUID–LIQUID INTERFACE

Let α and β be the two immiscible liquids that are in contact with each other. The distribution of species i between these two phases is expressed in terms of the partition coefficient as

$$K_i^{\alpha\beta} = \frac{c_i^\alpha}{c_i^\beta} \tag{2.236}$$

Octanol [$CH_3(CH_2)_7OH$] and water are partially immiscible, and the distribution of an organic compound i between these two phases is known as the *octanol–water partition coefficient*, K_i^{ow}, i.e.,

$$K_i^{ow} = \frac{c_i^o}{c_i^w} \tag{2.237}$$

Since K_i^{ow} values may range from 10^{-4} to 10^8 (encompassing 12 orders of magnitude), it is usually reported as $\log K_i^{ow}$.

Cells are mainly made of lipids, and they are generally modeled as a lipid bilayer model, with a long hydrophobic (water disliking) chain and a polar hydrophilic (water liking) end. The reason for choosing n-octanol is the fact that it exhibits both a hydrophobic and a hydrophilic character and its carbon/oxygen ratio is similar to that of lipids. In other words, n-octanol mimics the structure and properties of cells and organisms.

Since the octanol–water partition coefficient quantifies how a substance distributes itself between lipid and water, it is extensively used to describe lipophilic (lipid liking) and hydrophilic properties of a particular substance. In that respect, it is one of the key physical/chemical properties, such as vapor pressure and solubility in water, used to assess the impact of agricultural and industrial chemicals on the environment. For example, polychlorinated biphenyls (PCBs) have low solubilities in water and high octanol–water partition coefficients. If PCBs are accidentally released into a lake, then they are most probably found in higher concentrations in the sediment layer.

2.7.4 OTHER BOUNDARY CONDITIONS

Species cannot penetrate through an impermeable boundary. As a result, the molar flux and the concentration gradient are equal to zero. Also keep in mind that the concentration gradient is zero at the centerline of symmetry.

Unlike temperature, concentration is not continuous at a phase interface, i.e., $c_i^\alpha \neq c_i^\beta$ at the $\alpha-\beta$ interface. However, mass/molar fluxes are equal to each other if there is no adsorption or chemical reaction at the interface.

As stated in Section 2.2.2, the heterogeneous reaction rate expression appears as a boundary condition and it is represented by Eq. (2.114).

The terms "perfect sink" and "infinite source" are frequently used in the mass transfer literature. The term *perfect sink* implies that the concentration of the diffusing substance is zero. *Infinite source*, on the other hand, implies that the concentration does not change with time.

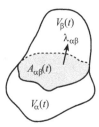

Figure 2.13   Material volume containing α and β phases.

2.7.5 JUMP BOUNDARY CONDITION

Consider a material volume $V_m(t)$ containing α and β phases separated by a singular surface $A_{\alpha\beta}(t) = A_{\beta\alpha}(t)$ as shown in Figure 2.13.[20] The velocity of the dividing surface is $\mathbf{w}$. Let $\lambda_{\alpha\beta}$ be the unit normal vector on $A_{\alpha\beta}$ pointing from the α-phase into the β-phase. Note that $\lambda_{\alpha\beta} = -\lambda_{\beta\alpha}$. Whitaker (1992) developed the species mass jump condition at a singular surface as

$$\frac{d}{dt}\int_{A_{\alpha\beta}(t)} \widehat{c}_i \, dA = \int_{A_{\alpha\beta}(t)} \left[c_i^\alpha(\mathbf{v}_i^\alpha - \mathbf{w}) \cdot \lambda_{\alpha\beta} + c_i^\beta(\mathbf{v}_i^\beta - \mathbf{w}) \cdot \lambda_{\beta\alpha} \right] dA + \int_{A_{\alpha\beta}(t)} \widehat{\mathcal{R}}_i \, dA, \quad (2.238)$$

where $\widehat{c}_i$ is the *excess surface concentration* (or simply the surface concentration) in mol/m^2 and $\widehat{\mathcal{R}}_i$ is the *excess surface rate of reaction* (or heterogeneous reaction rate) in $\text{mol}/\text{m}^2.\text{s}$. To proceed further, the surface transport theorem is needed to interchange the order of differentiation and integration in the term on the left side of Eq. (2.238). For simplicity, let us assume that the interface area $A_{\alpha\beta}$ is time independent. Under this condition, Eq. (2.238) reduces to

$$\boxed{\frac{\partial \widehat{c}_i}{\partial t} = c_i^\alpha(\mathbf{v}_i^\alpha - \mathbf{w}) \cdot \lambda_{\alpha\beta} + c_i^\beta(\mathbf{v}_i^\beta - \mathbf{w}) \cdot \lambda_{\beta\alpha} + \widehat{\mathcal{R}}_i} \quad \text{on } A_{\alpha\beta} = A_{\beta\alpha} \quad (2.239)$$

The summation of Eq. (2.239) over all species present in the system gives the *overall jump mass balance* at a phase interface in the form

$$\boxed{\frac{\partial \widehat{c}}{\partial t} = c^\alpha \left[(\mathbf{v}^*)^\alpha - \mathbf{w} \right] \cdot \lambda_{\alpha\beta} + c^\beta \left[(\mathbf{v}^*)^\beta - \mathbf{w} \right] \cdot \lambda_{\beta\alpha} + \sum_{i=1}^{N} \widehat{\mathcal{R}}_i} \quad \text{on } A_{\alpha\beta} = A_{\beta\alpha} \quad (2.240)$$

Problems

2.1 For a binary system of species, A and B show that

$$\mathbf{J}_A^{\blacksquare} = c \overline{V}_B \frac{M}{M_A M_B} \mathbf{j}_A$$

2.2 Show that

$$[\mathbf{j}] = \left[\mathbf{B}^{m\blacksquare} \right] \left[\mathbf{j}^{\blacksquare} \right],$$

---

[20]While moving at medium velocity, a *material volume* either expands or contracts so as to keep the total mass contained in it constant. A surface is said to be *singular* if it is discontinuous with respect to one or more quantities, such as velocity and density.

where the transformation matrix $[\mathbf{B}^{m\blacksquare}]$ is given by

$$[\mathbf{B}^{m\blacksquare}] = \begin{pmatrix} 1 & 0 & \cdots & 0 \\ 0 & 1 & \cdots & 0 \\ \vdots & \vdots & \vdots & \vdots \\ 0 & 0 & \cdots & 1 \end{pmatrix} - \begin{pmatrix} \omega_1 \\ \omega_2 \\ \vdots \\ \omega_{\mathcal{N}-1} \end{pmatrix} \cdot \begin{pmatrix} 1 - \dfrac{M_{\mathcal{N}}}{\overline{V}_{\mathcal{N}}} \dfrac{\overline{V}_1}{M_1} \\[2ex] 1 - \dfrac{M_{\mathcal{N}}}{\overline{V}_{\mathcal{N}}} \dfrac{\overline{V}_2}{M_2} \\[2ex] \vdots \\[2ex] 1 - \dfrac{M_{\mathcal{N}}}{\overline{V}_{\mathcal{N}}} \dfrac{\overline{V}_{\mathcal{N}-1}}{M_{\mathcal{N}-1}} \end{pmatrix}^{\mathrm{T}}$$

2.3 Apply the Sherman–Morrison formula to the transformation matrix $[\mathbf{B}^{m\blacksquare}]$ given in Problem 2.2 and show that

$$[\mathbf{j}^{\blacksquare}] = [\mathbf{B}^{\blacksquare m}][\mathbf{j}]$$

with

$$[\mathbf{B}^{\blacksquare m}] = [\mathbf{B}^{m\blacksquare}]^{-1} = \begin{pmatrix} 1 & 0 & \cdots & 0 \\ 0 & 1 & \cdots & 0 \\ \vdots & \vdots & \vdots & \vdots \\ 0 & 0 & \cdots & 1 \end{pmatrix} - \dfrac{M}{\widetilde{V}_{mix}} \begin{pmatrix} \omega_1 \\ \omega_2 \\ \vdots \\ \omega_{\mathcal{N}-1} \end{pmatrix} \cdot \begin{pmatrix} \dfrac{\overline{V}_1}{M_1} - \dfrac{\overline{V}_{\mathcal{N}}}{M_{\mathcal{N}}} \\[2ex] \dfrac{\overline{V}_2}{M_2} - \dfrac{\overline{V}_{\mathcal{N}}}{M_{\mathcal{N}}} \\[2ex] \vdots \\[2ex] \dfrac{\overline{V}_{\mathcal{N}-1}}{M_{\mathcal{N}-1}} - \dfrac{\overline{V}_{\mathcal{N}}}{M_{\mathcal{N}}} \end{pmatrix}^{\mathrm{T}},$$

where $\widetilde{V}_{mix}$ is defined by Eq. (2.83).

2.4 a) Show that

$$[\mathbf{j}] = [\mathbf{H}^{m*}][\mathbf{J}^*], \tag{1}$$

where the transformation matrix $[\mathbf{H}^{m*}]$ is given by

$$[\mathbf{H}^{m*}] = \begin{pmatrix} M_1 & 0 & \cdots & 0 \\ 0 & M_2 & \cdots & 0 \\ \vdots & \vdots & \vdots & \vdots \\ 0 & 0 & \cdots & M_{\mathcal{N}-1} \end{pmatrix} - \begin{pmatrix} \omega_1 \\ \omega_2 \\ \vdots \\ \omega_{\mathcal{N}-1} \end{pmatrix} \cdot \begin{pmatrix} M_1 - M_{\mathcal{N}} \\ M_2 - M_{\mathcal{N}} \\ \vdots \\ M_{\mathcal{N}-1} - M_{\mathcal{N}} \end{pmatrix}^{\mathrm{T}} \tag{2}$$

b) For a binary system of species A and B, show that Eq. (1) simplifies to

$$\mathbf{j}_A = \frac{M_A M_B}{M} \mathbf{J}_A^* \tag{3}$$

How can one calculate $\mathbf{j}_B$?

c) Note from Eq. (2.7) that

$$\begin{pmatrix} \omega_1 \\ \omega_2 \\ \vdots \\ \omega_{\mathcal{N}-1} \end{pmatrix} = \begin{pmatrix} \dfrac{x_1 M_1}{M} \\[2ex] \dfrac{x_2 M_2}{M} \\[2ex] \vdots \\[2ex] \dfrac{x_{\mathcal{N}-1} M_{\mathcal{N}-1}}{M} \end{pmatrix} \tag{4}$$

Substitute Eq. (4) into Eq. (2) to conclude that

$$[\mathbf{H}^{m*}] = \begin{pmatrix} M_1 & 0 & \cdots & 0 \\ 0 & M_2 & \cdots & 0 \\ \vdots & \vdots & \vdots & \vdots \\ 0 & 0 & \cdots & M_{\mathcal{N}-1} \end{pmatrix} - \begin{pmatrix} x_1 M_1 \\ x_2 M_2 \\ \vdots \\ x_{\mathcal{N}-1} M_{\mathcal{N}-1} \end{pmatrix} \cdot \begin{pmatrix} \dfrac{M_1 - M_{\mathcal{N}}}{M} \\ \dfrac{M_2 - M_{\mathcal{N}}}{M} \\ \vdots \\ \dfrac{M_{\mathcal{N}-1} - M_{\mathcal{N}}}{M} \end{pmatrix}^{\mathrm{T}} \tag{5}$$

2.5 Show that

$$[\mathbf{J}^*] = [\mathbf{H}^{*m}][\mathbf{j}],$$

where

$$[\mathbf{H}^{*m}] = \begin{pmatrix} \dfrac{1}{M_1} & 0 & \cdots & 0 \\ 0 & \dfrac{1}{M_2} & \cdots & 0 \\ \vdots & \vdots & \vdots & \vdots \\ 0 & 0 & \cdots & \dfrac{1}{M_{\mathcal{N}-1}} \end{pmatrix} - \begin{pmatrix} x_1 \\ x_2 \\ \vdots \\ x_{\mathcal{N}-1} \end{pmatrix} \cdot \begin{pmatrix} \dfrac{1}{M_1} - \dfrac{1}{M_{\mathcal{N}}} \\ \dfrac{1}{M_2} - \dfrac{1}{M_{\mathcal{N}}} \\ \vdots \\ \dfrac{1}{M_{\mathcal{N}-1}} - \dfrac{1}{M_{\mathcal{N}}} \end{pmatrix}^{\mathrm{T}}$$

Calculate $\mathbf{J}_i^*$ using the following data:

Species	y_i	$\mathbf{j}_i \times 10^4$ $(g/cm^2.s)$
H_2	0.12	1.830
CO	0.16	2.124
CO_2	0.20	1.151
O_2	0.15	-1.965
N_2	0.37	-3.140

(Answer: $8.074 \times 10^{-5}, -5.797 \times 10^{-6}, -1.411 \times 10^{-5}, -1.868 \times 10^{-5}, -4.215 \times 10^{-5}\,\text{mol/cm}^2.\text{s}$)

2.6 Show that

$$[\mathbf{J}^*] = [\mathbf{G}^{*m}][\mathbf{J}], \tag{1}$$

where the transformation matrix $[\mathbf{G}^{*m}]$ is given by

$$[\mathbf{G}^{*m}] = \begin{pmatrix} 1 & 0 & \cdots & 0 \\ 0 & 1 & \cdots & 0 \\ \vdots & \vdots & \vdots & \vdots \\ 0 & 0 & \cdots & 1 \end{pmatrix} - \begin{pmatrix} x_1 \\ x_2 \\ \vdots \\ x_{\mathcal{N}-1} \end{pmatrix} \cdot \begin{pmatrix} 1 - \dfrac{x_{\mathcal{N}}}{\omega_{\mathcal{N}}}\dfrac{\omega_1}{x_1} \\ 1 - \dfrac{x_{\mathcal{N}}}{\omega_{\mathcal{N}}}\dfrac{\omega_2}{x_2} \\ \vdots \\ 1 - \dfrac{x_{\mathcal{N}}}{\omega_{\mathcal{N}}}\dfrac{\omega_{\mathcal{N}-1}}{x_{\mathcal{N}-1}} \end{pmatrix}^{\mathrm{T}}$$

Calculate $\mathbf{J}_i^*$ using the following data:

Species	y_i	$\mathbf{J}_i \times 10^5$ $(\mathrm{mol/cm^2.s})$
H_2	0.412	0.823
H_2O	0.187	-1.913
CO	0.169	1.212
CO_2	0.177	-1.580
CH_4	0.056	0.629

(Answer: 3.855×10^{-6}, -2.112×10^{-5}, 1.033×10^{-5}, -7.679×10^{-6}, $1.461 \times 10^{-5}\,\mathrm{mol/cm^2.s}$)

2.7 At constant temperature and pressure, the Gibbs–Duhem equation relates the partial molar properties of species in a mixture as follows:

$$\sum_{k=1}^{\mathcal{N}} x_k\, d\overline{\varphi}_k = 0 \tag{1}$$

a) For a binary system consisting of species A and B, show that Eq. (1) reduces to

$$c_A\, d\overline{V}_A + c_B\, d\overline{V}_B = 0 \tag{2}$$

b) Since the volume fractions sum to unity, show that

$$c_A\, d\overline{V}_A + \overline{V}_A\, dc_A + c_B\, d\overline{V}_B + \overline{V}_B\, dc_B = 0 \tag{3}$$

c) Combine Eqs. (2) and (3) to obtain

$$\overline{V}_A\, dc_A + \overline{V}_B\, dc_B = 0 \tag{4}$$

and conclude that

$$\overline{V}_A \nabla c_A + \overline{V}_B \nabla c_B = 0 \tag{5}$$

2.8 The following speed data were collected on a two-lane highway heading outbound:

Vehicle Type	Average Weight (kg)	Average Speed (km/h)	% of Vehicles
Standard Car	2,000	120	55
Big Utility Car	4,500	100	27
Motorized Two-Wheeler	180	60	5
Heavy Vehicle	20,000	90	13

During the rush hour, the total number of vehicles passing through the observation point in an hour was measured as 1600.

a) Calculate the fluxes (in vehicles/lane.h) of vehicles.
b) Calculate the mass fluxes (in kg/lane.h) of vehicles.
c) Calculate the mass concentration (in kg/lane.km) of vehicles.
c) Calculate the mass-average speed of vehicles.

2.9 Show that

$$\mathbf{v}^* - \mathbf{v} = \sum_{k=1}^{\mathcal{N}} \left(\frac{M}{M_k} - 1 \right) \omega_k \mathbf{v}_k = \sum_{k=1}^{\mathcal{N}} \left(1 - \frac{M_k}{M} \right) x_k \mathbf{v}_k$$

When are mass- and molar-average velocities almost equal to each other?

2.10 Show that

$$\mathbf{v}^{\blacksquare} - \mathbf{v}^* = \sum_{k=1}^{\mathcal{N}-1} \left(\overline{V}_k - \overline{V}_\mathcal{N} \right) \mathbf{J}_k^* = \frac{1}{c} \sum_{k=1}^{\mathcal{N}-1} \left(\frac{\overline{V}_k}{\overline{V}_\mathcal{N}} - 1 \right) \mathbf{J}_k^{\blacksquare} \tag{1}$$

For a binary system consisting of species A and B, show that Eq. (1) reduces to

$$\mathbf{v}^{\blacksquare} - \mathbf{v}^* = \left(\overline{V}_A - \overline{V}_B \right) \mathbf{J}_A^* = \frac{\left(\overline{V}_A - \overline{V}_B \right)}{c \overline{V}_B} \mathbf{J}_A^{\blacksquare} \tag{2}$$

2.11 Estimate the diffusion coefficient for a binary mixture of argon (A) and oxygen (B) at 400K and 1atm using

a) The Chapman–Enskog theory,
b) The Fuller–Schettler–Giddings correlation,
c) The equation given by Marrero and Mason (1972) in the form

$$\mathcal{D}_{AB} P = 9.77 \times 10^{-6} T^{1.736} \ \left(\text{cm}^2/\text{s} \right) . \text{atm}$$

(Answer: a) $0.325 \, \text{cm}^2/\text{s}$, b) $0.334 \, \text{cm}^2/\text{s}$, c) $0.321 \, \text{cm}^2/\text{s}$)

2.12 The vitreous (also called vitreous humor) is a transparent, gelatinous substance that fills the space between the lens and the retina in the eye. It is 99% water, the rest being a mixture of collagen, proteins, salts, and sugar. Vitrectomy is a surgical procedure used to replace the vitreous with water or silicone oil. Discuss the advantages and disadvantages of using water and silicone oil as a replacement in terms of oxygen transport within the eye.

2.13 Estimate the diffusion coefficient of sulfur dioxide (A) in water (B) at 298 K and 1 atm using

a) The Wilke–Chang equation,
b) The Modified Tyn–Calus equation.

(Answer: a) $1.75 \times 10^{-5} \, \text{cm}^2/\text{s}$, b) $1.26 \times 10^{-5} \, \text{cm}^2/\text{s}$)

2.14 The temperature dependence of diffusion coefficients in liquids is generally expressed in the form of an Arrhenius relation, i.e.,

$$\mathcal{D}_{AB} = C_1 \exp \left(-\frac{C_2}{T} \right)$$

Use the following data provided by Snijder et al. (1995) for the diffusion of N_2O in toluene and evaluate the constants C_1 and C_2.

T (K)	$\mathcal{D}_{AB} \times 10^9 \ (\text{m}^2/\text{s})$
298.0	5.02
307.9	5.70
317.7	6.36
333.0	7.49
348.0	8.70

(Answer: $C_1 = 227.51 \times 10^{-9}$ and $C_2 = 1136.1$)

2.15 Estimate the infinitely dilute diffusion coefficient of ethanol (A) in water (B) at 298 K and 1 atm using the Wilke–Chang equation. Hills et al. (2011) reported the value as $1.23 \times 10^{-5} \text{cm}^2/\text{s}$.

(Answer: $1.403 \times 10^{-5} \text{cm}^2/\text{s}$)

2.16 Use the Stokes–Einstein equation to calculate

a) The infinitely dilute diffusion coefficient of ethanol (A) in water (B) at 313 K and 1 atm,
b) The infinitely dilute diffusion coefficient of water (B) in ethanol (A) at 313 K and 1 atm.

Discuss the possible sources of error in the calculations.

DATA:

Component	σ (Å)	μ (cP)
Ethanol	2.641	0.834
Water	4.530	0.655

The experimental values are given by Tyn and Calus (1975b) as

$$\mathcal{D}_{AB}^{\infty} = 1.70 \times 10^{-9}\,\text{m}^2/\text{s} \quad \text{and} \quad \mathcal{D}_{BA}^{\infty} = 1.64 \times 10^{-9}\,\text{m}^2/\text{s}$$

(Answer: a) $1.55 \times 10^{-9}\,\text{m}^2/\text{s}$, b) $2.08 \times 10^{-9}\,\text{m}^2/\text{s}$)

REFERENCES

Bird R. B., W. E. Stewart and E. N. Lightfoot. 2007. *Transport Phenomena*, 2nd edn. New York: Wiley.

Bondi, A. 1964. van der Waals volumes and radii. *J. Phys.Chem.* 68(3):441–51.

Burchard, J. K. and H. L. Toor. 1962. Diffusion in an ideal mixture of three completely miscible non-electrolytic liquids – Toluene, chlorobenzene, bromobenzene. *J. Phys. Chem.* 66(10):2015–22.

Duncan, J. B. and H. L. Toor. 1962. An experimental study of three component gas diffusion. *AIChE J.* 8(1):38–41.

Edward, J. T. 1970. Molecular volumes and the Stokes-Einstein equation. *J. Chem. Ed.* 47(4):261–70.

Einstein, A. 1905. Über die von der molekularkinetischen Theorie der Wärme geforderte Bewegung von in ruhenden Flüssigkeiten suspendierten Teilchen. *Ann. Physik.* 17:549–60.

Fick, A. 1995. On liquid diffusion. *J. Memb. Sci.* 100(1):33–38.

Fuller, E. N., P. D. Schettler and J. C. Giddings. 1966. A new method for prediction of binary gas-phase diffusion coefficients. *Ind. Eng. Chem.* 58(5):19–27.

Fuller, E. N., K. Ensley and J. C. Giddings. 1969. Diffusion of halogenated hydrocarbons in helium – The effect of structure on collision cross sections. *J. Phys. Chem.* 73(11):3679–85.

Hills, E. E., M. H. Abraham, A. Hersey and C. D. Bevan. 2011. Diffusion coefficients in ethanol and in water at 298K: Linear free energy relationships. *J. Fluid Phase Equilib.* 303:45–55.

Himmelblau, D. M. 1964. Diffusion of dissolved gases in liquids. *Chem. Rev.* 64(5): 527–50.

Job, G. and F. Herrmann. 2006. Chemical potential – A quantity in search of recognition. *Eur. J. Phys.* 27:353–71.

Johnson, P. A. and A. L. Babb. 1956. Liquid diffusion of non-electrolytes. *Chem. Rev.* 56(3):387–453.

Marrero, T. R. and E. A. Mason. 1972. Gaseous diffusion coefficients. *J. Phys. Chem. Ref. Data* 1(1):3–118.

Neufeld, P. D., A. R. Janzen and R. A. Aziz. 1972. Empirical equations to calculate 16 of the transport collision integrals $\Omega^{(l,s)*}$ for the Lennard-Jones (12-6) potential. *J. Chem. Phys.* 57(3):1100–2.

Philibert, J. 2006. One and a half century of diffusion: Fick, Einstein, before and beyond. *Diffusion Fund.* 4:6.1–6.19. http://ul.qucosa.de/fileadmin/data/qucosa/documents/19442/diff_fund_4%282006%296.pdf.

Pluen, A., P. A. Netti, R. K. Jain and D.A. Berk. 1999. Diffusion of macromolecules in agarose gels: Comparison of linear and globular configurations. *Biophys. J.* 77:542–52.

Poling, B. E., J. M. Prausnitz and J. P. O'Connell. 2001. *The Properties of Gases and Liquids*, 5th edn. New York: McGraw-Hill.

Sander, R. 2015. Compilation of Henry's law constants (version 4.0) for water as solvent. *Atmos. Chem. Phys.* 15:4399–4981. https://atmos-chem-phys.net/15/4399/2015/acp-15-4399-2015.pdf.

Siepmann, J., F. Lecomte and R. Bodmeier. 1999. Diffusion-controlled drug delivery systems: Calculation of the required composition to achieve desired release profiles. *J. Control. Release* 60:379–89.

Slattery, J. C. 1999. *Advanced Transport Phenomena*. Cambridge: Cambridge University Press.

Snijder, E. D., M. J. M. te Riele, G. F. Versteeg and V. P. M. van Swaaij. 1995. Diffusion coefficients of CO, CO_2, N_2O, and N_2 in ethanol and toluene. *J. Chem. Eng. Data* 40(1):37–39.

Tosun, I. 2013. *The Thermodynamics of Phase and Reaction equilibria*. Amsterdam: Elsevier.

Tyn, M. T. and W. F. Calus. 1975a. Diffusion coefficients in dilute binary liquid mixtures. *J. Chem. Eng. Data* 20(1):106–9.

Tyn, M. T. and W. F. Calus. 1975b. Temperature and concentration dependence of mutual diffusion coefficients of some binary liquid systems. *J. Chem. Eng. Data* 20(3):310–16.

Whitaker, S. 1992. The species mass jump condition at a singular surface. *Chem. Eng. Sci.* 47(7):1677–85.

Wilke, C. R. and P. Chang. 1995. Correlation of diffusion coefficients in dilute solutions. *AIChE J.* 1(2):264–70.

3 Foundations of Diffusion in Multicomponent Mixtures

When the number of species present in a mixture exceeds two, mass transport by diffusion is described by either a generalized Fick's law or Maxwell–Stefan (MS) equations.[1] This chapter provides insight into both of these approaches.

A generalized Fick's law is simply the extension of Fick's law for a binary system to a multicomponent system. Depending on how diffusive fluxes are defined with respect to the reference velocity frame, fluxes are related to the gradients of mass fraction, mole fraction, and molar concentration. In this case, however, the flux of a specific species is due not only to its own concentration gradient but also the concentration gradients of other species present in the mixture. As a result, the equations relating fluxes to concentration gradients are expressed in matrix notation with the Fick diffusion coefficient matrix being the proportionality factor. The transformation of Fick diffusion coefficient matrices from one velocity reference frame to another is given in Section 3.1.

A generalized Fick's law is only valid when the gradient of partial molar Gibbs energy is the sole driving force for diffusion. In the case of other driving forces, MS equations provide an alternative. Different forms of MS equations are presented in Section 3.2. These nonlinear equations separate mass transfer from thermodynamics by introducing a thermodynamic correction factor. As a result, MS diffusion coefficients are less concentration dependent than Fick diffusion coefficients.

Equations for calculation of the thermodynamic factor based on activity coefficient models and fugacity coefficient are presented in Section 3.3.

The link between MS and Fick diffusion coefficients is the thermodynamic factor. The equations relating these quantities are given in Section 3.4. Calculation of Fick diffusion coefficients from given MS diffusion coefficients, or *vice versa*, is provided by example problems.

Experimental data on diffusion coefficients are scarce. Section 3.5 is devoted to the frequently used prediction models for diffusion coefficients. In that respect, Vignes and Darken equations are presented.

Section 3.6 provides governing equations for multicomponent dilute gas mixtures.

3.1 GENERALIZED FICK'S LAW

For a binary system, diffusive fluxes relative to mass-, molar-, and volume-average velocities are defined by Eqs. (2.147), (2.155), and (2.163), respectively. The same diffusion coefficient, $\mathcal{D}_{AB}$, is used in these equations and $\mathcal{D}_{AB} = \mathcal{D}_{BA}$. In the case of multicomponent systems, however, different sets of diffusion coefficients are used depending on how diffusive fluxes are defined with respect to the reference velocity frames and they are different from one another.

3.1.1 DIFFUSIVE FLUX EXPRESSIONS

In a mixture of $\mathcal{N}$ species, Eq. (2.48) states that $(\mathcal{N} - 1)$ independent molar fluxes with reference to molar-average velocity exist. Thus, the generalization for diffusive molar flux relative to molar-average velocity is expressed as a linear combination of mole fraction gradients in the form of

$$\mathbf{J}_i^* = -c \sum_{k=1}^{\mathcal{N}-1} \mathcal{D}_{ik}^* \nabla x_k, \tag{3.1}$$

---

[1] Readers interested in the history of multicomponent diffusion theory may refer to Bird and Klingenberg (2013).

where $\mathcal{D}_{ik}^*$ represent Fick (or Fickian) diffusion coefficients with reference to molar-average velocity. In matrix notation, Eq. (3.1) is expressed in the form

$$[\mathbf{J}^*] = -c\,[\mathcal{D}^*]\,[\nabla x], \tag{3.2}$$

where $[\mathcal{D}^*]$ is a square matrix of order $(\mathcal{N} - 1)$ and $[\mathbf{J}^*]$ and $[\nabla x]$ are $(\mathcal{N} - 1)$ column vectors. Thus, in a mixture consisting of $\mathcal{N}$ species, $(\mathcal{N} - 1)^2$ Fick diffusion coefficients are required. The elements of $[\mathcal{D}^*]$ are not symmetric, i.e., $\mathcal{D}_{ij}^* \neq \mathcal{D}_{ji}^*$, but they are concentration dependent.

For a ternary system, for example, Eq. (3.1) is expressed as

$$\begin{aligned}
\mathbf{J}_1^* &= -c\,\mathcal{D}_{11}^* \nabla x_1 - c\,\mathcal{D}_{12}^* \nabla x_2 \\
\mathbf{J}_2^* &= -c\,\mathcal{D}_{21}^* \nabla x_1 - c\,\mathcal{D}_{22}^* \nabla x_2
\end{aligned} \tag{3.3}$$

In matrix notation, Eq. (3.3) is written in the form

$$\begin{pmatrix} \mathbf{J}_1^* \\ \mathbf{J}_2^* \end{pmatrix} = -c \begin{pmatrix} \mathcal{D}_{11}^* & \mathcal{D}_{12}^* \\ \mathcal{D}_{21}^* & \mathcal{D}_{22}^* \end{pmatrix} \begin{pmatrix} \nabla x_1 \\ \nabla x_2 \end{pmatrix} \tag{3.4}$$

The diagonal elements, $\mathcal{D}_{ii}^*$, relate the diffusive molar flux of species i to its own mole fraction gradient, ∇x_i. On the other hand, off-diagonal elements, $\mathcal{D}_{ik}^*$ ($i \neq k$), relate the diffusive molar flux of species i to the mole fraction gradient of species k, ∇x_k. Elements of the Fick diffusion coefficient matrix may take negative values[2]. Diagonal diffusion coefficients are usually (but not necessarily) greater than off-diagonal ones. Since Eq. (3.1) is written for species 1 and 2 (so-called *solutes*), the remaining one (species 3) is called a *solvent*, and its diffusive molar flux is calculated from $\mathbf{J}_3^* = 1 - (\mathbf{J}_1^* + \mathbf{J}_2^*)$. Although the species in the largest amount is usually chosen as the solvent, the choice of solvent is arbitrary. It should be kept in mind that the components of $[\mathcal{D}^*]$ may change depending on the choice of solvent.[3]

Similarly, the diffusive mass flux relative to mass-average velocity is expressed as

$$\mathbf{j}_i = -\rho \sum_{k=1}^{\mathcal{N}-1} \mathcal{D}_{ik}^m \nabla \omega_k, \tag{3.5}$$

where $\mathcal{D}_{ik}^m$ represent Fick diffusion coefficients with reference to mass-average velocity. In matrix notation, Eq. (3.5) is expressed in the form

$$[\mathbf{j}] = -\rho\,[\mathcal{D}^m]\,[\nabla \omega] \tag{3.6}$$

The diffusive molar flux relative to volume-average velocity is expressed as

$$\mathbf{J}_i^\blacksquare = -\sum_{k=1}^{\mathcal{N}-1} \mathcal{D}_{ik}^\blacksquare \nabla c_k, \tag{3.7}$$

where $\mathcal{D}_{ik}^\blacksquare$ represent Fick diffusion coefficients with reference to volume-average velocity. In matrix notation, Eq. (3.7) is expressed in the form

$$[\mathbf{J}^\blacksquare] = -[\mathcal{D}^\blacksquare]\,[\nabla c] \tag{3.8}$$

---

[2]This implies that $[\mathcal{D}^*]$ is not positive definite.

[3]See Problem 3.2.

As can be seen from the above equations, different sets of diffusion coefficients are used depending on the reference velocity frame used in defining diffusive fluxes. While diffusive mass fluxes are directly proportional to mass fraction gradient, diffusive molar fluxes are proportional to either mole fraction gradient or molar concentration gradient. Therefore, to transform diffusion coefficients from one reference velocity frame into another, it is necessary to relate ∇x_i to $\nabla \omega_i$ and ∇c_i to ∇x_i (or *vice versa*).

• **Transformation of ∇x_i to $\nabla \omega_i$**

Using Eq. (2.7), the gradient of mass fraction is expressed in the form

$$\nabla \omega_i = \nabla \left(\frac{M_i}{M} x_i \right) = \frac{M_i}{M} \nabla x_i - \frac{x_i M_i}{M^2} \nabla M = \frac{M_i}{M^2} (M \nabla x_i - x_i \nabla M) \tag{3.9}$$

The term ∇M can be calculated from Eq. (2.8) as

$$\nabla M = \sum_{k=1}^{\mathcal{N}} M_k \nabla x_k \qquad\qquad = \sum_{k=1}^{\mathcal{N}-1} M_k \nabla x_k + M_{\mathcal{N}} \nabla x_{\mathcal{N}} \tag{3.10}$$

Note that

$$\sum_{k=1}^{\mathcal{N}} x_k = 1 \quad \Rightarrow \quad \sum_{k=1}^{\mathcal{N}} \nabla x_k = 0 \quad \Rightarrow \quad \boxed{\nabla x_{\mathcal{N}} = -\sum_{k=1}^{\mathcal{N}-1} \nabla x_k} \tag{3.11}$$

Substitution of Eq. (3.11) into Eq. (3.10) yields

$$\nabla M = \sum_{k=1}^{\mathcal{N}-1} (M_k - M_{\mathcal{N}}) \nabla x_k \tag{3.12}$$

The term ∇x_i can be expressed as

$$\nabla x_i = \sum_{k=1}^{\mathcal{N}-1} \delta_{ik} \nabla x_k \tag{3.13}$$

Substitution of Eqs. (3.12) and (3.13) into Eq. (3.9) gives

$$\boxed{\nabla \omega_i = \frac{M_i}{M^2} \sum_{k=1}^{\mathcal{N}-1} \left[M \delta_{ik} - x_i (M_k - M_{\mathcal{N}}) \right] \nabla x_k} \tag{3.14}$$

For a binary system, Eq. (3.14) reduces to Eq. (2.152). In matrix notation, Eq. (3.14) is written as

$$\boxed{[\nabla \omega] = [\mathbf{L}^{\omega x}] [\nabla x],} \tag{3.15}$$

where the transformation matrix $[\mathbf{L}^{\omega x}]$ is given by

$$[\mathbf{L}^{\omega x}] = \begin{pmatrix} \dfrac{M_1}{M} & 0 & \cdots & 0 \\ 0 & \dfrac{M_2}{M} & \cdots & 0 \\ \vdots & \vdots & \vdots & \vdots \\ 0 & 0 & \cdots & \dfrac{M_{\mathcal{N}-1}}{M} \end{pmatrix} - \begin{pmatrix} x_1 M_1 \\ x_2 M_2 \\ \vdots \\ x_{\mathcal{N}-1} M_{\mathcal{N}-1} \end{pmatrix} \cdot \begin{pmatrix} \dfrac{M_1 - M_{\mathcal{N}}}{M^2} \\ \dfrac{M_2 - M_{\mathcal{N}}}{M^2} \\ \vdots \\ \dfrac{M_{\mathcal{N}-1} - M_{\mathcal{N}}}{M^2} \end{pmatrix}^{\mathrm{T}} \tag{3.16}$$

• Transformation of $\nabla \omega_i$ to ∇x_i

Using Eq. (2.7), the gradient of mole fraction is expressed in the form

$$\nabla x_i = \nabla \left(\frac{M}{M_i} \omega_i \right) = \frac{M}{M_i} \nabla \omega_i + \frac{\omega_i}{M_i} \nabla M = \frac{M^2}{M_i} \left(\frac{1}{M} \nabla \omega_i + \frac{\omega_i}{M^2} \nabla M \right) \tag{3.17}$$

The term ∇M can be calculated from Eq. (2.8) as

$$\begin{aligned} \nabla M &= \nabla \left(\sum_{k=1}^{\mathcal{N}} \frac{\omega_k}{M_k} \right)^{-1} = - \left(\sum_{k=1}^{\mathcal{N}} \frac{\omega_k}{M_k} \right)^{-2} \sum_{k=1}^{\mathcal{N}} \frac{1}{M_k} \nabla \omega_k \\ &= -M^2 \left(\sum_{k=1}^{\mathcal{N}-1} \frac{1}{M_k} \nabla \omega_k + \frac{1}{M_{\mathcal{N}}} \nabla \omega_{\mathcal{N}} \right) \end{aligned} \tag{3.18}$$

Note that

$$\sum_{k=1}^{\mathcal{N}} \omega_k = 1 \quad \Rightarrow \quad \sum_{k=1}^{\mathcal{N}} \nabla \omega_k = 0 \quad \Rightarrow \quad \boxed{\nabla \omega_{\mathcal{N}} = - \sum_{k=1}^{\mathcal{N}-1} \nabla \omega_k} \tag{3.19}$$

Substitution of Eq. (3.19) into Eq. (3.18) yields

$$\nabla M = -M^2 \sum_{k=1}^{\mathcal{N}-1} \left(\frac{1}{M_k} - \frac{1}{M_{\mathcal{N}}} \right) \nabla \omega_k \tag{3.20}$$

The term $\nabla \omega_i$ can be expressed as

$$\nabla \omega_i = \sum_{k=1}^{\mathcal{N}-1} \delta_{ik} \nabla \omega_k \tag{3.21}$$

Substitution of Eqs. (3.20) and (3.21) into Eq. (3.17) gives

$$\boxed{\nabla x_i = \frac{M^2}{M_i} \sum_{k=1}^{\mathcal{N}-1} \left[\frac{1}{M} \delta_{ik} - \omega_i \left(\frac{1}{M_k} - \frac{1}{M_{\mathcal{N}}} \right) \right] \nabla \omega_k} \tag{3.22}$$

In matrix notation, Eq. (3.22) is written as

$$\boxed{[\nabla x] = [\mathbf{L}^{x\omega}] [\nabla \omega],} \tag{3.23}$$

where the transformation matrix $[\mathbf{L}^{x\omega}]$ is given by

$$[\mathbf{L}^{x\omega}] = \begin{pmatrix} \dfrac{M}{M_1} & 0 & \cdots & 0 \\ 0 & \dfrac{M}{M_2} & \cdots & 0 \\ \vdots & \vdots & \vdots & \vdots \\ 0 & 0 & \cdots & \dfrac{M}{M_{\mathcal{N}-1}} \end{pmatrix} - \begin{pmatrix} \dfrac{\omega_1}{M_1} \\ \dfrac{\omega_2}{M_2} \\ \vdots \\ \dfrac{\omega_{\mathcal{N}-1}}{M_{\mathcal{N}-1}} \end{pmatrix} \cdot \begin{pmatrix} \dfrac{M^2}{M_1} - \dfrac{M^2}{M_{\mathcal{N}}} \\ \dfrac{M^2}{M_2} - \dfrac{M^2}{M_{\mathcal{N}}} \\ \vdots \\ \dfrac{M^2}{M_{\mathcal{N}-1}} - \dfrac{M^2}{M_{\mathcal{N}}} \end{pmatrix}^{\mathrm{T}} \tag{3.24}$$

• **Transformation of ∇c_i to ∇x_i**

The gradient of molar concentration of species i is

$$\nabla c_i = \nabla(cx_i) = c\nabla x_i + x_i \nabla c \tag{3.25}$$

Since volume fractions sum to unity, the total molar concentration can be expressed in the form

$$\sum_{k=1}^{\mathcal{N}} c_k \overline{V}_k = 1 \quad \Rightarrow \quad c\sum_{k=1}^{\mathcal{N}} x_k \overline{V}_k = 1 \quad \Rightarrow \quad \boxed{c = \frac{1}{\widetilde{V}_{mix}} = \frac{1}{\displaystyle\sum_{k=1}^{\mathcal{N}} x_k \overline{V}_k}} \tag{3.26}$$

Therefore, the gradient of the total molar concentration is

$$\begin{aligned} \nabla c &= -\frac{1}{\left(\displaystyle\sum_{k=1}^{\mathcal{N}} x_k \overline{V}_k\right)^2} \sum_{k=1}^{\mathcal{N}} \overline{V}_k \nabla x_k = -c^2 \sum_{k=1}^{\mathcal{N}} \overline{V}_k \nabla x_k \\ &= -c^2 \left(\sum_{k=1}^{\mathcal{N}-1} \overline{V}_k \nabla x_k + \overline{V}_{\mathcal{N}} \nabla x_{\mathcal{N}}\right) \end{aligned} \tag{3.27}$$

The use of Eq. (3.11) reduces Eq. (3.27) to

$$\nabla c = -c^2 \sum_{k=1}^{\mathcal{N}-1} \left(\overline{V}_k - \overline{V}_{\mathcal{N}}\right) \nabla x_k \tag{3.28}$$

Substitution of Eq. (3.28) into Eq. (3.25) and using

$$\nabla x_i = \sum_{k=1}^{\mathcal{N}-1} \delta_{ik} \nabla x_k \tag{3.29}$$

lead to

$$\nabla c_i = c\sum_{k=1}^{\mathcal{N}-1} \left[\delta_{ik} - cx_i\left(\overline{V}_k - \overline{V}_{\mathcal{N}}\right)\right]\nabla x_k = c\sum_{k=1}^{\mathcal{N}-1} \left[\delta_{ik} - x_i\left(\frac{\overline{V}_k - \overline{V}_{\mathcal{N}}}{\widetilde{V}_{mix}}\right)\right]\nabla x_k \tag{3.30}$$

In matrix notation, Eq. (3.30) is expressed as

$$\boxed{[\nabla c] = c\,[\mathbf{G}^{\blacksquare*}]\,[\nabla x],} \tag{3.31}$$

where $[\mathbf{G}^{\blacksquare*}]$ is defined by Eq. (2.82).

• **Transformation of ∇c_i to ∇x_i**

It is left as an exercise to the student to show that

$$\boxed{[\nabla x] = \frac{1}{c}\,[\mathbf{G}^{*\blacksquare}]\,[\nabla c],} \tag{3.32}$$

where $[\mathbf{G}^{*\blacksquare}]$ is defined by Eq. (2.78).

3.1.2 TRANSFORMATION OF FICK DIFFUSION COEFFICIENTS

• Transformation of $\mathcal{D}^m$ to $\mathcal{D}^*$

From Problem 2.4

$$[\mathbf{j}] = [\mathbf{H}^{m*}][\mathbf{J}^*] \qquad (3.33)$$

Substitution of Eq. (3.33) into Eq. (3.6) and using $\rho = cM$ yield

$$[\mathbf{H}^{m*}][\mathbf{J}^*] = -c[\mathcal{D}^m]M[\nabla\omega] \qquad (3.34)$$

Replacing $[\nabla\omega]$ in favor of $[\nabla x]$ by using Eq. (3.15) gives

$$[\mathbf{H}^{m*}][\mathbf{J}^*] = -c[\mathcal{D}^m]M[\mathbf{L}^{\omega x}][\nabla x] \qquad (3.35)$$

Multiplication of Eq. (3.35) from the left side by $[\mathbf{H}^{m*}]^{-1} = [\mathbf{H}^{*m}]$ gives

$$[\mathbf{J}^*] = -c[\mathbf{H}^{*m}][\mathcal{D}^m]M[\mathbf{L}^{\omega x}][\nabla x] \qquad (3.36)$$

Comparison of Eq. (3.36) with Eq. (3.2) results in

$$[\mathcal{D}^*] = [\mathbf{H}^{*m}][\mathcal{D}^m]M[\mathbf{L}^{\omega x}] \qquad (3.37)$$

or

$$[\mathcal{D}^*] = [\mathbf{H}^{*m}][\mathcal{D}^m][\mathbf{S}], \qquad (3.38)$$

where

$$[\mathbf{H}^{*m}] = \begin{pmatrix} \dfrac{1}{M_1} & 0 & \cdots & 0 \\ 0 & \dfrac{1}{M_2} & \cdots & 0 \\ \vdots & \vdots & \vdots & \vdots \\ 0 & 0 & \cdots & \dfrac{1}{M_{\mathcal{N}-1}} \end{pmatrix} - \begin{pmatrix} x_1 \\ x_2 \\ \vdots \\ x_{\mathcal{N}-1} \end{pmatrix} \cdot \begin{pmatrix} \dfrac{1}{M_1} - \dfrac{1}{M_{\mathcal{N}}} \\ \dfrac{1}{M_2} - \dfrac{1}{M_{\mathcal{N}}} \\ \vdots \\ \dfrac{1}{M_{\mathcal{N}-1}} - \dfrac{1}{M_{\mathcal{N}}} \end{pmatrix}^{\mathrm{T}} \qquad (3.39)$$

and

$$[\mathbf{S}] = M[\mathbf{L}^{\omega x}] = \begin{pmatrix} M_1 & 0 & \cdots & 0 \\ 0 & M_2 & \cdots & 0 \\ \vdots & \vdots & \vdots & \vdots \\ 0 & 0 & \cdots & M_{\mathcal{N}-1} \end{pmatrix} - \begin{pmatrix} x_1 M_1 \\ x_2 M_2 \\ \vdots \\ x_{\mathcal{N}-1} M_{\mathcal{N}-1} \end{pmatrix} \cdot \begin{pmatrix} \dfrac{M_1 - M_{\mathcal{N}}}{M} \\ \dfrac{M_2 - M_{\mathcal{N}}}{M} \\ \vdots \\ \dfrac{M_{\mathcal{N}-1} - M_{\mathcal{N}}}{M} \end{pmatrix}^{\mathrm{T}} \qquad (3.40)$$

Note from Eq. (5) of Problem 2.4 that $[\mathbf{S}] = [\mathbf{H}^{m*}] = [\mathbf{H}^{*m}]^{-1}$. Thus, Eq. (3.38) takes the final form of

$$\boxed{[\mathcal{D}^*] = [\mathbf{H}^{*m}][\mathcal{D}^m][\mathbf{H}^{*m}]^{-1}} \qquad (3.41)$$

• Transformation of $\mathcal{D}^*$ to $\mathcal{D}^m$

It is left as an exercise to the student to show that

$$\boxed{[\mathcal{D}^m] = [\mathbf{H}^{*m}]^{-1}[\mathcal{D}^*][\mathbf{H}^{*m}]} \qquad (3.42)$$

• Transformation of $\mathcal{D}^{\blacksquare}$ to $\mathcal{D}^*$

From Eq. (2.77)

$$[\mathbf{J}^*] = [\mathbf{G}^{*\blacksquare}][\mathbf{J}^{\blacksquare}] \tag{3.43}$$

Substitution of Eq. (3.8) into Eq. (3.43) yields

$$[\mathbf{J}^*] = -[\mathbf{G}^{*\blacksquare}][\mathcal{D}^{\blacksquare}][\nabla c] \tag{3.44}$$

Replacing $[\nabla c]$ in favor of $[\nabla x]$ by using Eq. (3.31) gives

$$[\mathbf{J}^*] = -c[\mathbf{G}^{*\blacksquare}][\mathcal{D}^{\blacksquare}][\mathbf{G}^{\blacksquare *}][\nabla x] \tag{3.45}$$

Comparison of Eq. (3.45) with Eq. (3.2) results in

$$\boxed{[\mathcal{D}^*] = [\mathbf{G}^{*\blacksquare}][\mathcal{D}^{\blacksquare}][\mathbf{G}^{\blacksquare *}] = [\mathbf{G}^{*\blacksquare}][\mathcal{D}^{\blacksquare}][\mathbf{G}^{*\blacksquare}]^{-1},} \tag{3.46}$$

where $[\mathbf{G}^{*\blacksquare}]$ is defined by Eq. (2.78).

• Transformation of $\mathcal{D}^{\blacksquare}$ to $\mathcal{D}^*$

It is left as an exercise to the student to show that

$$\boxed{[\mathcal{D}^{\blacksquare}] = [\mathbf{G}^{*\blacksquare}]^{-1}[\mathcal{D}^*][\mathbf{G}^{*\blacksquare}]} \tag{3.47}$$

3.1.3 PROPERTIES OF FICK DIFFUSION COEFFICIENT MATRICES

Reported experimental Fick diffusion coefficients are mostly measured with respect to the volume-average velocity. Once the elements of $[\mathcal{D}^{\blacksquare}]$ are experimentally determined, the values of $[\mathcal{D}^*]$ are calculated by using Eq. (3.46). Then the use of Eq. (3.42) gives the values of $[\mathcal{D}^m]$.

Cullinan (1965) showed that the eigenvalues of the Fick diffusion coefficient matrices are the same.[4] The constraints imposed by the second law of thermodynamics on the elements of the Fick diffusion coefficient matrices are given by Miller et al. (1986) as follows.

In a ternary system, there are two eigenvalues, λ_1 and λ_2. These eigenvalues are related to the invariants of the diffusion coefficient matrix $[\mathcal{D}]$ as[5]

$$\text{tr}[\mathcal{D}] = \lambda_1 + \lambda_2 > 0 \tag{3.48}$$

$$|\mathcal{D}| = \lambda_1 \lambda_2 > 0, \tag{3.49}$$

where "tr" and $|\mathcal{D}|$ stand for the *trace* and the *determinant* of the matrix $[\mathcal{D}]$, respectively. According to Eq. (3.48), even if one of the diagonal elements is negative, summation of the diagonal elements must be positive.

The eigenvalues can be determined from Eqs. (3.48) and (3.49) as

$$\lambda_{1,2} = \frac{\text{tr}[\mathcal{D}] \pm \sqrt{\Delta}}{2}, \tag{3.50}$$

where the discriminant Δ is defined by

$$\Delta = (\text{tr}[\mathcal{D}])^2 - 4|\mathcal{D}| = (\lambda_1 - \lambda_2)^2 \tag{3.51}$$

---

[4]If the eigenvalues of two matrices are the same, this does not imply that the elements of the two matrices have identical values.

[5]$[\mathcal{D}]$ stands for $[\mathcal{D}^{\blacksquare}]$, $[\mathcal{D}^*]$, or $[\mathcal{D}^m]$. The *invariants* of $[\mathcal{D}]$ are the scalars formed using the elements of $[\mathcal{D}]$ that are independent of the choice of the reference velocity frame (see Section A.4.2 in Appendix A).

For a quaternary system, the eigenvalues are related to the invariants of the diffusion coefficient matrix as

$$\text{tr}\,[\mathcal{D}] = \lambda_1 + \lambda_2 + \lambda_3 > 0 \tag{3.52}$$

$$\frac{(\text{tr}\,[\mathcal{D}])^2 - \text{tr}\,[\mathcal{D}^2]}{2} = \lambda_1\lambda_2 + \lambda_2\lambda_3 + \lambda_3\lambda_1 > 0 \tag{3.53}$$

$$|\mathcal{D}| = \lambda_1\,\lambda_2\,\lambda_3 > 0 \tag{3.54}$$

The term $\mathcal{D}^2$ on the left side of Eq. (3.53) implies $[\mathcal{D}]\cdot[\mathcal{D}]$.

Example 3.1 For a ternary liquid mixture containing 29.89 mol % acetone (1), 34.90% benzene (2), and 35.21% carbon tetrachloride (3) at 298K, Cullinan and Toor (1965) reported the following diffusion coefficients relative to the volume-average velocity:

$$\mathcal{D}^\blacksquare = \begin{pmatrix} 1.887 & -0.213 \\ -0.037 & 2.255 \end{pmatrix} \times 10^{-5}\,(\text{cm}^2/\text{s})$$

The partial molar volumes are given as

$$\overline{V}_1 = 74.05\,\text{cm}^3/\text{mol} \qquad \overline{V}_2 = 89.41\,\text{cm}^3/\text{mol} \qquad \overline{V}_3 = 97.09\,\text{cm}^3/\text{mol}$$

Calculations of the diffusion coefficients relative to the molar- and mass-average velocities are shown in the Mathcad worksheet given below. Note that the eigenvalues of the diffusion coefficient matrices are independent of the reference velocity frame.

ORIGIN:= 1

$$x := \begin{pmatrix} 0.2989 \\ 0.3490 \\ 0.3521 \end{pmatrix} \qquad V := \begin{pmatrix} 74.05 \\ 89.41 \\ 97.09 \end{pmatrix} \qquad \text{Dvolume} := \begin{pmatrix} 1.887 & -0.213 \\ -0.037 & 2.255 \end{pmatrix}\cdot 10^{-5} \qquad M := \begin{pmatrix} 58.08 \\ 78.11 \\ 153.82 \end{pmatrix}$$

$$G := \left[\begin{pmatrix} 1 & 0 \\ 0 & 1 \end{pmatrix} - \begin{pmatrix} x_1 \\ x_2 \end{pmatrix} \cdot \begin{pmatrix} 1 - \dfrac{V_1}{V_3} \\ 1 - \dfrac{V_2}{V_3} \end{pmatrix}^{\!T}\right] = \begin{pmatrix} 0.929 & -0.024 \\ -0.083 & 0.972 \end{pmatrix} \qquad \text{Eq. (2.78)}$$

$$\text{Dmole} := G\cdot\text{Dvolume}\cdot G^{-1} = \begin{pmatrix} 1.869\times 10^{-5} & -2.129\times 10^{-6} \\ -4.313\times 10^{-8} & 2.273\times 10^{-5} \end{pmatrix} \qquad \text{Eq. (3.46)}$$

$$H := \left[\begin{pmatrix} \dfrac{1}{M_1} & 0 \\ 0 & \dfrac{1}{M_2} \end{pmatrix} - \begin{pmatrix} x_1 \\ x_2 \end{pmatrix}\cdot \begin{pmatrix} \dfrac{1}{M_1} - \dfrac{1}{M_3} \\ \dfrac{1}{M_2} - \dfrac{1}{M_3} \end{pmatrix}^{\!T}\right] = \begin{pmatrix} 0.014 & -1.883\times 10^{-3} \\ -3.74\times 10^{-3} & 0.011 \end{pmatrix} \qquad \text{Eq. (3.39)}$$

$$\text{Dmass} := H^{-1}\cdot\text{Dmole}\cdot H = \begin{pmatrix} 1.908\times 10^{-5} & -1.12\times 10^{-6} \\ -1.346\times 10^{-6} & 2.234\times 10^{-5} \end{pmatrix} \qquad \text{Eq. (3.42)}$$

$$\text{eigenvals}\,(\text{Dvolume}) = \begin{pmatrix} 1.867\times 10^{-5} \\ 2.275\times 10^{-5} \end{pmatrix} \qquad \text{eigenvals}\,(\text{Dmole}) = \begin{pmatrix} 1.867\times 10^{-5} \\ 2.275\times 10^{-5} \end{pmatrix} \qquad \text{eigenvals}\,(\text{Dmass}) = \begin{pmatrix} 1.867\times 10^{-5} \\ 2.275\times 10^{-5} \end{pmatrix}$$

Mathcad worksheet of Example 3.1.

3.2 MS EQUATIONS

The equations describing the diffusion of gases in binary mixtures were developed by Maxwell (1866) based on the kinetic theory of gases. Later, these equations were generalized by Stefan (1871) for multicomponent mixtures. Thus, in the literature, the resulting equations are called either *Maxwell–Stefan equations* or *Stefan–Maxwell equations*. Since the pioneering work was done by Maxwell, it seems more appropriate to name them Maxwell–Stefan equations.

The thermodynamics of irreversible processes leads to an expression for the generalized diffusional driving forces, $\mathbf{d}_i$, as (Taylor and Krishna, 1993; Curtiss and Bird, 1999)

$$cRT\mathbf{d}_i = c_i \nabla_{T,P}\overline{G}_i + (c_i\overline{V}_i - \omega_i)\nabla P - \rho_i\left(\widehat{\mathbf{F}}_i - \sum_{k=1}^{\mathcal{N}}\omega_k\widehat{\mathbf{F}}_k\right), \tag{3.55}$$

where $\widehat{\mathbf{F}}_i$ is the external body force per unit mass acting on species i. The term $\nabla_{T,P}$ implies that the derivative is to be taken at constant T and P. The generalized diffusional driving forces[6] satisfy the following constraint:

$$\sum_{k=1}^{\mathcal{N}}\mathbf{d}_k = 0 \tag{3.56}$$

The conservation of momentum for the collisions between molecules in a multicomponent system leads to the following expression for the generalized diffusional driving forces (Taylor and Krishna, 1993):

$$\mathbf{d}_i = \sum_{k=1}^{\mathcal{N}}\frac{x_i x_k(\mathbf{v}_k - \mathbf{v}_i)}{\text{Ð}_{ik}}, \tag{3.57}$$

which is known as the *MS equations*. The terms Ð_{ik} are called *MS diffusion coefficients*, and they are symmetric,[7] i.e., $\text{Ð}_{ik} = \text{Ð}_{ki}$, all positive, and independent of the reference velocity frame. Like the Fick diffusion coefficient, the SI unit of the MS diffusion coefficient is m^2/s. Equation (3.57) simply states that the driving force on species i is equal to the sum of friction forces between i and other species k. Thus, the MS diffusion coefficient may be interpreted as the reciprocal drag (or friction) coefficient between species i and k. Since the right side of Eq. (3.57) equals zero when $k = i$ ($\mathbf{v}_k = \mathbf{v}_i$), Eq. (3.57) is expressed in the form

$$\mathbf{d}_i = \sum_{\substack{k=1 \\ k \neq i}}^{\mathcal{N}}\frac{x_i x_k(\mathbf{v}_k - \mathbf{v}_i)}{\text{Ð}_{ik}} \tag{3.58}$$

In an $\mathcal{N}$-component system, there are $\mathcal{N}(\mathcal{N} - 1)/2$ MS diffusion coefficients. Alternative forms of the MS equations can be derived by relating the velocity difference on the right side of Eq. (3.58) to different types of fluxes.

• MS equations in terms of diffusive molar fluxes relative to molar-average velocity

The diffusive molar flux of species i relative to the molar-average velocity is given by

$$\mathbf{J}_i^* = c_i(\mathbf{v}_i - \mathbf{v}^*) \qquad \Rightarrow \qquad \mathbf{v}_i - \mathbf{v}^* = \frac{\mathbf{J}_i^*}{c\,x_i} \tag{3.59}$$

---

[6]The unit of $\mathbf{d}_i$ is reciprocal length.

[7]This is dictated by the *Onsager reciprocal relations*.

Similarly, for species k

$$\mathbf{v}_k - \mathbf{v}^* = \frac{\mathbf{J}_k^*}{c\,x_k} \tag{3.60}$$

Subtraction of Eq. (3.59) from Eq. (3.60) gives

$$\mathbf{v}_k - \mathbf{v}_i = \frac{1}{c}\left(\frac{\mathbf{J}_k^*}{x_k} - \frac{\mathbf{J}_i^*}{x_i}\right) \tag{3.61}$$

Substitution of Eq. (3.61) into Eq. (3.58) leads to

$$\boxed{\mathbf{d}_i = \sum_{\substack{k=1 \\ k \neq i}}^{\mathcal{N}} \frac{x_i \mathbf{J}_k^* - x_k \mathbf{J}_i^*}{c\,\mathrm{\text{Đ}}_{ik}}} \tag{3.62}$$

- **MS equations in terms of total molar fluxes**

The total molar flux of species i is

$$\mathbf{N}_i = c_i\,\mathbf{v}_i \qquad \Rightarrow \qquad \mathbf{v}_i = \frac{\mathbf{N}_i}{c_i} \tag{3.63}$$

Similarly, for species k

$$\mathbf{v}_k = \frac{\mathbf{N}_k}{c_k} \tag{3.64}$$

Subtraction of Eq. (3.63) from Eq. (3.64) gives

$$\mathbf{v}_k - \mathbf{v}_i = \frac{\mathbf{N}_k}{c_k} - \frac{\mathbf{N}_i}{c_i} = \frac{1}{c}\left(\frac{x_i \mathbf{N}_k - x_k \mathbf{N}_i}{x_k\,x_i}\right) \tag{3.65}$$

Substitution of Eq. (3.65) into Eq. (3.58) leads to

$$\boxed{\mathbf{d}_i = \sum_{\substack{k=1 \\ k \neq i}}^{\mathcal{N}} \frac{x_i \mathbf{N}_k - x_k \mathbf{N}_i}{c\,\mathrm{\text{Đ}}_{ik}}} \tag{3.66}$$

3.2.1   ISOTHERMAL DIFFUSION IN THE ABSENCE OF EXTERNAL BODY FORCES

When the gradient of partial molar Gibbs energy is the sole driving force for diffusion, Eq. (3.55) simplifies to

$$\mathbf{d}_i = \frac{x_i}{RT}\nabla_{T,P}\overline{G}_i \tag{3.67}$$

Partial molar Gibbs energy is dependent on temperature, pressure, and composition. Since T and P are kept constant during differentiation, Eq. (3.67) is expressed as

$$\mathbf{d}_i = \frac{x_i}{RT}\sum_{k=1}^{\mathcal{N}-1}\left(\frac{\partial \overline{G}_i}{\partial x_k}\right)_{T,P,x_{j\neq k}}\nabla x_k \tag{3.68}$$

The subscripts on the partial derivative mean that temperature, pressure, and mole fractions of all components other than k are kept constant. To proceed one step further, it is necessary to express partial molar Gibbs energy in terms of either the activity coefficient or fugacity coefficient.

• Partial molar Gibbs energy in terms of the activity coefficient

In the case of liquid mixtures, nonideality is reflected by the activity coefficient, γ_i, term in the definition of partial molar Gibbs energy in the form

$$\overline{G}_i(T,P,x_i) = \widetilde{G}_i^o(T,P^o) + RT \ln \left[x_i \gamma_i(T,P,x_i) \right], \tag{3.69}$$

where $\widetilde{G}_i^o$ is the molar Gibbs energy of pure i at standard conditions.[8] Various models, such as two- and three-suffix Margules, van Laar, nonrandom two-liquid (NRTL), Wilson, and unified activity coefficient (UNIFAC), are available for the evaluation of the activity coefficient. Differentiation of Eq. (3.69) with respect to x_k gives

$$\left(\frac{\partial \overline{G}_i}{\partial x_k} \right)_{T,P,x_{j \neq k}} = \frac{RT}{x_i} \left(\frac{\partial x_i}{\partial x_k} + \frac{x_i}{\gamma_i} \frac{\partial \gamma_i}{\partial x_k} \right) = \frac{RT}{x_i} \left(\delta_{ik} + x_i \frac{\partial \ln \gamma_i}{\partial x_k} \right) \tag{3.70}$$

The so-called *thermodynamic factor*, Γ_{ik}, accounts for the deviation from ideal mixture behavior and is defined by

$$\boxed{\Gamma_{ik} = \delta_{ik} + x_i \left(\frac{\partial \ln \gamma_i}{\partial x_k} \right)_{T,P,x_{j \neq k}}} \tag{3.71}$$

so that Eq. (3.70) takes the following form:

$$\left(\frac{\partial \overline{G}_i}{\partial x_k} \right)_{T,P,x_{j \neq k}} = \frac{RT}{x_i} \Gamma_{ik} \tag{3.72}$$

• Partial molar Gibbs energy in terms of the fugacity coefficient

In the case of gas mixtures, partial molar Gibbs energy is expressed as

$$\overline{G}_i(T,P,x_i) = \lambda_i(T) + RT \ln \left[x_i P \widehat{\phi}_i(T,P,x_i) \right], \tag{3.73}$$

in which the fugacity coefficient, $\widehat{\phi}_i$, takes care of the deviation from ideal gas behavior. Fugacity coefficients are calculated from cubic equations of state, such as van der Waals, Redlich–Kwong, Soave–Redlich–Kwong, and Peng–Robinson. Differentiation of Eq. (3.73) with respect to x_k gives

$$\left(\frac{\partial \overline{G}_i}{\partial x_k} \right)_{T,P,x_{j \neq k}} = \frac{RT}{x_i} \left(\frac{\partial x_i}{\partial x_k} + \frac{x_i}{\widehat{\phi}_i} \frac{\partial \widehat{\phi}_i}{\partial x_k} \right) = \frac{RT}{x_i} \left(\delta_{ik} + x_i \frac{\partial \ln \widehat{\phi}_i}{\partial x_k} \right) \tag{3.74}$$

The form of Eq. (3.72) is still preserved if the thermodynamic factor is defined as

$$\boxed{\Gamma_{ik} = \delta_{ik} + x_i \left(\frac{\partial \ln \widehat{\phi}_i}{\partial x_k} \right)_{T,P,x_{j \neq k}}} \tag{3.75}$$

---

[8] The superscript ^{o} indicates the standard state conditions. The standard state temperature is taken as the temperature of the system, T. The standard state pressure (P^o) is usually taken as 1 bar.

Matrix representation of the driving force for diffusion

Substitution of Eq. (3.72) into Eq. (3.68) gives

$$
\mathbf{d}_i = \sum_{k=1}^{\mathcal{N}-1} \Gamma_{ik} \nabla x_k
\tag{3.76}
$$

so that the MS equations, Eqs. (3.62) and (3.66), take the following forms:

$$
\sum_{k=1}^{\mathcal{N}-1} \Gamma_{ik} \nabla x_k = \sum_{\substack{k=1 \\ k \neq i}}^{\mathcal{N}} \frac{x_i \mathbf{J}_k^* - x_k \mathbf{J}_i^*}{c \, \text{Đ}_{ik}}
\tag{3.77}
$$

$$
\sum_{k=1}^{\mathcal{N}-1} \Gamma_{ik} \nabla x_k = \sum_{\substack{k=1 \\ k \neq i}}^{\mathcal{N}} \frac{x_i \mathbf{N}_k - x_k \mathbf{N}_i}{c \, \text{Đ}_{ik}}
\tag{3.78}
$$

Introduction of the thermodynamic factor, Γ_{ik}, separates thermodynamics from mass transfer. Since both of these factors are embedded in Fick diffusion coefficients, MS diffusion coefficients are less concentration dependent than Fick diffusion coefficients.

In matrix notation, Eq. (3.76) is expressed as

$$
[\mathbf{d}] = [\Gamma] [\nabla x]
\tag{3.79}
$$

Note that $[\Gamma]$ is not symmetric and its elements may take negative values. For ideal mixtures, activity and fugacity coefficients are unity and $[\Gamma]$ reduces to an identity matrix $[\mathbf{I}]$. Thus, Eq. (3.79) becomes

$$
[\mathbf{d}] = [\nabla x] \quad \text{Ideal mixture}
\tag{3.80}
$$

3.3 CALCULATION OF THE THERMODYNAMIC FACTOR

Equations (3.71) and (3.75) indicate that the calculation of the thermodynamic factor, Γ, requires differentiation of either the activity or fugacity coefficient with respect to mole fraction. Moreover, the thermodynamic factor can also be predicted by molecular simulations.[9] The formulas for calculation of the thermodynamic factor based on various activity and fugacity coefficient models will be developed in the following section.

3.3.1 THERMODYNAMIC FACTOR BASED ON THE ACTIVITY COEFFICIENT

• **Binary mixtures**

For a binary system of species 1 and 2, the thermodynamic factor defined by Eq. (3.71) reduces to

$$
\Gamma = 1 + x_1 \left(\frac{\partial \ln \gamma_1}{\partial x_1} \right)_{T,P} = 1 + x_2 \left(\frac{\partial \ln \gamma_2}{\partial x_2} \right)_{T,P}
\tag{3.81}
$$

---

[9]For example, thermodynamic factors can be predicted using the conductor-like screening model-segment activity coefficient (COSMO-SAC) theory. It is a quantum-mechanically-based predictive model for activity coefficients (Hsieh et al., 2010).

Calculation of the thermodynamic factor based on some activity coefficient models available in the literature is given below.

Two-suffix (one-constant) Margules model

The activity coefficient is given by

$$\ln \gamma_1 = A x_2^2, \tag{3.82}$$

where the parameter A is dependent on temperature and pressure. The use of Eq. (3.82) in Eq. (3.81) gives the thermodynamic factor as

$$\boxed{\Gamma = 1 - 2A x_1 x_2} \tag{3.83}$$

Three-suffix (two-constant) Margules model

The activity coefficient is given by

$$\ln \gamma_1 = x_2^2 \left(A + 3B - 4B x_2 \right), \tag{3.84}$$

where the parameters A and B are dependent on temperature and pressure. The use of Eq. (3.84) in Eq. (3.81) gives the thermodynamic factor as

$$\boxed{\Gamma = 1 - 2x_1 x_2 \left[A - 3B(x_2 - x_1) \right]} \tag{3.85}$$

van Laar model

The activity coefficient is given by

$$\ln \gamma_1 = \frac{A}{\left(1 + \dfrac{A}{B} \dfrac{x_1}{x_2} \right)^2}, \tag{3.86}$$

where the parameters A and B are dependent on temperature and pressure. The use of Eq. (3.86) in Eq. (3.81) gives the thermodynamic factor as

$$\boxed{\Gamma = 1 - 2A^2 B^2 \frac{x_1 x_2}{(A x_1 + B x_2)^3}} \tag{3.87}$$

Wilson model

The Wilson equation is used when the components in the liquid phase are completely miscible over the whole composition range. It works well for mixtures of highly polar compounds, i.e., alcohol and water, and mixtures of hydrocarbons. The activity coefficient is given as

$$\ln \gamma_1 = - \left[\ln \left(x_1 + \Lambda_{12} x_2 \right) + x_2 \left(\frac{\Lambda_{21}}{x_2 + \Lambda_{21} x_1} - \frac{\Lambda_{12}}{x_1 + \Lambda_{12} x_2} \right) \right] \tag{3.88}$$

The parameters Λ_{12} and Λ_{21} in Eq. (3.88) are usually expressed in the form

$$\Lambda_{12} = \frac{\widetilde{V}_2}{\widetilde{V}_1} \exp\left(-\frac{\lambda_{12} - \lambda_{11}}{RT} \right) \quad \text{and} \quad \Lambda_{21} = \frac{\widetilde{V}_1}{\widetilde{V}_2} \exp\left(-\frac{\lambda_{21} - \lambda_{22}}{RT} \right), \tag{3.89}$$

where λ_{ij}'s are the energy parameters associated with the interaction between molecules i and j and $\widetilde{V}_i$ is the molar volume of pure liquid i. In most applications, the parameters $(\lambda_{12} - \lambda_{11})$ and $(\lambda_{21} - \lambda_{22})$ are considered independent of temperature.

The use of Eq. (3.88) in Eq. (3.81) gives the thermodynamic factor as

$$\Gamma = 1 + x_1 \left[\frac{\Lambda_{21}^2}{(x_2 + \Lambda_{21} x_1)^2} + \frac{(\Lambda_{12} - 1)^2 x_2 - 1}{(x_1 + \Lambda_{12} x_2)^2} \right] \tag{3.90}$$

NRTL model

When the system is highly nonideal and polar, the NRTL model is used, in which the activity coefficient is given by

$$\ln \gamma_1 = x_2^2 \left[\tau_{21} \left(\frac{G_{21}}{x_1 + G_{21} x_2} \right)^2 + \frac{\tau_{12} G_{12}}{(x_2 + G_{12} x_1)^2} \right], \tag{3.91}$$

where

$$G_{12} = \exp\left(-\alpha \tau_{12}\right) \qquad \text{and} \qquad G_{21} = \exp\left(-\alpha \tau_{21}\right) \tag{3.92}$$

The parameters τ_{12} and τ_{21} are expressed in terms of the energy parameters, g_{ij}, in the form

$$\tau_{12} = \frac{g_{12} - g_{22}}{RT} \qquad \text{and} \qquad \tau_{21} = \frac{g_{21} - g_{11}}{RT} \tag{3.93}$$

The use of the NRTL equation requires two temperature-dependent parameters, τ_{12} and τ_{21}, in addition to a nonrandomness parameter, α. Comparison with the experimental vapor–liquid equilibrium data indicates that α values change between 0.2 and 0.47. Thus, in the absence of information, it is generally recommended to take $\alpha = 0.3$ in the calculations.

The use of Eq. (3.91) in Eq. (3.81) gives the thermodynamic factor as

$$\Gamma = 1 - 2 x_1 x_2 \left[\frac{G_{12}^2 \tau_{12}}{(x_2 + G_{12} x_1)^3} + \frac{G_{21}^2 \tau_{21}}{(x_1 + G_{21} x_2)^3} \right] \tag{3.94}$$

Example 3.2 Zhang et al. (2015) reported the following NRTL parameters for a binary mixture of water (1) and glycerol (2):

$$\tau_{12} = -1.0486 + \frac{669.79}{T} \qquad \tau_{21} = 0.5754 - \frac{527.01}{T} \qquad \alpha = 0.3$$

Calculation of the thermodynamic factor for a mixture containing 83.64 mol % water at 298.15 K is given in the Mathcad worksheet shown below.

ORIGIN:= 1

$T := 298.15$ $\qquad$ $x := \begin{pmatrix} 0.8364 \\ 0.1636 \end{pmatrix}$

$\Gamma :=$ | $\tau 12 \leftarrow -1.0486 + \dfrac{669.79}{T}$

$\qquad$ $\tau 21 \leftarrow 0.5754 - \dfrac{527.01}{T}$

$\qquad$ $\alpha \leftarrow 0.3$

$\qquad$ $G12 \leftarrow \exp(-\alpha \cdot \tau 12)$

$\qquad$ $G21 \leftarrow \exp(-\alpha \cdot \tau 21)$

$\qquad$ $\Gamma \leftarrow 1 - 2 x_1 \cdot x_2 \cdot \left[\dfrac{G12^2 \cdot \tau 12}{\left(x_2 + G12 x_1\right)^3} + \dfrac{G21^2 \cdot \tau 21}{\left(x_1 + G21 \cdot x_2\right)^3} \right]$

$\qquad$ Γ

$\Gamma = 1.162$

Mathcad worksheet of Example 3.2.

• Multicomponent mixtures

Experimental determination of activity coefficients requires vapor–liquid and liquid–liquid equilibrium data. In that respect, most of the published data are for binary mixtures. Hence, efforts have been directed to extend available binary models to multicomponent systems so that the resulting equations require only the data for the binary subsystems.

Wilson model

The Wilson model for a multicomponent mixture is given by

$$\ln \gamma_i = 1 - \ln \left(\sum_{j=1}^{\mathcal{N}} \Lambda_{ij} x_j \right) - \sum_{m=1}^{\mathcal{N}} \left(\frac{\Lambda_{mi} x_m}{\sum_{j=1}^{\mathcal{N}} \Lambda_{mj} x_j} \right), \tag{3.95}$$

where

$$\Lambda_{ij} = \frac{\widetilde{V}_j}{\widetilde{V}_i} \exp\left(-\frac{\lambda_{ij} - \lambda_{ii}}{RT} \right) \qquad \text{with} \qquad \Lambda_{ii} = 1 \tag{3.96}$$

The thermodynamic factor is given by (Taylor and Krishna, 1993)

$$\boxed{\Gamma_{ij} = \delta_{ij} + x_i \left(Q_{ij} - Q_{i\mathcal{N}} \right),} \tag{3.97}$$

where

$$Q_{ij} = -\frac{\Lambda_{ij}}{S_i} - \frac{\Lambda_{ji}}{S_j} + \sum_{k=1}^{\mathcal{N}} \frac{x_k \Lambda_{ki} \Lambda_{kj}}{S_k^2},$$ (3.98)

in which

$$S_i = \sum_{j=1}^{\mathcal{N}} x_j \Lambda_{ij}$$ (3.99)

The subroutine "Multicomponent – Wilson" shown in Figure H.1 of Appendix H calculates the thermodynamic factor.

Example 3.3 Let us calculate the thermodynamic factor for a ternary liquid mixture consisting of 15 mol% chloroform (1), 15% methanol (2), and 70% benzene (3) at 298.15 K. The mixture is represented by the Wilson model with the following parameters (Kurihara et al., 1998):

$i-j$	$\lambda_{ij} - \lambda_{ii}$ (J/mol)	$\lambda_{ji} - \lambda_{jj}$ (J/mol)
$1-2$	-1492.36	7509.93
$1-3$	-181.72	-401.78
$2-3$	7476.31	730.83

The molar volumes are given as

$$\widetilde{V}_1 = 80.68 \, \text{cm}^3/\text{mol} \qquad \widetilde{V}_2 = 40.74 \, \text{cm}^3/\text{mol} \qquad \widetilde{V}_3 = 89.41 \, \text{cm}^3/\text{mol}$$

The Mathcad worksheet is given below.

ORIGIN:= 1

$R := 8.314 \qquad T := 298.15 \qquad x := \begin{pmatrix} 0.15 \\ 0.15 \\ 0.70 \end{pmatrix} \qquad V := \begin{pmatrix} 80.68 \\ 40.74 \\ 89.41 \end{pmatrix} \qquad N := 3$

$$\Lambda := \begin{pmatrix} 1 & \dfrac{V_2}{V_1}\cdot\exp\left(\dfrac{1492.36}{R\cdot T}\right) & \dfrac{V_3}{V_1}\cdot\exp\left(\dfrac{181.72}{R\cdot T}\right) \\ \dfrac{V_1}{V_2}\cdot\exp\left(\dfrac{-7509.93}{R\cdot T}\right) & 1 & \dfrac{V_3}{V_2}\cdot\exp\left(\dfrac{-7476.31}{R\cdot T}\right) \\ \dfrac{V_1}{V_3}\cdot\exp\left(\dfrac{401.78}{R\cdot T}\right) & \dfrac{V_2}{V_3}\cdot\exp\left(\dfrac{-730.83}{R\cdot T}\right) & 1 \end{pmatrix} = \begin{pmatrix} 1 & 0.922 & 1.192 \\ 0.096 & 1 & 0.108 \\ 1.061 & 0.339 & 1 \end{pmatrix}$$

→ Reference:C:\Users\tosun\Desktop\Subroutines\Multicomponent - Wilson.xmcd

$$\Gamma = \begin{pmatrix} 1.071 & 0.091 \\ -0.065 & 0.188 \end{pmatrix}$$

Mathcad worksheet of Example 3.3.

NRTL model

The NRTL model for a multicomponent mixture is given by

$$\ln \gamma_i = \frac{\sum\limits_{j=1}^{N} \tau_{ji} G_{ji} x_j}{\sum\limits_{m=1}^{N} G_{mi} x_m} + \sum\limits_{j=1}^{N} \frac{G_{ij} x_j}{\sum\limits_{m=1}^{N} G_{mj} x_m} \left(\tau_{ij} - \frac{\sum\limits_{r=1}^{N} \tau_{rj} G_{rj} x_r}{\sum\limits_{m=1}^{N} G_{mj} x_m} \right),$$

(3.100)

where

$$\tau_{ij} = \frac{g_{ij} - g_{jj}}{RT} \qquad G_{ij} = \exp(-\alpha_{ij} \tau_{ij}) \qquad \alpha_{ij} = \alpha_{ji}$$

(3.101)

The thermodynamic factor is given by (Taylor and Krishna, 1993)

$$\boxed{\Gamma_{ij} = \delta_{ij} + x_i (Q_{ij} - Q_{i\mathcal{N}}),}$$

(3.102)

where

$$Q_{ij} = \varepsilon_{ij} + \varepsilon_{ji} - \sum\limits_{k=1}^{N} \frac{x_k (G_{ik} \varepsilon_{jk} + G_{jk} \varepsilon_{ik})}{S_k},$$

(3.103)

in which

$$S_i = \sum\limits_{j=1}^{N} x_j G_{ji} \qquad C_i = \sum\limits_{j=1}^{N} x_j G_{ji} \tau_{ji} \qquad \varepsilon_{ij} = \frac{G_{ij}}{S_j} \left(\tau_{ij} - \frac{C_j}{S_j} \right)$$

(3.104)

The subroutine "Multicomponent – NRTL" shown in Figure H.2 of Appendix H calculates the thermodynamic factor.

Example 3.4 Let us calculate the thermodynamic factor for a ternary liquid mixture consisting of 10 mol% acetone (1), 30% methanol (2), and 60% benzene (3) at 298.15 K. The mixture is represented by the NRTL model with the following parameters (Kurihara et al., 1998):

$i-j$	$g_{ij} - g_{jj}$ (J/mol)	$g_{ji} - g_{ii}$ (J/mol)	α_{ij}
1 − 2	770.15	1023.18	0.1099
1 − 3	− 156.80	1572.56	0.4307
2 − 3	3352.10	5003.95	0.5020

From the Mathcad worksheet, the thermodynamic factor is calculated as

$$\Gamma = \begin{pmatrix} 1.014 & -0.017 \\ -0.307 & 0.216 \end{pmatrix}$$

ORIGIN:= 1

$$g := \begin{pmatrix} 0 & 770.15 & -156.80 \\ 1023.18 & 0 & 3352.10 \\ 1572.56 & 5003.95 & 0 \end{pmatrix} \qquad \alpha := \begin{pmatrix} 0 & 0.1099 & 0.4307 \\ 0.1099 & 0 & 0.5020 \\ 0.4307 & 0.5020 & 0 \end{pmatrix} \qquad x := \begin{pmatrix} 0.1 \\ 0.3 \\ 0.6 \end{pmatrix}$$

$$R := 8.314 \qquad T := 298.15 \qquad N := 3 \qquad \vec{\tau} := \frac{g}{R \cdot T}$$

$$\vec{G} := \exp(-\alpha \cdot \tau)$$

→| Reference:C:\Users\tosun\Desktop\Subroutines\Multicomponent - NRTL.xmcd

$$\Gamma = \begin{pmatrix} 1.014 & -0.017 \\ -0.307 & 0.216 \end{pmatrix}$$

Mathcad worksheet of Example 3.4.

UNIQUAC model

The UNIQUAC (UNIversal QUAsi-Chemical) model enables the prediction of activity coefficients without experimental data.[10] The starting point is to consider the excess Gibbs energy as the sum of combinatorial and residual contributions. The equations to calculate the thermodynamic factor based on this model are given by Taylor and Krishna (1993).

3.3.2 THERMODYNAMIC FACTOR BASED ON THE FUGACITY COEFFICIENT

For a binary system of species 1 and 2, the thermodynamic factor defined by Eq. (3.75) reduces to

$$\Gamma = 1 + x_1 \left(\frac{\partial \ln \widehat{\phi}_1}{\partial x_1} \right)_{T,P} \tag{3.105}$$

Fugacity coefficients are calculated from the cubic equations of state capable of describing substances in both liquid and vapor states. Among the various cubic equations of state, the Peng–Robinson equation of state (Peng and Robinson, 1976) is the most popular. It is one of the most widely used correlations in chemical engineering.

In terms of the compressibility factor of a mixture, Z, the Peng–Robinson equation of state is described by

$$Z^3 + pZ^2 + qZ + r = 0, \tag{3.106}$$

where

$$p = B - 1 \qquad q = A - 2B - 3B^2 \qquad r = B^3 + B^2 - AB \tag{3.107}$$

---

[10] Activity coefficients can also be predicted theoretically by group contribution models, such as UNIFAC, Modified UNIFAC, and analytical solutions of groups (ASOG).

The dimensionless mixture parameters A and B are expressed according to the van der Waals (or quadratic) mixing rule as

$$A = \sum_{i=1}^{2} \sum_{j=1}^{2} x_i x_j A_{ij} \quad \text{and} \quad B = \sum_{i=1}^{2} x_i B_i, \tag{3.108}$$

where x_i represents the mole fraction of species i.

The terms A_{ii} (or A_{jj}) and B_i are the pure component parameters defined by

$$A_{ii} = 0.45724 \left(\frac{P_r}{T_r^2} \right)_i \alpha_i \quad \text{and} \quad B_i = 0.07780 \left(\frac{P_r}{T_r} \right)_i, \tag{3.109}$$

where P_r and T_r are *reduced pressure* and *reduced temperature*, defined by

$$P_r = \frac{P}{P_c} \quad \text{and} \quad T_r = \frac{T}{T_c}, \tag{3.110}$$

in which P_c and T_c are *critical pressure* and *critical temperature*, respectively. The term α_i is given as

$$\alpha_i = \left[1 + \left(0.37464 + 1.54226 \, \omega_i - 0.26992 \, \omega_i^2 \right) \left(1 - \sqrt{T_{r_i}} \right) \right]^2, \tag{3.111}$$

where ω_i is the acentric factor of species i. It quantifies the degree of polarity of a molecule, i.e., how asymmetric it is. Critical constants and acentric factors of pure compounds are given in Appendix F.

The *unlike interaction parameter* A_{ij} is related to the pure component parameters as

$$A_{ij} = \left(1 - k_{ij} \right) \sqrt{A_{ii} A_{jj}}, \tag{3.112}$$

where k_{ij} is the adjustable binary interaction parameter with a symmetric property, i.e., $k_{ij} = k_{ji}$.

The subroutine "Root" shown in Figure H.3 of Appendix H calculates the roots of Eq. (3.106), while the subroutine "Mixture" shown in Figure H.4 of Appendix H calculates the compressibility factor, Z, as well as the dimensionless parameters A and B for the mixture.

The fugacity coefficient for the Peng–Robinson equation of state is given by (Tosun, 2013)

$$\ln \hat{\phi}_1 = \frac{B_1}{B} (Z - 1) - \ln (Z - B)$$
$$- \frac{A}{\sqrt{8} B} \left[\frac{2 (x_1 A_{11} + x_2 A_{12})}{A} - \frac{B_1}{B} \right] \ln \left[\frac{Z + (1 + \sqrt{2}) B}{Z + (1 - \sqrt{2}) B} \right] \tag{3.113}$$

Differentiation of Eq. (3.113) with respect to x_1 gives (Tuan et al., 1999)

$$\Xi = \frac{\partial \ln \hat{\phi}_1}{\partial x_1} = \frac{B_1 \Theta}{B} - \frac{B_1 (B_1 - B_2)(Z - 1)}{B^2} - \frac{\Theta - B_1 + B_2}{Z - B}$$
$$+ \left\{ \frac{A_{12} B_1 - A_{11} B_2}{\sqrt{2} B^2} + \frac{AB_1}{\sqrt{8} B^2} \left[\frac{\Omega}{A} - \frac{2 (B_1 - B_2)}{B} \right] \right\} \ln \left[\frac{Z + (1 + \sqrt{2}) B}{Z + (1 - \sqrt{2}) B} \right]$$
$$+ \left[\frac{2 (x_1 A_{11} + x_2 A_{12})}{B} - \frac{AB_1}{B^2} \right] \frac{B \Theta - Z (B_1 - B_2)}{\left[Z + (1 + \sqrt{2}) B \right] \left[Z + (1 - \sqrt{2}) B \right]}, \tag{3.114}$$

where

$$\Omega = 2 \left[x_1 A_{11} + (x_2 - x_1) A_{12} - x_2 A_{22} \right] \tag{3.115}$$

$$\Theta = \frac{(B_1 - B_2)\left[A - B(2 + 3B) + Z(6B + 2 - Z)\right] - \Omega(Z - B)}{A - B(2 + 3B) + Z(2B - 2 + 3Z)} \tag{3.116}$$

Thus, Eq. (3.105) becomes

$$\boxed{\Gamma = 1 + x_1\,\Xi} \tag{3.117}$$

Example 3.5 Tuan et al. (1999) reported Fick diffusion coefficients of methyl oleate (1) in supercritical carbon dioxide (2). The critical properties and the acentric factor for methyl oleate are given as

$$T_c = 764.0\,\mathrm{K} \qquad P_c = 12.80\,\mathrm{bar} \qquad \omega = 1.0494$$

The mixture is represented by the Peng–Robinson equation of state with $k_{12} = 0.063$. For a mixture containing 0.817 mol % methyl oleate at 313.15 K and 115 bar, the thermodynamic factor is calculated as $\Gamma = 0.4217$ as shown in the Mathcad worksheet.

Mathcad worksheet of Example 3.5.

3.4 MS EQUATIONS IN THE FORM OF GENERALIZED FICK EQUATIONS

The MS equation given by Eq. (3.77) is nonlinear. Therefore, it is much more appealing to express it in the form of the generalized Fick equation, Eq. (3.2). In this way, it is possible to relate MS diffusion coefficients to Fick diffusion coefficients.

Equation (3.77) can be expressed as

$$c\sum_{k=1}^{\mathcal{N}-1}\Gamma_{ik}\nabla x_k = x_i\sum_{k=1}^{\mathcal{N}}\frac{\mathbf{J}_k^*}{\text{\DH}_{ik}} - \mathbf{J}_i^*\sum_{k=1}^{\mathcal{N}}\frac{x_k}{\text{\DH}_{ik}}$$

$$= x_i\sum_{k=1}^{\mathcal{N}-1}\frac{\mathbf{J}_k^*}{\text{\DH}_{ik}} + x_i\frac{\mathbf{J}_{\mathcal{N}}^*}{\text{\DH}_{i\mathcal{N}}} - \mathbf{J}_i^*\sum_{k=1}^{\mathcal{N}}\frac{x_k}{\text{\DH}_{ik}} \tag{3.118}$$

The use of Eq. (2.50) in Eq. (3.118) yields

$$c \sum_{k=1}^{\mathcal{N}-1} \Gamma_{ik} \nabla x_k = x_i \sum_{k=1}^{\mathcal{N}-1} \left(\frac{1}{Đ_{ik}} - \frac{1}{Đ_{i\mathcal{N}}} \right) \mathbf{J}_k^* - \mathbf{J}_i^* \sum_{k=1}^{\mathcal{N}} \frac{x_k}{Đ_{ik}} \tag{3.119}$$

Rearrangement of Eq. (3.119) in the form

$$c \sum_{k=1}^{\mathcal{N}-1} \Gamma_{ik} \nabla x_k = x_i \sum_{\substack{k=1 \\ k \neq i}}^{\mathcal{N}-1} \left(\frac{1}{Đ_{ik}} - \frac{1}{Đ_{i\mathcal{N}}} \right) \mathbf{J}_k^* + x_i \left(\frac{1}{Đ_{ii}} - \frac{1}{Đ_{i\mathcal{N}}} \right) \mathbf{J}_i^* - \mathbf{J}_i^* \sum_{\substack{k=1 \\ k \neq i}}^{\mathcal{N}} \frac{x_k}{Đ_{ik}} - \mathbf{J}_i^* \frac{x_i}{Đ_{ii}} \tag{3.120}$$

leads to

$$c \sum_{k=1}^{\mathcal{N}-1} \Gamma_{ik} \nabla x_k = x_i \sum_{\substack{k=1 \\ k \neq i}}^{\mathcal{N}-1} \left(\frac{1}{Đ_{ik}} - \frac{1}{Đ_{i\mathcal{N}}} \right) \mathbf{J}_k^* - \left(\frac{x_i}{Đ_{i\mathcal{N}}} + \sum_{\substack{k=1 \\ k \neq i}}^{\mathcal{N}} \frac{x_k}{Đ_{ik}} \right) \mathbf{J}_i^* \tag{3.121}$$

If we define the matrix $\mathbf{B}$ with components

$$B_{ii} = \frac{x_i}{Đ_{i\mathcal{N}}} + \sum_{\substack{k=1 \\ k \neq i}}^{\mathcal{N}} \frac{x_k}{Đ_{ik}} \qquad \text{and} \qquad B_{ik} = x_i \left(\frac{1}{Đ_{i\mathcal{N}}} - \frac{1}{Đ_{ik}} \right) \quad i \neq k \tag{3.122}$$

Eq. (3.121) becomes

$$c \sum_{k=1}^{\mathcal{N}-1} \Gamma_{ik} \nabla x_k = - \left(B_{ii} \mathbf{J}_i^* + \sum_{\substack{k=1 \\ k \neq i}}^{\mathcal{N}-1} B_{ik} \mathbf{J}_k^* \right) \qquad i = 1, 2, \ldots, \mathcal{N} - 1 \tag{3.123}$$

In matrix notation, Eq. (3.123) is expressed as

$$-c \left[\Gamma \right] \left[\nabla x \right] = \left[\mathbf{B} \right] \left[\mathbf{J}^* \right] \tag{3.124}$$

Multiplication of Eq. (3.124) by the inverse of the matrix $\mathbf{B}$, $\mathbf{B}^{-1}$ from the left side yields

$$\left[\mathbf{J}^* \right] = -c \left[\mathbf{B} \right]^{-1} \left[\Gamma \right] \left[\nabla x \right] \tag{3.125}$$

Comparison of Eq. (3.125) with Eq. (3.2) implies that

$$\left[\mathcal{D}^* \right] = \left[\mathbf{B} \right]^{-1} \left[\Gamma \right] \tag{3.126}$$

For an ideal mixture, $[\Gamma] = [\mathbf{I}]$ and Eq. (3.126) reduces to

$$\boxed{\left[\mathcal{D}^* \right] = \left[\mathbf{B} \right]^{-1}} \quad \text{Ideal mixture} \tag{3.127}$$

3.4.1 BINARY MIXTURE

In the case of a binary mixture, the matrix $[\mathbf{B}]$ reduces to a single element B_{11}. The use of Eq. (3.122) gives B_{11} as

$$B_{11} = \frac{x_1}{Đ_{12}} + \frac{x_2}{Đ_{12}} = \frac{1}{Đ_{12}} \tag{3.128}$$

Since binary Fick diffusion coefficients are independent of the reference velocity frame, i.e., $\mathcal{D}_{12}^* = \mathcal{D}_{12}^m = \mathcal{D}_{12}^\blacksquare = \mathcal{D}_{12}$, Eq. (3.126) results in

$$\boxed{\mathcal{D}_{12} = Đ_{12}\,\Gamma}$$ (3.129)

For ideal mixtures, $\Gamma = 1$ and Fick diffusion coefficients are equal to MS diffusion coefficients.

Example 3.6 Rehfeldt and Stichlmair (2010) reported the binary Fick diffusion coefficients for a mixture of acetone (1) and water (2) at 298.15 K as a function of composition as follows:

x_1	0.004	0.1	0.3	0.5	0.7	0.9	0.975
$\mathcal{D}_{12} \times 10^9$ (m^2/s)	1.25	0.80	0.63	0.83	1.63	3.44	4.62

The system is represented by the Wilson equation with the following parameters:

$$\lambda_{12} - \lambda_{11} = 504.046\,\text{J/mol} \quad \text{and} \quad \lambda_{21} - \lambda_{22} = 4966.011\,\text{J/mol}$$

The molar volumes of pure liquids are given as

$$\widetilde{V}_1 = 74.04\,\text{cm}^3/\text{mol} \quad \text{and} \quad \widetilde{V}_2 = 18.07\,\text{cm}^3/\text{mol}$$

ORIGIN:= 1

$$\text{Dfick} := \begin{pmatrix} 1.25 \\ 0.80 \\ 0.63 \\ 0.83 \\ 1.63 \\ 3.44 \\ 4.62 \end{pmatrix} \cdot 10^{-9} \qquad x1 := \begin{pmatrix} 0.004 \\ 0.1 \\ 0.3 \\ 0.5 \\ 0.7 \\ 0.9 \\ 0.975 \end{pmatrix} \qquad V := \begin{pmatrix} 74.04 \\ 18.07 \end{pmatrix} \qquad T := 298.15 \qquad R := 8.314$$

x2 := 1 − x1

$$\Lambda12 := \frac{V_2}{V_1}\cdot\exp\left(\frac{-504.046}{R\cdot T}\right) = 0.199 \qquad \Lambda21 := \frac{V_1}{V_2}\cdot\exp\left(\frac{-4966.011}{R\cdot T}\right) = 0.553 \qquad \text{Eq. (3.89)}$$

$$\Gamma := \left[1 + x1\cdot\left[\frac{\Lambda21^2}{(x2 + \Lambda21\cdot x1)^2} + \frac{(\Lambda12 - 1)^2\cdot x2 - 1}{(x1 + \Lambda12\cdot x2)^2}\right]\right] \qquad \text{Eq. (3.90)}$$

$$\Gamma^T = (0.966\ \ 0.491\ \ 0.266\ \ 0.309\ \ 0.474\ \ 0.775\ \ 0.938)$$

$$\text{Dms} := \frac{\overrightarrow{\text{Dfick}}}{\Gamma} \qquad \text{Eq. (3.129)}$$

$$\text{Dms}^T = \left(1.294 \times 10^{-9}\ \ 1.628 \times 10^{-9}\ \ 2.368 \times 10^{-9}\ \ 2.69 \times 10^{-9}\ \ 3.44 \times 10^{-9}\ \ 4.439 \times 10^{-9}\ \ 4.927 \times 10^{-9}\right)$$

Mathcad worksheet of Example 3.6.

The MS diffusion coefficients are calculated as shown in the Mathcad worksheet, and both diffusion coefficients are plotted as a function of mole fraction of acetone in the figure below. Note that $Đ_{12} > \mathcal{D}_{12}$ since the thermodynamic factor is less than unity in this specific example. In the limit as $x_i \to 1$, the thermodynamic factor goes to unity and both diffusion coefficients are equal to each other.

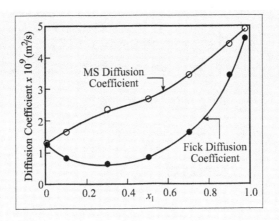

3.4.2 TERNARY MIXTURE

The use of Eq. (3.122) gives the components of the matrix $[\mathbf{B}]$ as

$$[\mathbf{B}] = \begin{pmatrix} \dfrac{x_1 + x_3}{\text{Đ}_{13}} + \dfrac{x_2}{\text{Đ}_{12}} & x_1\left(\dfrac{1}{\text{Đ}_{13}} - \dfrac{1}{\text{Đ}_{12}}\right) \\[3mm] x_2\left(\dfrac{1}{\text{Đ}_{23}} - \dfrac{1}{\text{Đ}_{12}}\right) & \dfrac{x_1}{\text{Đ}_{12}} + \dfrac{x_2 + x_3}{\text{Đ}_{23}} \end{pmatrix} \tag{3.130}$$

Thus, Eq. (3.126) relates the MS diffusion coefficients to the Fick diffusion coefficients in the form

$$\begin{pmatrix} \mathcal{D}_{11}^* & \mathcal{D}_{12}^* \\ \mathcal{D}_{21}^* & \mathcal{D}_{22}^* \end{pmatrix} = [\mathbf{B}]^{-1} \cdot \begin{pmatrix} \Gamma_{11} & \Gamma_{12} \\ \Gamma_{21} & \Gamma_{22} \end{pmatrix}, \tag{3.131}$$

where the inverse of $[\mathbf{B}]$ is given by

$$[\mathbf{B}]^{-1} = \frac{\begin{pmatrix} \text{Đ}_{13}\left[x_1\text{Đ}_{23} + (1 - x_1)\text{Đ}_{12}\right] & x_1\text{Đ}_{23}\left(\text{Đ}_{13} - \text{Đ}_{12}\right) \\[3mm] x_2\text{Đ}_{13}\left(\text{Đ}_{23} - \text{Đ}_{12}\right) & \text{Đ}_{23}\left[x_2\text{Đ}_{13} + (1 - x_2)\text{Đ}_{12}\right] \end{pmatrix}}{x_1\text{Đ}_{23} + x_2\text{Đ}_{13} + x_3\text{Đ}_{12}} \tag{3.132}$$

For a ternary system, there are three MS diffusion coefficients and four Fick diffusion coefficients. Therefore, calculation of the Fick diffusion coefficients from the MS diffusion coefficients using Eq. (3.131) is straightforward.

Example 3.7 For a ternary gas mixture of methane (1), argon (2), and hydrogen (3), Krishna (2016) reported the following MS diffusion coefficients at 307 K:

$$Đ_{12} = 2.16 \times 10^{-5} \, \text{m}^2/\text{s} \qquad Đ_{13} = 7.72 \times 10^{-5} \, \text{m}^2/\text{s} \qquad Đ_{23} = 8.33 \times 10^{-5} \, \text{m}^2/\text{s}$$

Taking $[\Gamma] = [\mathbf{I}]$, Eqs. (3.131) and (3.132) simplify to

$$\begin{pmatrix} \mathcal{D}_{11}^* & \mathcal{D}_{12}^* \\ \mathcal{D}_{21}^* & \mathcal{D}_{22}^* \end{pmatrix} = \frac{\begin{pmatrix} Đ_{13} \left[y_1 Đ_{23} + (1 - y_1) Đ_{12} \right] & y_1 Đ_{23} (Đ_{13} - Đ_{12}) \\ y_2 Đ_{13} (Đ_{23} - Đ_{12}) & Đ_{23} \left[y_2 Đ_{13} + (1 - y_2) Đ_{12} \right] \end{pmatrix}}{y_1 Đ_{23} + y_2 Đ_{13} + y_3 Đ_{12}}$$

For a gas mixture with the composition of $y_1 = 0.2575$, $y_2 = 0.4970$, and $y_3 = 0.2455$, the calculations of the Fick diffusion coefficients with reference to molar-average velocity are given in the Mathcad worksheet shown below:

ORIGIN:= 1

$$\text{Dms} := \begin{pmatrix} 2.16 \\ 7.72 \\ 8.33 \end{pmatrix} \cdot 10^{-5} \qquad y := \begin{pmatrix} 0.2575 \\ 0.4970 \\ 0.2455 \end{pmatrix}$$

$$D := \frac{\begin{bmatrix} \text{Dms}_2 \cdot \left[y_1 \cdot \text{Dms}_3 + \left(1 - y_1 \right) \cdot \text{Dms}_1 \right] & y_1 \cdot \text{Dms}_3 \cdot \left(\text{Dms}_2 - \text{Dms}_1 \right) \\ y_2 \cdot \text{Dms}_2 \cdot \left(\text{Dms}_3 - \text{Dms}_1 \right) & \text{Dms}_3 \cdot \left[y_2 \cdot \text{Dms}_2 + \left(1 - y_2 \right) \cdot \text{Dms}_1 \right] \end{bmatrix}}{y_1 \cdot \text{Dms}_3 + y_2 \cdot \text{Dms}_2 + y_3 \cdot \text{Dms}_1}$$

$$D = \begin{pmatrix} 4.444 \times 10^{-5} & 1.831 \times 10^{-5} \\ 3.635 \times 10^{-5} & 6.298 \times 10^{-5} \end{pmatrix}$$

Mathcad worksheet of Example 3.7.

The calculation of the MS diffusion coefficients from the Fick diffusion coefficients, however, is more complicated since we have four equations and three unknowns. In this case, the first step is to calculate $[\mathbf{B}]$

$$[\mathbf{B}] = [\Gamma] \cdot [\mathcal{D}^*]^{-1}, \tag{3.133}$$

from which the elements of $[\mathbf{B}]$ can be expressed as a column matrix as

$$\begin{pmatrix} B_{11} \\ B_{12} \\ B_{21} \\ B_{22} \end{pmatrix} = \frac{1}{|\mathcal{D}^*|} \begin{pmatrix} 0 & 0 & -\Gamma_{12} & \Gamma_{11} \\ \Gamma_{12} & -\Gamma_{11} & 0 & 0 \\ 0 & 0 & -\Gamma_{22} & \Gamma_{21} \\ \Gamma_{22} & -\Gamma_{12} & 0 & 0 \end{pmatrix} \begin{pmatrix} \mathcal{D}_{11}^* \\ \mathcal{D}_{12}^* \\ \mathcal{D}_{21}^* \\ \mathcal{D}_{22}^* \end{pmatrix} \tag{3.134}$$

The next step is to rearrange Eq. (3.130) in the form

$$
\underbrace{\begin{pmatrix} B_{11} \\ B_{12} \\ B_{21} \\ B_{22} \end{pmatrix}}_{[\mathbf{Y}]} = \underbrace{\begin{pmatrix} x_2 & x_1 + x_3 & 0 \\ -x_1 & x_1 & 0 \\ -x_2 & 0 & x_2 \\ x_1 & 0 & x_2 + x_3 \end{pmatrix}}_{[\mathbf{X}]} \cdot \begin{pmatrix} \dfrac{1}{Đ_{12}} \\[2mm] \dfrac{1}{Đ_{13}} \\[2mm] \dfrac{1}{Đ_{23}} \end{pmatrix}
\tag{3.135}
$$

The MS diffusion coefficients can be calculated from the above equation by the method of least squares. For this purpose, Eq. (3.135) should be multiplied by $[\mathbf{X}]^{\mathrm{T}}$ from the left side. Rearrangement gives the MS diffusion coefficients as

$$
\boxed{\begin{pmatrix} Đ_{12} \\ Đ_{13} \\ Đ_{23} \end{pmatrix} = \frac{1}{\left([\mathbf{X}]^{\mathrm{T}} \cdot [\mathbf{X}] \right)^{-1} \cdot [\mathbf{X}]^{\mathrm{T}} \cdot [\mathbf{Y}]}}
\tag{3.136}
$$

See Problem 3.8 for an alternative approach for calculating the MS diffusion coefficients from the Fick diffusion coefficients.

Example 3.8   A ternary mixture containing 50 mol % 1-propanol (1), 25% 1-chlorobutane (2), and 25% n-heptane (3) is at 298.15 K. Elements of the Fick diffusion coefficient matrix are reported by Rehfeldt and Stichlmair (2010) as

$$
[\mathcal{D}^*] = \begin{pmatrix} 0.5306 & -0.5840 \\ 0.4683 & 2.2920 \end{pmatrix} \times 10^{-9}\,\mathrm{m^2/s}
$$

The mixture is represented by the Wilson model with the following parameters:

$i-j$	$\lambda_{ij} - \lambda_{ii}$ (J/mol)	$\lambda_{ji} - \lambda_{jj}$ (J/mol)
$1-2$	4980.55	570.71
$1-3$	7294.05	703.40
$2-3$	1244.46	-175.51

The molar volumes are given as

$$
\widetilde{V}_1 = 75.10\,\mathrm{cm^3/mol} \qquad \widetilde{V}_2 = 105.08\,\mathrm{cm^3/mol} \qquad \widetilde{V}_3 = 147.46\,\mathrm{cm^3/mol}
$$

From the Mathcad worksheet shown below, the MS diffusion coefficients are calculated as

$$
Đ_{12} = 4.152 \times 10^{-9}\,\mathrm{m^2/s} \qquad Đ_{13} = 2.549 \times 10^{-9}\,\mathrm{m^2/s} \qquad Đ_{23} = 1.529 \times 10^{-9}\,\mathrm{m^2/s}
$$

To check whether these values are correct, let us reverse the calculations. Using the calculated MS diffusion coefficients, the inverse of matrix $[\mathbf{B}]$ is calculated from Eq. (3.132) as

$$
[\mathbf{B}]^{-1} = \begin{pmatrix} 2.968 & -0.5023 \\ -0.685 & 2.351 \end{pmatrix} \times 10^{-9}
$$

Thus, from Eq. (3.126)

$$
[\mathcal{D}^*] = \begin{pmatrix} 2.968 & -0.5023 \\ -0.685 & 2.351 \end{pmatrix} \times 10^{-9} \cdot \begin{pmatrix} 0.221 & -0.096 \\ 0.273 & 0.911 \end{pmatrix} = \begin{pmatrix} 0.519 & -0.743 \\ 0.490 & 2.208 \end{pmatrix} \times 10^{-9}\,\mathrm{m^2/s}
$$

ORIGIN:= 1

$R := 8.314$ $T := 298.15$ $N := 3$

$$x := \begin{pmatrix} 0.5 \\ 0.25 \\ 0.25 \end{pmatrix} \qquad V := \begin{pmatrix} 75.10 \\ 105.08 \\ 147.47 \end{pmatrix} \qquad Dfick := \begin{pmatrix} 0.5306 & -0.584 \\ 0.4683 & 2.292 \end{pmatrix} \cdot 10^{-9}$$

$$\Lambda := \begin{pmatrix} 1 & \dfrac{V_2}{V_1}\cdot\exp\left(\dfrac{-4980.550}{R\cdot T}\right) & \dfrac{V_3}{V_1}\cdot\exp\left(\dfrac{-7294.051}{R\cdot T}\right) \\[2mm] \dfrac{V_1}{V_2}\cdot\exp\left(\dfrac{-570.706}{R\cdot T}\right) & 1 & \dfrac{V_3}{V_2}\cdot\exp\left(\dfrac{-1244.455}{R\cdot T}\right) \\[2mm] \dfrac{V_1}{V_3}\cdot\exp\left(\dfrac{-703.402}{R\cdot T}\right) & \dfrac{V_2}{V_3}\cdot\exp\left(\dfrac{175.515}{R\cdot T}\right) & 1 \end{pmatrix} = \begin{pmatrix} 1 & 0.188 & 0.104 \\ 0.568 & 1 & 0.849 \\ 0.383 & 0.765 & 1 \end{pmatrix}$$

→ Reference:C:\Users\tosun\Desktop\Subroutines\Multicomponent - Wilson.xmcd

$$\Gamma = \begin{pmatrix} 0.221 & -0.096 \\ 0.273 & 0.911 \end{pmatrix}$$

$$B := \Gamma \cdot Dfick^{-1} = \begin{pmatrix} 3.699 \times 10^8 & 5.248 \times 10^7 \\ 1.343 \times 10^8 & 4.319 \times 10^8 \end{pmatrix}$$

$$Y := \begin{pmatrix} B_{1,1} \\ B_{1,2} \\ B_{2,1} \\ B_{2,2} \end{pmatrix} \qquad X := \begin{pmatrix} x_2 & x_1 + x_3 & 0 \\ -x_1 & x_1 & 0 \\ -x_2 & 0 & x_2 \\ x_1 & 0 & x_2 + x_3 \end{pmatrix}$$

$$Dms := \dfrac{1}{\left(X^T \cdot X\right)^{-1} \cdot X^T \cdot Y} = \begin{pmatrix} 4.152 \times 10^{-9} \\ 2.549 \times 10^{-9} \\ 1.529 \times 10^{-9} \end{pmatrix}$$

Mathcad worksheet of Example 3.8.

• Limiting cases

Case (i): MS diffusivities are nearly equal to each other

In a mixture consisting of almost identical species, MS diffusivities are equal to each other, i.e.,

$$Đ_{12} \simeq Đ_{13} \simeq Đ_{23} = Đ_m \tag{3.137}$$

Thus, the inverse of the matrix $[\mathbf{B}]$, Eq. (3.132), simplifies to

$$[\mathbf{B}]^{-1} = Đ_m [\mathbf{I}] \tag{3.138}$$

Case (ii): Concentration of species 1 is dilute

In this case, $x_1 \simeq 0$ and Eq. (3.132) simplifies to

$$[\mathbf{B}]^{-1} = \frac{\begin{pmatrix} Đ_{12}Đ_{13} & 0 \\ x_2 Đ_{13}(Đ_{23} - Đ_{12}) & Đ_{23}(x_2 Đ_{13} + x_3 Đ_{12}) \end{pmatrix}}{x_2 Đ_{13} + x_3 Đ_{12}} \tag{3.139}$$

3.4.3 QUATERNARY MIXTURE

The use of Eq. (3.122) gives the components of the matrix $[\mathbf{B}]$ as

$$[\mathbf{B}] = \begin{pmatrix} \dfrac{x_1 + x_4}{Đ_{14}} + \dfrac{x_2}{Đ_{12}} + \dfrac{x_3}{Đ_{13}} & -x_1\left(\dfrac{1}{Đ_{12}} - \dfrac{1}{Đ_{14}}\right) & -x_1\left(\dfrac{1}{Đ_{13}} - \dfrac{1}{Đ_{14}}\right) \\ -x_2\left(\dfrac{1}{Đ_{12}} - \dfrac{1}{Đ_{24}}\right) & \dfrac{x_2 + x_4}{Đ_{24}} + \dfrac{x_1}{Đ_{12}} + \dfrac{x_3}{Đ_{23}} & -x_2\left(\dfrac{1}{Đ_{23}} - \dfrac{1}{Đ_{24}}\right) \\ -x_3\left(\dfrac{1}{Đ_{13}} - \dfrac{1}{Đ_{34}}\right) & -x_3\left(\dfrac{1}{Đ_{23}} - \dfrac{1}{Đ_{34}}\right) & \dfrac{x_3 + x_4}{Đ_{34}} + \dfrac{x_1}{Đ_{13}} + \dfrac{x_2}{Đ_{23}} \end{pmatrix} \tag{3.140}$$

Thus, Eq. (3.126) relates the MS diffusion coefficients to the Fick diffusion coefficients in the form

$$\begin{pmatrix} \mathcal{D}^*_{11} & \mathcal{D}^*_{12} & \mathcal{D}^*_{13} \\ \mathcal{D}^*_{21} & \mathcal{D}^*_{22} & \mathcal{D}^*_{23} \\ \mathcal{D}^*_{31} & \mathcal{D}^*_{32} & \mathcal{D}^*_{33} \end{pmatrix} = [\mathbf{B}]^{-1} \cdot \begin{pmatrix} \Gamma_{11} & \Gamma_{12} & \Gamma_{13} \\ \Gamma_{21} & \Gamma_{22} & \Gamma_{23} \\ \Gamma_{31} & \Gamma_{32} & \Gamma_{33} \end{pmatrix} \tag{3.141}$$

For a quaternary system, there are six MS diffusion coefficients and nine Fick diffusion coefficients. Therefore, calculation of the Fick diffusion coefficients from the MS diffusion coefficients using Eq. (3.141) is straightforward.

The calculation of the MS diffusion coefficients from the Fick diffusion coefficients is again more complicated since the number of equations exceeds the number of unknowns. For this purpose, the first step is to calculate the elements of the matrix $[\mathbf{B}]$ using Eq. (3.133). Then Eq. (3.140) should be rearranged in the form

$$\underbrace{\begin{pmatrix} B_{11} \\ B_{12} \\ B_{13} \\ B_{21} \\ B_{22} \\ B_{23} \\ B_{31} \\ B_{32} \\ B_{33} \end{pmatrix}}_{[\mathbf{Y}]} = \underbrace{\begin{pmatrix} x_2 & x_3 & x_1 + x_4 & 0 & 0 & 0 \\ -x_1 & 0 & x_1 & 0 & 0 & 0 \\ 0 & -x_1 & x_1 & 0 & 0 & 0 \\ -x_2 & 0 & 0 & 0 & x_2 & 0 \\ x_1 & 0 & 0 & x_3 & x_2 + x_4 & 0 \\ 0 & 0 & 0 & -x_2 & x_2 & 0 \\ 0 & -x_3 & 0 & 0 & 0 & x_3 \\ 0 & 0 & 0 & -x_3 & 0 & x_3 \\ 0 & x_1 & 0 & x_2 & 0 & x_3 + x_4 \end{pmatrix}}_{[\mathbf{X}]} \cdot \begin{pmatrix} \dfrac{1}{Đ_{12}} \\ \dfrac{1}{Đ_{13}} \\ \dfrac{1}{Đ_{14}} \\ \dfrac{1}{Đ_{23}} \\ \dfrac{1}{Đ_{24}} \\ \dfrac{1}{Đ_{34}} \end{pmatrix} \tag{3.142}$$

Multiplication of Eq. (3.142) by $[\mathbf{X}]^{\mathrm{T}}$ from the left side and rearrangement yield

$$
\begin{pmatrix} Đ_{12} \\ Đ_{13} \\ Đ_{14} \\ Đ_{23} \\ Đ_{24} \\ Đ_{34} \end{pmatrix} = \frac{1}{\left([\mathbf{X}]^{\mathrm{T}} \cdot [\mathbf{X}]\right)^{-1} \cdot [\mathbf{X}]^{\mathrm{T}} \cdot [\mathbf{Y}]}
\tag{3.143}
$$

See Problem 3.9 for an alternative approach for calculating the MS diffusion coefficients from the Fick diffusion coefficients.

3.5 PREDICTION OF DIFFUSION COEFFICIENTS

MS diffusion coefficients are related to the gradient of partial molar Gibbs energy, a quantity that is impossible to measure experimentally. Fick diffusion coefficients, on the other hand, can be measured experimentally. Various experimental techniques (diaphragm measurement technique, conductance method, Taylor dispersion technique, nuclear magnetic resonance (NMR) spectroscopy, Gouy interferometric method, dynamic light scattering (DLS), Raman spectroscopy, and microfluidics) used for the measurement of diffusion coefficients are summarized by Peters et al. (2016). In the case of liquids, Fick diffusion coefficients are dependent on concentration as well as temperature and pressure. This necessitates extensive experimental effort in the laboratory. In the literature, most of the available data are for binary mixtures. Since accurate measurement of diffusion coefficients for ternary and quaternary mixtures is rather time consuming and expensive if not impossible, experimental data are scarce.[11] Once Fick diffusion coefficients are known, MS diffusion coefficients can be determined as shown in Example 3.6 by choosing an appropriate activity coefficient model.

Theoretical calculations of Fick and MS diffusion coefficients are possible by molecular dynamics simulations. These calculations, however, require large amounts of CPU time.

Therefore, efforts have been directed to develop models for the prediction of diffusion coefficients using a minimum number of experimentally or theoretically determined parameters. Coverage of all the predictive models available in the literature is beyond the scope of this text.[12] In the following section, two of the most commonly used models will be briefly given.

3.5.1 VIGNES EQUATION

Fick ($\mathcal{D}^m$, $\mathcal{D}^*$, $\mathcal{D}^\blacksquare$) and MS ($Đ$) diffusion coefficients are identical at the infinite dilution limit. The diffusion coefficient of component i infinitely diluted in component j is expressed as

$$
\mathcal{D}_{ij}^{\infty} = D_{ij}^{x_i \to 0}
\tag{3.144}
$$

For a binary mixture, Vignes (1966) proposed the following logarithmic average to evaluate MS diffusion coefficients in concentrated solutions based on the infinite dilution diffusion coefficients:

$$
\boxed{Đ_{ij} = (\mathcal{D}_{ij}^{\infty})^{x_j} (\mathcal{D}_{ji}^{\infty})^{x_i}}
\tag{3.145}
$$

---

[11]The literature survey conducted by Mutoru and Firoozabadi (2011) reveals experimental data for 94 ternary and 13 quaternary systems.

[12]Hierarchy of predictive models for diffusion coefficients is presented by Bardow et al. (2009).

Kooijman and Taylor (1991) generalized the Vignes equation to multicomponent mixtures as[13]

$$\text{Đ}_{ij} = (\mathcal{D}_{ij}^{\infty})^{x_j} (\mathcal{D}_{ji}^{\infty})^{x_i} \prod_{\substack{k=1 \\ k \neq i,j}}^{\mathcal{N}} (\mathcal{D}_{ik}^{\infty} \mathcal{D}_{jk}^{\infty})^{x_k/2} \qquad i,j = 1,2...,\mathcal{N} \text{ and } i \neq j \qquad (3.146)$$

Infinite dilution diffusion coefficients are determined from (1) correlations given in Chapter 2, i.e., the Wilke–Chang equation, (2) experimental measurements, and (3) molecular simulations. Once they are known, MS and Fick diffusion coefficients are calculated as follows:

- Use Eq. (3.146) to calculate Đ_{ij} values.
- Use Eq. (3.132) to evaluate the components of $[\mathbf{B}]^{-1}$.
- Depending on the activity coefficient model, evaluate $[\Gamma]$.
- Use Eq. (3.126) to calculate the components of $[\mathcal{D}^*]$.
- Use Eqs. (3.42) and (3.47) to calculate the components of $[\mathcal{D}^m]$ and $[\mathcal{D}^{\blacksquare}]$, respectively.

Example 3.9 For a binary mixture of acetone (1) and 1-butanol (2) at 298.15 K, Rehfeldt and Stichlmair (2010) reported the infinite dilution diffusion coefficients as

$$\mathcal{D}_{12}^{\infty} = 0.94 \times 10^{-9} \text{m}^2/\text{s} \qquad \mathcal{D}_{21}^{\infty} = 2.79 \times 10^{-9} \text{m}^2/\text{s}$$

The system is represented by the Wilson model with the following parameters:

$$\lambda_{12} - \lambda_{11} = -59.526 \text{J/mol} \qquad \lambda_{21} - \lambda_{22} = 1381.892 \text{J/mol}$$

The molar volumes are given as

$$\widetilde{V}_1 = 74.04 \text{cm}^3/\text{mol} \qquad \widetilde{V}_2 = 92.00 \text{cm}^3/\text{mol}$$

According to Eq. (3.145), the MS diffusion coefficients are expressed as a function of composition in the form

$$\text{Đ}_{12} \times 10^9 = 0.94^{x_2} 2.79^{x_1} \qquad (1)$$

The MS diffusion coefficients calculated from Eq. (1) are given in the second column of the table shown below. The third column shows the thermodynamic factor calculated from Eq. (3.90). The Fick diffusion coefficients calculated from Eq. (3.129) are given in the fourth column and compared with the experimental values.

x_1	$\text{Đ}_{12} \times 10^9$ (m^2/s)	Γ	$\mathcal{D}_{12} \times 10^9$ (m^2/s) Calculated	Experimental
0.1	1.048	0.964	1.01	1.00
0.2	1.168	0.927	1.08	1.07
0.3	1.303	0.890	1.16	1.13
0.4	1.453	0.856	1.24	1.29
0.5	1.619	0.826	1.34	1.38
0.6	1.806	0.805	1.45	1.49
0.7	2.013	0.799	1.61	1.72
0.8	2.244	0.817	1.83	1.85
0.9	2.502	0.875	2.19	2.43

---

[13]It should be pointed out that Eq. (3.146) is not the only equation used to predict Đ_{ij} values based on the Vignes model. For other Vignes-based formulas, see Wesselingh and Bollen (1997), Krishna and van Baten (2005), and Rehfeldt and Stichlmair (2007).

Example 3.10 Using the experimental data of Alimadadian and Colver (1976), Kooijman and Taylor (1991) reported the following infinite dilution diffusion coefficients for a ternary mixture of acetone (1), benzene (2), and methanol (3) at 298.15K:

$$\mathcal{D}_{12}^{\infty} = 3.0368 \times 10^{-9} \text{m}^2/\text{s} \qquad \mathcal{D}_{21}^{\infty} = 4.2778 \times 10^{-9} \text{m}^2/\text{s}$$

$$\mathcal{D}_{13}^{\infty} = 2.6009 \times 10^{-9} \text{m}^2/\text{s} \qquad \mathcal{D}_{31}^{\infty} = 4.7951 \times 10^{-9} \text{m}^2/\text{s}$$

$$\mathcal{D}_{23}^{\infty} = 2.4159 \times 10^{-9} \text{m}^2/\text{s} \qquad \mathcal{D}_{32}^{\infty} = 3.6480 \times 10^{-9} \text{m}^2/\text{s}$$

The mixture is represented by the NRTL model with the following parameters:

$i-j$	$g_{ij} - g_{jj}$ (J/mol)	$g_{ji} - g_{ii}$ (J/mol)	α_{ij}
1 − 2	− 1009.49	3416.75	0.2998
1 − 3	3397.88	1309.50	0.2942
2 − 3	5699.92	3621.53	0.5023

ORIGIN := 1

$$\text{Dinf} := \begin{pmatrix} 0 & 3.0368 & 2.6009 \\ 4.2778 & 0 & 2.4159 \\ 4.7951 & 3.6480 & 0 \end{pmatrix} \cdot 10^{-9} \qquad x := \begin{pmatrix} 0.2060 \\ 0.5480 \\ 0.2460 \end{pmatrix} \qquad \alpha := \begin{pmatrix} 0 & 0.2998 & 0.2942 \\ 0.2998 & 0 & 0.5023 \\ 0.2942 & 0.5023 & 0 \end{pmatrix}$$

$N := 3 \qquad R := 8.314 \qquad R := 8.314 \qquad T := 298.15$

$$g := \begin{pmatrix} 0 & -1009.49 & 3397.88 \\ 3416.75 & 0 & 5699.92 \\ 1309.50 & 3621.53 & 0 \end{pmatrix}$$

$$\tau := \frac{\overrightarrow{g}}{R \cdot T} = \begin{pmatrix} 0 & -0.407 & 1.371 \\ 1.378 & 0 & 2.299 \\ 0.528 & 1.461 & 0 \end{pmatrix}$$

$$G := \overrightarrow{\exp(-\alpha \cdot \tau)} = \begin{pmatrix} 1 & 1.13 & 0.668 \\ 0.662 & 1 & 0.315 \\ 0.856 & 0.48 & 1 \end{pmatrix}$$

$$\text{Dms} := \begin{bmatrix} \left(\text{Dinf}_{1,2}\right)^{x_2} \cdot \left(\text{Dinf}_{2,1}\right)^{x_1} \cdot \left(\text{Dinf}_{1,3} \cdot \text{Dinf}_{2,3}\right)^{\frac{x_3}{2}} \\ \left(\text{Dinf}_{1,3}\right)^{x_3} \cdot \left(\text{Dinf}_{3,1}\right)^{x_1} \cdot \left(\text{Dinf}_{1,2} \cdot \text{Dinf}_{3,2}\right)^{\frac{x_2}{2}} \\ \left(\text{Dinf}_{2,3}\right)^{x_3} \cdot \left(\text{Dinf}_{3,2}\right)^{x_2} \cdot \left(\text{Dinf}_{2,1} \cdot \text{Dinf}_{3,1}\right)^{\frac{x_1}{2}} \end{bmatrix} = \begin{pmatrix} 3.1087 \times 10^{-9} \\ 3.3771 \times 10^{-9} \\ 3.4465 \times 10^{-9} \end{pmatrix}$$ Eq. (3.146)

$$\text{Binverse} := \frac{\begin{bmatrix} \text{Dms}_2 \cdot \left[x_1 \cdot \text{Dms}_3 + \left(1 - x_1\right) \cdot \text{Dms}_1 \right] & x_1 \cdot \text{Dms}_3 \cdot \left(\text{Dms}_2 - \text{Dms}_1\right) \\ x_2 \cdot \text{Dms}_2 \cdot \left(\text{Dms}_3 - \text{Dms}_1\right) & \text{Dms}_3 \cdot \left[x_2 \cdot \text{Dms}_2 + \left(1 - x_2\right) \cdot \text{Dms}_1 \right] \end{bmatrix}}{x_1 \cdot \text{Dms}_3 + x_2 \cdot \text{Dms}_2 + x_3 \cdot \text{Dms}_1} = \begin{pmatrix} 3.228 \times 10^{-9} & 5.732 \times 10^{-11} \\ 1.88 \times 10^{-10} & 3.374 \times 10^{-9} \end{pmatrix}$$ Eq. (3.132)

⊡ Reference:C:\Users\tosun\Desktop\Subroutines\Multicomponent - NRTL.xmcd

$$\Gamma = \begin{pmatrix} 0.728 & -0.074 \\ -0.437 & 0.257 \end{pmatrix}$$

$$\text{Dfick} := \text{Binverse} \cdot \Gamma = \begin{pmatrix} 2.325 \times 10^{-9} & -2.245 \times 10^{-10} \\ -1.338 \times 10^{-9} & 8.539 \times 10^{-10} \end{pmatrix}$$ Eq. (3.126)

Mathcad worksheet of Example 3.10.

For a mixture having a composition of $x_1 = 0.2060$, $x_2 = 0.5480$, and $x_3 = 0.2460$, the Fick diffusion coefficient matrix is calculated as

$$[\mathcal{D}^*]^{\text{calc}} = \begin{pmatrix} 2.325 & -0.2245 \\ -1.338 & 0.8539 \end{pmatrix} \times 10^{-9} \, \text{m}^2/\text{s}$$

When compared with the reported Fick matrix by Kooijman and Taylor (2010), i.e.,

$$[\mathcal{D}^*] = \begin{pmatrix} 3.2882 & 0.2711 \\ -0.3408 & 2.1788 \end{pmatrix} \times 10^{-9} \, \text{m}^2/\text{s}$$

the predictions of the Vignes equation seem unsatisfactory for this system.

3.5.2 DARKEN EQUATION

The equation proposed by Darken (1948) for binary mixtures considers MS diffusivities to vary linearly with composition,[14] i.e.,

$$Đ_{ij} = x_j \, \mathcal{D}_{i,self} + x_i \, \mathcal{D}_{j,self}, \tag{3.147}$$

where $\mathcal{D}_{i,self}$ and $\mathcal{D}_{j,self}$ are *self- diffusion coefficients* of species i and j, respectively. In the absence of driving forces, molecules move with random Brownian motion. The self- diffusion coefficient is a measure of this motion and is dependent on composition. Self-diffusion coefficients are either measured by experiments[15] or estimated by molecular dynamics simulations. Self-diffusion coefficients are defined not only for pure species but also for each species in a mixture.

The self-diffusion coefficients in Eq. (3.147) must be the values at the same mixture composition. Since these values are scarce, application of the Darken equation is limited. To overcome the limitations of the Darken equation, Liu et al. (2011) first generalized the Darken equation to multicomponent mixtures in the form

$$Đ_{ij} = \mathcal{D}_{i,self} \, \mathcal{D}_{j,self} \sum_{k=1}^{\mathcal{N}} \frac{x_k}{\mathcal{D}_{k,self}} \tag{3.148}$$

and then proposed the following equation to estimate the self-diffusion coefficient of species i in the mixture from the self-diffusion coefficients at infinite dilution, $\mathcal{D}_{i,self}^{x_k \to 1}$, as

$$\frac{1}{\mathcal{D}_{i,self}} = \sum_{k=1}^{\mathcal{N}} \frac{x_k}{\mathcal{D}_{i,self}^{x_k \to 1}} \tag{3.149}$$

Note that $\mathcal{D}_{i,self}^{x_k \to 1}$ is the diffusion coefficient of component i infinitely diluted in component k, i.e., $\mathcal{D}_{ik}^{\infty}$, and $\mathcal{D}_{i,self}^{x_i \to 1}$ is the self-diffusion coefficient of the pure component i.

---

[14]The Darken equation is not an empirical mixing rule. For the rigorous development of Eq. (3.147), see Liu et al. (2011).

[15]For self-diffusion coefficients of pure substances, see Winkelmann (2017).

Example 3.11 Kooijman and Taylor (1991) reported the following infinite dilution diffusion coefficients for a ternary mixture of acetone (1), benzene (2), and methanol (3) at 298.15 K:

$$\mathcal{D}_{12}^{\infty} = 3.0368 \times 10^{-9} \text{m}^2/\text{s} \qquad \mathcal{D}_{13}^{\infty} = 2.6009 \times 10^{-9} \text{m}^2/\text{s}$$

$$\mathcal{D}_{21}^{\infty} = 4.2778 \times 10^{-9} \text{m}^2/\text{s} \qquad \mathcal{D}_{23}^{\infty} = 2.4159 \times 10^{-9} \text{m}^2/\text{s}$$

$$\mathcal{D}_{31}^{\infty} = 4.7951 \times 10^{-9} \text{m}^2/\text{s} \qquad \mathcal{D}_{32}^{\infty} = 3.6480 \times 10^{-9} \text{m}^2/\text{s}$$

The pure component self-diffusion coefficients for acetone, benzene, and methanol are 4.8×10^{-9}, 2.3×10^{-9}, and $2.27 \times 10^{-9} \text{m}^2/\text{s}$, respectively.

For a ternary system, the components of the MS diffusion coefficients are shown in the table below:

$Đ_{ij}$	Vignes [Eq. (3.146)]	Darken [Eq. (3.148)]
$Đ_{12}$	$(\mathcal{D}_{12}^{\infty})^{x_2} (\mathcal{D}_{21}^{\infty})^{x_1} (\mathcal{D}_{13}^{\infty}\mathcal{D}_{23}^{\infty})^{x_3/2}$	$\mathcal{D}_{1,self}\mathcal{D}_{2,self}\left(\dfrac{x_1}{\mathcal{D}_{1,self}} + \dfrac{x_2}{\mathcal{D}_{2,self}} + \dfrac{x_3}{\mathcal{D}_{3,self}}\right)$
$Đ_{13}$	$(\mathcal{D}_{13}^{\infty})^{x_3} (\mathcal{D}_{31}^{\infty})^{x_1} (\mathcal{D}_{12}^{\infty}\mathcal{D}_{32}^{\infty})^{x_2/2}$	$\mathcal{D}_{1,self}\mathcal{D}_{3,self}\left(\dfrac{x_1}{\mathcal{D}_{1,self}} + \dfrac{x_2}{\mathcal{D}_{2,self}} + \dfrac{x_3}{\mathcal{D}_{3,self}}\right)$
$Đ_{23}$	$(\mathcal{D}_{23}^{\infty})^{x_3} (\mathcal{D}_{32}^{\infty})^{x_2} (\mathcal{D}_{21}^{\infty}\mathcal{D}_{31}^{\infty})^{x_1/2}$	$\mathcal{D}_{2,self}\mathcal{D}_{3,self}\left(\dfrac{x_1}{\mathcal{D}_{1,self}} + \dfrac{x_2}{\mathcal{D}_{2,self}} + \dfrac{x_3}{\mathcal{D}_{3,self}}\right)$

The self-diffusion coefficients are calculated from

$$\mathcal{D}_{1,self} = \left(\frac{x_1}{\mathcal{D}_{1,self}^{x_1 \to 1}} + \frac{x_2}{\mathcal{D}_{12}^{\infty}} + \frac{x_3}{\mathcal{D}_{13}^{\infty}}\right)^{-1}$$

$$\mathcal{D}_{2,self} = \left(\frac{x_1}{\mathcal{D}_{21}^{\infty}} + \frac{x_2}{\mathcal{D}_{2,self}^{x_2 \to 1}} + \frac{x_3}{\mathcal{D}_{23}^{\infty}}\right)^{-1}$$

$$\mathcal{D}_{3,self} = \left(\frac{x_1}{\mathcal{D}_{31}^{\infty}} + \frac{x_2}{\mathcal{D}_{32}^{\infty}} + \frac{x_3}{\mathcal{D}_{3,self}^{x_3 \to 1}}\right)^{-1}$$

The values of the MS diffusion coefficients based on both models are shown in the table below.

x_1	x_2	x_3	$Đ_{12} \times 10^9 \text{m}^2/\text{s}$		$Đ_{13} \times 10^9 \text{m}^2/\text{s}$		$Đ_{23} \times 10^9 \text{m}^2/\text{s}$	
			Vignes	Darken	Vignes	Darken	Vignes	Darken
0.766	0.114	0.120	3.8584	3.6533	4.2741	4.1693	4.0978	3.6443
0.400	0.500	0.100	3.4167	3.1432	3.7579	4.1860	3.8171	3.4034
0.206	0.548	0.246	3.1087	2.8551	3.3771	3.6759	3.4465	3.0104
0.150	0.298	0.552	2.8757	2.7178	3.0683	2.9999	3.0016	2.6069

It should be pointed out that both Vignes and Darken equations yield monotonically increasing or decreasing values of the MS diffusion coefficients as a function of composition. In reality, MS diffusion coefficients may exhibit a minimum or maximum, especially for highly nonideal mixtures.

3.6   GOVERNING EQUATIONS FOR DILUTE GAS MIXTURES

Multicomponent gas mixtures at low to moderate pressures can be considered ideal. Under these circumstances, $\mathbf{d}_i = \nabla y_i$ and $Đ_{ik} = \mathcal{D}_{ik}$ and Eq. (3.62) becomes

$$c\nabla y_i = y_i \sum_{\substack{k=1 \\ k \neq i}}^{\mathcal{N}} \frac{\mathbf{J}_k^*}{\mathcal{D}_{ik}} - \mathbf{J}_i^* \sum_{\substack{k=1 \\ k \neq i}}^{\mathcal{N}} \frac{y_k}{\mathcal{D}_{ik}} \tag{3.150}$$

When the mixture is dilute, in other words, trace amounts of solutes are present in a dominant component of the mixture, i.e., solvent, it is plausible to make the simplification

$$\mathbf{J}_i^* \sum_{\substack{k=1 \\ k \neq i}}^{\mathcal{N}} \frac{y_k}{\mathcal{D}_{ik}} \gg y_i \sum_{\substack{k=1 \\ k \neq i}}^{\mathcal{N}} \frac{\mathbf{J}_k^*}{\mathcal{D}_{ik}} \tag{3.151}$$

on the basis that $y_i \ll 1$ so that Eq. (3.150) simplifies to

$$c\nabla y_i = -\mathbf{J}_i^* \sum_{\substack{k=1 \\ k \neq i}}^{\mathcal{N}} \frac{y_k}{\mathcal{D}_{ik}} \tag{3.152}$$

If the *effective binary diffusion coefficient* of species i in a mixture, $\mathcal{D}_{im}$, is defined as

$$\boxed{\frac{1}{\mathcal{D}_{im}} = \sum_{\substack{k=1 \\ k \neq i}}^{\mathcal{N}} \frac{y_k}{\mathcal{D}_{ik}}} \tag{3.153}$$

Eq. (3.152) takes the form

$$\mathbf{J}_i^* = -c\mathcal{D}_{im}\nabla y_i \tag{3.154}$$

The use of Eq. (3.154) in Eq. (2.32) gives the total molar flux as

$$\boxed{\mathbf{N}_i = -c\mathcal{D}_{im}\nabla y_i + y_i \sum_{k=1}^{\mathcal{N}} \mathbf{N}_k} \qquad y_i \ll 1 \tag{3.155}$$

3.6.1   SPECIAL CASE FOR $\mathbf{N}_k = 0$ ($i \neq k$)

When component i diffuses through a stagnant mixture, Eq. (3.66) simplifies to

$$\nabla y_i = -\frac{\mathbf{N}_i}{c} \sum_{\substack{k=1 \\ k \neq i}}^{\mathcal{N}} \frac{y_k}{\mathcal{D}_{ik}} \tag{3.156}$$

On the other hand, Eq. (3.155) becomes

$$\mathbf{N}_i = -c\mathcal{D}_{im}\nabla y_i + y_i\mathbf{N}_i \qquad \Rightarrow \qquad \nabla y_i = -\frac{\mathbf{N}_i}{c}\frac{1-y_i}{\mathcal{D}_{im}} \tag{3.157}$$

Substitution of Eq. (3.157) into Eq. (3.156) leads to

$$\boxed{\mathcal{D}_{im} = \frac{1-y_i}{\displaystyle\sum_{\substack{k=1 \\ k \neq i}}^{\mathcal{N}} \frac{y_k}{\mathcal{D}_{ik}}}} \tag{3.158}$$

Problems

3.1 For a ternary liquid mixture containing 27.81 mol % methanol (1), 57.08% isobutanol (2), and 15.11% 1-propanol (3) at 303.15 K, Shuck and Toor (1963) reported the following diffusion coefficients relative to the volume-average velocity:

$$[\mathcal{D}^\bullet] = \begin{pmatrix} 0.765 & 0.027 \\ -0.039 & 0.624 \end{pmatrix} \times 10^{-5}\,cm^2/s$$

The partial molar volumes are given as

$$\overline{V}_1 = 40.73\,cm^3/mol \qquad \overline{V}_2 = 92.91\,cm^3/mol \qquad \overline{V}_3 = 75.14\,cm^3/mol$$

The molecular weights are

$$M_1 = 32.04\,g/mol \qquad M_2 = 74.12\,g/mol \qquad M_3 = 60.10\,g/mol$$

a) Show that the diffusion coefficients relative to the molar-average velocity are given as

$$[\mathcal{D}^*] = \begin{pmatrix} 0.7658 & 0.0125 \\ -0.0932 & 0.6232 \end{pmatrix} \times 10^{-5}\,cm^2/s$$

b) Show that the diffusion coefficients relative to the mass-average velocity are given as

$$[\mathcal{D}^m] = \begin{pmatrix} 0.7648 & 0.0116 \\ -0.0885 & 0.6242 \end{pmatrix} \times 10^{-5}\,cm^2/s$$

c) Show that the eigenvalues of the diffusion coefficient matrices are independent of the reference velocity frame.

3.2 For a ternary system containing 26.98 mol % water (1), 18.97% chloroform (2), and 54.05% acetic acid (3), Vitagliano et al. (1978) considered acetic acid as the solvent and reported the following Fick diffusion coefficients relative to the volume-average velocity at 298.15 K:

$$[\mathcal{D}_3^\bullet] = \begin{bmatrix} (\mathcal{D}_{11}^\bullet)_3 & (\mathcal{D}_{12}^\bullet)_3 \\ (\mathcal{D}_{21}^\bullet)_3 & (\mathcal{D}_{22}^\bullet)_3 \end{bmatrix} = \begin{pmatrix} 0.498 & 0.321 \\ 0.295 & 0.983 \end{pmatrix} \times 10^{-5}\,cm^2/s,$$

where the subscript 3 indicates the solvent (acetic acid). Thus, Eq. (3.7) is written for the solutes (water and chloroform) as

$$\mathbf{J}_1^\bullet = (\mathcal{D}_{11}^\bullet)_3\,\nabla c_1 + (\mathcal{D}_{12}^\bullet)_3\,\nabla c_2 \tag{1}$$

$$\mathbf{J}_2^\bullet = (\mathcal{D}_{21}^\bullet)_3\,\nabla c_1 + (\mathcal{D}_{22}^\bullet)_3\,\nabla c_2 \tag{2}$$

a) Since the choice of solvent is arbitrary, let chloroform be the solvent. In this case, Eq. (3.7) is written for the solutes (water and acetic acid) as

$$\mathbf{J}_1^\bullet = (\mathcal{D}_{11}^\bullet)_2\,\nabla c_1 + (\mathcal{D}_{13}^\bullet)_2\,\nabla c_3 \tag{3}$$

$$\mathbf{J}_3^\bullet = (\mathcal{D}_{31}^\bullet)_2\,\nabla c_1 + (\mathcal{D}_{33}^\bullet)_2\,\nabla c_3 \tag{4}$$

From Problem 2.7

$$\nabla c_2 = -\frac{\overline{V}_1}{\overline{V}_2}\nabla c_1 - \frac{\overline{V}_3}{\overline{V}_2}\nabla c_3 \tag{5}$$

Substitute Eq. (5) into Eq. (1) to obtain

$$\mathbf{J}_1^\bullet = \left[(\mathcal{D}_{11}^\bullet)_3 - \frac{\overline{V}_1}{\overline{V}_2}(\mathcal{D}_{12}^\bullet)_3\right]\nabla c_1 - \frac{\overline{V}_3}{\overline{V}_2}(\mathcal{D}_{12}^\bullet)_3\,\nabla c_3 \tag{6}$$

Compare Eqs. (3) and (6) to conclude that

$$(\mathcal{D}_{11}^{\blacksquare})_2 = (\mathcal{D}_{11}^{\blacksquare})_3 - \frac{\overline{V}_1}{\overline{V}_2}(\mathcal{D}_{12}^{\blacksquare})_3 \qquad \text{and} \qquad (\mathcal{D}_{13}^{\blacksquare})_2 = -\frac{\overline{V}_3}{\overline{V}_2}(\mathcal{D}_{12}^{\blacksquare})_3 \tag{7}$$

From Eq. (2.54)

$$\mathbf{J}_2^{\blacksquare} = -\frac{\overline{V}_1}{\overline{V}_2}\mathbf{J}_1^{\blacksquare} - \frac{\overline{V}_3}{\overline{V}_2}\mathbf{J}_3^{\blacksquare} \tag{8}$$

Substitute Eqs. (2.54) and (3) into Eq. (2) and compare the resulting equation with Eq. (4) to conclude that

$$(\mathcal{D}_{31}^{\blacksquare})_2 = \frac{\overline{V}_1}{\overline{V}_3}\left[-(\mathcal{D}_{11}^{\blacksquare})_3 + \frac{\overline{V}_1}{\overline{V}_2}(\mathcal{D}_{12}^{\blacksquare})_3 - \frac{\overline{V}_2}{\overline{V}_1}(\mathcal{D}_{21}^{\blacksquare})_3 + (\mathcal{D}_{22}^{\blacksquare})_3\right] \tag{9}$$

and

$$(\mathcal{D}_{33}^{\blacksquare})_2 = \frac{\overline{V}_1}{\overline{V}_2}(\mathcal{D}_{12}^{\blacksquare})_3 + (\mathcal{D}_{22}^{\blacksquare})_3 \tag{10}$$

b) The partial molar volumes are given as

$$\overline{V}_1 = 18.07\,\text{cm}^3/\text{mol} \qquad \overline{V}_2 = 80.64\,\text{cm}^3/\text{mol} \qquad \overline{V}_3 = 57.52\,\text{cm}^3/\text{mol}$$

Show that the components of the diffusion coefficient matrix are

$$[\mathcal{D}_2^{\blacksquare}] = \begin{bmatrix} (\mathcal{D}_{11}^{\blacksquare})_2 & (\mathcal{D}_{13}^{\blacksquare})_2 \\ (\mathcal{D}_{31}^{\blacksquare})_2 & (\mathcal{D}_{33}^{\blacksquare})_2 \end{bmatrix} = \begin{pmatrix} 0.426 & -0.229 \\ -0.239 & 1.055 \end{pmatrix} \times 10^{-5}\,\text{cm}^2/\text{s}$$

c) Repeat the procedure given in part (a) if water is chosen as the solvent and show that the components of the matrix are

$$[\mathcal{D}_1^{\blacksquare}] = \begin{bmatrix} (\mathcal{D}_{22}^{\blacksquare})_1 & (\mathcal{D}_{23}^{\blacksquare})_1 \\ (\mathcal{D}_{32}^{\blacksquare})_1 & (\mathcal{D}_{33}^{\blacksquare})_1 \end{bmatrix} = \begin{pmatrix} -0.334 & -0.939 \\ 1.065 & 1.814 \end{pmatrix} \times 10^{-5}\,\text{cm}^2/\text{s},$$

leading to a negative value for the main diffusion coefficient. Note that although $\mathcal{D}_{ii}^{\blacksquare}$ may take negative values, the summation of diagonal elements is greater than zero as stated by Eq. (3.48).

d) Show that the traces, determinants, and eigenvalues of the matrices $[\mathcal{D}_1^{\blacksquare}]$, $[\mathcal{D}_2^{\blacksquare}]$, and $[\mathcal{D}_3^{\blacksquare}]$ are equal to each other.

3.3 From Problem 3.2

$$(\mathcal{D}_{11}^{\blacksquare})_2 = (\mathcal{D}_{11}^{\blacksquare})_3 - \frac{\overline{V}_1}{\overline{V}_2}(\mathcal{D}_{12}^{\blacksquare})_3 \tag{1}$$

$$(\mathcal{D}_{13}^{\blacksquare})_2 = -\frac{\overline{V}_3}{\overline{V}_2}(\mathcal{D}_{12}^{\blacksquare})_3 \tag{2}$$

Volume fractions sum to unity, i.e.,

$$c_1\overline{V}_1 + c_2\overline{V}_2 + c_3\overline{V}_3 = 1 \tag{3}$$

Show that the simultaneous solution of Eqs. (1)–(3) leads to the following expressions for the partial molar volumes:

$$\overline{V}_1 = \frac{(\mathcal{D}_{11}^{\blacksquare})_3 - (\mathcal{D}_{11}^{\blacksquare})_2}{c_1\left[(\mathcal{D}_{11}^{\blacksquare})_3 - (\mathcal{D}_{11}^{\blacksquare})_2\right] + c_2(\mathcal{D}_{12}^{\blacksquare})_3 - c_3(\mathcal{D}_{13}^{\blacksquare})_2} \tag{4}$$

$$\overline{V}_2 = \frac{(\mathcal{D}_{12}^\blacksquare)_3}{c_1\left[(\mathcal{D}_{11}^\blacksquare)_3 - (\mathcal{D}_{11}^\blacksquare)_2\right] + c_2(\mathcal{D}_{12}^\blacksquare)_3 - c_3(\mathcal{D}_{13}^\blacksquare)_2} \tag{5}$$

$$\overline{V}_3 = -\frac{(\mathcal{D}_{13}^\blacksquare)_2}{c_1\left[(\mathcal{D}_{11}^\blacksquare)_3 - (\mathcal{D}_{11}^\blacksquare)_2\right] + c_2(\mathcal{D}_{12}^\blacksquare)_3 - c_3(\mathcal{D}_{13}^\blacksquare)_2} \tag{6}$$

Therefore, partial molar volumes can be calculated once diffusion coefficients are experimentally measured.

3.4 A binary liquid mixture of acetone (1) and n-butanol (2) at 298.15 K is represented by the Wilson model with the following parameters:

$$\lambda_{12} - \lambda_{11} = -59.526 \, \text{J/mol} \qquad \lambda_{21} - \lambda_{22} = 1381.892 \, \text{J/mol}$$

The molar volumes of pure components are

$$\widetilde{V}_1 = 74.05 \, \text{cm}^3/\text{mol} \qquad \widetilde{V}_2 = 91.97 \, \text{cm}^3/\text{mol}$$

Show that the values of the thermodynamic factor as a function of composition are given by

x_1	0.1	0.2	0.3	0.4	0.5	0.6	0.7	0.8	0.9
Γ	0.964	0.927	0.890	0.856	0.826	0.805	0.799	0.817	0.875

3.5 A ternary liquid mixture consists of 27.3 mol % toluene (1), 60.2% ethanol (2), and 12.5% water (3) at 298 K. The mixture is represented by the NRTL model with the following parameters:

$i-j$	τ_{ij}	τ_{ji}	α_{ij}
$1-2$	1.938	0.6	0.529
$1-3$	15.219	7.529	0.2
$2-3$	-0.0978	2.096	0.293

Show that the thermodynamic factor is given by

$$\Gamma = \begin{pmatrix} 0.17 & -0.321 \\ 0.42 & 1.147 \end{pmatrix}$$

3.6 Rehfeldt and Stichlmair (2010) reported the binary Fick diffusion coefficient as $2.40 \times 10^{-9} \, \text{m}^2/\text{s}$ for a mixture containing 80 mol % acetone (1) and 20% 1-propanol (2) at 298.15 K. The system is represented by the Wilson equation with the following parameters:

$$\lambda_{12} - \lambda_{11} = 811.905 \, \text{J/mol} \qquad \text{and} \qquad \lambda_{21} - \lambda_{22} = 770.316 \, \text{J/mol}$$

The molar volumes of pure liquids are given as

$$\widetilde{V}_1 = 74.04 \, \text{cm}^3/\text{mol} \qquad \text{and} \qquad \widetilde{V}_2 = 75.12 \, \text{cm}^3/\text{mol}$$

Calculate the MS diffusion coefficient.
(**Answer:** $2.97 \times 10^{-9} \, \text{m}^2/\text{s}$)

3.7 The following MS diffusion coefficients are reported by Guevara-Carrion et al. (2016) for a ternary mixture of 40.4 mol % water (1), 40% methanol, and 19.6% ethanol at 298.15 K using molecular simulations:

$$\text{Đ}_{12} = 1.530 \times 10^{-9} \, \text{m}^2/\text{s} \qquad \text{Đ}_{13} = 1.282 \times 10^{-9} \, \text{m}^2/\text{s} \qquad \text{Đ}_{23} = 1.023 \times 10^{-9} \, \text{m}^2/\text{s}$$

The system is represented by the Wilson equation with the parameters

$$\Lambda = \begin{pmatrix} 1 & 1.02 & 0.80 \\ 0.22 & 1 & 1.01 \\ 0.1 & 1.03 & 1 \end{pmatrix}$$

The molar volumes are given as

$$\tilde{V}_1 = 18.07\,\text{cm}^3/\text{mol} \qquad \tilde{V}_2 = 40.85\,\text{cm}^3/\text{mol} \qquad \tilde{V}_3 = 58.38\,\text{cm}^3/\text{mol}$$

Show that the elements of the Fick diffusion coefficient matrix are

$$[\mathcal{D}^*] = \begin{pmatrix} 0.6984 & -0.2593 \\ 0.2105 & 1.339 \end{pmatrix} \times 10^{-9}\,\text{m}^2/\text{s}$$

3.8 For a ternary system, the MS diffusion coefficients can be obtained from the Fick diffusion coefficients by using Eq. (3.136). Now let us develop an alternative procedure as follows:

a) Using Eq. (3.134), the following matrix identities can be written as

$$\begin{pmatrix} B_{11} \\ B_{12} \end{pmatrix} = \begin{pmatrix} x_2 & x_1 + x_3 \\ -x_1 & x_1 \end{pmatrix} \cdot \begin{pmatrix} \dfrac{1}{Đ_{12}} \\ \dfrac{1}{Đ_{13}} \end{pmatrix} \tag{1}$$

and

$$\begin{pmatrix} B_{21} \\ B_{22} \end{pmatrix} = \begin{pmatrix} -x_2 & x_2 \\ x_1 & x_2 + x_3 \end{pmatrix} \cdot \begin{pmatrix} \dfrac{1}{Đ_{12}} \\ \dfrac{1}{Đ_{23}} \end{pmatrix} \tag{2}$$

b) Show that

$$\begin{pmatrix} \dfrac{1}{Đ_{12}} \\ \dfrac{1}{Đ_{13}} \end{pmatrix} = \begin{pmatrix} 1 & -\dfrac{x_1 + x_3}{x_1} \\ 1 & \dfrac{x_2}{x_1} \end{pmatrix} \cdot \begin{pmatrix} B_{11} \\ B_{12} \end{pmatrix} \tag{3}$$

and

$$\begin{pmatrix} \dfrac{1}{Đ_{12}} \\ \dfrac{1}{Đ_{23}} \end{pmatrix} = \begin{pmatrix} -\dfrac{x_2 + x_3}{x_2} & 1 \\ \dfrac{x_1}{x_2} & 1 \end{pmatrix} \cdot \begin{pmatrix} B_{21} \\ B_{22} \end{pmatrix} \tag{4}$$

Thus, conclude that

$$Đ_{12} = \dfrac{1}{B_{11} - \left(\dfrac{x_1 + x_3}{x_1}\right) B_{12}} = \dfrac{1}{B_{22} - \left(\dfrac{x_2 + x_3}{x_2}\right) B_{21}} \tag{5}$$

$$Đ_{13} = \dfrac{1}{B_{11} + \left(\dfrac{x_2}{x_1}\right) B_{12}} \tag{6}$$

$$Đ_{23} = \dfrac{1}{B_{22} + \left(\dfrac{x_1}{x_2}\right) B_{21}} \tag{7}$$

These equations are also developed by Krishna and van Baten (2005) using a different approach.

c) Using the experimental data of Cullinan and Toor (1965), Kooijman and Taylor (1991) reported the following infinite dilution diffusion coefficients for a ternary mixture of acetone (1), benzene (2), and carbon tetrachloride (3) at 298.15 K:

$$\mathcal{D}_{12}^{\infty} = 2.75 \times 10^{-9} \text{m}^2/\text{s} \qquad \mathcal{D}_{13}^{\infty} = 1.70 \times 10^{-9} \text{m}^2/\text{s}$$

$$\mathcal{D}_{21}^{\infty} = 2.75 \times 10^{-9} \text{m}^2/\text{s} \qquad \mathcal{D}_{23}^{\infty} = 1.42 \times 10^{-9} \text{m}^2/\text{s}$$

$$\mathcal{D}_{31}^{\infty} = 3.57 \times 10^{-9} \text{m}^2/\text{s} \qquad \mathcal{D}_{32}^{\infty} = 1.91 \times 10^{-9} \text{m}^2/\text{s}$$

The mixture is represented by the NRTL model with the following parameters:

$i-j$	τ_{ij}	τ_{ji}	α_{ij}
$1-2$	-0.46504	0.74632	0.2
$1-3$	-0.42790	1.5931	0.2
$2-3$	-0.51821	0.7338	0.2

For a mixture having a composition of $x_1 = 0.1497, x_2 = 0.6984$, and $x_3 = 0.1519$, the Fick diffusion coefficient matrix is given by

$$[\mathcal{D}^*] = \begin{pmatrix} 1.9652 & 0.0137 \\ -0.1522 & 1.9248 \end{pmatrix} \times 10^{-9} \text{ m}^2/\text{s}$$

Show that the MS diffusion coefficients calculated from Eq. (3.136) as well as the equations given in this problem, i.e., (5)–(7), are given as follows:

$Đ_{ij} \times 10^9 \ (\text{m}^2/\text{s})$	Eq. (3.136)	Eqs. (5)–(7)
$Đ_{12}$	2.0962	1.9719 and 2.1631
$Đ_{13}$	3.5394	4.2992
$Đ_{23}$	1.7874	1.8016

Note that the two different expressions for $Đ_{12}$ in Eq. (5) yield different values.

d) Use the calculated values of the MS diffusion coefficients, and back calculate the Fick diffusion coefficient matrix for both cases.

3.9 Let us apply the procedure explained in Problem 3.8 to quaternary systems.

a) Using Eq. (3.142), the following matrix identities can be written as

$$\begin{pmatrix} B_{11} \\ B_{12} \\ B_{13} \end{pmatrix} = \begin{pmatrix} x_2 & x_3 & x_1 + x_4 \\ -x_1 & 0 & x_1 \\ 0 & -x_1 & x_1 \end{pmatrix} \begin{pmatrix} \dfrac{1}{Đ_{12}} \\ \dfrac{1}{Đ_{13}} \\ \dfrac{1}{Đ_{14}} \end{pmatrix} \qquad (1)$$

$$\begin{pmatrix} B_{21} \\ B_{22} \\ B_{23} \end{pmatrix} = \begin{pmatrix} -x_2 & 0 & x_2 \\ x_1 & x_3 & x_2 + x_4 \\ 0 & -x_2 & x_2 \end{pmatrix} \cdot \begin{pmatrix} \dfrac{1}{Đ_{12}} \\ \dfrac{1}{Đ_{23}} \\ \dfrac{1}{Đ_{24}} \end{pmatrix} \qquad (2)$$

$$
\begin{pmatrix} B_{31} \\ B_{32} \\ B_{33} \end{pmatrix} = \begin{pmatrix} -x_3 & 0 & x_3 \\ 0 & -x_3 & x_3 \\ x_1 & x_2 & x_3 + x_4 \end{pmatrix} \cdot \begin{pmatrix} \dfrac{1}{\DJ_{13}} \\ \dfrac{1}{\DJ_{23}} \\ \dfrac{1}{\DJ_{34}} \end{pmatrix} \tag{3}
$$

b) Solve Eqs. (1)–(3) for the MS diffusion coefficients and show that

$$
\DJ_{12} = \frac{1}{B_{11} + \left(\dfrac{x_2 - 1}{x_1}\right) B_{12} + \dfrac{x_3}{x_1} B_{13}} = \frac{1}{\left(\dfrac{x_1 - 1}{x_2}\right) B_{21} + B_{22} + \dfrac{x_3}{x_2} B_{23}}
$$

$$
\DJ_{13} = \frac{1}{B_{11} + \dfrac{x_2}{x_1} B_{12} + \left(\dfrac{x_3 - 1}{x_1}\right) B_{13}} = \frac{1}{\left(\dfrac{x_1 - 1}{x_3}\right) B_{31} + \dfrac{x_2}{x_3} B_{32} + B_{33}}
$$

$$
\DJ_{14} = \frac{1}{B_{11} + \dfrac{x_2}{x_1} B_{12} + \dfrac{x_3}{x_1} B_{13}}
$$

$$
\DJ_{23} = \frac{1}{\dfrac{x_1}{x_2} B_{21} + B_{22} + \left(\dfrac{x_3 - 1}{x_2}\right) B_{23}} = \frac{1}{\dfrac{x_1}{x_3} B_{31} + \left(\dfrac{x_2 - 1}{x_3}\right) B_{32} + B_{33}}
$$

$$
\DJ_{24} = \frac{1}{\dfrac{x_1}{x_2} B_{21} + B_{22} + \dfrac{x_3}{x_2} B_{23}}
$$

$$
\DJ_{34} = \frac{1}{\dfrac{x_1}{x_3} B_{31} + \dfrac{x_2}{x_3} B_{32} + B_{33}}
$$

3.10 For a binary mixture of acetone (1) and water (2) at 298.15 K, Rehfeldt and Stichlmair (2010) reported the infinite dilution diffusion coefficients as

$$
\mathcal{D}_{12}^\infty = 1.28 \times 10^{-9} \mathrm{m}^2/\mathrm{s} \qquad \mathcal{D}_{21}^\infty = 5.08 \times 10^{-9} \mathrm{m}^2/\mathrm{s}
$$

Using the data given in Example 3.6 and the Vignes equation, calculate the Fick diffusion coefficient for a mixture containing 70 mol % acetone. The reported value is $1.63 \times 10^{-9} \mathrm{m}^2/\mathrm{s}$.

(Answer: $1.592 \times 10^{-9} \mathrm{m}^2/\mathrm{s}$)

3.11 Wesselingh and Krishna (1990) proposed the following equation for the application of the Vignes equation to multicomponent mixtures:

$$
\DJ_{ij} = (\mathcal{D}_{ij}^\infty)^{x_j} (\mathcal{D}_{ji}^\infty)^{x_i} \prod_{\substack{k=1 \\ k \neq i,j}}^{\mathcal{N}} (\mathcal{D}_{ij}^\infty \mathcal{D}_{ji}^\infty)^{x_k/2} \tag{1}
$$

a) For a ternary system, show that Eq. (1) simplifies to

$$
\DJ_{ij} = (\mathcal{D}_{ij}^\infty)^{(1+x_j-x_i)/2} (\mathcal{D}_{ji}^\infty)^{(1+x_i-x_j)/2} \tag{2}
$$

b) For a ternary mixture of acetone (1), benzene (2), and carbon tetrachloride (3) at 298.15K, the infinite dilution diffusion coefficients are given in Problem 3.8. For a mixture having a composition of $x_1 = 0.6$, $x_2 = 0.3$, and $x_3 = 0.1$, calculate the MS diffusion coefficients using Eq. (2) and compare them with the values calculated from Eq. (3.146).

3.12 The following infinite dilution diffusion coefficients are reported for a ternary mixture of methanol (1), 1-butanol (2), and 1-propanol (3) at 298.15K (Rehfeldt and Stichlmair, 2010):

$$\mathcal{D}_{12}^{\infty} = 0.48 \times 10^{-9} \mathrm{m^2/s} \qquad \mathcal{D}_{13}^{\infty} = 0.68 \times 10^{-9} \mathrm{m^2/s}$$
$$\mathcal{D}_{21}^{\infty} = 1.30 \times 10^{-9} \mathrm{m^2/s} \qquad \mathcal{D}_{23}^{\infty} = 0.51 \times 10^{-9} \mathrm{m^2/s}$$
$$\mathcal{D}_{31}^{\infty} = 1.37 \times 10^{-9} \mathrm{m^2/s} \qquad \mathcal{D}_{32}^{\infty} = 0.40 \times 10^{-9} \mathrm{m^2/s}$$

The mixture is represented by the Wilson model with the following parameters:

$i-j$	$\lambda_{ij} - \lambda_{ii}$ (J/mol)	$\lambda_{ji} - \lambda_{jj}$ (J/mol)
$1-2$	831.34	414.28
$1-3$	5141.49	-3318.89
$2-3$	1915.02	-953.37

The molar volumes are given as

$$\widetilde{V}_1 = 40.74 \, \mathrm{cm^3/mol} \qquad \widetilde{V}_2 = 92.00 \, \mathrm{cm^3/mol} \qquad \widetilde{V}_1 = 75.10 \, \mathrm{cm^3/mol}$$

For a mixture having a composition of $x_1 = 0.3$, $x_2 = 0.1$, and $x_3 = 0.6$, show that

$$[\mathcal{D}^*] = \begin{pmatrix} 0.7591 & 0.0434 \\ 0.0078 & 0.6968 \end{pmatrix} \times 10^{-9} \ \mathrm{m^2/s}$$

The Fick matrix reported by Rehfeldt and Stichlmair (2010) is

$$[\mathcal{D}^*] = \begin{pmatrix} 0.6509 & -0.0002 \\ -0.3862 & 0.6348 \end{pmatrix} \times 10^{-9} \ \mathrm{m^2/s}$$

3.13 Liu et al. (2011) proposed the following equation for the application of the Vignes equation to multicomponent mixtures:

$$Đ_{ij} = (\mathcal{D}_{ij}^{\infty})^{x_j} (\mathcal{D}_{ji}^{\infty})^{x_i} \prod_{\substack{k=1 \\ k \neq i,j}}^{\mathcal{N}} \left(\frac{\mathcal{D}_{ik}^{\infty} \mathcal{D}_{jk}^{\infty}}{\mathcal{D}_{k,self}^{x_k \rightarrow 1}} \right)^{x_k} \tag{1}$$

For a quaternary system, they also reported the following values of the diffusion coefficients in reduced units:

$$\mathcal{D}_{12}^{\infty} = 0.99 \qquad \mathcal{D}_{13}^{\infty} = 0.90 \qquad \mathcal{D}_{14}^{\infty} = 0.82 \qquad \mathcal{D}_{1,self}^{x_1 \rightarrow 1} = 1.41$$

$$\mathcal{D}_{21}^{\infty} = 1.17 \qquad \mathcal{D}_{23}^{\infty} = 0.54 \qquad \mathcal{D}_{24}^{\infty} = 0.47 \qquad \mathcal{D}_{2,self}^{x_2 \rightarrow 1} = 0.64$$

$$\mathcal{D}_{31}^{\infty} = 1.10 \qquad \mathcal{D}_{32}^{\infty} = 0.56 \qquad \mathcal{D}_{34}^{\infty} = 0.37 \qquad \mathcal{D}_{3,self}^{x_3 \rightarrow 1} = 0.45$$

$$\mathcal{D}_{41}^{\infty} = 1.06 \qquad \mathcal{D}_{42}^{\infty} = 0.51 \qquad \mathcal{D}_{43}^{\infty} = 0.38 \qquad \mathcal{D}_{4,self}^{x_4 \rightarrow 1} = 0.32$$

For a mixture having a composition of $x_1 = 0.1$, $x_2 = 0.2$, $x_3 = 0.56$, and $x_4 = 0.14$, show that the components of the MS diffusion coefficients calculated by Eq. (1) and the Darken equation, Eq. (3.148), are given as follows:

$Đ_{ij}$	Eq. (1)	Darken
$Đ_{12}$	1.086	1.055
$Đ_{13}$	0.918	0.883
$Đ_{14}$	0.800	0.762
$Đ_{23}$	0.574	0.543
$Đ_{24}$	0.500	0.469
$Đ_{34}$	0.423	0.392

REFERENCES

Alimadadian, A. and C. P. A. Colver. 1976. A new technique for the measurement of ternary diffusion coefficients in liquid systems. *Can. J. Chem. Eng.* 54:208–13.

Bardow, A., E. Kriesten, M. A. Voda, F. Casanova, B. Blümich and W. Marquardt. 2009. Prediction of multicomponent mutual diffusion in liquids: Model discrimination using NMR data. *Fluid Phase Equilibr.* 278:27–35.

Bird, R. B. and D. J. Klingenberg. 2013. Multicomponent diffusion – A brief review. *Adv. Water Res.* 62:238–42.

Cullinan, H. T. 1965. Analysis of the flux equations of multicomponent diffusion. *Ind. Eng. Chem. Fund.* 4(2):133–9.

Cullinan, H. T. and H. L. Toor. 1965. Diffusion in the three-component liquid system: Acetone–benzene–carbon tetrachloride. *J. Phys. Chem.* 69(11):3941–49.

Curtiss, C. F. and R. B. Bird. 1999. Multicomponent diffusion. *Ind. Eng. Chem. Res.* 38:2515–22; errata, 2001. 40:1791.

Darken, L. S. 1948. Diffusion, mobility and their interrelation through free energy in binary metallic systems. *Trans. Inst. Min. Metall. Eng.* 175:184–201.

Derlacki, Z. J., A. J. Easteal, A. V. J. Edge, L. A. Woolf and Z. Roksandic. 1985. Diffusion coefficients of methanol and water and the mutual diffusion coefficient in methanol-water solutions at 278 and 298K. *J. Phys. Chem.* 89(24):5318–22.

Guevara-Carrion, G., Y. Gaponenko, T. Janzen, J. Vrabec and V. Shevtsova. 2016. Diffusion in multicomponent liquids: From microscopic to macroscopic scales. *J. Phys. Chem. B.* 120:12193–210.

Hsieh, C. M., S. I. Sandler and S. T. Lin. 2010. Improvements of COSMO-SAC for vapor–liquid and liquid–liquid equilibrium predictions. *Fluid Phase Equilibr.* 297:90–7.

Kooijman, H. A. and R. Taylor. 1991. Estimation of diffusion coefficients in multicomponent liquid systems. *Ind. Eng. Chem. Res.* 30(6):1217–22.

Krishna, R. 2016. Diffusing uphill with James Clerk Maxwell and Josef Stefan. 2016. *Curr. Opin. Chem. Eng.* 12:106–19.

Krishna, R. and J. M. van Baten. 2005. The Darken relation for multicomponent diffusion in liquid mixtures of linear alkanes: An investigation using molecular dynamics (MD) simulations. *Ind. Eng. Chem. Res.* 44:6939–47.

Kurihara, K., H. Hori and K. Kojima. 1998. Vapor–liquid data for acetone+methanol+benzene, chloroform+methanol+benzene, and constituent binary systems at 101.3kPa. *J. Chem. Eng. Data* 43:264–69.

Liu, X., T. J. H. Vlugt and A. Bardow. 2011. Predictive Darken equation for Maxwell–Stefan diffusivities in multicomponent mixtures. *Ind. Eng. Chem. Res.* 50(17):10350–8.

Liu, X., A. Martin-Calvo, E. McGarrity, S. K. Schnell, S. Calero, J. M. Simon, D. Bedeaux, S. Kjelstrup, A. Bardow and T. J. H. Vlugt. 2012. Fick diffusion coefficients in ternary liquid systems from equilibrium molecular dynamics simulations. *Ind. Eng. Chem. Res.* 51(30):10247–58.

Maxwell, J. C. 1866. On the dynamic theory of gases. *Phil. Trans. R. Soc.* 157:49–88.

Miller, D. G., V. Vitagliano and R. Sartorio. 1986. Some comments on multicomponent diffusion: Negative main term diffusion coefficients, second law constraints, solvent choices, and reference frame transformations. *J. Phys. Chem.* 90(8):1509–19.

Mutoru, J. W. and A. Firoozabadi. 2011. Form of multicomponent Fickian diffusion coefficients matrix. *J. Chem. Thermodyn.* 43(8):1192–1203.

Peng, D. Y. and D. B. Robinson. 1976. A new two-constant equation of state. *Ind. Eng. Chem. Fund.* 15(1):59–64.

Peters, C., L. Wolff, T. J. H. Vlugt and A. Bardow. 2016. Diffusion in liquids: Experiments, molecular dynamics, and engineering models. In *Experimental Thermodynamics Volume X: Non-Equilibrium Thermodynamics with Applications*, eds. D. Bedeaux, S. K. Kjelstrup and J. V. Sengers, 78–104. Croydon: Royal Society of Chemistry.

Rehfeldt, S. and J. Stichlmair. 2007. Measurement and calculation of multicomponent diffusion coefficients in liquids. *Fluid Phase Equil.* 256(1):99–104.

Rehfeldt, S. and J. Stichlmair. 2010. Measurement and prediction of multicomponent diffusion coefficients in four ternary liquid systems. *Fluid Phase Equilibr.* 290:1–14.

Shuck, F. O. and H. L. Toor. 1963. Diffusion in the three component liquid system: Methyl alcohol–n-Propyl alcohol–Isobutyl alcohol. *J. Phys. Chem.* 67(3):540–5.

Stefan, J. 1871. Über das Gleichgewicht und die Bewegung insbesondere die diffusion von Gasgemengen. *Akad. Wiss. Wien* 63:63–124.

Taylor, R. and R. Krishna. 1993. *Multicomponent Mass Transfer*. New York: Wiley.

Tosun, I. 2013. *The Thermodynamics of Phase and Reaction Equilibria*. Amsterdam: Elsevier.

Tuan, D. Q., J. A., Zollweg and S. S. H. Rizvi. 1999. Concentration dependence of the diffusion coefficient of lipid in supercritical carbon dioxide. *Ind. Eng. Chem. Res.* 38(7):2787–93.

Vignes, A. 1966. Diffusion in binary solutions – Variation of diffusion coefficient with composition. *Ind. Eng. Chem. Fund.* 5(2):189–99.

Vitagliano, V., R. Sartorio, S. Scala and D. Spaduzzi. 1978. Diffusion in a ternary system and the critical mixing point. *J. Solution Chem.* 7(8):605–21.

Wesselingh, J. A. and A. M. Bollen. 1997. Multicomponent diffusivities from the free volume theory. *Chem. Eng. Res. Des.* 75(6):590–602.

Wesselingh, J. A. and R. Krishna. 1990. *Elements of Mass Transfer*. Chichester: Ellis Horwood.

Winkelmann, J. 2017. *Diffusion in Gases, Liquids and Electrolytes – Part 1: Pure Liquids and Solute in Solvent*, ed. M. D. Lechner. Berlin: Springer.

Zhang, L., B. Yang and W. Zhang. 2015. Vapor–liquid equilibrium of water+ethanol+glycerol: Experimental measurement and modeling for ethanol dehydration by extractive distillation. *J. Chem. Eng. Data* 60(6):1892–9.

4 Mass Transfer in Binary Systems without Bulk Flow: Steady-State Examples

This chapter deals with steady-state examples of mass transfer for binary systems in the case of no bulk flow. The solution procedure for such problems can be summarized as follows:

- Define your system.
- If possible, draw a simple sketch.
- List your plausible assumptions.
- Use Table 2.3 and simplify the species continuity equation.
- Using Eqs. (2.164)–(2.166), express the appropriate total mass/molar flux expression.
- Substitute the total mass/molar flux expression into the species continuity equation to obtain the governing equation.
- Write down the boundary conditions.
- Convert the governing equation and its associated boundary conditions into dimensionless form.
- Solve the governing equation.
- If possible, investigate the limiting cases and compare the results with the known solutions.

4.1 DIFFUSION OF FLUIDS THROUGH SOLIDS AND/OR MEMBRANES[1]

In the case of mass transfer of fluids through solids and/or membranes, the order of magnitude of the diffusive flux is much greater than that of the convective flux, i.e.,

$$O\left(-c\mathcal{D}_{AB}\nabla x_A\right) \gg O\left[x_A\left(\mathbf{N}_A + \mathbf{N}_B\right)\right] \tag{4.1}$$

Thus, Eq. (2.165) simplifies to

$$\boxed{\mathbf{N}_A = -c\mathcal{D}_{AB}\nabla x_A} \tag{4.2}$$

4.1.1 DIFFUSION IN CARTESIAN COORDINATES

Consider steady one-dimensional diffusion of species A in the z-direction through a rectangular slab (species B) of thickness L as shown in Figure 4.1. Mole fractions of species A in the solid phase at $z = 0$ and $z = L$ are x_{A_o} and x_{A_L}, respectively, with $x_{A_o} > x_{A_L}$. We are interested in the molar transfer rate of species A through the slab.

Let us assume that the total molar concentration and the diffusion coefficient are constant. Postulating $N_{A_z} = N_{A_z}(z)$ and $N_{A_x} = N_{A_y} = 0$, the equation of continuity for species A, Eq. (A) of Table 2.3, simplifies to

$$\frac{dN_{A_z}}{dz} = 0 \quad \Rightarrow \quad N_{A_z} = \text{constant} \tag{4.3}$$

---

[1] Membranes, either porous or nonporous, are selective barriers between two phases; they allow the transfer of desired species from one phase to another. Mainly four types of membranes (polymeric, metallic, ceramic, and liquid) are used in industrial applications.

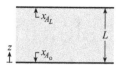

Figure 4.1 Diffusion through a rectangular slab.

On the other hand, Eq. (4.2) reduces to

$$N_{A_z} = -c\mathcal{D}_{AB}\frac{dx_A}{dz}$$ (4.4)

Since c and $\mathcal{D}_{AB}$ are constant, substitution of Eq. (4.4) into Eq. (4.3) gives

$$\frac{d}{dz}\left(\frac{dx_A}{dz}\right) = 0$$ (4.5)

The boundary conditions are

$$\text{at}\quad z = 0\qquad x_A = x_{A_o}$$ (4.6)

$$\text{at}\quad z = L\qquad x_A = x_{A_L}$$ (4.7)

The solution of Eq. (4.5) leads to the following linear concentration distribution:

$$\boxed{\frac{x_{A_o} - x_A}{x_{A_o} - x_{A_L}} = \frac{z}{L}}$$ (4.8)

The molar flux of species A is calculated from Eq. (4.4) as follows:

$$\boxed{N_{A_z} = c\mathcal{D}_{AB}\left(\frac{x_{A_o} - x_{A_L}}{L}\right) = \mathcal{D}_{AB}\left(\frac{c_{A_o} - c_{A_L}}{L}\right)}$$ (4.9)

The molar transfer rate of species A is

$$\boxed{\mathcal{W}_A = AN_{A_z} = A\mathcal{D}_{AB}\left(\frac{c_{A_o} - c_{A_L}}{L}\right),}$$ (4.10)

where A is the slab area.

• Electrical circuit analogy

Using the analogy with Ohm's law, i.e., current = voltage/resistance, it is customary in the literature to express the rate equation in the form

$$\text{Rate} = \frac{\text{Driving force}}{\text{Resistance}}$$ (4.11)

Note that Eq. (4.10) can be expressed as

$$\mathcal{W}_A = \frac{c_{A_o} - c_{A_L}}{\dfrac{L}{A\mathcal{D}_{AB}}}$$ (4.12)

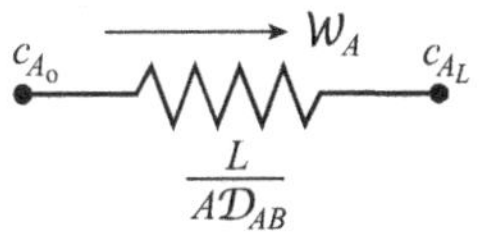

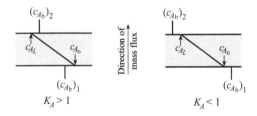

Figure 4.2 Electrical circuit analogy for Eq. (4.12).

Comparison of Eq. (4.12) with Eq. (4.11) indicates that

$$\text{Driving force} = c_{A_o} - c_{A_L} \tag{4.13}$$

$$\boxed{\text{Resistance} = \frac{L}{A\mathcal{D}_{AB}} = \frac{\text{Thickness}}{(\text{Area})(\text{Diffusion coefficient})}} \tag{4.14}$$

Hence, the electrical circuit analogy of a rectangular slab can be represented as shown in Figure 4.2.

• Transfer rate in terms of bulk fluid properties

Let $(c_{A_b})_1$ and $(c_{A_b})_2$ be the bulk concentrations of fluids adjacent to the surfaces at $z = 0$ and $z = L$, respectively. Since it is much easier to measure bulk concentrations, it is then necessary to relate c_{A_o} and c_{A_L} to $(c_{A_b})_1$ and $(c_{A_b})_2$.

Case (i): $Bi_M > 40$

In this case, the resistances to mass transfer in the fluid phases are negligible. In other words, there is no variation in concentration within the bulk phases. Under equilibrium conditions, a partition coefficient K_A relates the concentrations of species A within the solid at the interfaces to bulk concentrations as

$$c_{A_o} = K_A (c_{A_b})_1 \quad \text{and} \quad c_{A_L} = K_A (c_{A_b})_2, \tag{4.15}$$

in which partition coefficients for the surfaces located at $z = 0$ and $z = L$ are considered the same. Depending on whether $K_A > 1$ or $K_A < 1$, the representative concentration distributions are shown in Figure 4.3.

The use of Eq. (4.15) in Eq. (4.10) results in

$$\boxed{\mathcal{W}_A = A K_A \mathcal{D}_{AB} \left[\frac{(c_{A_b})_1 - (c_{A_b})_2}{L} \right]} \tag{4.16}$$

and the resulting electrical circuit analogy is depicted in Figure 4.4.

Figure 4.3 Representative concentration distributions depending on the value of the partition coefficient when $Bi_M > 40$.

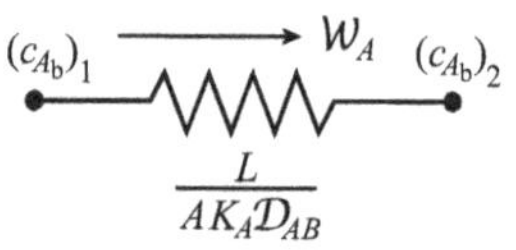

Figure 4.4 Electrical circuit analogy for Eq. (4.16).

Example 4.1 Consider diffusion of a gas through a polymeric film. Expressing concentrations in Eq. (4.16) in terms of partial pressures using Eq. (2.235) yields

$$W_A = AK_A \mathcal{D}_{AB} S_A \left(\frac{\overline{P}_{A_1} - \overline{P}_{A_2}}{L} \right) \tag{1}$$

In the membrane literature, the partition coefficient, the diffusion coefficient, and the solubility coefficient are lumped into the term *permeability*, P_M, such that

$$P_M = K_A \mathcal{D}_{AB} S_A \tag{2}$$

Thus, Eq. (1) reduces to

$$W_A = AP_M \left(\frac{\overline{P}_{A_1} - \overline{P}_{A_2}}{L} \right) = \frac{\overline{P}_{A_1} - \overline{P}_{A_2}}{\dfrac{L}{AP_M}}, \tag{3}$$

where the term L/AP_M can be interpreted as the resistance of a polymer film. From Eq. (2), the unit of permeability is

$$P_M \; [=] \; \frac{(\text{Mole})\,(\text{Length})}{(\text{Time})\,(\text{Area})\,(\text{Pressure})} \tag{4}$$

Sometimes Eq. (3) is expressed in terms of the volumetric flow rate, $\dot{Q}_A$, as

$$\dot{Q}_A = AP_M^* \left(\frac{\overline{P}_{A_1} - \overline{P}_{A_2}}{L} \right) \tag{5}$$

In this case, the unit of P_M^* is given by

$$P_M^* \; [=] \; \frac{[\text{Volume (STP)}]\,(\text{Length})}{(\text{Time})\,(\text{Area})\,(\text{Pressure})} \tag{6}$$

In the literature, P_M^* values are generally expressed in terms of *"barrer,"* defined by

$$1\,\text{barrer} = 10^{-10} \frac{\left[\text{cm}^3\,(\text{STP})\right]\,(\text{cm})}{(\text{s})\,(\text{cm}^2)\,(\text{cmHg})} \tag{7}$$

Case (*ii*): $0.1 < \text{Bi}_\text{M} < 40$

In this case, the representative concentration distributions are shown in Figure 4.5, and the concentrations of species A within the solid at the interfaces are expressed as

$$c_{A_o} = K_A c_{A_o}^{\text{f}} \quad\text{and}\quad c_{A_L} = K_A c_{A_L}^{\text{f}} \tag{4.17}$$

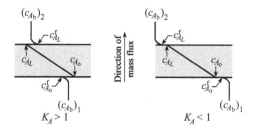

Figure 4.5 Representative concentration distributions depending on the value of the partition coefficient when $0.1 < \mathrm{Bi_M} < 40$.

Substitution of Eq. (4.17) into Eq. (4.10) yields

$$\mathcal{W}_A = AN_{A_z} = AK_A\mathcal{D}_{AB}\left(\frac{c_{A_o}^{\mathrm{f}} - c_{A_L}^{\mathrm{f}}}{L}\right) \tag{4.18}$$

According to Newton's law of mass transfer, Eq. (1.30), the molar transfer rate of species A from the bulk fluid placed at the bottom to the surface at $z = 0$ is equal to that from the surface at $z = L$ to the bulk fluid placed at the top and is given by

$$\mathcal{W}_A = Ak_{c_1}\left[(c_{A_b})_1 - c_{A_o}^{\mathrm{f}}\right] = Ak_{c_2}\left[c_{A_L}^{\mathrm{f}} - (c_{A_b})_2\right], \tag{4.19}$$

where k_c represents the average mass transfer coefficient. Equations (4.18) and (4.19) can be rearranged in the form

$$(c_{A_b})_1 - c_{A_o}^{\mathrm{f}} = \mathcal{W}_A\left(\frac{1}{Ak_{c_1}}\right) \tag{4.20}$$

$$c_{A_o}^{\mathrm{f}} - c_{A_L}^{\mathrm{f}} = \mathcal{W}_A\left(\frac{L}{AK_A\mathcal{D}_{AB}}\right) \tag{4.21}$$

$$c_{A_L}^{\mathrm{f}} - (c_{A_b})_2 = \mathcal{W}_A\left(\frac{1}{Ak_{c_2}}\right) \tag{4.22}$$

Addition of Eqs. (4.20)–(4.22) gives the molar transfer rate of species A as

$$\mathcal{W}_A = \frac{(c_{A_b})_1 - (c_{A_b})_2}{\dfrac{1}{Ak_{c_1}} + \dfrac{L}{AK_A\mathcal{D}_{AB}} + \dfrac{1}{Ak_{c_2}}}, \tag{4.23}$$

in which the terms in the denominator indicate that the resistances are in series. The electrical circuit analogy for this case is given in Figure 4.6. When $k_c \to \infty$, the resistance $1/Ak_c \to 0$. In other words, high mass transfer coefficients lead to no resistance within the bulk fluid phase. Consequently, Eq. (4.23) simplifies to Eq. (4.16).

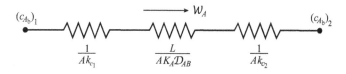

Figure 4.6 Electrical circuit analogy for Eq. (4.23).

Example 4.2 Consider transfer of species i from the concentrated solution to the dilute solution through two nonporous membranes under steady conditions as shown in the figure below. Equation (4.8) implies that the concentration distributions are linear. Let us assume $Bi_M > 40$ so that the resistances to mass transfer in the concentrated and dilute solutions are negligible. According to Eq. (4.12), the molar transfer rate of species i through membrane A is

$$\mathcal{W}_i = \frac{c_i^A\big|_{z=0} - c_i^A\big|_{z=L_A}}{\dfrac{L_A}{A\mathcal{D}_A}}, \tag{1}$$

where $\mathcal{D}_A$ is the effective diffusion coefficient of species i in membrane A.

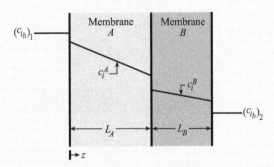

Partition coefficient K_i^A relates the concentrations of species i at $z = 0$ as

$$c_i^A\big|_{z=0} = K_i^A (c_{i_b})_1 \tag{2}$$

Substitution of Eq. (2) into Eq. (1) and rearrangement yield

$$(c_{i_b})_1 - \frac{c_i^A\big|_{z=L_A}}{K_i^A} = \mathcal{W}_i \left(\frac{L_A}{A K_i^A \mathcal{D}_A} \right) \tag{3}$$

Under steady conditions, the molar transfer rate of species i remains constant. Thus, the molar transfer rate of species i through membrane B is

$$\mathcal{W}_i = \frac{c_i^B\big|_{z=L_A} - c_i^B\big|_{z=L_A+L_B}}{\dfrac{L_B}{A\mathcal{D}_B}}, \tag{4}$$

where $\mathcal{D}_B$ is the effective diffusion coefficient of species i in membrane B. Partition coefficient K_i^B relates the concentrations of species i at $z = L_A + L_B$ as

$$c_i^B\big|_{z=L_A+L_B} = K_i^B (c_{i_b})_2 \tag{5}$$

Substitution of Eq. (5) into Eq. (4) and rearrangement give

$$\frac{c_i^B\big|_{z=L_A}}{K_i^B} - (c_{i_b})_2 = \mathcal{W}_i \left(\frac{L_B}{A K_i^B \mathcal{D}_B} \right) \tag{6}$$

The boundary condition at $z = L_A$ is given by

$$\frac{c_i^A\big|_{z=L_A}}{K_i^A} = \frac{c_i^B\big|_{z=L_A}}{K_i^B} \tag{7}$$

Therefore, addition of Eqs. (4) and (6) results in

$$\mathcal{W}_i = \frac{(c_{i_b})_1 - (c_{i_b})_2}{\dfrac{1}{A}\left(\dfrac{L_A}{K_i^A \mathcal{D}_A} + \dfrac{L_B}{K_i^B \mathcal{D}_B}\right)} \tag{8}$$

Thus, for diffusion through multilayered materials in series, Eq. (8) can be generalized as

$$\mathcal{W}_i = \frac{(c_{i_b})_1 - (c_{i_b})_2}{\dfrac{1}{A}\displaystyle\sum_{k=1}^{m}\dfrac{L_k}{K_i^k \mathcal{D}_k}}, \tag{9}$$

where k represents the layer number.

4.1.2 DIFFUSION IN CYLINDRICAL COORDINATES

Consider steady one-dimensional diffusion of species A in the radial direction through the walls of a hollow cylinder (species B) with inner and outer radii of R_i and R_o, respectively, as shown in Figure 4.7. Mole fractions of species A in the solid phase at $r = R_i$ and $r = R_o$ are x_{A_i} and x_{A_o}, respectively, with $x_{A_i} > x_{A_o}$. We are interested in the molar transfer rate of species A through the walls of the cylinder.

Let us assume that the total molar concentration and the diffusion coefficient are constant. Postulating $N_{A_r} = N_{A_r}(r)$ and $N_{A_\theta} = N_{A_z} = 0$, the equation of continuity for species A, Eq. (B) of Table 2.3, simplifies to

$$\frac{d}{dr}(r N_{A_r}) = 0 \tag{4.24}$$

On the other hand, Eq. (4.2) reduces to

$$N_{A_r} = -c \mathcal{D}_{AB} \frac{dx_A}{dr} \tag{4.25}$$

Since c and $\mathcal{D}_{AB}$ are constant, substitution of Eq. (4.25) into Eq. (4.24) gives

$$\frac{d}{dr}\left(r \frac{dx_A}{dr}\right) = 0 \tag{4.26}$$

The boundary conditions are

$$\text{at} \quad r = R_i \qquad x_A = x_{A_i} \tag{4.27}$$

$$\text{at} \quad z = R_o \qquad x_A = x_{A_o} \tag{4.28}$$

The solution of Eq. (4.26) gives the concentration distribution as

$$\boxed{\frac{x_{A_i} - x_A}{x_{A_i} - x_{A_o}} = \frac{\ln(r/R_i)}{\ln(R_o/R_i)}} \tag{4.29}$$

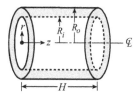

Figure 4.7 Diffusion through a hollow cylinder.

The molar flux of species A is calculated from Eq. (4.25) as

$$N_{A_r} = c \mathcal{D}_{AB} \left[\frac{x_{A_i} - x_{A_o}}{\ln(R_o/R_i)} \right] \frac{1}{r} = \mathcal{D}_{AB} \left[\frac{c_{A_i} - c_{A_o}}{\ln(R_o/R_i)} \right] \frac{1}{r} \tag{4.30}$$

The molar transfer rate of species A is

$$\mathcal{W}_A = 2\pi R_i H \, N_{A_r}|_{r=R_i} = 2\pi R_o H \, N_{A_r}|_{r=R_o} = 2\pi H \mathcal{D}_{AB} \left[\frac{c_{A_i} - c_{A_o}}{\ln(R_o/R_i)} \right] \tag{4.31}$$

• Electrical Circuit Analogy

Rearrangement of Eq. (4.31) gives

$$\mathcal{W}_A = \frac{c_{A_i} - c_{A_o}}{\dfrac{\ln(R_o/R_i)}{2\pi H \mathcal{D}_{AB}}}, \tag{4.32}$$

in which the denominator can be regarded as the resistance, i.e.,

$$\text{Resistance} = \frac{\ln(R_o/R_i)}{2\pi H \mathcal{D}_{AB}} \tag{4.33}$$

At first, it looks as if the resistance expressions for the Cartesian and cylindrical coordinates are different from each other. However, the similarities between Eqs. (4.14) and (4.33) can be shown by the following analysis.

The *logarithmic mean area*, A_{LM}, is defined as

$$A_{LM} = \frac{A_o - A_i}{\ln(A_o/A_i)} = \frac{2\pi H (R_o - R_i)}{\ln(R_o/R_i)} \tag{4.34}$$

Substitution of Eq. (4.34) into Eq. (4.33) gives

$$\text{Resistance} = \frac{R_o - R_i}{A_{LM} \mathcal{D}_{AB}} = \frac{\text{Thickness}}{(\text{Area})(\text{Diffusion coefficient})}, \tag{4.35}$$

which has the same form as Eq. (4.14). Thus, Eq. (4.32) is expressed as

$$\mathcal{W}_A = \frac{c_{A_i} - c_{A_o}}{\dfrac{R_o - R_i}{A_{LM} \mathcal{D}_{AB}}} \tag{4.36}$$

The electrical circuit analogy of the cylindrical wall is shown in Figure 4.8.

When the ratio of the radius of the inner pipe to that of the outer pipe is close to unity, i.e., $R_i \to R_o$, a concentric annulus may be considered a thin plane slit and its curvature can be neglected. In this case, the logarithmic and arithmetic areas are almost equal to each other and Eq. (4.36) reduces to Eq. (4.12).

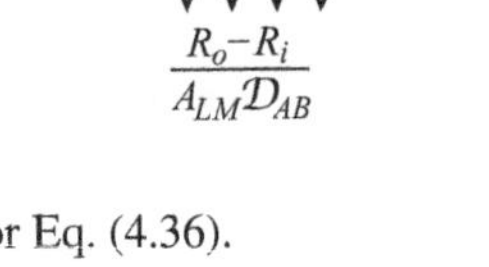

Figure 4.8 Electrical circuit analogy for Eq. (4.36).

• Transfer Rate in Terms of Bulk Fluid Properties

The use of Eq. (4.31) in the calculation of the molar transfer rate of species A requires the surface values c_{A_i} and c_{A_o} to be known or measured. In common practice, the bulk concentrations of the fluids adjoining the surfaces at $r = R_i$ and $r = R_o$, i.e., $(c_{A_b})_i$ and $(c_{A_b})_o$, are known. It is then necessary to relate c_{A_i} and c_{A_o} to $(c_{A_b})_i$ and $(c_{A_b})_o$.

Let us consider a more general case of $0.1 < \mathrm{Bi_M} < 40$. The concentrations of species A within the solid at the interfaces are expressed as

$$c_{A_i} = K_A\, c_{A_i}^{\mathrm{f}} \qquad \text{and} \qquad c_{A_o} = K_A\, c_{A_o}^{\mathrm{f}} \tag{4.37}$$

Substitution of Eq. (4.37) into Eq. (4.31) yields

$$\mathcal{W}_A = 2\pi H K_A \mathcal{D}_{AB} \left[\frac{c_{A_i}^{\mathrm{f}} - c_{A_o}^{\mathrm{f}}}{\ln(R_o/R_i)} \right] \tag{4.38}$$

On the other hand, application of Newton's law of mass transfer gives

$$\mathcal{W}_A = A_i k_{c_i} \left[(c_{A_b})_i - c_{A_i}^{\mathrm{f}} \right] = A_o k_{c_o} \left[c_{A_o}^{\mathrm{f}} - (c_{A_b})_o \right], \tag{4.39}$$

where the surface areas A_i and A_o are expressed in the form

$$A_i = 2\pi R_i H \qquad \text{and} \qquad A_o = 2\pi R_o H \tag{4.40}$$

Equations (4.38) and (4.39) can be rearranged in the form

$$(c_{A_b})_i - c_{A_i}^{\mathrm{f}} = \mathcal{W}_A \left(\frac{1}{A_i k_{c_i}} \right) \tag{4.41}$$

$$c_{A_i}^{\mathrm{f}} - c_{A_o}^{\mathrm{f}} = \mathcal{W}_A \left(\frac{\ln(R_o/R_i)}{2\pi H K_A \mathcal{D}_{AB}} \right) = \mathcal{W}_A \left(\frac{R_o - R_i}{A_{LM} K_A \, \mathcal{D}_{AB}} \right) \tag{4.42}$$

$$c_{A_L}^{\mathrm{f}} - (c_{A_b})_o = \mathcal{W}_A \left(\frac{1}{A_o k_{c_o}} \right) \tag{4.43}$$

Addition of Eqs. (4.41)–(4.43) gives the molar transfer rate of species A as

$$\boxed{\mathcal{W}_A = \frac{(c_{A_b})_i - (c_{A_b})_o}{\dfrac{1}{A_i k_{c_i}} + \dfrac{R_o - R_i}{A_{LM} K_A \, \mathcal{D}_{AB}} + \dfrac{1}{A_o k_{c_o}}},} \tag{4.44}$$

in which the terms in the denominator indicate that the resistances are in series. The electrical circuit analogy for this case is given in Figure 4.9.

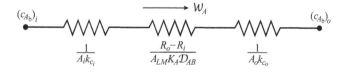

Figure 4.9   Electrical circuit analogy for Eq. (4.43).

Example 4.3 All carbonated beverages, i.e., Coca Cola, Sprite, Fanta, etc., are bottled under pressure to increase the carbon dioxide dissolved in solution. The CO_2 in the soda forms carbonic acid, which counteracts the sweet taste of the drink. Consider diffusion of CO_2 through the walls of a 1.5 L cola bottle made of polyethylene terephthalate (PET). Approximate the bottle as a cylinder, and assume that the inner surface of the bottle is saturated with CO_2 while the concentration at the outer surface is almost zero. Calculate the loss of CO_2 in 12h through the lateral surface of the bottle under steady conditions using the following data:

- Pressure of CO_2 in a closed bottle = 3 bar
- Height of bottle = 23.5 cm
- Inner diameter of bottle = 9.5 cm
- Thickness of the PET bottle wall = 0.3 mm
- Diffusion coefficient of CO_2 in PET = $2 \times 10^{-9}\,cm^2/s$
- Solubility coefficient of CO_2 in PET = $1.7\,m^3(STP)/m^3$ of PET.bar

Solution

The molar flow rate of CO_2 (species A) through the lateral surface of the PET bottle (species B) is given by Eq. (4.31) as

$$W_A = 2\pi H \mathcal{D}_{AB} \left[\frac{c_{A_i} - c_{A_o}}{\ln(R_o/R_i)} \right] \tag{1}$$

The molar concentration of CO_2 at the inner surface, c_{A_i}, is calculated from Eq. (2.235) as

$$c_{A_i} = \left[\frac{1.7\,m^3(STP)/m^3.bar}{22.4\,m^3(STP)/kmol} \right] (3\,bar) = 0.228\,kmol/m^3 = 0.228 \times 10^{-3}\,mol/cm^3$$

Substitution of the values into Eq. (1) leads to

$$W_A = 2\pi(23.5)(2 \times 10^{-9}) \left[\frac{0.228 \times 10^{-3} - 0}{\ln\left(\dfrac{4.75 + 0.03}{4.75}\right)} \right] = 1.07 \times 10^{-8}\,mol/s$$

Therefore, the loss of CO_2 in 12h is

$$\text{Loss of } CO_2 = (1.07 \times 10^{-8})(44)(12 \times 3600) = 0.02\,g$$

4.1.3 DIFFUSION IN SPHERICAL COORDINATES

Consider steady one-dimensional diffusion of species A in the radial direction through the walls of a hollow sphere (species B) with inner and outer radii of R_i and R_o, respectively, as shown in Figure 4.10. Mole fractions of species A in the solid phase at $r = R_i$ and $r = R_o$ are x_{A_i} and x_{A_o}, respectively, with $x_{A_i} > x_{A_o}$. We are interested in the molar transfer rate of species A through the walls of the sphere.

Let us assume that the total molar concentration and the diffusion coefficient are constant. Postulating $N_{A_r} = N_{A_r}(r)$ and $N_{A_\theta} = N_{A_\phi} = 0$, the equation of continuity for species A, Eq. (C) of Table 2.3, simplifies to

$$\frac{d}{dr}\left(r^2 N_{A_r} \right) = 0 \tag{4.45}$$

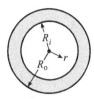

Figure 4.10 Diffusion through a hollow sphere.

On the other hand, Eq. (4.2) reduces to

$$N_{A_r} = -c\mathcal{D}_{AB}\frac{dx_A}{dr} \tag{4.46}$$

Since c and $\mathcal{D}_{AB}$ are constant, substitution of Eq. (4.46) into Eq. (4.45) gives

$$\frac{d}{dr}\left(r^2\frac{dx_A}{dr}\right) = 0 \tag{4.47}$$

The boundary conditions are

$$\text{at}\quad r = R_i\qquad x_A = x_{A_i} \tag{4.48}$$
$$\text{at}\quad z = R_o\qquad x_A = x_{A_o} \tag{4.49}$$

The solution of Eq. (4.47) gives the concentration distribution as

$$\boxed{\frac{x_{A_i} - x_A}{x_{A_i} - x_{A_o}} = \frac{(1/R_i) - (1/r)}{(1/R_i) - (1/R_o)}} \tag{4.50}$$

The molar flux of species A is calculated from Eq. (4.46) as

$$\boxed{N_{A_r} = c\mathcal{D}_{AB}\left[\frac{x_{A_i} - x_{A_o}}{(1/R_i) - (1/R_o)}\right]\frac{1}{r^2} = \mathcal{D}_{AB}\left[\frac{c_{A_i} - c_{A_o}}{(1/R_i) - (1/R_o)}\right]\frac{1}{r^2}} \tag{4.51}$$

The molar transfer rate of species A is

$$\boxed{\mathcal{W}_A = 4\pi R_i^2\,N_{A_r}|_{r=R_i} = 4\pi R_o^2\,N_{A_r}|_{r=R_o} = 4\pi\mathcal{D}_{AB}\left[\frac{c_{A_i} - c_{A_o}}{(1/R_i) - (1/R_o)}\right]} \tag{4.52}$$

• Electrical Circuit Analogy

Rearrangement of Eq. (4.52) gives

$$\mathcal{W}_A = \frac{c_{A_i} - c_{A_o}}{\dfrac{(1/R_i) - (1/R_o)}{4\pi\mathcal{D}_{AB}}}, \tag{4.53}$$

in which the denominator can be regarded as the resistance, i.e.,

$$\text{Resistance} = \frac{(1/R_i) - (1/R_o)}{4\pi\mathcal{D}_{AB}} \tag{4.54}$$

The *geometric mean area*, A_{GM}, is defined as

$$A_{GM} = \sqrt{A_i A_o} = \sqrt{(4\pi R_i^2)(4\pi R_o^2)} = 4\pi R_i R_o \tag{4.55}$$

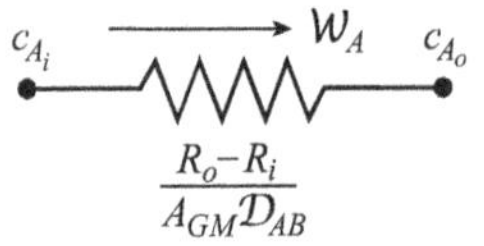

Figure 4.11   Electrical circuit analogy for Eq. (4.57).

so that Eq. (4.54) becomes

$$\boxed{\text{Resistance} = \frac{R_o - R_i}{A_{GM}\, \mathcal{D}_{AB}} = \frac{\text{Thickness}}{(\text{Area})\,(\text{Diffusion coefficient})},}$$
(4.56)

which has the same form as Eq. (4.14). Thus, Eq. (4.53) is expressed as

$$W_A = \frac{c_{A_i} - c_{A_o}}{\dfrac{R_o - R_i}{A_{GM}\, \mathcal{D}_{AB}}}$$
(4.57)

The electrical circuit analogy of the spherical wall is shown in Figure 4.11.

• Transfer Rate in Terms of Bulk Fluid Properties

The use of Eq. (4.52) in the calculation of the molar transfer rate of species A requires the surface values c_{A_i} and c_{A_o} to be known or measured. In common practice, the bulk concentrations of the adjoining fluids to the surfaces at $r = R_i$ and $r = R_o$, i.e., $(c_{A_b})_i$ and $(c_{A_b})_o$, are known. It is then necessary to relate c_{A_i} and c_{A_o} to $(c_{A_b})_i$ and $(c_{A_b})_o$. The procedure for the spherical case is similar to that for the cylindrical case and is left as an exercise for students. The result is

$$\boxed{W_A = \frac{(c_{A_b})_i - (c_{A_b})_o}{\dfrac{1}{A_i k_{c_i}} + \dfrac{R_0 - R_i}{A_{GM} K_A \mathcal{D}_{AB}} + \dfrac{1}{A_o k_{c_o}}},}$$
(4.58)

where

$$A_i = 4\pi R_i^2 \qquad \text{and} \qquad A_o = 4\pi R_o^2$$
(4.59)

Example 4.4   A spherical neoprene container (species B) of inside radius $R_i = 30\,\text{cm}$ and outside radius $R_o = 35\,\text{cm}$ contains hydrogen gas (species A) at 2.5 bar and 298 K. The diffusion coefficient and the solubility coefficient of hydrogen in neoprene are $1.8 \times 10^{-10}\,\text{m}^2/\text{s}$ and $2.37 \times 10^{-3}\,\text{kmol/m}^3.\text{bar}$, respectively. Calculate the initial rate of loss of hydrogen from the container.

Solution

The use of Eq. (2.235) in Eq. (4.52) yields

$$W_A = 4\pi \mathcal{D}_{AB} S_A \left[\frac{\overline{P}_{A_i} - \overline{P}_{A_o}}{(1/R_i) - (1/R_o)} \right]$$
(1)

The partial pressure of hydrogen at the outer surface of the container is practically zero, i.e., $\overline{P}_{A_o} = 0$. Substitution of the numerical values into Eq. (1) gives

$$W_A = 4\pi(1.8 \times 10^{-10})(2.37 \times 10^{-3})\left[\frac{2.5}{(1/0.3) - (1/0.35)} \right] = 2.814 \times 10^{-11}\,\text{kmol/s}$$

4.2 EQUIMOLAR COUNTERDIFFUSION

Two very large tanks are connected by a capillary tube of radius R and length L as shown in Figure 4.12. Both tanks contain gases A and B with compositions $y_A^L > y_A^R$ and $y_B^R > y_B^L$. The pressure and temperature throughout the system are uniform. We are interested in the concentration profile and the molar fluxes of gases A and B through the capillary tube. The problem will be analyzed with the following assumptions:

- Since the volumes of the tanks are very large compared to the capillary volume, concentrations in the tanks do not change with time. As a result, steady-state conditions prevail.
- Species A and B form an ideal gas mixture. Thus, the total molar concentration of the gas mixture in the capillary, $c = n/V = P/RT$, is constant.
- The diffusion coefficient is constant.
- There is no chemical reaction between species A and B.

Let us postulate one-dimensional transport with $N_{A_z} = N_{A_z}(z)$ and $N_{B_z} = N_{B_z}(z)$. Since the total pressure remains constant, the total number of moles in the capillary does not change. This implies that equimolar counterdiffusion takes place within the capillary and for every mole of species A diffusing in the positive z-direction, one mole of species B diffuses back in the negative z-direction,[2] i.e.,

$$N_{A_z} = -N_{B_z} \tag{4.60}$$

As a result, the molar-average velocity, v_z^*, is zero. The equation of continuity for species A, Eq. (B) of Table 2.3, simplifies to

$$\frac{dN_{A_z}}{dz} = 0 \qquad \Rightarrow \qquad N_{A_z} = \text{constant} \tag{4.61}$$

On the other hand, the expression for the total molar flux of species A, i.e., Eq. (2.165), becomes

$$N_{A_z} = -c\mathcal{D}_{AB}\frac{dy_A}{dz} \tag{4.62}$$

Substitution of Eq. (4.62) into Eq. (4.61) gives

$$\frac{d}{dz}\left(\frac{dy_A}{dz}\right) = 0 \tag{4.63}$$

The boundary conditions are

$$\text{at} \quad z = 0 \qquad y_A = y_A^L \tag{4.64}$$

$$\text{at} \quad z = L \qquad y_A = y_A^R \tag{4.65}$$

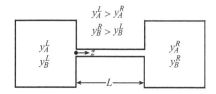

Figure 4.12 Equimolar counterdiffusion through a capillary tube.

---

[2]In other words, since species A diffuses more rapidly from species B in the positive z-direction, there must be a compensating flow of species B in the negative z-direction so as to prevent accumulation of all species on one side.

The solution of Eq. (4.63) leads to the following linear concentration distribution within the capillary:

$$\boxed{\frac{y_A^L - y_A}{y_A^L - y_A^R} = \frac{z}{L}}$$

(4.66)

The molar flux of species A is calculated from Eq. (4.62) as

$$\boxed{N_{A_z} = c\,\mathcal{D}_{AB}\left(\frac{y_A^L - y_A^R}{L}\right)}$$

(4.67)

Note that the determination of the molar flux does not necessarily require the concentration distribution to be determined *a priori*. Since N_{A_z} is constant, Eq. (4.62) can be arranged as

$$N_{A_z}\int_0^L dz = -c\,\mathcal{D}_{AB}\int_{y_A^L}^{y_A^R} dy_A$$

(4.68)

Integration of Eq. (4.68) also leads to Eq. (4.67).

Although the molar-average velocity is zero, the mass-average velocity is given by

$$v_z = \frac{n_{A_z} + n_{B_z}}{\rho} = \frac{N_{A_z}M_A + N_{B_z}M_B}{cM} = \frac{N_{A_z}(M_A - M_B)}{c\,(y_A M_A + y_B M_B)}$$

(4.69)

Example 4.5 Calculate the initial molar flow rate of species A through the capillary tube, 40 cm long and 6 mm in diameter, for the following conditions:

$$P = 1\,\text{bar} \qquad T = 298\,\text{K} \qquad \mathcal{D}_{AB} = 4.5 \times 10^{-5}\,\text{m}^2/\text{s}$$

$$y_A^L = 0.8 \qquad y_A^R = 0.4$$

Solution

The total molar concentration is

$$c = \frac{P}{RT} = \frac{1}{(8.314 \times 10^{-5})(298)} = 40.363\,\text{mol/m}^3$$

The molar flux is calculated from Eq. (4.67) as

$$N_{A_z} = (40.363)(4.5 \times 10^{-5})\left(\frac{0.8 - 0.4}{0.4}\right) = 1.816 \times 10^{-3}\,\text{mol/m}^2\text{.s}$$

The molar transfer rate is

$$\mathcal{W}_A = A N_{A_z} = \frac{\pi(6 \times 10^{-3})^2}{4}(1.816 \times 10^{-3}) = 5.135 \times 10^{-8}\,\text{mol/s}$$

4.2.1 EQUIMOLAR COUNTERDIFFUSION IN A TAPERED CONICAL DUCT

Instead of a capillary tube, suppose that the two large tanks in the previous section are connected by a truncated conical duct as shown in Figure 4.13. Since the total pressure remains constant, the total number of moles in the conical duct does not change. This implies that equimolar counterdiffusion takes place within the conical duct and the molar-average velocity is zero. If the taper angle is small,

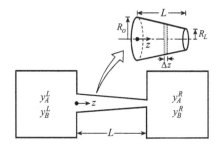

Figure 4.13 Diffusion through a slightly tapered conical duct.

mass transport can be considered one-dimensional in the z-direction with the only nonzero molar flux component, N_{A_z}, given by

$$N_{A_z} = -c\mathcal{D}_{AB}\frac{dy_A}{dz} \tag{4.70}$$

In this case, however, the area perpendicular to the direction of molar flux is not constant but changes in the axial direction. The conservation statement for the mass of species A, i.e.,

$$\text{(Rate of mass of } A \text{ in)} - \text{(Rate of mass of } A \text{ out)} = 0 \tag{4.71}$$

is written over a differential volume element of thickness Δz, as shown in Figure 4.13, as

$$(AN_{A_z})\big|_z - (AN_{A_z})\big|_{z+\Delta z} = 0 \tag{4.72}$$

Dividing Eq. (4.72) by Δz and taking the limit as $\Delta z \to 0$ give

$$\lim_{\Delta z \to 0} \frac{(AN_{A_z})\big|_z - (AN_{A_z})\big|_{z+\Delta z}}{\Delta z} = 0 \tag{4.73}$$

or

$$\frac{d(AN_{A_z})}{dz} = 0 \tag{4.74}$$

Since flux times area gives the molar transfer rate of species A, $\mathcal{W}_A$, it is possible to conclude that

$$AN_{A_z} = \text{constant} = \mathcal{W}_A, \tag{4.75}$$

in which the area A is perpendicular to the direction of mass flux. The variation in the radius of the cone as a function of the axial direction is represented by

$$R = R_o - \left(\frac{R_o - R_L}{L}\right)z \tag{4.76}$$

so that the area is

$$A = \pi\left[R_o - \left(\frac{R_o - R_L}{L}\right)z\right]^2 \tag{4.77}$$

Substitution of Eqs. (4.70) and (4.77) into Eq. (4.75) and integration give

$$-c\mathcal{D}_{AB}\int_{y_A^L}^{y_A^R} dy_A = \mathcal{W}_A\int_0^L \frac{dz}{\pi\left[R_o - \left(\frac{R_o - R_L}{L}\right)z\right]^2} \tag{4.78}$$

or

$$W_A = \pi R_o R_L c \mathcal{D}_{AB} \left(\frac{y_A^L - y_A^R}{L} \right) \tag{4.79}$$

Note that the starting point in this problem was not the equation of continuity for species A. The application of the so-called *shell balance approach* yields Eq. (4.74). In fact, the equation of continuity is always the starting point for problems involving mass transfer as long as the coordinate system is compatible with the geometry of the problem. The approach presented here is an approximation that holds when R_o/R_L is not very different from unity. For exact analysis of the problem, the term $\nabla \cdot \mathbf{N}_A$ should be expressed in the conical coordinate system (Moon and Spencer, 1961).

4.3   EVAPORATION OF A LIQUID IN A CAPILLARY TUBE

Consider a pure liquid A in a capillary tube of diameter D as shown in Figure 4.14. As evaporation takes place, liquid A is slowly added from the bottom of the capillary tube so as to keep the liquid–gas interface constant. We are interested in the molar rate of evaporation of species A from the liquid surface into a gas mixture of A and B. The problem will be analyzed with the following assumptions:

- Steady-state conditions prevail.
- Species A and B form an ideal gas mixture.
- Species B has negligible solubility in liquid A.
- The entire system is maintained at constant temperature and pressure, i.e., the total molar concentration in the gas phase, $c = P/RT$, is constant.
- The diffusion coefficient is constant.
- There is no chemical reaction between species A and B.

Postulating one-dimensional mass transport with $N_{A_r} = N_{A_\theta} = 0$ and $N_{A_z} = N_{A_z}(z)$, the equation of continuity for species A, Eq. (B) of Table 2.3, simplifies to

$$\frac{dN_{A_z}}{dz} = 0 \quad \Rightarrow \quad N_{A_z} = \text{constant} \quad 0 \le z \le L \tag{4.80}$$

Similarly, for species B

$$\frac{dN_{B_z}}{dz} = 0 \quad \Rightarrow \quad N_{B_z} = \text{constant} \quad 0 \le z \le L \tag{4.81}$$

Since species B is insoluble in liquid A, $N_{B_z}|_{z=0} = 0$. This implies that

$$N_{B_z} = 0 \quad \text{for} \quad 0 \le z \le L \tag{4.82}$$

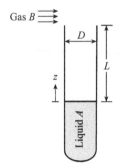

Figure 4.14   Evaporation from a capillary tube.

Thus, the total molar flux of species A, given by Eq. (2.165),

$$N_{A_z} = -c\mathcal{D}_{AB}\frac{dy_A}{dz} + y_A\left(N_{A_z} + N_{B_z}\right), \tag{4.83}$$

simplifies to

$$N_{A_z} = -c\mathcal{D}_{AB}\frac{dy_A}{dz} + y_A N_{A_z} \tag{4.84}$$

Solving for N_{A_z} yields

$$N_{A_z} = -\frac{c\mathcal{D}_{AB}}{1-y_A}\frac{dy_A}{dz} \tag{4.85}$$

Since N_{A_z}, c, and $\mathcal{D}_{AB}$ are constants, one can write

$$\frac{1}{1-y_A}\frac{dy_A}{dz} = \text{constant} = -C_1, \tag{4.86}$$

where the minus sign in front of the constant C_1 is used for mathematical convenience. Integration of Eq. (4.86) results in

$$\ln(1-y_A) = C_1 z + C_2 \tag{4.87}$$

According to Eq. (2.215), the boundary condition at $z = 0$ is given by

$$\text{at} \quad z = 0 \quad y_A = y_{A_o} = \frac{P_A^{vap}}{P} \tag{4.88}$$

At the top of the tube, it is plausible to assume that the mole fraction of species A is practically zero, i.e.,

$$\text{at} \quad z = L \quad y_A = 0 \tag{4.89}$$

Thus, the constants C_1 and C_2 are evaluated as

$$C_1 = \frac{1}{L}\ln\left(\frac{1}{1-y_{A_o}}\right) \quad \text{and} \quad C_2 = \ln(1-y_{A_o}) \tag{4.90}$$

Substitution of the constants into Eq. (4.87) gives the concentration distribution in the form

$$\boxed{y_A = 1 - (1-y_{A_o})^{1-(z/L)}} \tag{4.91}$$

The use of Eq. (4.86) in Eq. (4.85) gives the molar flux of species A as

$$\boxed{N_{A_z} = c\mathcal{D}_{AB}C_1 = \frac{c\mathcal{D}_{AB}}{L}\ln\left(\frac{1}{1-y_{A_o}}\right)} \tag{4.92}$$

Note that the determination of flux expression does not necessarily require the concentration distribution to be determined *a priori*. Since N_{A_z} is constant, Eq. (4.85) can be arranged as

$$N_{A_z}\int_0^L dz = -c\mathcal{D}_{AB}\int_{y_{A_o}}^0 \frac{dy_A}{1-y_A} \tag{4.93}$$

Integration of Eq. (4.93) also leads to Eq. (4.92).

Before proceeding further, it is necessary to clarify one important point. Examination of the total flux expression given by Eq. (4.84) indicates that the convective term, i.e., $y_A N_{A_z}$, is not zero. At first, it may seem strange to a student to see this example in a chapter entitled "Mass Transfer in Binary Systems *without Bulk Flow*." The tricky part of mass transfer problems is that there is no need to have a bulk flow of the mixture as a result of external means, such as pressure drop, in order to have a nonzero convective flux term in the total flux expressions, i.e., Eqs. (2.164)–(2.166). In this example, although there is no bulk flow in the region $0 \le z \le L$, diffusion creates its own convection. As stated in Section 2.4, this phenomenon is called *diffusion-induced convection* and it is a characteristic of mass transfer. In the case of heat transfer, for example, conduction does not generate its own convection.

4.3.1 LIMITING CASE FOR SMALL VALUES OF y_{A_o}

The approximation $\ln(1-x) \simeq -x$ holds when x is small. Therefore, for small values of y_{A_o}, it is possible to write the term

$$\ln\left(\frac{1}{1-y_{A_o}}\right) = -\ln(1-y_{A_o}) \simeq y_{A_o} \qquad (4.94)$$

so that Eq. (4.92) simplifies to

$$N_{A_z} = \frac{c\mathcal{D}_{AB} y_{A_o}}{L}, \qquad (4.95)$$

which corresponds to the case in which the convective molar flux is considered negligible, i.e., Eq. (4.9). The effect of y_{A_o} on the variation in the mole fraction of species A as a function of position is shown in Figure 4.15. While it is safe to neglect the convective term when $y_{A_o} < 0.2$, it should be taken into consideration for larger values of y_{A_o}.

4.3.2 VELOCITIES

The molar-average velocity is given by

$$v_z^* = \frac{N_{A_z} + N_{B_z}}{c} = \frac{N_{A_z}}{c} = \frac{\mathcal{D}_{AB}}{L} \ln\left(\frac{1}{1-y_{A_o}}\right), \qquad (4.96)$$

which is constant.

The mass-average velocity, on the other hand, is dependent on position and is given by

$$v_z = \frac{n_{A_z} + n_{B_z}}{\rho} = \frac{N_{A_z} M_A}{cM} = \frac{\mathcal{D}_{AB}}{L} \ln\left(\frac{1}{1-y_{A_o}}\right) \frac{M_A}{[M_B + y_A (M_A - M_B)]} \qquad (4.97)$$

This result leads to the following interesting conclusions:

- The mass-average velocity is determined on the basis of a solution to a diffusion problem rather than the equation of motion.
- The no-slip boundary condition at the capillary tube surface is violated.

For a more thorough analysis of this problem, see Whitaker (1991).

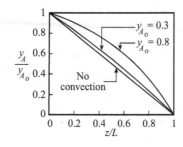

Figure 4.15   Mole fraction distribution as a function of position with y_{A_o} as a parameter.

4.3.3 TOTAL MOLAR FLUX OF SPECIES *B*

Since species *B* is insoluble in liquid *A*, we concluded that $N_{B_z} = 0$ in Eq. (4.82). Does this imply that the gas film above the liquid is stagnant? The molar flux of *B* is

$$N_{B_z} = -c\mathcal{D}_{AB}\frac{dy_B}{dz} + y_B N_{A_z} = \underbrace{c\mathcal{D}_{AB}\frac{dy_A}{dz}}_{-(1-y_A)N_{A_z}\,[\text{Eq. (4.85)}]} + (1-y_A)N_{A_z} = 0 \qquad (4.98)$$

The total molar flux of species *B* is zero NOT as a result of a "stagnant" gas film above liquid *A*. As can be seen from Eq. (4.98), the diffusive and convective fluxes of species *B* are equal in magnitude but opposite in direction. Thus, the total molar flux of species *B* turns out to be zero. This phenomenon is similar to the case in which a person's position is fixed while walking on a treadmill.

4.4 DIFFUSION THROUGH A STAGNANT LIQUID

Consider steady one-dimensional diffusion of liquid *A* through a stagnant film of liquid *B* with thickness *L* as shown in Figure 4.16. The mole fractions of *A* at $z = 0$ and $z = L$ are known. We are interested in the molar transfer rate of species *A* through the liquid film of *B*.

Postulating one-dimensional mass transport with $N_{A_z} = N_{A_z}(z)$ and $N_{A_x} = N_{A_y} = 0$, the equation of continuity for species *A*, Eq. (A) of Table 2.3, simplifies to

$$\frac{dN_{A_z}}{dz} = 0 \qquad \Rightarrow \qquad N_{A_z} = \text{constant} \qquad (4.99)$$

To proceed further, it is necessary to express the total molar flux of species *A*, i.e., N_{A_z}, either by Eq. (2.165) or by Eq. (2.166).

4.4.1 ANALYSIS BASED ON THE MOLAR-AVERAGE VELOCITY

According to Eq. (2.165), the total molar flux of species *A* is given as

$$N_{A_z} = -c\mathcal{D}_{AB}\frac{dx_A}{dz} + x_A\left(N_{A_z} + N_{B_z}\right) \qquad (4.100)$$

Since species *B* is stagnant, $N_{B_z} = 0$ and Eq. (4.100) simplifies to

$$N_{A_z} = -\frac{c\mathcal{D}_{AB}}{1-x_A}\frac{dx_A}{dz} \qquad (4.101)$$

The total molar concentration, *c*, is not constant but dependent on the mole fractions of species *A* and *B*. Assuming ideal mixture behavior, i.e., $\overline{V}_i = \widetilde{V}_i$, the total molar concentration is expressed as

$$c = \frac{1}{\widetilde{V}_{mix}} = \frac{1}{x_A\widetilde{V}_A + x_B\widetilde{V}_B} \qquad (4.102)$$

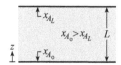

Figure 4.16 Diffusion of liquid *A* through a stagnant liquid film *B*.

Expressing x_B in terms of x_A, i.e., $x_B = 1 - x_A$, yields

$$c = \frac{1}{\widetilde{V}_B + (\widetilde{V}_A - \widetilde{V}_B)x_A} \tag{4.103}$$

If $\mathcal{D}_{AB}$ is considered constant,[3] combination of Eqs. (4.101) and (4.105) leads to

$$N_{A_z} \int_0^L dz = -\mathcal{D}_{AB} \int_{x_{A_o}}^{x_{A_L}} \frac{dx_A}{\left[\widetilde{V}_B + (\widetilde{V}_A - \widetilde{V}_B)x_A\right](1 - x_A)} \tag{4.104}$$

Integration of Eq. (4.104) results in

$$\begin{aligned}
N_{A_z} &= \frac{\mathcal{D}_{AB}}{L\widetilde{V}_A}\left\{ \ln\left(\frac{1 - x_{A_L}}{1 - x_{A_o}}\right) - \ln\left[\frac{\widetilde{V}_B + (\widetilde{V}_A - \widetilde{V}_B)x_{A_L}}{\widetilde{V}_B + (\widetilde{V}_A - \widetilde{V}_B)x_{A_o}}\right]\right\} \\
&= \frac{\mathcal{D}_{AB}}{L\widetilde{V}_A}\left[\ln\left(\frac{x_{B_L}}{x_{B_o}}\right) - \ln\left(\frac{c_o}{c_L}\right)\right] = \frac{\mathcal{D}_{AB}}{L\widetilde{V}_A}\ln\left(\frac{c_{B_L}}{c_{B_o}}\right),
\end{aligned} \tag{4.105}$$

where c_o and c_L are the values of the total molar concentration at $z = 0$ and $z = L$, respectively.

4.4.2 ANALYSIS BASED ON THE VOLUME-AVERAGE VELOCITY

From Eq. (2.166), the total molar flux of species A is given as

$$N_{A_z} = -\mathcal{D}_{AB}\frac{dc_A}{dz} + c_A\left(\overline{V}_A N_{A_z} + \overline{V}_B N_{B_z}\right) \tag{4.106}$$

Since $N_{B_z} = 0$ and $\overline{V}_A = \widetilde{V}_A$, Eq. (4.106) simplifies to

$$N_{A_z} = -\frac{\mathcal{D}_{AB}}{1 - \widetilde{V}_A c_A}\frac{dc_A}{dz} \tag{4.107}$$

If $\mathcal{D}_{AB}$ is considered constant, rearrangement of Eq. (4.107) results in

$$N_{A_z} \int_0^L dz = -\mathcal{D}_{AB} \int_{c_{A_o}}^{c_{A_L}} \frac{dc_A}{1 - \widetilde{V}_A c_A} \tag{4.108}$$

Integration of Eq. (4.108) leads to

$$N_{A_z} = \frac{\mathcal{D}_{AB}}{L\widetilde{V}_A}\ln\left(\frac{1 - \widetilde{V}_A c_{A_L}}{1 - \widetilde{V}_A c_{A_o}}\right) \tag{4.109}$$

The use of the identity from Eq. (4.102), i.e.,

$$1 - \widetilde{V}_A c_A = \widetilde{V}_B c_B \tag{4.110}$$

simplifies Eq. (4.109) to

$$N_{A_z} = \frac{\mathcal{D}_{AB}}{L\widetilde{V}_A}\ln\left(\frac{c_{B_L}}{c_{B_o}}\right), \tag{4.111}$$

which is identical with Eq. (4.5).

---

[3]Diffusion coefficients in liquids are strong functions of concentration. Thus, this assumption may lead to erroneous results.

4.4.3 VELOCITIES

The use of Eq. (2.23) gives the mass-average velocity as

$$v_z^* = \frac{N_{A_z}}{c} \tag{4.112}$$

Substitution of Eqs. (4.103) and (4.111) into Eq. (4.112) gives

$$\boxed{v_z^* = \left(\frac{\widetilde{V}_B}{\widetilde{V}_A} x_B + x_A\right) \frac{\mathcal{D}_{AB}}{L} \ln\left(\frac{c_{B_L}}{c_{B_o}}\right)} \tag{4.113}$$

The volume-average velocity is obtained from Eq. (2.24) as

$$v_z^\blacksquare = \widetilde{V}_A N_{A_z} \tag{4.114}$$

Substitution of Eq. (4.111) into Eq. (4.114) yields

$$\boxed{v_z^\blacksquare = \frac{\mathcal{D}_{AB}}{L} \ln\left(\frac{c_{B_L}}{c_{B_o}}\right)} \tag{4.115}$$

In this specific example, while $v_z^\blacksquare$ remains constant, v_z^* changes as a function of composition.

Example 4.6 Toluene (A) is diffusing through a 1.5-mm-thick stagnant bromobenzene (B) film at 298 K. If $x_{A_o} = 0.30$ and $x_{A_L} = 0.05$, determine the molar flux of toluene under steady conditions. Burchard and Toor (1962) reported the diffusion coefficient as

$$\mathcal{D}_{AB} \times 10^5 = 1.411 + 0.856 x_A,$$

where $\mathcal{D}_{AB}$ is in cm^2/s. At 298 K

$$\rho_A = 865\,\text{kg/m}^3 \qquad \text{and} \qquad \rho_B = 1488.2\,\text{kg/m}^3$$

Solution

From Appendix F

$$M_A = 92.138\,\text{kg/kmol} \qquad \text{and} \qquad M_B = 157.008\,\text{kg/kmol}$$

Since $\mathcal{D}_{AB}$ is a function of concentration, Eq. (4.105) cannot be used to calculate the molar flux of toluene. Let us express the diffusion coefficient as

$$\mathcal{D}_{AB} = \alpha + \beta x_A \tag{1}$$

In this case, Eq. (4.104) should be arranged in the form of

$$N_{A_z} \int_0^L dz = -\int_{x_{A_o}}^{x_{A_L}} \frac{\alpha + \beta x_A}{\left[\widetilde{V}_B + (\widetilde{V}_A - \widetilde{V}_B)x_A\right](1 - x_A)} dx_A \tag{2}$$

Integration of Eq. (2) results in

$$N_{A_z} = \frac{\alpha + \beta}{L\widetilde{V}_A} \ln\left(\frac{x_{B_L}}{x_{B_o}}\right) + \frac{1}{L\widetilde{V}_A}\left(\frac{\beta \widetilde{V}_B}{\widetilde{V}_A - \widetilde{V}_B} - \alpha\right) \ln\left(\frac{c_o}{c_L}\right) \tag{3}$$

Note that when $\alpha = \mathcal{D}_{AB}$ and $\beta = 0$, Eq. (3) reduces to Eq. (4.105). The molar volumes of species A and B are

$$\widetilde{V}_A = \frac{M_A}{\rho_A} = \frac{92.138}{0.865} = 106.5\,\text{cm}^3/\text{mol}$$

$$\widetilde{V}_B = \frac{M_B}{\rho_B} = \frac{157.008}{1.4882} = 105.5\,\text{cm}^3/\text{mol}$$

The values of the total molar concentration at $z = 0$ and $z = L$ are calculated from Eq. (4.103) as

$$c_o = \frac{1}{105.5 + (106.5 - 105.5)(0.3)} = 9.45 \times 10^{-3}\,\text{mol/cm}^3$$

$$c_L = \frac{1}{105.5 + (106.5 - 105.5)(0.05)} = 9.47 \times 10^{-3}\,\text{mol/cm}^3$$

Therefore, the use of Eq. (3) gives the molar flux of toluene through the bromobenzene layer as

$$N_{A_z} = \frac{(1.411 + 0.856) \times 10^{-5}}{(0.15)(106.5)} \ln\left(\frac{0.95}{0.70}\right)$$

$$+ \frac{10^{-5}}{(0.15)(106.5)} \left[\frac{(0.856)(105.5)}{106.5 - 105.5} - 1.411\right] \ln\left(\frac{9.45}{9.47}\right) = 3.145 \times 10^{-7}\,\text{mol/cm}^2.\text{s}$$

Comment: Let us resolve the problem by using two types of simplifying assumptions:

• Case (i): The average value of the diffusion coefficient is

$$\langle \mathcal{D}_{AB} \rangle = \frac{\displaystyle\int_{x_{A_o}}^{x_{A_L}} (\alpha + \beta x_A)\, dx_A}{\displaystyle\int_{x_{A_o}}^{x_{A_L}} dx_A} = \alpha + \frac{\beta}{2}(x_{A_L} + x_{A_o})$$

$$= \left[1.411 + \frac{0.856}{2}(0.05 + 0.30)\right] \times 10^{-5} = 1.561 \times 10^{-5}\,\text{cm}^2/\text{s}$$

The use of Eq. (4.105) with the average value of the diffusion coefficient gives

$$N_{A_z} = \frac{\langle \mathcal{D}_{AB} \rangle}{L \widetilde{V}_A} \ln\left(\frac{c_{B_L}}{c_{B_o}}\right)$$

$$= \frac{1.561 \times 10^{-5}}{(0.15)(106.5)} \ln\left[\frac{(9.47 \times 10^{-3})(0.95)}{(9.45 \times 10^{-3})(0.70)}\right] = 3.005 \times 10^{-7}\,\text{mol/cm}^2.\text{s}$$

The error introduced by assuming the diffusion coefficient to be a constant at its average value is

$$\text{Error} = \left(\frac{3.005 - 3.145}{3.145}\right) \times 100 = -4.6\%$$

• Case (ii): Since c_o and c_L do not differ much, let us assume that the total molar concentration is constant at the average value of

$$\langle c \rangle = \frac{(9.45 + 9.47) \times 10^{-3}}{2} = 9.46 \times 10^{-3}\,\text{mol/cm}^3$$

Rearrangement of Eq. (4.104) leads to

$$N_{A_z} \int_0^L dz = -\langle c \rangle \int_{x_{A_o}}^{x_{A_L}} \frac{\alpha + \beta x_A}{1 - x_A}\, dx_A$$

Integration gives

$$
\begin{aligned}
N_{A_z} &= \frac{\langle c \rangle}{L} \left[(\alpha + \beta) \ln \left(\frac{x_{B_L}}{x_{B_o}} \right) + \beta \left(x_{B_o} - x_{B_L} \right) \right] \\
&= \frac{9.46 \times 10^{-3}}{0.15} \left[(1.411 + 0.856) \ln \left(\frac{0.95}{0.70} \right) + (0.856)(0.7 - 0.95) \right] \times 10^{-5} \\
&= 3.016 \times 10^{-7} \, \mathrm{mol/cm^2.s}
\end{aligned}
$$

The error is

$$
\text{Error} = \left(\frac{3.016 - 3.145}{3.145} \right) \times 100 = -4.1\%
$$

4.5 DIFFUSION WITH A HETEROGENEOUS REACTION

An ideal gas A diffuses at steady-state in the positive z-direction through a hypothetical flat stagnant gas film of thickness δ as shown in Figure 4.17. The gas composition at $z = 0$, i.e., y_{A_o}, is known. At $z = \delta$ there is a solid catalyst surface at which A undergoes the following irreversible first-order heterogeneous dimerization reaction:

$$
2A \to B
$$

We are interested in determination of the molar flux of species A through the gas film.

Let us assume that the total molar concentration and the diffusion coefficient are constant. Postulating one-dimensional mass transport with $N_{A_z} = N_{A_z}(z)$ and $N_{A_x} = N_{A_y} = 0$, the equation of continuity for species A, Eq. (A) of Table 2.3, simplifies to

$$
\frac{dN_{A_z}}{dz} = 0 \quad \Rightarrow \quad N_{A_z} = \text{constant} \tag{4.116}
$$

Note that $\mathcal{R}_A = 0$ since the reaction is heterogeneous. On the other hand, the total molar flux of species A, Eq. (2.165), is expressed as

$$
N_{A_z} = -c \mathcal{D}_{AB} \frac{dy_A}{dz} + y_A \left(N_{A_z} + N_{B_z} \right) \tag{4.117}
$$

The stoichiometry of the chemical reaction implies that for every 2 moles of A diffusing in the positive z-direction 1 mole of B diffuses back in the negative z-direction. According to Eq. (2.115), the relationship between the fluxes can be expressed as

$$
\frac{1}{2} N_{A_z} = -N_{B_z} \tag{4.118}
$$

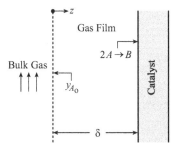

Figure 4.17 Heterogeneous reaction on a catalyst surface.

The use of Eq. (4.118) in Eq. (4.117) gives

$$N_{A_z} = -\frac{c\mathcal{D}_{AB}}{1-0.5y_A}\frac{dy_A}{dz} \tag{4.119}$$

Since N_{A_z} is constant, Eq. (4.119) can be rearranged as

$$N_{A_z}\int_0^\delta dz = -c\mathcal{D}_{AB}\int_{y_{A_o}}^{y_{A_\delta}}\frac{dy_A}{1-0.5y_A} \tag{4.120}$$

or

$$N_{A_z} = \frac{2c\mathcal{D}_{AB}}{\delta}\ln\left(\frac{1-0.5y_{A_\delta}}{1-0.5y_{A_o}}\right) \tag{4.121}$$

Although y_{A_o} is a known quantity, the mole fraction of species A in the gas phase at the catalytic surface, y_{A_δ}, is unknown and must be determined from the boundary condition. From Eq. (2.114), the rate of reaction is expressed as

$$\text{at} \quad z=\delta \qquad N_{A_z} = k_1''c_A = k_1''cy_A, \tag{4.122}$$

where k_1'' is the surface reaction rate constant. Therefore, y_{A_δ} is expressed from Eq. (4.122) as

$$y_{A_\delta} = \frac{N_{A_z}}{ck_1''} \tag{4.123}$$

Substitution of Eq. (4.123) into Eq. (4.121) results in

$$\boxed{N_{A_z} = \frac{2c\mathcal{D}_{AB}}{\delta}\ln\left[\frac{1-0.5\left(N_{A_z}/ck_1''\right)}{1-0.5y_{A_o}}\right],} \tag{4.124}$$

which is a transcendental equation in N_{A_z}. It is interesting to investigate two limiting cases of Eq. (4.124).

• Limiting case when k_1'' is large

Since $\ln(1-x)\simeq -x$ for small values of x,

$$\ln\left[1-0.5\left(N_{A_z}/ck_1''\right)\right] \simeq -0.5\left(N_{A_z}/ck_1''\right) \tag{4.125}$$

so that Eq. (4.124) reduces to

$$N_{A_z} = 2ck_1''\left(1+\frac{\delta k_1''}{\mathcal{D}_{AB}}\right)^{-1}\ln\left(\frac{1}{1-0.5y_{A_o}}\right) \tag{4.126}$$

The dimensionless term $\delta k_1''/\mathcal{D}_{AB}$ in Eq. (4.126) is called the *Thiele modulus*, and it quantifies the ratio of the rate of surface reaction to the rate of diffusion.

• Limiting case when $k_1'' = \infty$

When $k_1'' = \infty$, the reaction is instantaneous. In other words, once species A reaches the catalytic surface, it is immediately converted to species B so that $y_{A_\delta} = 0$. For $k_1'' = \infty$, Eq. (4.124) reduces to

$$N_{A_z} = \frac{2c\mathcal{D}_{AB}}{\delta}\ln\left(\frac{1}{1-0.5y_{A_o}}\right) \tag{4.127}$$

Note that Eq. (4.127) can also be obtained from Eq. (4.121) by letting $y_{A_\delta} = 0$.

4.5.1 VELOCITIES

The molar-average velocity is given by

$$\boxed{v_z^* = \frac{N_{A_z} + N_{B_z}}{c} = \frac{1}{2}\frac{N_{A_z}}{c}}$$
(4.128)

Since both N_{A_z} and c are constants, v_z^* remains constant for $0 \le z \le \delta$.

On the other hand, the mass-average velocity is

$$v_z = \frac{M_A N_{A_z} + M_B N_{B_z}}{\rho} = \frac{N_{A_z}(M_A - 0.5 M_B)}{\rho}$$
(4.129)

As a result of the dimerization reaction, $M_A = 0.5 M_B$ and Eq. (4.129) leads to

$$\boxed{v_z = 0}$$
(4.130)

Thus, if one of the characteristic velocities is zero, this does not necessarily imply that the other characteristic velocities are also zero.

Example 4.7 A cylindrical tube of diameter D and length L is closed at one end. While the closed end is coated with a solid species S, the open end is exposed to a gas mixture consisting of species A, B, C, and D with compositions y_A^*, y_B^*, y_C^*, and y_D^*, respectively, as shown in the figure below. Species A undergoes the following rapid heterogeneous reaction at $z = 0$:

$$3S(s) + 5/2A(g) \rightarrow 2B(g) + C(g)$$

We are interested in the rate of consumption of species A under steady conditions.

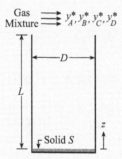

The problem will be analyzed with the following assumptions:

- Since there are four species present, the problem will be analyzed by using Eq. (3.155), i.e.,

$$\mathbf{N}_A = -c\mathcal{D}_{Am}\nabla y_A + y_A(\mathbf{N}_A + \mathbf{N}_B + \mathbf{N}_C + \mathbf{N}_D),$$
(1)

  where the effective binary diffusion coefficient of species A in the mixture, $\mathcal{D}_{Am}$, is given by Eq. (3.153).
- Species A, B, C, and D form an ideal gas mixture.
- The entire system is maintained at constant temperature and pressure. Thus, the total molar concentration is constant.
- $\mathcal{D}_{Am}$ is constant.
- The position of the catalyst surface does not change with time.
- Species A, B, C, and D do not diffuse into the solid S.

Postulating one-dimensional mass transport with $N_{A_r} = N_{A_\theta} = 0$ and $N_{A_z} = N_{A_z}(z)$, the equation of continuity for species A, Eq. (B) of Table 2.3, simplifies to

$$\frac{dN_{A_z}}{dz} = 0 \quad \Rightarrow \quad N_{A_z} = \text{constant} \quad 0 \le z \le L \tag{2}$$

Similarly, we can show that the molar fluxes of species B, C, and D are all constant. According to Eq. (2.115), the relationship between the fluxes can be expressed as

$$-\frac{2}{5} N_{A_z} = \frac{1}{2} N_{B_z} = N_{C_z} \tag{3}$$

Since species D is inert, $N_{D_z} = 0$ and Eq. (1) is expressed as

$$N_{A_z} = -c\mathcal{D}_{Am} \frac{dy_A}{dz} + y_A \left(N_{A_z} + N_{B_z} + N_{C_z}\right) \tag{4}$$

The use of Eq. (3) in Eq. (4) and rearrangement result in

$$N_{A_z} \int_0^L dz = -c\mathcal{D}_{Am} \int_0^{y_A^*} \frac{dy_A}{1 + 0.2\, y_A} \tag{5}$$

Integration of Eq. (5) leads to

$$N_{A_z} = -\frac{c\mathcal{D}_{Am}}{L} \ln(1 + 0.2 y_A^*), \tag{6}$$

where the minus sign indicates that species A diffuses in the negative z-direction. Therefore, the molar rate of consumption of species A is given by

$$\mathcal{W}_A = \frac{\pi D^2 c \mathcal{D}_{Am}}{4L} \ln(1 + 0.2 y_A^*)$$

4.6   DIFFUSION AND REACTION IN A CYLINDRICAL CATALYST PORE

Consider an idealized single cylindrical pore of radius R and length L in a catalyst particle as shown in Figure 4.18. The bulk gas stream has a species A concentration of c_{A_b}. Species A diffuses through a hypothetical stagnant gas film, and its concentration at the pore mouth, i.e., $z = 0$, is c_{A_o}. As species A diffuses into the catalyst pore, it undergoes the first-order irreversible reaction

$$A \to B$$

on the interior lateral surface of the catalyst. However, no reaction takes place on the surface at $z = L$. We are interested in the molar rate of conversion of species A under steady-state conditions.

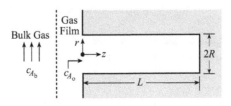

Figure 4.18   Diffusion and reaction in a cylindrical pore.

Let us assume that the system is isothermal and the diffusion coefficient is constant. As a result of symmetry, $N_{A_\theta} = 0$. Postulating $N_{A_r} = N_{A_r}(r, z)$ and $N_{A_z} = N_{A_z}(r, z)$, the equation of continuity for species A, Eq. (B) of Table 2.3, simplifies to

$$\frac{1}{r} \frac{\partial}{\partial r} (r N_{A_r}) + \frac{\partial N_{A_z}}{\partial z} = 0 \tag{4.131}$$

Since the temperature is constant and there is no volume change due to the reaction, the pressure and hence the total molar concentration, c, remain constant. Moreover, the stoichiometry of the reaction indicates that $\mathbf{N}_A = -\mathbf{N}_B$. Thus, $\mathbf{v}^* = 0$ and the components of the molar flux are expressed as

$$N_{A_r} = -\mathcal{D}_{AB} \frac{\partial c_A}{\partial r} \tag{4.132}$$

$$N_{A_z} = -\mathcal{D}_{AB} \frac{\partial c_A}{\partial z} \tag{4.133}$$

Substitution of Eqs. (4.132) and (4.133) into Eq. (4.131) gives the governing equation as

$$\frac{1}{r} \frac{\partial}{\partial r} \left(r \frac{\partial c_A}{\partial r} \right) + \frac{\partial^2 c_A}{\partial z^2} = 0 \tag{4.134}$$

The boundary conditions associated with Eq. (4.134) are

$$\text{at} \quad r = 0 \qquad \frac{\partial c_A}{\partial r} = 0 \tag{4.135}$$

$$\text{at} \quad r = R \qquad -\mathcal{D}_{AB} \frac{\partial c_A}{\partial r} = k_1'' c_A \tag{4.136}$$

$$\text{at} \quad z = 0 \qquad c_A = c_{A_o} \tag{4.137}$$

$$\text{at} \quad z = L \qquad \frac{\partial c_A}{\partial z} = 0 \tag{4.138}$$

The term k_1'' in Eq. (4.136) is the first-order surface reaction rate constant and has the dimensions of m/s. Equation (4.138) implies that the flux of species A is zero since there is no mass transfer through the surface at $z = L$.

If the measuring instrument, i.e., the concentration probe, is not sensitive enough to detect concentration variations in the radial direction, then it is necessary to change the scale of the problem to match that of the measuring device. In other words, it is necessary to average the governing equation up to the scale of the concentration measuring probe.

The area-averaged concentration for species A is defined by

$$\langle c_A \rangle = \frac{\int_0^{2\pi} \int_0^R c_A \, r \, dr \, d\theta}{\int_0^{2\pi} \int_0^R r \, dr \, d\theta} = \frac{2}{R^2} \int_0^R c_A \, r \, dr \tag{4.139}$$

Although the local concentration, c_A, is dependent on r and z, the area-averaged concentration, $\langle c_A \rangle$, depends only on z.

Area averaging is performed by integrating Eq. (4.134) over the cross-sectional area of the pore. The result is

$$\int_0^{2\pi} \int_0^R \frac{1}{r} \frac{\partial}{\partial r} \left(r \frac{\partial c_A}{\partial r} \right) r \, dr \, d\theta + \int_0^{2\pi} \int_0^R \frac{\partial^2 c_A}{\partial z^2} r \, dr \, d\theta = 0 \tag{4.140}$$

Since c_A does not depend on θ, Eq. (4.140) simplifies to

$$\int_0^R \frac{1}{r} \frac{\partial}{\partial r} \left(r \frac{\partial c_A}{\partial r} \right) r\,dr + \int_0^R \frac{\partial^2 c_A}{\partial z^2} r\,dr = 0 \tag{4.141}$$

The first term in Eq. (4.141) is

$$\int_0^R \frac{1}{r} \frac{\partial}{\partial r} \left(r \frac{\partial c_A}{\partial r} \right) r\,dr = \left(r \frac{\partial c_A}{\partial r} \right) \Big|_{r=0}^{r=R} = R \frac{\partial c_A}{\partial r} \Big|_{r=R} \tag{4.142}$$

The use of Eq. (4.136) in Eq. (4.142) yields

$$\int_0^R \frac{1}{r} \frac{\partial}{\partial r} \left(r \frac{\partial c_A}{\partial r} \right) r\,dr = -\frac{k_1'' R}{\mathcal{D}_{AB}} c_A \big|_{r=R} \tag{4.143}$$

Since the limits of the integration are constant, the order of differentiation and integration in the second term of Eq. (4.141) can be interchanged to obtain

$$\int_0^R \frac{\partial^2 c_A}{\partial z^2} r\,dr = \frac{d^2}{dz^2} \left(\int_0^R c_A r\,dr \right) \tag{4.144}$$

The use of Eq. (4.139) in Eq. (4.144) gives

$$\int_0^R \frac{\partial^2 c_A}{\partial z^2} r\,dr = \frac{R^2}{2} \frac{d^2 \langle c_A \rangle}{dz^2} \tag{4.145}$$

Substitution of Eqs. (4.143) and (4.145) into Eq. (4.141) and rearrangement yield

$$\mathcal{D}_{AB} \frac{d^2 \langle c_A \rangle}{dz^2} - \frac{2}{R} k_1'' c_A \big|_{r=R} = 0, \tag{4.146}$$

which is much simpler than Eq. (4.134). However, it contains two dependent variables, $\langle c_A \rangle$ and $c_A|_{r=R}$, which are at two different scales. When $\mathrm{Bi_M} \ll 1$, it is plausible to assume

$$c_A|_{r=R} \simeq \langle c_A \rangle \tag{4.147}$$

so that Eq. (4.146) takes the form

$$\mathcal{D}_{AB} \frac{d^2 \langle c_A \rangle}{dz^2} - \frac{2}{R} k_1'' \langle c_A \rangle = 0 \tag{4.148}$$

Integration of Eqs. (4.137) and (4.138) over the cross-sectional area of the pore gives the boundary conditions associated with Eq. (4.148) as

$$\text{at} \quad z = 0 \qquad \langle c_A \rangle = c_{A_o} \tag{4.149}$$

$$\text{at} \quad z = L \qquad \frac{d \langle c_A \rangle}{dz} = 0 \tag{4.150}$$

Equations (4.134) and (4.148) are at two different scales. Equation (4.148) is obtained by averaging Eq. (4.134) over the cross-sectional area perpendicular to the direction of mass flux. As a result, the boundary condition, i.e., the heterogeneous reaction rate expression, appears in the conservation statement.[4] The accuracy of the measurements dictates the equation to work with since the scale of the measurements should be compatible with the scale of the equation.

---

[4] The heterogeneous reaction rate expression and the transfer coefficients at the phase interfaces, i.e., friction factor, heat transfer coefficient, and mass transfer coefficient, should appear in the boundary conditions. If these quantities appear in the governing equations, this implies that these equations are averaged over either the area or volume of the system. In this case, dependent variables represent averaged quantities and not local values.

Note that the term $2/R$ in Eq. (4.148) is the catalyst surface area per unit volume, i.e.,

$$\frac{2}{R} = \frac{2\pi RL}{\pi R^2 L} = a_v = \frac{\text{Catalyst surface area}}{\text{Pore volume}} \tag{4.151}$$

Since the heterogeneous reaction rate expression has the unit of moles/(area)(time), multiplication of this term by a_v converts the unit to moles/(volume)(time).

The first and second terms in Eq. (4.148) represent mass transfer by diffusion and heterogeneous reaction, respectively. The order of magnitude estimates of these terms are

$$\text{Rate of diffusion} \sim O\left(\mathcal{D}_{AB}\frac{c_{A_o}}{L^2}\right) \tag{4.152}$$

$$\text{Rate of heterogeneous reaction} \sim O\left(\frac{2k_1'' c_{A_o}}{R}\right) \tag{4.153}$$

The *Thiele modulus* or the *Damköhler number*,[5] Λ, quantifies the ratio of the rate of the heterogeneous reaction to the rate of diffusion and is given by

$$\Lambda^2 = \frac{\text{Rate of heterogeneous reaction}}{\text{Rate of diffusion}} = \frac{2k_1'' c_{A_o}/R}{\mathcal{D}_{AB}c_{A_o}/L^2} = \frac{2k_1'' L^2}{\mathcal{D}_{AB}} \tag{4.154}$$

Before solving Eq. (4.148), it is convenient to express the governing equation and the boundary conditions in dimensionless form. Introduction of the dimensionless quantities

$$\theta = \frac{\langle c_A \rangle}{c_{A_o}} \quad \text{and} \quad \xi = \frac{z}{L} \tag{4.155}$$

reduces Eqs. (4.148)–(4.150) to

$$\frac{d^2\theta}{d\xi^2} - \Lambda^2 \theta = 0 \tag{4.156}$$

$$\text{at} \quad \xi = 0 \quad \theta = 1 \tag{4.157}$$

$$\text{at} \quad \xi = 1 \quad \frac{d\theta}{d\xi} = 0 \tag{4.158}$$

Equation (4.156) is similar to Eq. (D.39) in Appendix D. Thus, the solution is

$$\theta = \frac{\cosh\Lambda\cosh(\Lambda\xi) - \sinh\Lambda\sinh(\Lambda\xi)}{\cosh\Lambda} \tag{4.159}$$

The use of the identity

$$\cosh(x - y) = \cosh x \cosh y - \sinh x \sinh y \tag{4.160}$$

reduces the solution to the form

$$\boxed{\theta = \frac{\cosh\left[\Lambda(1-\xi)\right]}{\cosh\Lambda}} \tag{4.161}$$

The molar flow rate of species A entering the pore through the surface at $z = 0$ is

$$\boxed{\mathcal{W}_A = \pi R^2 \left(-\mathcal{D}_{AB}\frac{d\langle c_A \rangle}{dz}\bigg|_{z=0}\right) = \frac{\pi R^2 \mathcal{D}_{AB} c_{A_o} \Lambda \tanh\Lambda}{L}} \tag{4.162}$$

---

[5]While the Thiele modulus is preferred in the analysis of mass transport in a porous medium, the Damköhler number is used for packed bed analysis.

4.6.1   EFFECTIVENESS FACTOR

The *effectiveness factor* is defined as the ratio of the apparent rate of conversion to the rate if the entire internal surface were exposed to the concentration c_{A_o}. Under steady conditions

$$\begin{pmatrix} \text{Rate of moles of species } A \text{ entering} \\ \text{the pore through the surface at } z = 0 \end{pmatrix} = \begin{pmatrix} \text{Rate of conversion of species } A \text{ to} \\ \text{species } B \text{ at the catalytic surface} \end{pmatrix} \quad (4.163)$$

Thus, Eq. (4.162) also represents the apparent rate of conversion. The effectiveness factor, η, is then defined as

$$\eta = \frac{\pi R^2 \mathcal{D}_{AB} c_{A_o} \Lambda \tanh \Lambda / L}{2\pi R L k_1'' c_{A_o}} = \frac{\tanh \Lambda}{\Lambda} \quad (4.164)$$

The variation in the effectiveness factor as a function of the Thiele modulus is shown in Figure 4.19.

• Limiting case when $\Lambda \to 0$

As the Thiele modulus approaches zero, the rate of diffusion becomes much larger than the rate of reaction. The Taylor series expansion of η in terms of Λ gives

$$\eta = 1 - \frac{1}{3}\Lambda^2 + \frac{2}{15}\Lambda^4 - \frac{17}{315}\Lambda^6 + \dots \quad (4.165)$$

Therefore, η approaches unity as $\Lambda \to 0$, indicating that the entire surface is exposed to a reactant.

• Limiting case when $\Lambda \to \infty$

Large values of the Thiele modulus correspond to cases in which the diffusion rate is very slow and the surface reaction is very rapid. Under these conditions, the effectiveness factor becomes

$$\eta = \frac{1}{\Lambda} \quad (4.166)$$

This implies that a good part of the catalyst surface is starved for a reactant and hence not effective. As $\Lambda \to \infty$, η approaches zero.

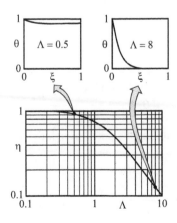

Figure 4.19   Variation in the effectiveness factor, η, as a function of the Thiele modulus, Λ, (Tosun, 2007).

4.7 DIFFUSION AND REACTION IN A SPHERICAL CATALYST

Species A diffuses into a spherical porous catalyst particle of radius R and undergoes a first-order irreversible reaction on the interior surface of the catalyst. The concentration of species A at the outer surface of the catalyst, c_{A_R}, is known. We are interested in the molar rate of depletion of species A under steady conditions. The problem will be analyzed with the following assumptions:

- Isothermal conditions prevail.
- Convective flux is negligible with respect to the molecular flux.
- The total concentration is constant.

In the previous example, the catalyst pore is idealized as a perfect cylindrical pore. In reality, the geometry within a porous catalyst particle is rather complex. In this case, it is necessary to average the species continuity equation over the volume of the catalyst particle. For the sake of simplicity, the details of the derivation will be skipped and the final form of the averaged equation of continuity for species A will be expressed as

$$\frac{\partial c_A}{\partial t} + \nabla \cdot \mathbf{N}_A = \overline{\mathcal{R}}_A, \tag{4.167}$$

where c_A and $\mathbf{N}_A$ stand for average concentration and average total molar flux, respectively. By averaging we generate a continuum in which we treat the heterogeneous reaction as if it were homogeneous. Thus, the term $\overline{\mathcal{R}}_A$ represents the rate of generation of species A per unit volume, defined by

$$\overline{\mathcal{R}}_A = a_v(-k_1'' c_A), \tag{4.168}$$

where a_v is the catalyst surface area per unit volume of catalyst volume. For the problem at hand, Eq. (4.167) simplifies to

$$\frac{1}{r^2} \frac{d}{dr}(r^2 N_{A_r}) = -a_v k_1'' c_A \tag{4.169}$$

The averaged form of the total molar flux is

$$N_{A_r} = -\mathcal{D}_{eff} \frac{dc_A}{dr}, \tag{4.170}$$

in which the convective part is neglected. The term $\mathcal{D}_{eff}$ is the *effective diffusion coefficient,* depending not only on temperature and pressure but also on the interior geometry of the catalyst. Substitution of Eq. (4.170) into Eq. (4.169) results in

$$\frac{\mathcal{D}_{eff}}{r^2} \frac{d}{dr}\left(r^2 \frac{dc_A}{dr} \right) = a_v k_1'' c_A \tag{4.171}$$

The boundary conditions associated with Eq. (4.171) are

$$\text{at} \quad r = 0 \qquad \frac{dc_A}{dr} = 0 \quad \text{or} \quad c_A \text{ is finite} \tag{4.172}$$

$$\text{at} \quad r = R \qquad c_A = c_{A_R} \tag{4.173}$$

The order of magnitude estimates of the terms in Eq. (4.171) are

$$\text{Rate of diffusion} \sim O\left(\mathcal{D}_{eff} \frac{c_{A_R}}{R^2} \right) \tag{4.174}$$

$$\text{Rate of reaction} \sim O\left(a_v k_1'' c_{A_R} \right) \tag{4.175}$$

Thus, the *Thiele modulus* for this problem is defined by

$$\Lambda^2 = \frac{\text{Rate of reaction}}{\text{Rate of diffusion}} = \frac{a_v k_1'' c_{A_R}}{\mathcal{D}_{eff}\, c_{A_R}/R^2} = \frac{a_v k_1'' R^2}{\mathcal{D}_{eff}} \tag{4.176}$$

Before solving Eq. (4.171), it is convenient to express the governing equation and the boundary conditions in dimensionless form. Introduction of the dimensionless quantities

$$\theta = \frac{c_A}{c_{A_R}} \qquad \text{and} \qquad \xi = \frac{r}{R} \tag{4.177}$$

reduces Eqs. (4.171)–(4.173) to

$$\frac{1}{\xi^2}\frac{d}{d\xi}\left(\xi^2 \frac{d\theta}{d\xi}\right) - \Lambda^2 \theta = 0 \tag{4.178}$$

$$\text{at} \quad \xi = 0 \qquad \frac{d\theta}{d\xi} = 0 \tag{4.179}$$

$$\text{at} \quad \xi = 1 \qquad \theta = 1 \tag{4.180}$$

The transformation

$$\theta = \frac{u(\xi)}{\xi} \tag{4.181}$$

converts spherical coordinates to Cartesian coordinates so that Eqs. (4.178)–(4.180) take the form

$$\frac{d^2 u}{d\xi^2} - \Lambda^2 u = 0 \tag{4.182}$$

$$\text{at} \quad \xi = 0 \qquad u = 0 \tag{4.183}$$

$$\text{at} \quad \xi = 1 \qquad u = 1 \tag{4.184}$$

The solution is given by

$$u = \frac{\sinh(\Lambda \xi)}{\sinh \Lambda} \tag{4.185}$$

The use of Eq. (4.185) in Eq. (4.181) gives the concentration distribution as

$$\boxed{\frac{c_A}{c_{A_R}} = \frac{R}{r}\,\frac{\sinh\left[\Lambda(r/R)\right]}{\sinh \Lambda}} \tag{4.186}$$

The molar flow rate of species A entering the catalyst particle through the surface at $r = R$ is

$$\boxed{\mathcal{W}_A = 4\pi R^2 \left(-\mathcal{D}_{eff}\left.\frac{dc_A}{dr}\right|_{r=R}\right) = 4\pi R \mathcal{D}_{eff}\, c_{A_R}(1 - \Lambda \coth \Lambda)} \tag{4.187}$$

4.7.1 EFFECTIVENESS FACTOR

As stated in Section 4.6.1, the effectiveness factor is the ratio of the apparent rate of conversion to the rate if the entire interior surface of the catalyst particle were uniformly exposed to the concentration c_{A_R}. Under steady conditions

$$\left(\begin{array}{c}\text{Rate of moles of species } A \text{ entering}\\ \text{the catalyst through the surface at } r = R\end{array}\right) = \left(\begin{array}{c}\text{Rate of conversion of species } A\\ \text{at the catalytic surface}\end{array}\right) \tag{4.188}$$

Thus, Eq. (4.187) also represents the apparent rate of conversion. The effectiveness factor, η, is then defined as

$$\boxed{\eta = \frac{4\pi R \mathcal{D}_{eff}\, c_{A_R}(1 - \Lambda\coth\Lambda)}{\left(\dfrac{4}{3}\pi R^3\right)\left(-a_v k_1'' c_{A_R}\right)} = \frac{3}{\Lambda^2}(\Lambda\coth\Lambda - 1)}$$

(4.189)

The variation in the effectiveness factor as a function of the Thiele modulus is shown in Figure 4.20.

• Limiting case when $\Lambda \to 0$

As the Thiele modulus approaches zero, the rate of diffusion becomes much larger than the rate of reaction. The Taylor series expansion of $\coth\Lambda$ is given by

$$\coth\eta = \frac{1}{\Lambda} + \frac{\Lambda}{3} - \frac{\Lambda^3}{45} + \frac{2\Lambda^5}{945} + \dots$$

(4.190)

Substitution of Eq. (4.190) into Eq. (4.189) gives

$$\eta = 1 - \frac{\Lambda}{15} + \frac{2\Lambda^4}{315} + \dots$$

(4.191)

Therefore, η approaches unity as $\Lambda \to 0$, indicating that the entire interior surface is exposed to a reactant.

• Limiting case when $\Lambda \to \infty$

Large values of the Thiele modulus correspond to cases in which the diffusion rate is very slow and the surface reaction is very rapid. Rearrangement of Eq. (4.189) gives

$$\eta = \frac{3\coth\Lambda}{\Lambda} - \frac{3}{\Lambda^2}$$

(4.192)

When Λ is large, $\coth\Lambda \to 1$ and Eq. (4.192) reduces to

$$\eta = \frac{3}{\Lambda}$$

(4.193)

This implies that a good part of the catalyst interior surface is starved for a reactant. In other words, species A cannot reach the center of the spherical catalyst particle. As $\Lambda \to \infty$, η approaches zero.

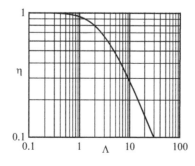

Figure 4.20 Variation in the effectiveness factor, η, as a function of the Thiele modulus, Λ.

4.8 DIFFUSION IN A LIQUID WITH A HOMOGENEOUS REACTION

Gas A dissolves in liquid B and diffuses into the liquid phase as shown in Figure 4.21. As it diffuses, species A undergoes the following irreversible chemical reaction with species B to form AB:

$$A + B \rightarrow AB$$

The rate of reaction is expressed by

$$\mathfrak{r} = k_1''' c_A \tag{4.194}$$

We are interested in determination of concentration distribution within the liquid phase and the rate of consumption of species A.

The problem will be analyzed with the following assumptions:

- Steady-state conditions prevail.
- The total concentration is constant, i.e.,

$$c = c_A + c_B + c_{AB} \simeq c_B = \text{constant} \tag{4.195}$$

- The concentration of AB does not interfere with the diffusion of A through B, i.e., A molecules, for the most part, hit molecules B, and hardly ever hit molecules AB. This is known as *pseudobinary behavior.*
- The convective flux is negligible with respect to the molecular flux.

Postulating one-dimensional mass transport with $N_{A_z} = N_{A_z}(z)$ and $N_{A_r} = N_{A_\theta} = 0$, the equation of continuity for species A, Eq. (B) of Table 2.3, simplifies to

$$\frac{dN_{A_z}}{dz} = \mathcal{R}_A \tag{4.196}$$

Since the convective molar flux is negligible, Eq. (2.165) gives the total molar flux as

$$N_{A_z} = -c \mathcal{D}_{AB} \frac{dx_A}{dz} = -\mathcal{D}_{AB} \frac{dc_A}{dz} \tag{4.197}$$

The use of Eq. (2.112) gives the rate of depletion of species A per unit volume as

$$\mathcal{R}_A = -k_1''' c_A \tag{4.198}$$

Substitution of Eqs. (4.197) and (4.198) into Eq. (4.196) yields the following governing equation:

$$\mathcal{D}_{AB} \frac{d^2 c_A}{dz^2} - k_1''' c_A = 0 \tag{4.199}$$

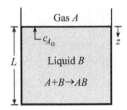

Figure 4.21   Diffusion and reaction in a liquid.

The boundary conditions associated with the problem are

$$\text{at} \quad z = 0 \qquad c_A = c_{A_o} \tag{4.200}$$

$$\text{at} \quad z = L \qquad \frac{dc_A}{dz} = 0 \tag{4.201}$$

The value of c_{A_o} in Eq. (4.200) can be determined from Henry's law, i.e., Eq. (2.223). The boundary condition given by Eq. (4.201) indicates that since species A cannot diffuse through the bottom of the container, i.e., an impermeable wall, the molar flux and the concentration gradient of species A are zero.

The first and second terms in Eq. (4.199) represent mass transfer by diffusion and homogeneous reaction, respectively. The order of magnitude estimates of these terms are

$$\text{Rate of diffusion} \sim O\left(\mathcal{D}_{AB} \frac{c_{A_o}}{L^2}\right) \tag{4.202}$$

$$\text{Rate of homogeneous reaction} \sim O\left(k_1''' c_{A_o}\right) \tag{4.203}$$

The Thiele modulus, Λ, quantifies the ratio of the rate of homogeneous reaction to the rate of diffusion and is given by

$$\Lambda^2 = \frac{\text{Rate of homogeneous reaction}}{\text{Rate of diffusion}} = \frac{k_1''' c_{A_o}}{\mathcal{D}_{AB} c_{A_o}/L^2} = \frac{k_1''' L^2}{\mathcal{D}_{AB}} \tag{4.204}$$

Before solving Eq. (4.199), it is convenient to express the governing equation and the boundary conditions in dimensionless form. Introduction of the dimensionless quantities

$$\theta = \frac{c_A}{c_{A_o}} \qquad \text{and} \qquad \xi = \frac{z}{L} \tag{4.205}$$

reduces Eqs. (4.199)–(4.201) to

$$\frac{d^2\theta}{d\xi^2} - \Lambda^2 \theta = 0 \tag{4.206}$$

$$\text{at} \quad \xi = 0 \qquad \theta = 1 \tag{4.207}$$

$$\text{at} \quad \xi = 1 \qquad \frac{d\theta}{d\xi} = 0 \tag{4.208}$$

Equations (4.206)–(4.208) are exactly the same as Eqs. (4.156)–(4.158). Thus, the solution is

$$\boxed{\theta = \frac{\cosh\left[\Lambda(1-\xi)\right]}{\cosh\Lambda}} \tag{4.209}$$

The molar flux of species A entering the liquid is

$$N_{A_z}\big|_{z=0} = -\mathcal{D}_{AB} \frac{dc_A}{dz}\bigg|_{z=0} = -\frac{\mathcal{D}_{AB}\, c_{A_o}}{L} \frac{d\theta}{d\xi}\bigg|_{\xi=0} \tag{4.210}$$

The use of Eq. (4.209) in Eq. (4.210) gives

$$\boxed{N_{A_z}\big|_{z=0} = \frac{\mathcal{D}_{AB}\, c_{A_o} \Lambda \tanh\Lambda}{L}} \tag{4.211}$$

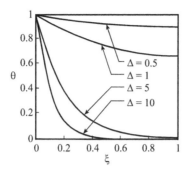

Figure 4.22   Variation in θ as a function of ξ, with Λ being a parameter.

Thus, the molar rate of species A entering the liquid is

$$\mathcal{W}_A = \frac{A\mathcal{D}_{AB}\,c_{A_o}\Lambda\tanh\Lambda}{L},\tag{4.212}$$

where A is the surface area of the liquid. Note that Eq. (4.212) also represents the rate of consumption of species A by the homogeneous chemical reaction.

It is interesting to observe how the Thiele modulus affects the concentration distribution. Figure 4.22 shows variation in θ as a function of ξ, with Λ being a parameter. For small values of Λ, i.e., rate of diffusion $\gg$ rate of reaction, most of species A diffuses through the liquid without undergoing a reaction and c_A has an appreciable value at the bottom of the container. On the other hand, for large values of Λ, i.e., rate of reaction $\gg$ rate of diffusion, as soon as species A enters the liquid phase, it undergoes a homogeneous reaction with species B. As a result, species A is depleted before it reaches the bottom of the container. Note that the slope of the tangent to the curve drawn at $\xi = 1$ should be zero, i.e., parallel to the ξ-axis, as a result of Eq. (4.201).

Example 4.8   Immobilized biocatalysts are extensively used in the chemical and pharmaceutical industries. They are also used as biosensors and in medical diagnoses and drug screening. Biocatalysts are produced by immobilizing enzymes on different supports, such as membranes, polymeric beads, and gels.

Consider a porous membrane, semi-infinite in the z-direction, containing an immobilized enzyme. Species A enters the membrane through the surface at $z = 0$ and as it diffuses into the membrane, it reacts with the enzyme. The molar rate of depletion of species A per unit volume is given by

$$\mathcal{R}_A = -\frac{k\,c_A}{k^* + c_A}\tag{1}$$

The concentration of species A at $z = 0$ is maintained constant at c_{A_o}. The membrane surface area is A, and the effective diffusion coefficient, $\mathcal{D}_{eff}$, is constant. Calculate the molar rate of consumption of species A under steady conditions.

Solution

Postulating one-dimensional mass transport with $N_{A_z} = N_{A_z}(z)$ and $N_{A_x} = N_{A_y} = 0$, the equation of continuity for species A, Eq. (A) of Table 2.3, simplifies to

$$\frac{dN_{A_z}}{dz} = \mathcal{R}_A\tag{2}$$

Neglecting the convective term within the membrane, the total molar flux of species A, Eq. (2.165), is expressed as

$$N_{A_z} = -\mathcal{D}_{eff} \frac{dc_A}{dz} \tag{3}$$

Substitution of Eqs. (1) and (3) into Eq. (2) gives the governing equation in the form

$$\mathcal{D}_{eff} \frac{d^2 c_A}{dz^2} = \frac{k c_A}{k^* + c_A} \tag{4}$$

The boundary conditions are

$$\text{at} \quad z = 0 \qquad c_A = c_{A_o} \tag{5}$$

$$\text{at} \quad z = \infty \qquad c_A = 0 \quad \text{and} \quad \frac{dc_A}{dz} = 0 \tag{6}$$

In terms of the dimensionless quantities

$$\theta = \frac{c_A}{c_{A_o}} \qquad \xi = \sqrt{\frac{k}{k^* \mathcal{D}_{eff}}}\, z \qquad \alpha = \frac{c_{A_o}}{k^*} \tag{7}$$

Eqs. (4)–(6) take the form

$$\frac{d^2 \theta}{d\xi^2} = \frac{\theta}{1 + \alpha\theta} \tag{8}$$

$$\text{at} \quad \xi = 0 \qquad \theta = 1 \tag{9}$$

$$\text{at} \quad \xi = \infty \qquad \theta = 0 \quad \text{and} \quad \frac{d\theta}{d\xi} = 0 \tag{10}$$

Multiplication of Eq. (8) by $d\theta/d\xi$ and making use of the identity

$$\frac{d}{d\xi}\left(\frac{d\theta}{d\xi}\right)^2 = 2 \frac{d\theta}{d\xi} \frac{d^2\theta}{d\xi^2} \tag{11}$$

lead to

$$\frac{d}{d\xi}\left(\frac{d\theta}{d\xi}\right)^2 = \frac{2\theta}{1 + \alpha\theta} \frac{d\theta}{d\xi} \tag{12}$$

Integration of Eq. (12) results in

$$\left(\frac{d\theta}{d\xi}\right)^2 = \frac{2}{\alpha^2}\left[\alpha\theta - \ln(1 + \alpha\theta)\right] + C, \tag{13}$$

where C is an integration constant. The boundary condition given by Eq. (10) indicates that $C = 0$. Thus,

$$\frac{d\theta}{d\xi} = \pm \sqrt{\frac{2}{\alpha^2}\left[\alpha\theta - \ln(1 + \alpha\theta)\right]} \tag{14}$$

Choosing the plus sign in Eq. (14) results in a negative value of N_{A_z} according to Eq. (3), indicating that species A diffuses in the negative z-direction. Therefore, the minus sign should be chosen to give

$$\frac{d\theta}{d\xi} = -\sqrt{\frac{2}{\alpha^2}\left[\alpha\theta - \ln(1 + \alpha\theta)\right]} \tag{15}$$

From an engineering point of view, we are not interested in solving Eq. (15) to obtain the concentration distribution but rather in estimating the molar flux of species A through the membrane surface at $z = 0$, i.e.,

$$N_{A_z}\big|_{z=0} = -\mathcal{D}_{eff} \frac{dc_A}{dz}\bigg|_{z=0} = -c_{A_o} \sqrt{\frac{k\mathcal{D}_{eff}}{k^*}} \frac{d\theta}{d\xi}\bigg|_{\xi=0} \tag{16}$$

Substitution of Eq. (15) into Eq. (16) yields

$$N_{A_z}\big|_{z=0} = \sqrt{2kk^*\mathcal{D}_{eff}\left[\frac{c_A}{k^*} - \ln\left(1 + \frac{c_A}{k^*}\right)\right]} \tag{17}$$

The molar rate of species A entering the membrane is

$$\mathcal{W}_A = A\sqrt{2kk^*\mathcal{D}_{eff}\left[\frac{c_A}{k^*} - \ln\left(1 + \frac{c_A}{k^*}\right)\right]}, \tag{18}$$

which also represents the molar rate of depletion of species A as a result of the homogeneous reaction.

Comment: The rate of reaction is expressed in terms of Monod (or Michaelis–Menten) type kinetics as reflected in Eq. (1), i.e.,

$$\mathfrak{r} = \frac{kc_A}{k^* + c_A} \tag{19}$$

When $k^* \gg c_A$, Eq. (19) reduces to the first-order reaction with $\mathfrak{r} = (k/k^*)c_A$. On the other hand, when $c_A \gg k^*$, Eq. (19) turns out to be the zeroth-order reaction, i.e., $\mathfrak{r} = k$.

Example 4.9 Microorganisms might adhere to biological or inanimate surfaces as *biofilms*, a generic name given to cell clusters held together by the slimy, glue-like substances they secrete. A typical example of a biofilm is the plaque that forms on your teeth. Consider a spherical biofilm (species B) of radius R surrounded by a solution having an antimicrobial agent (species A) concentration of c_{A_∞}. As species A diffuses into the biofilm, it undergoes an irreversible zeroth-order reaction. Postulating one-dimensional mass transport with $N_{A_r} = N_{A_r}(r)$ and $N_{A_\theta} = N_{A_\phi} = 0$, the equation of continuity for species A, Eq. (C) of Table 2.3, simplifies to

$$\frac{1}{r^2}\frac{d}{dr}\left(r^2 N_{A_r}\right) = \mathcal{R}_A = -k_o''', \tag{1}$$

where k_o''' is the zeroth-order rate constant. Neglecting the convective term within the biofilm, the total molar flux of species A, Eq. (2.165), is expressed as

$$N_{A_r} = -\mathcal{D}_{eff}\frac{dc_A}{dr} \tag{2}$$

Substitution of Eq. (2) into Eq. (1) gives the governing equation in the form

$$\frac{\mathcal{D}_{eff}}{r^2}\frac{d}{dr}\left(r^2\frac{dc_A}{dr}\right) = k_o''' \tag{3}$$

Let us introduce the following dimensionless quantities:

$$\theta = \frac{c_A}{K_A c_{A_\infty}} \qquad \xi = \frac{r}{R} \qquad \Lambda = \frac{k_o''' R^2}{K_A c_{A_\infty}\mathcal{D}_{eff}}, \tag{4}$$

where the term K_A is the partition coefficient. Under these circumstances, Eq. (3) becomes

$$\frac{1}{\xi^2}\frac{d}{d\xi}\left(\xi^2\frac{d\theta}{d\xi}\right)=\Lambda \tag{5}$$

The term Λ quantifies the ratio of the rate of reaction to the rate of diffusion. If Λ is large, species A will be depleted at some point, ξ_c, within the biofilm. At this location, not only will the concentration of species A be zero but also there will be no flux of species A through this point. Thus, the following boundary conditions can be written:

$$\text{at} \quad \xi=\xi_c \quad \theta=0 \tag{6}$$

$$\text{at} \quad \xi=\xi_c \quad \frac{d\theta}{d\xi}=0 \tag{7}$$

The solution of Eq. (5) subject to the boundary conditions given by Eqs. (6) and (7) is

$$\theta=\frac{\Lambda}{6}\xi^2+\frac{\Lambda}{3}\xi_c^3\frac{1}{\xi}-\frac{\Lambda}{2}\xi_c^2 \tag{8}$$

The dimensionless concentration at the surface of the biofilm is unity, i.e.,

$$\text{at} \quad \xi=1 \quad \theta=1 \tag{9}$$

Application of Eq. (9) gives

$$\xi_c^3-\frac{3}{2}\xi_c^2+\left(\frac{1}{2}-\frac{3}{\Lambda}\right)=0, \tag{10}$$

from which ξ_c can be determined.

Let us consider the case when $\xi_c=0$. This implies that the concentration is zero at the center of the biofilm and the corresponding radius of the biofilm, $R_{\min}$, represents the minimum radius to deplete all the species. From Eq. (10)

$$R_{\min}=\sqrt{\frac{6K_A c_{A_\infty}\mathcal{D}_{eff}}{k_o'''}} \tag{11}$$

Example 4.10 Since the cornea is the transparent part of the eye, it does not contain blood vessels. When the eyes are open, oxygen is supplied to the cornea from the surrounding air. When the eyes are closed, the capillaries of the palpebral conjunctiva provide the oxygen. In both cases, the mass transfer resistance of tear fluid is considered negligible. The rear surface of the cornea is in contact with the anterior chamber, in which aqueous humor is produced. The schematic diagram is shown below.

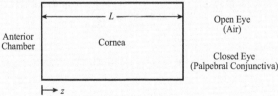

The rate of metabolic oxygen (species A) loss per unit volume is given as

$$\mathcal{R}_A=-\frac{Q_{\max}\overline{P}_A}{K+\overline{P}_A}, \tag{1}$$

where Q_{max} is the maximum volumetric oxygen consumption rate, K is the Monod constant, and $\overline{P}_A$ is the partial pressure[6] of oxygen. Considering one-dimensional diffusion in the cornea, the governing equation for oxygen is expressed as

$$\mathcal{D}_{AB}\frac{d^2 c_A}{dz^2} + \mathcal{R}_A = 0 \tag{2}$$

In terms of partial pressures, Eq. (2) takes the form

$$\mathcal{D}_{AB}S_A\frac{d^2\overline{P}_A}{dz^2} - \frac{Q_{max}\overline{P}_A}{K+\overline{P}_A} = 0, \tag{3}$$

where S_A is the solubility coefficient of oxygen in the cornea. Due to its nonlinear nature, Eq. (3) is solved with the help of Mathcad using the following parameters:

$$L = 500\,\mu m \quad \mathcal{D}_{AB} = 6\times 10^{-5}\,cm^2/s \quad S_A = 2.3\times 10^{-5}\,mL/cm^3.mmHg \quad K = 2.2\,mmHg$$

$$Q_{max} = 1.2\times 10^{-4}\,mL(STP)/cm^3.s \quad \overline{P}_A\big|_{z=0} = 24\,mmHg \quad \overline{P}_A\big|_{z=L} = 155\,mmHg \text{ (Open eye)}$$

Example 4.11   Consider continuous release of a pollutant (species A) into a stagnant medium (species B). Let Q be the mass released per unit cross-sectional area of the medium per unit time. The pollutant undergoes an irreversible first-order homogeneous chemical reaction. Assuming one-dimensional diffusion under steady conditions, the governing equation is

$$\mathcal{D}_{AB}\frac{d^2 c_A}{dz^2} - k_1''' c_A = 0 \tag{1}$$

If the source is located at $z = 0$, diffusion takes place over the domain $-\infty < z < \infty$ with the following boundary conditions:

$$\text{at } z = \pm\infty \qquad c_A = 0 \tag{2}$$

The solution of Eq. (1) is given by

$$c_A = C_1 \exp\left(\sqrt{k_1'''/\mathcal{D}_{AB}}\,z\right) + C_2 \exp\left(-\sqrt{k_1'''/\mathcal{D}_{AB}}\,z\right), \tag{3}$$

where C_1 and C_2 are constants. To satisfy the boundary conditions, it is necessary to divide the domain into two parts. In the region on the right side of the source, i.e., $0 < z < \infty$, the solution is

$$c_A^R = C_2 \exp\left(-\sqrt{k_1'''/\mathcal{D}_{AB}}\,z\right) \tag{4}$$

---

[6]In the medical literature, partial pressure is named tension.

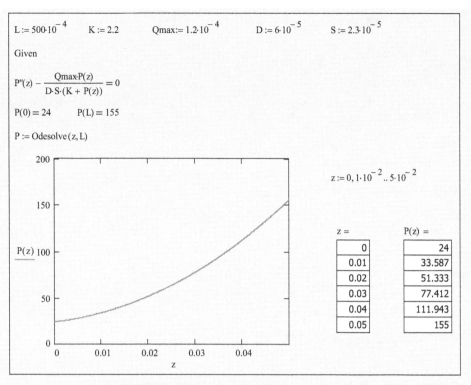

$L := 500 \cdot 10^{-4}$ $K := 2.2$ $Qmax := 1.2 \cdot 10^{-4}$ $D := 6 \cdot 10^{-5}$ $S := 2.3 \cdot 10^{-5}$

Given

$$P''(z) - \frac{Qmax \cdot P(z)}{D \cdot S \cdot (K + P(z))} = 0$$

$P(0) = 24$ $P(L) = 155$

$P := Odesolve(z, L)$

$z := 0, 1 \cdot 10^{-2} .. 5 \cdot 10^{-2}$

$z =$	$P(z) =$
0	24
0.01	33.587
0.02	51.333
0.03	77.412
0.04	111.943
0.05	155

Mathcad worksheet of Example 4.10.

In the region on the left side of the source, i.e., $-\infty < z < 0$, the solution is

$$c_A^L = C_1 \exp\left(\sqrt{k_1''' / \mathcal{D}_{AB}}\, z \right) \tag{5}$$

At the location of the source, concentrations are equal to each other

$$c_A^R \big|_{z=0} = c_A^L \big|_{z=0} \quad \Rightarrow \quad C_2 = C_1 = C \tag{6}$$

Once the mass is released into the medium, half of it will diffuse in the positive z-direction and the other half will diffuse in the negative z-direction. Thus, we can write

$$-\mathcal{D}_{AB} \frac{dc_A^R}{dz} \bigg|_{z=0} = \frac{Q}{2} \tag{7}$$

The use of Eq. (4) in Eq. (7) gives the constant C as

$$C = \frac{Q}{2\sqrt{k_1''' \mathcal{D}_{AB}}} \tag{8}$$

Thus, the concentration distribution is expressed in the form

$$c_A = \begin{cases} \dfrac{Q}{2\sqrt{k_1''' \mathcal{D}_{AB}}} \exp\left(-\sqrt{k_1''' / \mathcal{D}_{AB}}\, z \right) & 0 < z < \infty \\[4ex] \dfrac{Q}{2\sqrt{k_1''' \mathcal{D}_{AB}}} \exp\left(\sqrt{k_1''' / \mathcal{D}_{AB}}\, z \right) & -\infty < z < 0 \end{cases} \tag{9}$$

The maximum concentration occurs at $z = 0$, and it is given by

$$c_{A_{max}} = \frac{Q}{2\sqrt{k_1''' \mathcal{D}_{AB}}} \qquad (10)$$

A representative plot of $c_A/c_{A_{max}}$ versus position is shown in the figure below. The width, W, of the diffusing patch is defined as the length of the region that contains 95% of the species. Noting that

$$\int_0^{W/2} e^{-u}\, du = 0.95 \qquad \Rightarrow \qquad W \simeq 6$$

the width is given by

$$W = 6\sqrt{\frac{\mathcal{D}_{AB}}{k_1'''}}$$

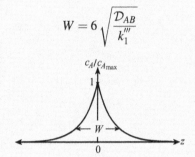

4.9 DIFFUSION WITH HETEROGENEOUS AND HOMOGENEOUS REACTIONS

Figure 4.23 shows a stagnant gas film, composed of species A and B, adjacent to a flat catalyst surface in which species A diffuses at steady-state through the film of thickness δ to the catalyst surface where the irreversible first-order heterogeneous reaction

$$A \rightarrow B$$

occurs. As species B leaves the surface, it decomposes by the following irreversible first-order homogeneous reaction:

$$B \rightarrow A$$

The compositions of species A and B at the outer edge of the film, y_{A_o} and y_{B_o}, are known. The entire system is maintained at constant temperature and pressure. We are interested in the molar flux of species A through the film.

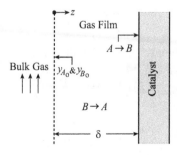

Figure 4.23 Diffusion with heterogeneous and homogeneous reactions.

Let us assume that the total molar concentration and the diffusion coefficient are constant. Postulating one-dimensional mass transport with $N_{A_z} = N_{A_z}(z)$ and $N_{B_z} = N_{B_z}(z)$, the equations of continuity for species A and B, Eq. (A) of Table 2.3, simplify to

$$\frac{dN_{A_z}}{dz} = \mathcal{R}_A \tag{4.213}$$

$$\frac{dN_{B_z}}{dz} = \mathcal{R}_B, \tag{4.214}$$

where

$$\mathcal{R}_A = k_1''' c_B = k_1''' c y_B \qquad \text{and} \qquad \mathcal{R}_B = -k_1''' c_B = -k_1''' c y_B \tag{4.215}$$

Noting that $\mathcal{R}_A = -\mathcal{R}_B$, addition of Eqs. (4.213) and (4.214) leads to

$$\frac{d}{dz}\left(N_{A_z} + N_{B_z}\right) = 0 \quad \Longrightarrow \quad N_{A_z} + N_{B_z} = \text{constant} \qquad 0 \le z \le \delta \tag{4.216}$$

The boundary conditions on the catalyst surface are expressed as

$$N_{A_z}\big|_{z=\delta} = k_1'' c_A\big|_{z=\delta} \qquad \text{and} \qquad N_{B_z}\big|_{z=\delta} = -k_1'' c_A\big|_{z=\delta} \tag{4.217}$$

Since $N_{A_z}\big|_{z=\delta} + N_{B_z}\big|_{z=\delta} = 0$, this implies that the constant in Eq. (4.216) is zero. Thus,

$$N_{A_z} + N_{B_z} = 0 \qquad 0 \le z \le \delta \tag{4.218}$$

In this problem, we need to solve either Eq. (4.213) or (4.214) since $y_A + y_B = 1$. From Eq. (2.165), the total molar flux of species B is given by

$$N_{B_z} = -c\mathcal{D}_{AB}\frac{dy_B}{dz} \tag{4.219}$$

Substitution of Eqs. (4.215) and (4.219) into Eq. (4.214) gives

$$\frac{d^2 y_B}{dz^2} - \left(\frac{k_1'''}{\mathcal{D}_{AB}}\right) y_B = 0 \tag{4.220}$$

The boundary conditions associated with the problem are

$$\text{at} \quad z = 0 \qquad y_B = y_{B_o} \tag{4.221}$$

$$\text{at} \quad z = \delta \qquad y_B = 1 + \frac{N_{B_z}\big|_{z=\delta}}{k_1'' c} \tag{4.222}$$

Introduction of the dimensionless quantities

$$\xi = \frac{z}{\delta} \qquad \text{and} \qquad \Lambda^2 = \frac{k_1''' \delta^2}{\mathcal{D}_{AB}} \tag{4.223}$$

reduces Eqs. (4.220)–(4.222) to

$$\frac{d^2 y_B}{d\xi^2} - \Lambda^2 y_B = 0 \tag{4.224}$$

$$\text{at} \quad \xi = 0 \qquad y_B = y_{B_o} \tag{4.225}$$

$$\text{at} \quad \xi = 1 \qquad y_B = 1 + \frac{N_{B_z}\big|_{\xi=1}}{k_1'' c} \tag{4.226}$$

Equation (4.224) is similar to Eq. (D.39) in Appendix D. Thus, the solution is

$$y_B = y_{B_o} \cosh(\Lambda\xi) + \left(1 - y_{B_o}\cosh\Lambda + \frac{N_{B_z}\big|_{\xi=1}}{k_1'' c}\right) \frac{\sinh(\Lambda\xi)}{\sinh\Lambda} \qquad (4.227)$$

The molar flux of species B, Eq. (4.219), in dimensionless form is given by

$$N_{B_z} = -\frac{c\mathcal{D}_{AB}}{\delta}\frac{dy_B}{d\xi} \qquad (4.228)$$

The molar flux of species B on the catalytic surface is

$$N_{B_z}\big|_{\xi=1} = -\frac{c\mathcal{D}_{AB}\Lambda}{\delta}\left[y_{B_o}\sinh\Lambda + \left(1 - y_{B_o}\cosh\Lambda + \frac{N_{B_z}\big|_{\xi=1}}{k_1'' c}\right)\frac{\cosh\Lambda}{\sinh\Lambda}\right] \qquad (4.229)$$

Solving for $N_{B_z}\big|_{\xi=1}$ yields

$$N_{B_z}\big|_{\xi=1} = \frac{\Lambda(y_{B_o} - \cosh\Lambda)}{\dfrac{\delta\sinh\Lambda}{c\mathcal{D}_{AB}} + \dfrac{\Lambda\cosh\Lambda}{k_1'' c}} \qquad (4.230)$$

Substitution of Eq. (4.230) into Eq. (4.227) leads to

$$\boxed{y_B = y_{B_o}\cosh(\Lambda\xi) + \left\{1 - y_{B_o}\cosh\Lambda + \left[\frac{y_{B_o} - \cosh\Lambda}{\Omega\,(\sinh\Lambda/\Lambda) + \cosh\Lambda}\right]\right\}\frac{\sinh(\Lambda\xi)}{\sinh\Lambda}}, \qquad (4.231)$$

where

$$\Omega = \frac{\delta k_1''}{\mathcal{D}_{AB}} \qquad (4.232)$$

The molar flux of species A at $\xi = 0$ is given by

$$N_{A_z}\big|_{\xi=0} = -N_{B_z}\big|_{\xi=0} = \frac{ck_1''}{\Omega}\frac{dy_B}{d\xi}\bigg|_{\xi=0} \qquad (4.233)$$

The use of Eq. (4.231) in Eq. (4.233) results in

$$\boxed{N_{A_z}\big|_{\xi=0} = \frac{ck_1''}{\Omega}\left(\frac{\Lambda}{\sinh\Lambda}\right)\left\{1 - y_{B_o}\cosh\Lambda + \left[\frac{y_{B_o} - \cosh\Lambda}{\Omega\,(\sinh\Lambda/\Lambda) + \cosh\Lambda}\right]\right\}} \qquad (4.234)$$

• **Limiting case when $k_1'' = \infty$**

When $k_1'' = \infty$ ($\Omega = \infty$), the reaction is instantaneous. In this case, Eqs. (4.231) and (4.234) become

$$y_B = y_{B_o}\cosh(\Lambda\xi) + (1 - y_{B_o}\cosh\Lambda)\frac{\sinh(\Lambda\xi)}{\sinh\Lambda} \qquad (4.235)$$

$$N_{A_z}\big|_{\xi=0} = \frac{c\mathcal{D}_{AB}}{\delta}(1 - y_{B_o}\cosh\Lambda) \qquad (4.236)$$

• Limiting case when $k_1''' = 0$

When $k_1''' = 0$ ($\Lambda = 0$), no homogeneous reaction takes place within the gas film. Under these circumstances, Eqs. (4.231) and (4.234) reduce to

$$y_B = y_{B_o} + (1 - y_{B_o}) \left(\frac{\Omega}{1+\Omega} \right) \xi \tag{4.237}$$

$$N_{A_z}\big|_{\xi=0} = \frac{k_1'' c_{A_o}}{1+\Omega} \tag{4.238}$$

PROBLEMS

4.1 Modified Atmosphere Packaging (MAP) is the process of adjusting the gas composition in the headspace of food packages to prolong shelf life. The gas mixture usually consists of carbon dioxide, nitrogen, and oxygen. Meat packages, for example, contain high concentrations of carbon dioxide to prevent the growth of microorganisms by suppressing microbial activity.

Consider one-dimensional diffusion of carbon dioxide through a new polymeric film $270\,\mu m$ thick under steady conditions. The partial pressure of carbon dioxide inside the package is $0.6\,atm$ and outside it is $0.03\,atm$. If $P_M^* = 19$ barrer, estimate the molar flux of carbon dioxide.

(Answer: $1.36 \times 10^{-10}\,mol/cm^2.s$)

4.2 Patients suffering from acute or chronic kidney malfunction need either a kidney transplant or dialysis. Dialysis is the process of removal of waste products and excess water from the blood. In the dialysis machine while blood flows through a tubular membrane, a liquid (dialysate) flows around the external surface of the membrane. Waste products diffuse through the walls of the membrane into the dialysate.

Consider the flow of blood through a cylindrical tubular membrane of $200\,\mu m$ internal diameter. The membrane has a wall thickness of $35\,\mu m$, and the concentration of urea on the inner surface of the membrane is $2.8\,mol/m^3$. Calculate the maximum molar flow rate of urea under steady conditions if the length of the membrane is $250\,mm$ and the diffusion coefficient of urea in the membrane is $3 \times 10^{-7}\,cm^2/s$.

(Answer: $4.4 \times 10^{-10}\,mol/s$)

4.3 Repeat the analysis given in Example 4.2 for two cylindrical membranes, A and B, and show that the molar transfer rate of species i is given by

$$\mathcal{W}_i = 2\pi H \frac{\left[(c_{i_b})_1 - (c_{i_b})_2 \right]}{\left[\dfrac{\ln(R^*/R_A)}{K_i^A \mathcal{D}_A} + \dfrac{\ln(R_B/R^*)}{K_i^B \mathcal{D}_B} \right]},$$

where R_A is the inner radius of membrane A, R^* is the outer radius of membrane A and the inner radius of membrane B, and R_B is the outer radius of membrane B. The solutions located in the regions $0 \leq r \leq R_A$ and $r \geq R_B$ have bulk concentrations of $(c_{i_b})_1$ and $(c_{i_b})_2$, respectively, with $(c_{i_b})_1 > (c_{i_b})_2$.

4.4 The effective use of a drug is achieved by its controlled release. Diffusion-controlled drug delivery systems are generally classified as reservoir systems and monolithic systems as shown in the figure below (Siepmann and Siepmann, 2008, 2012). Reservoir devices consist of a drug reservoir surrounded by a barrier material, which is usually a polymeric membrane. The drug is released into the surroundings by diffusion through this rate controlling membrane. In the monolithic systems, the drug is embedded in a polymeric matrix. The drug diffuses from the polymer matrix into the surroundings. Both systems may be in the shape of a slab, cylinder, or sphere.

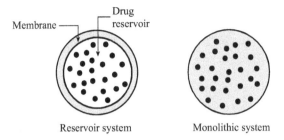

Reservoir system   Monolithic system

Consider a saturated solution containing a large excess of undissolved solute A (drug) encapsulated within a spherical polymeric membrane (B) of inner and outer radii of R_i and R_o, respectively. Note that the diffusion process does not affect the concentration within the reservoir as long as excess drug is present. Show that the maximum molar release rate of the drug is given by

$$\mathcal{W}_A = \frac{4\pi R_i R_o \mathcal{D}_{AB} K_A c_A^{eq}}{R_o - R_i},$$

where K_A is the partition coefficient and c_A^{eq} is the saturation solubility of A in the solution.

4.5 Two very large tanks are connected by capillary tubes with different diameters as shown in the figure below. Both tanks contain gases A and B with compositions $y_A^L > y_A^R$ and $y_B^R > y_B^L$. The pressure and temperature throughout the system are uniform. Show that the molar transfer rate of species A is given by

$$\mathcal{W}_A = \frac{\pi}{4}\left(\frac{L_1}{D_1^2} + \frac{L_2}{D_2^2}\right)^{-1} c\mathcal{D}_{AB}(y_A^L - y_A^R)$$

4.6 Consider diffusion with a heterogeneous chemical reaction as described in Section 4.5.

a) Rewrite Eq. (4.124) in terms of the dimensionless flux, $\overline{N}_A$, defined by

$$\overline{N}_A = \frac{N_{A_z}}{ck_1''}$$

and calculate its value for $y_{A_o} = 0.8$ and $\Lambda^2 = k_1'' \delta / \mathcal{D}_{AB} = 5$.

b) Show that the concentration distribution is given by

$$y_A = 2\left[1 - (1 - 0.5 y_{A_o})\exp\left(\frac{\overline{N}_A \Lambda^2}{2}\xi\right)\right],$$

where ξ is the dimensionless distance defined by $\xi = z/L$. Plot y_A versus ξ when $y_{A_o} = 0.8$ and $\Lambda^2 = 5$.

(Answer: a) 0.169)

4.7 Repeat the analysis given in Section 4.5 for the following first-order heterogeneous reaction:

$$A \rightarrow B$$

Show that the molar flux of species A through the gas film is given by

$$N_{A_z}\big|_{\xi=0} = \frac{k_1'' c_{A_o}}{1+\Omega},$$

where

$$\Omega = \frac{\delta k_1''}{\mathcal{D}_{AB}}$$

4.8 Repeat the analysis given in Section 4.6 for the zeroth-order reaction in the following way:

a) Show that the concentration distribution is given by

$$\theta = 1 + \Lambda^2 \left(\frac{\xi^2}{2} - \xi \right), \tag{1}$$

where the dimensionless quantities are defined by

$$\theta = \frac{\langle c_A \rangle}{c_{A_o}} \qquad \xi = \frac{z}{L} \qquad \Lambda = \sqrt{\frac{2 k_o'' L^2}{R \mathcal{D}_{AB} c_{A_o}}} \tag{2}$$

The solution given by Eq. (1) is valid only for $\Lambda \leq \sqrt{2}$. Why?

b) For $\Lambda > \sqrt{2}$, only a fraction ϕ $(0 < \phi < 1)$ of the surface is available for the chemical reaction. Under these circumstances, show that the concentration distribution is given by

$$\theta = 1 + \Lambda^2 \left(\frac{\xi^2}{2} - \phi \xi \right) \qquad 0 \leq \xi \leq \phi \tag{3}$$

4.9 Species A diffuses into a cylindrical catalyst pellet of radius R and length L $(L \gg R)$ in the radial direction and undergoes a first-order irreversible reaction on the interior surface of the catalyst. The concentration of species A at the outer surface of the cylinder, c_{A_R}, is known.

a) Start with Eq. (4.167) and show that the dimensionless governing equation and its boundary conditions are given as

$$\frac{d}{d\xi} \left(\xi \frac{d\theta}{d\xi} \right) - \Lambda^2 \theta = 0$$

$$\xi = 0 \qquad \frac{d\theta}{d\xi} = 0 \qquad \text{or} \qquad \theta \text{ is finite}$$

$$\xi = 1 \qquad \theta = 1,$$

where

$$\theta = \frac{c_A}{c_{A_R}} \qquad \xi = \frac{r}{R} \qquad \Lambda^2 = \frac{a_v k_1'' R^2}{\mathcal{D}_{eff}}$$

b) Show that the dimensionless concentration distribution is given by

$$\theta = \frac{I_0(\Lambda \xi)}{I_0(\Lambda)}$$

c) Show that the molar flow rate of species A entering the catalyst particle through the lateral surface is

$$\mathcal{W}_A = -2\pi L \mathcal{D}_{eff} c_{A_R} \Lambda \frac{I_1(\Lambda)}{I_0(\Lambda)}$$

What does the minus sign signify?

d) Show that the effectiveness factor is given by

$$\eta = \frac{2}{\Lambda} \frac{I_1(\Lambda)}{I_0(\Lambda)}$$

4.10 A conical capillary tube of length L is closed at one end. While the closed end is coated with a catalyst, the open end is exposed to a binary gas mixture of A and B having a constant composition of y_A^* as shown in the figure below.

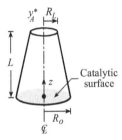

An irreversible first-order reaction, i.e.,

$$A \rightarrow B,$$

takes place on the catalyst surface. Assuming a rapid reaction, ideal gas mixture, isothermal condition, and constant total pressure along the capillary tube, show that the molar rate of consumption of species A under steady conditions, $\mathcal{W}_A$, is given by

$$\mathcal{W}_A = \frac{\pi R_o R_L c \mathcal{D}_{AB} y_A^*}{L}$$

4.11 Repeat Problem 4.10 for the reaction

$$A \rightarrow 2B$$

and show that the molar rate of consumption of species A under steady conditions, $\mathcal{W}_A$, is given by

$$\mathcal{W}_A = \frac{\pi R_o R_L c \mathcal{D}_{AB} \ln(1 + y_A^*)}{L}$$

In which reaction is the molar rate of consumption of species A greater? Why?

4.12 Tooth color is an important aspect of aesthetics. In that respect, dental whitening is a frequently used method to obtain sparkling white teeth. Dental whiteners are bleaching agents, such as hydrogen peroxide or carbamide peroxide, that diffuse into the tooth and react with stain molecules.

Human teeth mainly consist of two parts. The outer part of the tooth is called the enamel. The layer underneath the enamel is the dentin. Studies have shown that tooth color is predominantly determined by the properties of the dentin.

Consider one-dimensional diffusion of a bleaching agent (species A) through a dentin (species B) layer of thickness δ. As it diffuses, it also undergoes a first-order reaction with a rate constant k_1'''. While the concentration at $z = 0$ is c_{A_o}, its value drops to zero at $z = \delta$.

a) Show that the concentration distribution is given as

$$\theta = \frac{\sinh\left[\Lambda(1 - \xi)\right]}{\sinh\Lambda},$$

where the dimensionless quantities are defined by

$$\theta = \frac{c_A}{c_{A_o}} \qquad \xi = \frac{z}{\delta} \qquad \Lambda^2 = \frac{k_1'''\,\delta^2}{\mathcal{D}_{AB}},$$

b) Show that the molar flux of a bleaching agent entering the dentin layer is expressed in the form

$$N_{A_z}\big|_{z=0} = \left(\frac{\mathcal{D}_{AB}c_{A_o}}{\delta}\right)\Lambda\coth\Lambda$$

c) What happens when $\Lambda \to 0$?

4.13 Species A diffuses into a flat biofilm slab and undergoes a zeroth-order chemical reaction. The surface of the biofilm is exposed to a concentration of c_{A_∞}.

a) Show that the distance, z_c, at which species A is depleted is given by

$$z_c = \sqrt{\frac{2K_A c_{A_\infty}\mathcal{D}_{eff}}{k_o'''}},$$

where K_A is the partition coefficient.

b) Calculate the penetration depth of oxygen into a *Pseudomonas aeruginosa* biofilm using the following data[7]:

$$K_A = 1 \qquad c_{A_\infty} = 6\,\text{mg/L} \qquad \mathcal{D}_{eff} = 1.53 \times 10^{-5}\,\text{cm}^2/\text{s} \qquad k_o''' = 3.1\,\text{mg/L.s}$$

(Answer: $0.77\,\mu\text{m}$)

4.14 Consider the diffusion and reaction inside a spherical catalyst as given in Section 4.7. Solve Eq. (4.178) using the method of Laplace transform.

4.15 A long polymeric rod of radius R is subjected to high temperatures and ultraviolet light for a prolonged period. As a result, the following irreversible zeroth-order depolymerization reaction takes place within the rod:

$$P \to M + A$$

a) Under steady conditions, write down the governing equation for species A and its associated boundary conditions in terms of the following dimensionless quantities:

$$\theta = \frac{c_A}{c_A^{eq}} \qquad \xi = \frac{r}{R} \qquad \Lambda = \frac{k_o'''R^2}{4\mathcal{D}_{AB}c_A^{eq}},$$

---

[7]This problem is taken from Stewart (2003).

where k_o''' is the zeroth-order reaction rate constant in $\text{mol/m}^3.\text{s}$ and c_A^{eq} is the known equilibrium concentration of species A at the surface of the rod.

b) Show that the concentration distribution is given by

$$\theta = 1 + \Lambda(1 - \xi^2)$$

c) What would be the concentration distribution of species A when $\Lambda \ll 1$?

4.16 Krogh's cylinder[8] is generally used for the mathematical modeling of oxygen transport from blood to tissues. In this model, a tissue is considered to be composed of long cylindrical units, each surrounding a capillary in which blood flows. A schematic of a single Krogh's cylinder is shown in the figure below.

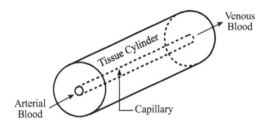

In the model, no exchange of oxygen is assumed between the adjacent cylindrical units.
a) Once the oxygen (species A) is transferred into the tissue, it diffuses radially and is depleted by an irreversible first-order reaction. For the geometry shown below, show that the governing equation and its boundary conditions are written as

$$\frac{\mathcal{D}_{AB}}{r} \frac{d}{dr} \left(r \frac{dc_A}{dr} \right) - k_1''' c_A = 0 \tag{1}$$

$$\text{at} \quad r = R_o \qquad c_A = K_A c_A^b \tag{2}$$

$$\text{at} \quad r = R_1 \qquad \frac{dc_A}{dr} = 0, \tag{3}$$

where c_A^b is the concentration of oxygen in the blood flowing through the capillary and K_A is the partition coefficient.

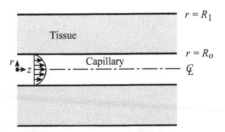

b) Using the dimensionless quantities

$$\theta = \frac{c_A}{K_A c_A^b} \qquad \xi = \frac{r}{R_o} \qquad \Lambda^2 = \frac{k_1''' R_o^2}{\mathcal{D}_{AB}} \qquad \kappa = \frac{R_i}{R_o} \tag{4}$$

---

[8]Schack August Steenberg Krogh, Danish physiologist, was the recipient of the Nobel Prize in Medicine in 1920.

express Eqs. (1)–(3) in dimensionless form.

c) Show that the concentration distribution is expressed as

$$\theta = C_1 I_o(\Lambda\xi) + C_2 K_o(\Lambda\xi),\tag{5}$$

where I_o and K_o are the modified Bessel functions of the first and second kind, respectively, of order zero, and the constants C_1 and C_2 are given by

$$C_1 = \frac{K_1(\Lambda\kappa)}{I_o(\Lambda)K_1(\Lambda\kappa) + I_1(\Lambda\kappa)K_o(\Lambda)}\tag{6}$$

$$C_2 = \frac{I_1(\Lambda\kappa)}{I_o(\Lambda)K_1(\Lambda\kappa) + I_1(\Lambda\kappa)K_o(\Lambda)}\tag{7}$$

d) If the oxygen concentration reaches a critical value, $c_{A_{cr}}$, below which the tissue dies at $r = R_{cr}$, a necrotic tissue will form in the region $R_{cr} \leq r \leq R_1$ as shown in the figure below.

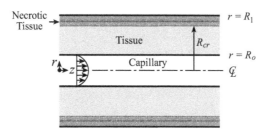

Obtain the concentration distribution for this case.

REFERENCES

Burchard, J. K. and H. L. Toor. 1962. Diffusion in an ideal mixture of three completely miscible non-electrolytic liquids–Toluene, chlorobenzene, bromobenzene. *J. Phys. Chem.* 66(10): 2015–22.

Kwon, K. C., T. H. Ibrahim, Y. K. Park and C. M. Simmons. 2002. Inexpensive and simple binary molecular diffusion experiments. *Chem. Eng. Ed.* 36(1): 68–73.

Moon, P. and D. E. Spencer. 1961. *Field Theory Handbook*. Berlin: Springer.

Siepmann, J. and F. Siepmann. 2008. Mathematical modeling of drug delivery. *Int. J. Pharm.* 264:328–43.

Siepmann, J. and F. Siepmann. 2012. Modeling of diffusion controlled drug delivery. *J. Control. Release* 161:351–62.

Stewart, P. S. 2003. Diffusion in biofilms. *J. Bacteriol.* 185(5):1485–91.

Tosun, I. 2007. Modeling in Transport Phenomena-A Conceptual Approach. 2nd edn. Amsterdam: Elsevier.

Whitaker, S. 1991. Role of the species momentum equation in the analysis of the Stefan diffusion tube. *Ind. Eng. Chem. Res.* 30(5):978–83.

5 Mass Transfer in Binary Systems without Bulk Flow: Pseudosteady-State Examples

In engineering analysis, the neglect of the unsteady-state term is often referred to as *pseudosteady-state* (or *quasi-steady-state*) approximation. In this chapter, first the criterion for using such approximation is developed and then its application to several cases is presented with example problems. The use of pseudosteady-state approximation requires the molar (or mass) flux of species to be known at the system boundary. If the molar flux expression cannot be obtained from the solution of the species continuity equation, then it is expressed with the help of Newton's law of mass transfer. This approach, however, introduces another unknown quantity, called the mass transfer coefficient, that can be obtained from the engineering correlations. Some of the available mass transfer correlations in different geometries are also presented.

5.1 PSEUDOSTEADY-STATE APPROXIMATION

The physical significance of each term in the equation of continuity for species A, Eq. (2.169), is given as

$$\underbrace{\frac{\partial c_A}{\partial t}}_{\substack{\text{Unsteady-state}\\ \text{(Accumulation)}}} + \underbrace{\mathbf{v} \cdot \nabla c_A}_{\text{Convection}} = \underbrace{\mathcal{D}_{AB} \nabla^2 c_A}_{\text{Diffusion}} + \underbrace{\mathcal{R}_A}_{\text{Reaction}} \qquad (5.1)$$

The order of magnitude estimates of the unsteady-state and diffusive terms are

$$\text{Unsteady-state term} \sim O\left[\frac{(\Delta c_A)_{ch}}{t_{ch}^D}\right] \qquad \text{Diffusive term} \sim O\left[\mathcal{D}_{AB}\frac{(\Delta c_A)_{ch}}{L_{ch}^2}\right], \qquad (5.2)$$

where $(\Delta c_A)_{ch}$, t_{ch}^D, and L_{ch} represent the characteristic concentration difference of species A, characteristic time for diffusion, and characteristic diffusion length, respectively. Since each process experiences an unsteady-state period before reaching steady-state conditions, during this transition period, unsteady-state and diffusive transport terms must have the same order of magnitude, i.e.,

$$O\left[\frac{(\Delta c)_{ch}}{t_{ch}^D}\right] = O\left[\mathcal{D}_{AB}\frac{(\Delta c)_{ch}}{L_{ch}^2}\right] \qquad (5.3)$$

Therefore, the time it takes for a given process to reach steady-state is

$$\boxed{t_{ch}^D = \frac{L_{ch}^2}{\mathcal{D}_{AB}}} \qquad (5.4)$$

The term t_{ch}^D is also referred to as the *diffusion timescale*. According to Eq. (5.4), diffusion time increases with the square of diffusion distance and is inversely proportional to the diffusion coefficient.

Example 5.1[1]   Most living organisms need oxygen for the oxidation of glucose to produce carbon dioxide and water with the concomitant release of chemical energy. The *Amoeba proteus* is a unicellular organism about $250\,\mu$m in diameter. It is commonly found on decaying bottom vegetation of freshwater ponds and streams. Taking the diffusion coefficient of oxygen in water as $1.8 \times 10^{-5}\text{cm}^2/$s, the time for oxygen to reach the center of an *Amoeba proteus* by diffusion is

$$t_{ch}^D = \frac{(125 \times 10^{-4})^2}{1.8 \times 10^{-5}} \simeq 9\text{s},$$

which is quite fast.

Now let us assume that the body of a rhino is spherical with a diameter of 1.5 m. In this case, the time for oxygen to reach the center of a rhino by diffusion is

$$t_{ch}^D = \frac{(75)^2}{1.8 \times 10^{-5}} = 3.125 \times 10^8\text{s} \simeq 10 \text{ years}$$

Therefore, diffusion alone cannot provide the necessary oxygen for a rhino's cells. The respiratory system provides the necessary oxygen by bulk flow. This is the reason why rhinos have the lungs and amoebas do not.

When the timescale of the system, t_{sys}, is much larger than the diffusion timescale, i.e.,

$$t_{sys} \gg \frac{L_{ch}^2}{\mathcal{D}_{AB}} \qquad \Longrightarrow \qquad \boxed{\frac{t_{sys}\mathcal{D}_{AB}}{L_{ch}^2} \gg 1,} \qquad (5.5)$$

it is plausible to neglect the unsteady-state (or accumulation) term, even though the process itself is unsteady. In engineering analysis, this is called *pseudosteady-state* approximation. The procedure for pseudosteady-state analysis is as follows:

- Neglect the unsteady state condition(s), and obtain the mass (or molar) flux at the interface either from the solution of the species continuity equation or from Newton's law of mass transfer.
- Assume that the resulting flux expression holds at any instant of time.
- Write the macroscopic mass balance for the species in question over the volume of the system of interest in the form

$$\begin{pmatrix} \text{Rate of} \\ \text{mass in} \end{pmatrix} - \begin{pmatrix} \text{Rate of} \\ \text{mass out} \end{pmatrix} + \begin{pmatrix} \text{Rate of mass} \\ \text{generation} \end{pmatrix} = \begin{pmatrix} \text{Rate of mass} \\ \text{accumulation} \end{pmatrix} \qquad (5.6)$$

- Insert the flux expression into Eq. (5.6), and solve the resulting ordinary differential equation.

5.2 MASS TRANSFER COEFFICIENT

In engineering problems related to mass transfer, we are interested in the amount (mass or mole) of a specific species transferred to or from the system of interest through its boundaries. Accomplishment of this task requires the following four-step procedure:

- Solve the species continuity equation to express the concentration of species as a function of position and time.

---

[1]The idea for this example was taken from Math Bench (*mathbench.umd.edu*).

- Differentiate the concentration distribution with respect to position, and evaluate its value at the system boundary to obtain an expression for the flux of species.
- Integrate the flux expression over the surface area of the system to obtain an expression for the flow rate of species through the boundaries.
- Integrate the flow rate over time to obtain the amount of species.

An analytical/numerical solution of the species continuity equation, however, is not possible most of the time. In that case, flux of species is determined with the help of Newton's law of mass transfer defined by Eq. (1.30). For species A, it is expressed as

$$N_A|_{int} = k_c (\Delta c_A)_{ch}, \tag{5.7}$$

where k_c is the mass transfer coefficient and $(\Delta c_A)_{ch}$ is the characteristic concentration difference for species A. The mass transfer coefficient is obtained from the experimental information, which is usually expressed in terms of engineering correlations. These correlations, however, are limited to a specific geometry, equipment configuration, boundary conditions, and substance.

5.2.1 PHYSICAL INTERPRETATION OF THE MASS TRANSFER COEFFICIENT

A uniform stream of fluid B, such as air, is flowing with a velocity v_∞ over a flat plate, the upper surface of which is coated with species A. The concentration of species A in the flowing stream is $c_{A\infty}$ and the concentration of species A at the surface of the plate is c_A^{eq} as shown in Figure 5.1.

The total molar flux of species A at the wall surface is the sum of the diffusive and convective fluxes, i.e.,

$$N_{A_x}|_{x=0} = -\mathcal{D}_{AB} \left. \frac{\partial c_A}{\partial x} \right|_{x=0} + c_A^{eq} v_x^*|_{x=0}, \tag{5.8}$$

where the molar-average velocity is given by

$$v_x^* = \frac{c_A v_{A_x} + c_B v_{B_x}}{c} \tag{5.9}$$

The value of $v_{B_x}|_{x=0}$ is zero due to the no-slip boundary condition at the wall. However, the transfer of species A from the wall to the flowing stream is possible only if $v_{A_x}|_{x=0}$ is nonzero. As a result, $v_x^* \neq 0$ and the convective term in Eq. (5.8) does not automatically vanish at the wall. Under the conditions of *low mass transfer rates*, it is plausible to assume

$$O\left(-\mathcal{D}_{AB} \left. \frac{\partial c_A}{\partial x} \right|_{x=0} \right) \gg O\left(c_A^{eq} v_x^*|_{x=0} \right) \tag{5.10}$$

and simplify Eq. (5.8) to

$$N_{A_x}|_{x=0} = -\mathcal{D}_{AB} \left. \frac{\partial c_A}{\partial x} \right|_{x=0} \tag{5.11}$$

For flow over a flat plate, Eq. (5.7) is written as

$$N_{A_x}|_{x=0} = k_c (c_A^{eq} - c_{A\infty}) \tag{5.12}$$

Combination of Eqs. (5.11) and (5.12) leads to

$$k_c = -\frac{\mathcal{D}_{AB}}{c_A^{eq} - c_{A\infty}} \left. \frac{\partial c_A}{\partial x} \right|_{x=0} \tag{5.13}$$

When the evaluation of the concentration gradient at the wall is not possible, the problem is idealized as shown in Figure 5.1. In the idealized case, which is known as the *film model*, the entire resistance

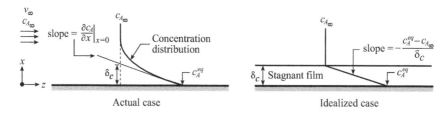

Figure 5.1 The film model for mass transfer.

to mass transfer is assumed to be confined to a stagnant film in the fluid next to the wall. The thickness of the film, δ_c, is such that it provides the same resistance to mass transfer by diffusion as the resistance that exists for the actual process. As a result, the concentration gradient in the film is constant and equal to

$$-\left.\frac{\partial c_A}{\partial x}\right|_{x=0} = \frac{c_A^{eq} - c_{A_\infty}}{\delta_c} \tag{5.14}$$

Substitution of Eq. (5.14) into Eq. (5.13) gives

$$\boxed{k_c = \frac{\mathcal{D}_{AB}}{\delta_c}} \tag{5.15}$$

5.2.2 OTHER DEFINITIONS OF MASS TRANSFER COEFFICIENTS

Cussler (1984), one of the major researchers in the area of mass transfer, complained about the way mass transfer is being taught by instructors and stated that

> "We take a relatively simple subject (mass transfer) and make it a nearly incomprehensible tangle of subscripts, superscripts, unit conversions, dimensionless correlations, correction factors, archaic graphs, and turgidly-written textbooks. We make a mess of it, so students think it is hard."

Since concentration can be defined in different ways, it is not surprising to come across different definitions of the mass transfer coefficient in the literature. Based on the differences in partial pressures and mole fractions, the molar flux can be expressed as

$$N_A|_{int} = k_p (\Delta \overline{P}_A)_{ch} \tag{5.16}$$

and

$$N_A|_{int} = k_x (\Delta x_A)_{ch} \tag{5.17}$$

The relationships between different definitions of mass transfer coefficients are given by

$$k_c = \begin{cases} k_p RT = \dfrac{k_x}{c} & \text{For a gas at constant } T \text{ \& } P \\[2ex] \dfrac{k_p \mathcal{H}_A M_{mix}}{\rho_{mix}} = \dfrac{k_x M_{mix}}{\rho_{mix}} & \text{For a dilute liquid mixture} \end{cases} \tag{5.18}$$

The mass transfer coefficient based on the difference in molar concentration, k_c, defined by Eq. (5.7) will be used throughout this book[2].

---

[2]The three problems presented by Cussler (1984) clearly show the advantage of using k_c as the mass transfer coefficient.

5.2.3 TWO-FILM THEORY

The two-film theory proposed by Lewis (1916) and Whitman (1923) is one of the oldest and most frequently used models for the transfer of solutes from the gas phase to the liquid phase. In this model, the entire resistance to mass transfer is assumed to lie in the two hypothetical films located on either side of the interface as shown in Figure 5.2. Within these two regions, mass transfer takes place only by diffusion under steady conditions.

The molar fluxes of species A in the gas and liquid phases are equal to each other at the interface, i.e.,

$$N_A = k_c^G(c_{A_b}^G - c_{A_{int}}^G) = k_c^L(c_{A_{int}}^L - c_{A_b}^L) \tag{5.19}$$

Equation (5.19) can be expressed as

$$\frac{N_A}{k_c^G} = c_{A_b}^G - c_{A_{int}}^G \tag{5.20}$$

and

$$\frac{N_A}{k_c^L} = c_{A_{int}}^L - c_{A_b}^L \tag{5.21}$$

Assuming thermodynamic equilibrium at the interface, we can relate the concentrations by the use of the partition coefficient in the form

$$K_A = \frac{c_{A_{int}}^G}{c_{A_{int}}^L} \tag{5.22}$$

Addition of Eqs. (5.19)–(5.21) leads to

$$\boxed{N_A = K_T(c_{A_b}^G - K_A c_{A_b}^L),} \tag{5.23}$$

where K_T is the *overall mass transfer coefficient*, defined by

$$\boxed{\frac{1}{K_T} = \frac{1}{k_c^G} + \frac{K_A}{k_c^L}} \tag{5.24}$$

From Eq. (5.23), we see that the appropriate driving force is $(c_{A_b}^G - K_A c_{A_b}^L)$ and not $(c_{A_b}^G - c_{A_b}^L)$. The reason for this is the fact that mass transfer should stop (or the driving force must be zero) when the system reaches equilibrium. Under equilibrium conditions, however, $c_{A_b}^G \neq c_{A_b}^L$.

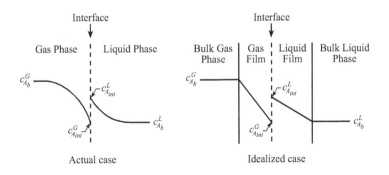

Figure 5.2 Two-film model.

5.3 MASS TRANSFER CORRELATIONS

Mass transfer correlations are given in the form of

$$\text{Sh} = \text{Sh}(\text{Re}, \text{Sc}), \tag{5.25}$$

where the dimensionless numbers are defined in terms of the characteristic length L_{ch} and the characteristic velocity v_{ch} as

$$\text{Sh} = \text{Sherwood number} = \frac{k_c L_{ch}}{\mathcal{D}_{AB}} \tag{5.26}$$

$$\text{Re} = \text{Reynolds number} = \frac{L_{ch} v_{ch} \rho}{\mu} \tag{5.27}$$

$$\text{Sc} = \text{Schmidt number} = \frac{\mu}{\rho \mathcal{D}_{AB}} \tag{5.28}$$

The properties, such as density, viscosity, and diffusion coefficient, that appear in these dimensionless numbers are dependent on temperature and concentration. Therefore, reference temperatures and concentrations should be defined for the evaluation of dimensionless numbers. *Bulk temperature/concentration* and *film temperature/concentration* are two commonly used approaches in the literature.

• Bulk temperature/concentration

For flow inside pipes, the *bulk temperature/concentration* at a particular location in the pipe is the average temperature/concentration if the fluid was thoroughly mixed, sometimes called the *mixing-cup temperature/concentration*. The bulk temperature and concentration are denoted by T_b and c_b, respectively, and are defined by

$$T_b = \frac{\iint_A v_n T \, dA}{\iint_A v_n \, dA} \quad \text{and} \quad c_b = \frac{\iint_A v_n c \, dA}{\iint_A v_n \, dA}, \tag{5.29}$$

where v_n is the component of velocity in the direction of mean flow and A is the area perpendicular to the mean flow.

For the case of flow past bodies immersed in an infinite fluid, the bulk temperature/concentration becomes the free stream temperature/concentration, i.e.,

$$\left. \begin{array}{l} T_b = T_\infty \\ c_b = c_\infty \end{array} \right\} \quad \text{For flow over submerged objects} \tag{5.30}$$

• Film temperature/concentration

The *film temperature and concentration* are denoted by T_f and c_f, respectively, and are defined as the arithmetic averages of the bulk and surface values, i.e.,

$$T_f = \frac{T_b + T_w}{2} \quad \text{and} \quad c_f = \frac{c_b + c_w}{2}, \tag{5.31}$$

where subscript w represents the conditions at the surface or the wall.

Some of the available mass transfer correlations depending on the system geometry are presented below.[3] The values obtained from these correlations are not exact; the error introduced in using

---

[3]The correlations given in Sections 5.3.1–5.3.5 are taken from Tosun (2007). Readers may refer to Cussler (2009) for the mass transfer correlations that are not covered here.

a correlation may be up to $\pm 25\%$. Sometimes more than one correlation may be applicable for the same problem. In these cases, different answers may be obtained depending on the correlation used in the calculations. It is ironic that we still use the correlations obtained at least 50 years ago using quite "primitive" instrumentation compared to existing sophisticated counterparts. In today's "publish or perish" era, researchers are much more interested in fitting "old" data to obtain "better" correlations rather than trying to generate "new" data leading to correlations with higher accuracy.

5.3.1 FLOW OVER A FLAT PLATE

A uniform fluid (species B) of velocity v_∞ and having a concentration of c_{A_∞} is flowing over the top of a flat plate of length L and width W. The top surface of the plate is coated with species A, which has a saturation solubility of c_A^{eq} in fluid B. Using several simplifying assumptions, Blasius (1908) solved the equations of change analytically and obtained the following expressions depending on the flow conditions:

$$\text{Sh} = \begin{cases} 0.664\,\text{Re}^{1/2}\,\text{Sc}^{1/3} & \text{Laminar} & \text{Re} \leq 500,000 \\[2mm] (0.037\,\text{Re}^{4/5} - 871)\,\text{Sc}^{1/3} & \text{Laminar \& Turbulent} & 5 \times 10^5 < \text{Re} < 10^8 \\[2mm] 0.037\,\text{Re}^{4/5}\,\text{Sc}^{1/3} & \text{Turbulent} & \text{Re} > 10^8 \end{cases} \tag{5.32}$$

The characteristic length and the characteristic velocity in the dimensionless numbers are taken as L and v_∞, respectively. All physical properties must be evaluated at the film temperature.

5.3.2 FLOW OVER A SINGLE SPHERE

The following two cases are possible for a single sphere (species A) of radius R immersed in an infinite fluid (species B): (*i*) sphere and fluid are both stationary, and (*ii*) sphere and/or fluid is moving.

• Sphere and fluid are stagnant

Consider the transfer of species A from a spherical solid, drop, or bubble to fluid B having a concentration of c_{A_∞}. The concentration distribution will be determined with the following assumptions:

(*i*)   Steady-state conditions prevail, i.e., mass transfer does not affect the radius.
(*ii*) The saturation solubility of A in fluid B at the outer surface of the sphere is c_A^{eq}.
(*iii*) The diffusion coefficient and the total molar concentration of the fluid are constant.

Postulating one-dimensional mass transport with $N_{A_r} = N_{A_r}(r)$ and $N_{A_\theta} = N_{A_\phi} = 0$, the equation of continuity for species A, Eq. (C) of Table 2.3, simplifies to

$$\frac{d(r^2 N_{A_r})}{dr} = 0 \quad \Rightarrow \quad r^2 N_{A_r} = \text{constant} = R^2\, N_{A_r}|_{r=R} \tag{5.33}$$

From Eq. (2.165), the total molar flux of species A in the r-direction is given by

$$N_{A_r} = -c\mathcal{D}_{AB}\frac{dx_A}{dr} + x_A\left(N_{A_r} + N_{B_r}\right) \tag{5.34}$$

If the convective term is neglected, Eq. (5.34) simplifies to

$$N_{A_r} = -\mathcal{D}_{AB}\frac{dc_A}{dr} \tag{5.35}$$

Substitution of Eq. (5.35) into Eq. (5.33) and rearrangement give

$$-\mathcal{D}_{AB} \int_{c_A^{eq}}^{c_{A\infty}} dc_A = R^2 \, N_{A_r}|_{r=R} \int_R^\infty \frac{dr}{r^2} \tag{5.36}$$

Carrying out the integration yields

$$N_{A_r}|_{r=R} = \frac{\mathcal{D}_{AB}(c_A^{eq} - c_{A\infty})}{R} \tag{5.37}$$

According to Newton's law of mass transfer, the molar flux of species A at the outer surface of the sphere is expressed in terms of the mass transfer coefficient as

$$N_{A_r}|_{r=R} = k_c(c_{A_w} - c_{A\infty}) \tag{5.38}$$

Equating Eqs. (5.37) and (5.38) leads to

$$\frac{k_c}{\mathcal{D}_{AB}} = \frac{1}{R} = \frac{2}{D} \tag{5.39}$$

Therefore, the Sherwood number is

$$\boxed{\mathrm{Sh} = \frac{k_c D}{\mathcal{D}_{AB}} = 2} \tag{5.40}$$

• Sphere and/or fluid is moving

In this case, we may encounter the following three cases: (i) sphere is stagnant, fluid flows over the sphere; (ii) fluid is stagnant, sphere moves through the fluid; and (iii) sphere and fluid are both moving. The characteristic velocity to be used in the dimensionless numbers is either the velocity of the fluid if the sphere is stagnant or the terminal velocity of the sphere if the fluid is stagnant. The characteristic length is the diameter of the sphere.

Ranz–Marshall Correlation

Ranz and Marshall (1952a, 1952b) proposed the following correlation for constant surface composition and low mass transfer rates:

$$\boxed{\mathrm{Sh} = 2 + 0.6 \, \mathrm{Re}^{1/2} \, \mathrm{Sc}^{1/3}} \tag{5.41}$$

Equation (5.41) is valid for

$$2 \leq \mathrm{Re} \leq 200 \qquad \text{and} \qquad 0.6 \leq \mathrm{Sc} \leq 2.7$$

and all physical properties must be evaluated at the film temperature. Note that when $\mathrm{Re} \to 0$, Eq. (5.41) reduces to Eq. (5.40).

Frossling Correlation

The correlation proposed by Frossling (1938),

$$\boxed{\mathrm{Sh} = 2 + 0.552 \, \mathrm{Re}^{1/2} \, \mathrm{Sc}^{1/3},} \tag{5.42}$$

is valid for

$$2 \leq \mathrm{Re} \leq 800 \qquad \text{and} \qquad 0.6 \leq \mathrm{Sc} \leq 2.7$$

Steinberger and Treybal (1960) modified the Frossling correlation as

$$\text{Sh} = 2 + 0.552\,\text{Re}^{0.53}\,\text{Sc}^{1/3}, \tag{5.43}$$

which is valid for

$$1500 \leq \text{Re} \leq 12{,}000 \quad \text{and} \quad 0.6 \leq \text{Sc} \leq 1.85$$

Steinberger–Treybal Correlation

The correlation originally proposed by Steinberger and Treybal (1960) includes a correction term for natural convection. The lack of experimental data, however, makes this term very difficult to calculate in most cases. The effect of natural convection becomes negligible when the Reynolds number is high and the Steinberger–Treybal correlation reduces to

$$\text{Sh} = 0.347\,\text{Re}^{0.62}\,\text{Sc}^{1/3} \tag{5.44}$$

Equation (5.44) is recommended for liquids when

$$2000 \leq \text{Re} \leq 16{,}900$$

5.3.3 FLOW OVER A SINGLE CYLINDER

Consider the flow of a fluid with a velocity of v_∞ over a circular cylinder of diameter D. The characteristic length and the characteristic velocity in the dimensionless numbers are taken as D and v_∞, respectively. All physical properties must be evaluated at the film temperature.

Bedingfield–Drew Correlation

Bedingfield and Drew (1950) proposed the following correlation for cross and parallel flow of gases to the cylinder of diameter D in which mass transfer to or from the ends of the cylinder is not considered:

$$\text{Sh} = 0.281\,\text{Re}^{1/2}\,\text{Sc}^{0.44} \tag{5.45}$$

Equation (5.45) is valid for

$$400 \leq \text{Re} \leq 25{,}000 \quad \text{and} \quad 0.6 \leq \text{Sc} \leq 2.6$$

Linton–Sherwood Correlation

The correlation proposed by Linton and Sherwood (1950) in the form

$$\text{Sh} = 0.281\,\text{Re}^{0.6}\,\text{Sc}^{1/3} \tag{5.46}$$

is suitable for liquids. Equation (5.46) is valid for

$$400 \leq \text{Re} \leq 25{,}000 \quad \text{and} \quad \text{Sc} \leq 3000$$

5.3.4 FLOW IN CIRCULAR PIPES

Mass transfer in cylindrical tubes is encountered in a variety of operations such as wetted wall columns, reverse osmosis, and cross-flow ultrafiltration. Mass transfer correlations depend on whether the flow is laminar or turbulent. The characteristic length and the characteristic velocity in the dimensionless numbers are taken as the diameter of the pipe and the average velocity, respectively. All physical properties must be evaluated at the mean bulk temperature.

• Laminar flow correlation

For laminar flow mass transfer in a circular tube with constant wall concentration

$$\mathrm{Sh} = 1.86 \left[\mathrm{Re}\,\mathrm{Sc}\,(D/L) \right]^{1/3} \tag{5.47}$$

Equation (5.47) is valid for

$$[\mathrm{Re}\,\mathrm{Sc}\,(D/L)]^{1/3} \geq 2$$

• Turbulent flow correlations

Gilliland–Sherwood Correlation

Gilliland and Sherwood (1934) correlated the experimental results obtained from wetted wall columns in the form

$$\mathrm{Sh} = 0.023\,\mathrm{Re}^{0.83}\,\mathrm{Sc}^{0.44}, \tag{5.48}$$

which is valid for

$$2000 \leq \mathrm{Re} \leq 35{,}000 \qquad \text{and} \qquad 0.6 \leq \mathrm{Sc} \leq 2.5$$

Linton–Sherwood correlation

The correlation proposed by Linton and Sherwood (1950) is given by

$$\mathrm{Sh} = 0.023\,\mathrm{Re}^{0.83}\,\mathrm{Sc}^{1/3} \tag{5.49}$$

Equation (5.49) is valid for

$$2000 \leq \mathrm{Re} \leq 70{,}000 \qquad \text{and} \qquad 0.6 \leq \mathrm{Sc} \leq 2500$$

5.3.5 FLOW IN PACKED BEDS

The chemical and energy industries deal predominantly with multiphase and multicomponent systems in which considerable attention is devoted to increasing the interfacial contact between the phases to enhance property transfers and chemical reactions at these extended surface interfaces. As a result, packed beds are extensively used in the chemical process industries. Some examples are gas absorption, catalytic reactors, and deep bed filtration.

Dwivedi and Upadhyay (1977) proposed a single correlation for both gases and liquids in packed and fluidized beds in terms of the j-factor as

$$\varepsilon\, j_{M_{pb}} = \frac{0.765}{(\mathrm{Re}_{pb}^*)^{0.82}} + \frac{0.365}{(\mathrm{Re}_{pb}^*)^{0.386}}, \tag{5.50}$$

which is valid for $0.01 \leq \mathrm{Re}_{pb}^* \leq 15{,}000$. While the term ε in Eq. (5.50) is the porosity (or void volume fraction) of the packed bed, the terms $j_{M_{pb}}$ and Re_{pb}^* are defined by

$$j_{M_{pb}} = \left(\frac{k_c}{v_o} \right) \mathrm{Sc}^{2/3} \qquad \text{and} \qquad \mathrm{Re}_{pb}^* = \frac{D_P v_o \rho}{\mu}, \tag{5.51}$$

where v_o is the superficial velocity[4] of the fluid passing through the packed bed and D_P is the diameter of the packing material.

---

[4]Superficial velocity is obtained by dividing the volumetric flow rate of the fluid passing through the packed bed by the total cross-sectional area of the packed bed.

5.3.6 SOLID–LIQUID SUSPENSIONS IN AGITATED TANKS

The rate of mass transfer from or to solid particles suspended in agitated liquids is dependent on many factors, such as impeller characteristics; particle size, shape, and concentration; and whether the tank is baffled or not. An excellent review on the topic is provided by Pangarkar et al. (2002). Numerous correlations proposed to evaluate the mass transfer coefficient can be classified into three groups based on the definition of the Reynolds number.

• Reynolds number based on Kolmogoroff's theory of isotropic turbulence

In this case, the Reynolds number is defined as

$$\text{Re}_K = \frac{D_p^{4/3} \varepsilon^{1/3} \rho}{\mu}, \tag{5.52}$$

where D_p is the particle diameter and ε represents the rate of energy dissipation defined by

$$\varepsilon = \frac{P}{M_L}, \tag{5.53}$$

in which P is the impeller power input and M_L is the mass of the liquid in the tank.

Asai et al. (1988) proposed the empirical correlation

$$\text{Sh} = \left[2^{5.8} + \left(0.61 \, \text{Re}_K^{0.58} \, \text{Sc}^{1/3} \right)^{5.8} \right]^{1/5.8}, \tag{5.54}$$

which is valid for

$$0.0229 \le \text{Re}_K \le 495 \qquad \text{and} \qquad 269 \le \text{Sc} \le 11,300$$

• Reynolds number based on slip velocity

Slip velocity is defined as the difference between bulk liquid velocity and the terminal settling velocity of particles. The correlation proposed by Miller (1971) is given by

$$\text{Sh} = 0.0267 \left(2 + 1.10 \, \text{Re}_s^{1/2} \, \text{Sc}^{1/3} \right) N^{0.626}, \tag{5.55}$$

where N is the impeller rotational speed in revolutions per minute (rpm) and Re_s is defined as

$$\text{Re}_s = \frac{D_p v_s \rho}{\mu}, \tag{5.56}$$

in which the slip velocity v_s is related to the terminal velocity v_t as

$$\frac{v_s}{v_t} = 0.644 \times 10^{-3} N^{1.239} \tag{5.57}$$

• Reynolds number based on impeller speed

In this case, two types of Reynolds number are encountered in the correlations: Reynolds number based on impeller diameter, Re_N, and Reynolds number based on tank diameter, Re_T. They are defined as

$$\text{Re}_N = \frac{N D_i^2 \rho}{\mu} \qquad \text{and} \qquad \text{Re}_T = \frac{N D_T^2 \rho}{\mu}, \tag{5.58}$$

where D_i is the impeller diameter, N is the impeller rotational speed, and D_T is the tank diameter. Kulov et al. (1983) proposed the correlation

$$\text{Sh} = 0.267\,\text{Re}_N^{3/4}\,\text{Sc}^{1/4}\,N_P^{1/4}\left(\frac{D_T^4}{VD_i}\right)^4, \tag{5.59}$$

where V is the volume of liquid in the tank and the power number, N_P, is defined by

$$N_P = \frac{P}{\rho N^3 D_i^5}, \tag{5.60}$$

in which P is the impeller power input. The characteristic length in the Sherwood number is taken as the tank diameter.

5.3.7 HOLLOW FIBER GEOMETRIES

Depending on the geometry, Wickramasinghe et al. (1992) provided the following correlations:

- **Flow inside hollow fibers**

$$\boxed{\text{Sh} = 1.62\,\text{Gz}} \qquad \text{Gz} > 4 \tag{5.61}$$

The dimensionless *Graetz number*, Gz, is defined by

$$\text{Gz} = \text{Re}\,\text{Sc}\left(\frac{d}{L}\right), \tag{5.62}$$

where d and L are the fiber diameter and fiber length, respectively. The characteristic length in the Reynolds number is the fiber diameter.

- **Flow outside and parallel to hollow fibers**

$$\boxed{\text{Sh} = 0.019\,\text{Gr}} \qquad \text{Gz} < 60 \tag{5.63}$$

The dimensionless *Graetz number*, Gz, is defined by

$$\text{Gz} = \text{Re}\,\text{Sc}\left(\frac{D_h}{L}\right), \tag{5.64}$$

where D_h is the *hydraulic equivalent diameter*, defined by

$$D_h = 4\left(\frac{\text{Flow area}}{\text{Wetted perimeter}}\right) \tag{5.65}$$

The characteristic length in the Reynolds number is the hydraulic equivalent diameter.

- **Flow outside and across hollow fibers**

$$\text{Sh} = \begin{cases} 0.15\,\text{Re}^{0.8}\,\text{Sc}^{0.33} & \text{Re} > 2.5 \\ 0.12\,\text{Re}\,\text{Sc}^{0.33} & \text{Re} < 2.5 \end{cases} \tag{5.66}$$

The Graetz number is defined by Eq. (5.64).

5.4 DIAPHRAGM CELL

One of the most classical and easiest ways of measuring binary diffusion coefficients in liquid systems is to use a diaphragm cell. A diaphragm cell consists of two well-stirred chambers of known volumes separated by a sintered glass diaphragm (or membrane) as shown in Figure 5.3. Solutions of different and known compositions are placed in the chambers, and the variations in concentrations are measured as a function of time.

For a membrane of thickness L separating two liquids with constant concentrations of c_A^L and c_A^R ($c_A^L > c_A^R$), the steady-state concentration distribution is shown to be linear in Section 4.1.1. The use of Eq. (4.16) gives the molar flux as

$$N_{A_z} = K_A \mathcal{D}_{AB} \left(\frac{c_A^L - c_A^R}{L} \right) \tag{5.67}$$

The first step in the pseudosteady-state analysis is to assume that the steady-state value of the molar flux holds at any instant of time. Thus,

$$N_{A_z}(t) = K_A \mathcal{D}_{AB} \left[\frac{c_A^L(t) - c_A^R(t)}{L} \right] \tag{5.68}$$

Choosing the left chamber as the system, the macroscopic mass balance for species A is

$$-\left(\begin{array}{c} \text{Rate of} \\ \text{mass } A \text{ out} \end{array} \right) = \left(\begin{array}{c} \text{Rate of accumulation} \\ \text{of mass } A \end{array} \right) \tag{5.69}$$

or

$$-\left[K_A \mathcal{D}_{AB} \left(\frac{c_A^L - c_A^R}{L} \right) \right] A = \frac{d}{dt} \left(V_L c_A^L \right), \tag{5.70}$$

where A is the effective cross-sectional area of the diaphragm and V_L is the volume of the chamber on the left. Rearrangement of Eq. (5.70) yields

$$\frac{dc_A^L}{dt} = -\frac{K_A \mathcal{D}_{AB} A}{L V_L} (c_A^L - c_A^R) \tag{5.71}$$

Now let us choose the right chamber as the system. The macroscopic mass balance for species A is expressed as

$$\left(\begin{array}{c} \text{Rate of} \\ \text{mass } A \text{ in} \end{array} \right) = \left(\begin{array}{c} \text{Rate of accumulation} \\ \text{of mass } A \end{array} \right) \tag{5.72}$$

or

$$\left[K_A \mathcal{D}_{AB} \left(\frac{c_A^L - c_A^R}{L} \right) \right] A = \frac{d}{dt} \left(V_R c_A^R \right), \tag{5.73}$$

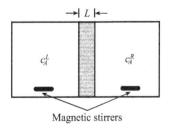

Figure 5.3 A diaphragm cell.

where V_R is the volume of the chamber on the right. Rearrangement of Eq. (5.73) gives

$$\frac{dc_A^R}{dt} = \frac{K_A \mathcal{D}_{AB} A}{L V_R}(c_A^L - c_A^R) \tag{5.74}$$

Subtraction of Eq. (5.74) from Eq. (5.71) gives

$$\frac{d(c_A^L - c_A^R)}{dt} = -\beta K_A \mathcal{D}_{AB}(c_A^L - c_A^R), \tag{5.75}$$

where β is the so-called *diaphragm cell constant*, defined by

$$\beta = \frac{A}{L}\left(\frac{1}{V_L} + \frac{1}{V_R}\right) \tag{5.76}$$

Integration gives

$$\int_{c_{A_o}^L - c_{A_o}^R}^{c_A^L - c_A^R} \frac{d(c_A^L - c_A^R)}{c_A^L - c_A^R} = -\beta K_A \mathcal{D}_{AB} \int_0^t dt \tag{5.77}$$

or

$$\mathcal{D}_{AB} = \frac{1}{\beta K_A t} \ln\left(\frac{c_{A_o}^L - c_{A_o}^R}{c_A^L - c_A^R}\right), \tag{5.78}$$

where $c_{A_o}^L$ and $c_{A_o}^R$ are the initial concentrations of species A in the left and right chambers, respectively. The value of $\mathcal{D}_{AB}$ calculated from Eq. (5.78) is called the *integral diffusion coefficient*. It is an average value for the concentration range.

5.4.1 VALIDITY OF THE PSEUDOSTEADY-STATE APPROXIMATION

The timescale of the system, t_{sys}, is

$$t_{sys} \sim O\left(\frac{1}{\beta K_A \mathcal{D}_{AB}}\right) \tag{5.79}$$

Substitution of Eq. (5.79) into Eq. (5.5) gives the criterion for the pseudosteady-state approximation as

$$A L K_A\left(\frac{1}{V_L} + \frac{1}{V_R}\right) \ll 1 \tag{5.80}$$

5.5 STEFAN DIFFUSION PROBLEM

One way of measuring the diffusion coefficients of vapors is to place a small amount of liquid in a vertical capillary, generally known as the Stefan diffusion tube, and to blow a gas stream of known composition across the top as shown in Figure 5.4. The diffusion coefficient can be estimated by observing the decrease in the liquid–gas interface as a function of time. This problem was solved in Section 4.3 by assuming that the liquid level does not change as a result of evaporation, and the molar transfer rate of species A was calculated by Eq. (4.92) as

$$N_{A_z} = \frac{c \mathcal{D}_{AB}}{L} \ln\left(\frac{1}{1 - y_{A_o}}\right) \tag{5.81}$$

Since the liquid level drops as a result of evaporation, the unsteady-state problem at hand will be solved by pseudosteady-state analysis.

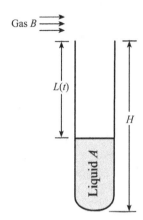

Figure 5.4 The Stefan diffusion tube.

The first step in pseudosteady-state analysis is to assume that the steady-state value of the molar flux holds at any instant, i.e.,

$$N_{A_z}(t) = \frac{cD_{AB}}{L(t)} \ln\left(\frac{1}{1 - y_{A_o}}\right) \tag{5.82}$$

Choosing liquid A within the capillary as a system, the macroscopic mass balance is expressed as

$$-\left(\begin{array}{c}\text{Rate of} \\ \text{mass } A \text{ out}\end{array}\right) = \left(\begin{array}{c}\text{Rate of accumulation} \\ \text{of mass } A\end{array}\right) \tag{5.83}$$

or

$$-\underbrace{\left[\frac{cD_{AB}}{L(t)} \ln\left(\frac{1}{1 - y_{A_o}}\right)\right]}_{N_{A_z}} AM_A = \frac{d}{dt}\left[(H - L)A\rho_A^L\right], \tag{5.84}$$

where ρ_A^L is the density of species A in the liquid phase, A is the cross-sectional area of the capillary, and M_A is the molecular weight of species A. Rearrangement of Eq. (5.84) gives

$$cD_{AB}M_A \ln\left(\frac{1}{1 - y_{A_o}}\right) \int_0^t dt = \rho_A^L \int_{L_o}^L L \, dL \tag{5.85}$$

or

$$L^2 = \left[\frac{2cD_{AB}M_A}{\rho_A^L} \ln\left(\frac{1}{1 - y_{A_o}}\right)\right] t + L_o^2 \tag{5.86}$$

Therefore, the diffusion coefficient is determined from the slope of the L^2 versus t plot.
Alternatively, rearrangement of Eq. (5.86) yields

$$\frac{t}{L - L_o} = \left[\frac{\rho_A^L}{2M_A c D_{AB} \ln\left(\frac{1}{1 - y_{A_o}}\right)}\right](L - L_o) - \frac{\rho_A^L L_o}{M_A c D_{AB} \ln\left(\frac{1}{1 - y_{A_o}}\right)} \tag{5.87}$$

In this case, the diffusion coefficient is determined from the slope of the $t/(L - L_o)$ versus $(L - L_o)$ plot. What is the advantage of using Eq. (5.87) over Eq. (5.86)?

Since continuous detection of the change in the liquid level is rather difficult and subject to experimental error, Kwon et al. (2002) placed the Stefan tube on a scale and recorded the mass of the liquid as a function of time. The relationship between the initial mass of the liquid, m_o, and the mass of the liquid at any given time, m, is given by

$$m - m_o = A \rho_A^L (L_o - L) \tag{5.88}$$

and Eq. (5.86) is expressed as

$$\boxed{\left(\frac{m_o - m}{A \rho_A^L} \right) \left(2L_o + \frac{m_o - m}{A \rho_A^L} \right) = \left[\frac{2}{\rho_A^L} c \mathcal{D}_{AB} M_A \ln \left(\frac{1}{1 - y_{A_o}} \right) \right] t} \tag{5.89}$$

When the term on the left side of Eq. (5.89) is plotted versus time, the diffusion coefficient is obtained from the slope of the resulting straight line.

5.5.1 SIMPLIFICATION FOR SMALL VALUES OF y_{A_o}

When $y_{A_o} < 0.2$, as stated in Section 4.3.1, the logarithmic term in Eqs. (5.86), (5.87), and (5.89) can be approximated as

$$\ln \left(\frac{1}{1 - y_{A_o}} \right) \simeq y_{A_o} \tag{5.90}$$

and these equations simplify to

$$L^2 = \left(\frac{2 P_A^{vap} \mathcal{D}_{AB}}{RT c_A^L} \right) t + L_o^2 \tag{5.91}$$

$$\frac{t}{L - L_o} = \left(\frac{RT c_A^L}{2 P_A^{vap} \mathcal{D}_{AB}} \right) (L - L_o) - \frac{RT c_A^L L_o}{P_A^{vap} \mathcal{D}_{AB}} \tag{5.92}$$

$$\left(\frac{m_o - m}{A \rho_A^L} \right) \left(2L_o + \frac{m_o - m}{A \rho_A^L} \right) = \left(\frac{2 P_A^{vap} \mathcal{D}_{AB}}{RT c_A^L} \right) t \tag{5.93}$$

5.5.2 VALIDITY OF THE PSEUDOSTEADY-STATE APPROXIMATION

The timescale of the system, t_{sys}, is

$$t_{sys} \sim O \left(\frac{RT c_A^L L_o^2}{2 P_A^{vap} \mathcal{D}_{AB}} \right) \tag{5.94}$$

Substitution of Eq. (5.94) into Eq. (5.5) gives the criterion for the pseudosteady-state approximation as

$$\boxed{\frac{RT c_A^L}{2 P_A^{vap}} \gg 1} \tag{5.95}$$

5.5.3 APPLICATION OF THE JUMP SPECIES CONTINUITY EQUATION

Now let us consider how to use the jump condition in the solution of mass transfer problems. Let α-phase be the pure liquid A and β-phase be the gaseous mixture of A and B. The term $\lambda_{\alpha\beta}$ represents the unit normal vector at the α–β interface pointing from the α-phase to the β-phase. In other words, $\lambda_{\alpha\beta} = -\lambda_{\beta\alpha} = \mathbf{e}_z$. The molar flux of species A, Eq. (5.82), is expressed as

$$N_{A_z}(t) = c_A^\beta \mathbf{v}_A^\beta \cdot \mathbf{e}_z = \frac{c_\beta \mathcal{D}_{AB}}{L(t)} \ln \left(\frac{1}{1 - y_{A_o}} \right) \tag{5.96}$$

With the help of Eq. (2.239), jump mass balances for species A and B are written in the forms

$$c_A^\alpha \left(\mathbf{v}_A^\alpha - \mathbf{w}\right) \cdot \mathbf{e}_z - c_A^\beta \left(\mathbf{v}_A^\beta - \mathbf{w}\right) \cdot \mathbf{e}_z = 0 \tag{5.97}$$

$$c_B^\alpha \left(\mathbf{v}_B^\alpha - \mathbf{w}\right) \cdot \mathbf{e}_z - c_B^\beta \left(\mathbf{v}_B^\beta - \mathbf{w}\right) \cdot \mathbf{e}_z = 0 \tag{5.98}$$

Since the α-phase does not contain species B, $c_B^\alpha = 0$. On the other hand, $\mathbf{v}_A^\alpha \cdot \mathbf{e}_z = 0$ since the α-phase is stagnant. Thus, Eqs. (5.97) and (5.98) simplify to

$$N_{A_z} = -c_A^\alpha \left(1 - \frac{c_A^\beta}{c_A^\alpha}\right) (\mathbf{w} \cdot \mathbf{e}_z) \tag{5.99}$$

$$N_{B_z} = c_B^\beta (\mathbf{w} \cdot \mathbf{e}_z) \tag{5.100}$$

As a result of the large difference between the liquid- and gas-phase concentrations, it is plausible to assume that $c_A^\beta / c_A^\alpha \simeq 0$. Noting that

$$\mathbf{w} \cdot \mathbf{e}_z = \frac{dL}{dt} \tag{5.101}$$

Eq. (5.99) becomes

$$\frac{dL}{dt} = -\frac{N_{A_z}}{c_A^\alpha} \tag{5.102}$$

Substitution of Eq. (5.96) into Eq. (5.102) yields

$$\frac{dL}{dt} = -\frac{c_\beta \mathcal{D}_{AB}}{c_A^\alpha L(t)} \ln\left(\frac{1}{1 - y_{A_o}}\right), \tag{5.103}$$

which is identical to Eq. (5.84) obtained from the macroscopic mass balance.

5.6 EVAPORATION OF A LIQUID DROPLET

Species A in the form of a liquid droplet of initial radius R_o is suspended in a stagnant gas B at a temperature T_∞. We are interested in the time it takes for the droplet to evaporate completely. The problem at hand is unsteady-state since the radius of the droplet is changing as a function of time. However, the problem will be solved by using the pseudosteady-state approximation.

Postulating one-dimensional mass transport with $N_{A_r} = N_{A_r}(r)$ and $N_{A_\theta} = N_{A_\phi} = 0$, the equation of continuity for species A, Eq. (C) of Table 2.3, under steady-state conditions simplifies to

$$\frac{d(r^2 N_{A_r})}{dr} = 0 \quad \Rightarrow \quad r^2 N_{A_r} = \text{constant} = R^2 \left. N_{A_r} \right|_{r=R} \tag{5.104}$$

From Eq. (2.165), the total molar flux of species A in the r-direction is given by

$$N_{A_r} = -c\mathcal{D}_{AB} \frac{dy_A}{dr} + y_A \left(N_{A_r} + N_{B_r}\right) \tag{5.105}$$

Since species B is stagnant, $N_{B_r} = 0$ and Eq. (5.105) becomes

$$N_{A_r} = -\frac{c\mathcal{D}_{AB}}{1 - y_A} \frac{dy_A}{dr} \tag{5.106}$$

Substitution of Eq. (5.106) into Eq. (5.104) and rearrangement give

$$-c\mathcal{D}_{AB} \int_{y_A^{eq}}^{0} \frac{dy_A}{1 - y_A} = R^2 \left. N_{A_r} \right|_{r=R} \int_{R}^{\infty} \frac{dr}{r^2}, \tag{5.107}$$

where y_A^{eq} is the saturation concentration of species A in B at $r = R$ in the gas phase, given by Eq. (2.215). Carrying out the integrations in Eq. (5.107) yields

$$N_{A_r}|_{r=R} = -\frac{c\mathcal{D}_{AB}}{R}\ln(1 - y_A^{eq}) \tag{5.108}$$

The pseudosteady-state approximation states that Eq. (5.108) holds at any instant of time, i.e.,

$$N_{A_r}|_{r=R}(t) = -\frac{c\mathcal{D}_{AB}}{R(t)}\ln(1 - y_A^{eq}) \tag{5.109}$$

Choosing the liquid droplet as a system, the macroscopic mass balance is expressed as

$$-\begin{pmatrix} \text{Rate of} \\ \text{mass } A \text{ out} \end{pmatrix} = \begin{pmatrix} \text{Rate of accumulation} \\ \text{of mass } A \end{pmatrix} \tag{5.110}$$

or

$$-4\pi R^2 \left[-\frac{c\mathcal{D}_{AB}}{R}\ln(1 - y_A^{eq}) \right] M_A = \frac{d}{dt}\left(\frac{4}{3}\pi R^3 \rho_A^L \right) \tag{5.111}$$

Equation (5.111) is rearranged as

$$\int_0^t dt = \frac{\rho_A^L}{c\mathcal{D}_{AB}M_A \ln(1 - y_A^{eq})} \int_{R_o}^0 R\, dR \tag{5.112}$$

or

$$\boxed{t = -\frac{\rho_A^L R_o^2}{2c\mathcal{D}_{AB}M_A \ln(1 - y_A^{eq})}} \tag{5.113}$$

5.6.1 SIMPLIFICATION FOR SMALL VALUES OF y_A^{eq}

For small values of y_A^{eq}, $\ln(1 - y_A^{eq}) \simeq -y_A^{eq}$. Substitution of $y_A^{eq} = P_A^{vap}/P$ and $c = P/RT_\infty$ into Eq. (5.113) leads to

$$t = \frac{RT_\infty \rho_A^L R_o^2}{2M_A P_A^{vap} \mathcal{D}_{AB}} \tag{5.114}$$

5.6.2 VALIDITY OF THE PSEUDOSTEADY-STATE APPROXIMATION

The timescale of the system, t_{sys}, is

$$t_{sys} \sim O\left(\frac{RT_\infty \rho_A^L R_o^2}{2M_A P_A^{vap} \mathcal{D}_{AB}} \right) \tag{5.115}$$

Substitution of Eq. (5.115) into Eq. (5.5) gives the criterion for the pseudosteady-state approximation as

$$\boxed{\frac{RT_\infty \rho_A^L}{2M_A P_A^{vap}} \gg 1} \tag{5.116}$$

5.7 SUBLIMATION OF A NAPHTHALENE SPHERE

A spherical naphthalene (species A) of initial radius R_o is suspended in air (species B) at a temperature of T_∞. We are interested in the time required for the naphthalene sphere to disappear completely as a result of sublimation.

Since the radius of the naphthalene sphere decreases as a result of sublimation, the problem at hand will be tackled with pseudosteady-state analysis. Choosing the naphthalene sphere as a system, the macroscopic mass balance is expressed as

$$- \left(\begin{array}{c} \text{Rate of} \\ \text{mass } A \text{ out} \end{array} \right) = \left(\begin{array}{c} \text{Rate of accumulation} \\ \text{of mass } A \end{array} \right) \tag{5.117}$$

or

$$- \left(4\pi R^2 \right) k_c \left(c_{A_w} - c_{A_\infty} \right) M_A = \frac{d}{dt} \left(\frac{4}{3} \pi R^3 \rho_A^S \right), \tag{5.118}$$

where c_A^{eq} and c_{A_∞} are the naphthalene concentrations on the surface of the sphere and in air, respectively. The term ρ_A^S stands for the density of solid naphthalene. Taking $c_{A_\infty} = 0$ and rearrangement give

$$t = \frac{\rho_A^S}{M_A c_A^{eq}} \int_0^{R_o} \frac{dR}{k_c} = \frac{\rho_A^S R_o}{M_A c_A^{eq}} \int_0^1 \frac{du}{k_c}, \tag{5.119}$$

where

$$u = \frac{R}{R_o} \tag{5.120}$$

To proceed further, we need to relate the mass transfer coefficient to the radius (or diameter) of the naphthalene.

5.7.1 STAGNANT AIR

In this case, Eq. (5.40) states that

$$\text{Sh} = \frac{k_c D}{\mathcal{D}_{AB}} = 2 \quad \Rightarrow \quad k_c = \frac{\mathcal{D}_{AB}}{R} = \left(\frac{\mathcal{D}_{AB}}{R_o} \right) \frac{1}{u} \tag{5.121}$$

Substitution of Eq. (5.121) into Eq. (5.119) and integration give

$$t = \frac{\rho_A^S R_o^2}{2 M_A c_A^{eq} \mathcal{D}_{AB}} = \frac{R T_\infty \rho_A^S R_o^2}{2 M_A P_A^{vap} \mathcal{D}_{AB}}, \tag{5.122}$$

which is similar to Eq. (5.114).

5.7.2 AIR MOVES AT A CERTAIN VELOCITY

The use of the Ranz–Marshall correlation, Eq. (5.41), gives

$$\frac{k_c D}{\mathcal{D}_{AB}} = 2 + 0.6 \left(\frac{D v_\infty \rho}{\mu} \right)^{1/2} \text{Sc}^{1/3} \tag{5.123}$$

or

$$k_c = \frac{\mathcal{D}_{AB}}{R_o} \frac{1 + \alpha \sqrt{u}}{u}, \tag{5.124}$$

where

$$\alpha = 0.3 \, \text{Re}_o^{1/2} \, \text{Sc}^{1/3}, \tag{5.125}$$

in which Re_o is the Reynolds number based on the initial radius of the sphere. Substitution of Eq. (5.124) into Eq. (5.119) yields

$$t = \frac{\rho_A^S R_o^2}{M_A c_A^{eq} \mathcal{D}_{AB}} \int_0^1 \frac{u}{1 + \alpha \sqrt{u}} du \qquad (5.126)$$

The integral in Eq. (5.126) can be evaluated as

$$\int_0^1 \frac{u}{1 + \alpha \sqrt{u}} du = \int_0^1 \left(\frac{\sqrt{u}}{\alpha} - \frac{1}{\alpha^2} + \frac{1}{\alpha^2} \frac{1}{1 + \alpha \sqrt{u}} \right) du$$

$$= \frac{2}{3\alpha} - \frac{1}{\alpha^2} + \frac{2}{\alpha^4} \left[\alpha - \ln(1 + \alpha) \right] \qquad (5.127)$$

so that the time required for the disappearance of the naphthalene sphere is

$$\boxed{t = \frac{\rho_A^S R_o^2}{M_A c_A^{eq} \mathcal{D}_{AB}} \left\{ \frac{2}{3\alpha} - \frac{1}{\alpha^2} + \frac{2}{\alpha^4} \left[\alpha - \ln(1 + \alpha) \right] \right\}} \qquad (5.128)$$

Note that when $\alpha \to 0$

$$\lim_{\alpha \to 0} \left\{ \frac{2}{3\alpha} - \frac{1}{\alpha^2} + \frac{2}{\alpha^4} \left[\alpha - \ln(1 + \alpha) \right] \right\} = \frac{1}{2} \qquad (5.129)$$

and Eq. (5.128) reduces to Eq. (5.122).

5.8 SHRINKING PARTICLE MODEL

The term "shrinking particle" implies that the loss in the mass of a particle leads to a decrease in its size. For a spherical particle of initial radius R_o, the decrease in the radius of the particle, R, is shown in Figure 5.5. The transfer of mass from the particle to the bulk fluid takes place through a fluid film surrounding the particle. The examples presented in Sections 5.5 and 5.6 are examples of the shrinking particle model. Dissolution of solid particles as well as solid–fluid noncatalytic reactions is generally modeled based on this approach. The following reactions are typical examples of the shrinking particle model:

$$\mathrm{C}(s) + \mathrm{O}_2(g) \to \mathrm{CO}_2(g)$$

$$2\,\mathrm{C}(s) + \mathrm{O}_2(g) \to 2\,\mathrm{CO}(g)$$

$$\mathrm{C}(s) + \mathrm{CO}_2(g) \to 2\,\mathrm{CO}(g)$$

Switchable solvents are nonionic liquids (an alcohol and an amine) that can be converted to ionic liquids (a salt in liquid form) upon exposure to an atmosphere of carbon dioxide and then switched back to the nonionic form when exposed to an inert gas, such as nitrogen or argon (Jessop et al.,

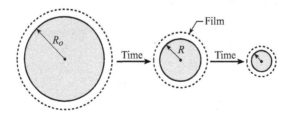

Figure 5.5 Shrinking particle model.

2005). Thus, the so-called "CO_2-switchable solvents" can be switched reversibly from one kind of liquid to a very different kind of liquid, i.e., from being hydrophobic to hydrophilic, simply by the addition or removal of carbon dioxide.

Nanta et al. (2018) studied dissolution of cellulose particles (species A) in a CO_2-switchable solvent (species B). Their analysis is based on the following assumptions:

- The cellulose particles are spherical with an initial radius of R_o.
- All CO_2 is absorbed in the liquid system, and the equilibrium concentration of CO_2 depends on the temperature and pressure of the system.
- The molar consumption rate of CO_2 controls the reaction of the CO_2-switchable solvent (CO_2-SWS).
- The flux of CO_2 in the ionic liquid mixture represents the diffusive molar flux of the CO_2-SWS to the cellulose surface.

The CO_2-SWS diffuses through the liquid film to the cellulose surface on which the following reaction takes place:

$$\text{Cellulose} + CO_2\text{-SWS} \rightarrow \text{Dissolved cellulose}$$

The flux of CO_2 can be expressed as

$$-N_{CO_2} = -N_B = k_c\left[(c_{CO_2})_b - (c_{CO_2})_w\right], \tag{5.130}$$

where $(c_{CO_2})_b$ is the bulk concentration of CO_2 and $(c_{CO_2})_w$ is the concentration of CO_2 at the cellulose surface. The minus sign in Eq. (5.130) is due to the fact that carbon dioxide diffuses in the negative r-direction. Since the reaction between CO_2-SWS and cellulose is instantaneous, Eq. (5.130) reduces to

$$N_B = -k_c\,(c_{CO_2})_b \tag{5.131}$$

From the stoichiometry of the reaction, every mole of CO_2-SWS reacts with 1 mole of cellulose particle, i.e., $N_A = -N_B$. Thus,

$$N_A = k_c\,(c_{CO_2})_b \tag{5.132}$$

The macroscopic mass balance for the cellulose particle is

$$-\begin{pmatrix} \text{Rate of} \\ \text{mass } A \text{ out} \end{pmatrix} = \begin{pmatrix} \text{Rate of accumulation} \\ \text{of mass } A \end{pmatrix} \tag{5.133}$$

or

$$-4\pi R^2 k_c\,(c_{CO_2})_b M_A = \frac{d}{dt}\left(\frac{4}{3}\pi R^3 \rho_A\right), \tag{5.134}$$

where ρ_A and M_A are the density and the molecular weight of cellulose, respectively. The time for the complete dissolution of the cellulose particles is determined from Eq. (5.134) as

$$t = \frac{\rho_A R_o}{(c_{CO_2})_b M_A}\int_0^1 \frac{du}{k_c}, \tag{5.135}$$

where the dimensionless parameter u is defined by

$$u = \frac{R}{R_o} \tag{5.136}$$

To relate the radius of cellulose particle, R, to the mass transfer coefficient, Nanta et al. (2018) used the Frossling correlation

$$\frac{k_c 2R}{\mathcal{D}_{AB}} = 2 + 0.6\,\text{Re}_N^{1/2}\,\text{Sc}^{1/3}, \tag{5.137}$$

where the Reynolds number is defined as a function of rotational speed N and the diameter of the magnetic agitator D_i in the form

$$\text{Re}_N = \frac{ND_i^2 \rho}{\mu} \tag{5.138}$$

Substitution of Eq. (5.137) into Eq. (5.135) and integration result in

$$t = \frac{\rho_A R_o^2}{2(c_{CO_2})_b M_A \mathcal{D}_{AB} \alpha}, \tag{5.139}$$

where

$$\alpha = 1 + 0.3\,\text{Re}_N^{1/2}\,\text{Sc}^{1/3} \tag{5.140}$$

Discuss the validity of using the Frossling correlation with the Reynolds number defined by Eq. (5.138).

5.9 SHRINKING CORE MODEL

A schematic diagram of the shrinking core model for a spherical solid particle is shown in Figure 5.6. The reaction takes place at the outer boundary of the unreacted solid. As a result, this boundary moves inward, leaving behind the product layer. Reactant species should diffuse not only through the film surrounding the particle but also through the product layer to reach the reaction surface. This model is used for the dissolution of solid particles, i.e., leaching of solid ores, as well as solid–fluid noncatalytic reactions, such as

$$\text{CaO}\,(s) + \text{CO}_2\,(g) \rightarrow \text{CaCO}_3\,(s)$$

$$\text{FeO}\,(s) + \text{H}_2\,(g) \rightarrow \text{Fe}\,(s) + \text{H}_2\text{O}\,(g)$$

5.9.1 RECTANGULAR GEOMETRY

Silicon is a widely used semiconductor material. It reacts with oxygen to form silicon dioxide (SiO_2), which acts as a protective layer. Oxidation of a slab of silicon by oxygen (species A) is schematically shown in Figure 5.7.

The molar flux of species A from the bulk gas to the SiO_2 surface is given by

$$N_{A_z} = k_c(c_{A_b} - c_{A_s}) \tag{5.141}$$

At $z = 0$, the concentrations c_{A_s} and c_{A_o} are related to each other by the use of Eq. (2.223), i.e.,

$$c_{A_o} = \frac{1}{\mathcal{H}_A^*}\overline{P}_{A_s} = \frac{RT}{\mathcal{H}_A^*}c_{A_s} \tag{5.142}$$

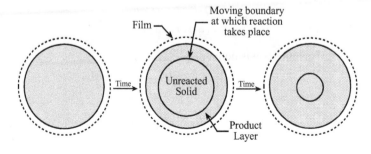

Figure 5.6   Shrinking core model.

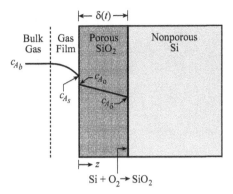

Figure 5.7 Oxidation of a silicon slab.

Substitution of Eq. (5.142) into Eq. (5.141) gives

$$N_{A_z} = k_c^* (c_{A_b}^* - c_{A_o}) \qquad \Rightarrow \qquad c_{A_b}^* - c_{A_o} = \frac{1}{k_c^*} N_{A_z}, \tag{5.143}$$

where

$$k_c^* = \frac{\mathcal{H}_A^*}{RT} k_c \qquad \text{and} \qquad c_{A_b}^* = \frac{RT}{\mathcal{H}_A^*} c_{A_b} \tag{5.144}$$

A pseudosteady-state approximation is used for modeling species A concentration in the SiO_2 layer. The use of Eq. (4.9) gives the steady-state molar flux of species A as

$$N_{A_z} = \frac{\mathcal{D}_{eff}(c_{A_o} - c_{A_\delta})}{\delta} \qquad \Rightarrow \qquad c_{A_o} - c_{A_\delta} = \frac{\delta}{\mathcal{D}_{eff}} N_{A_z} \tag{5.145}$$

The heterogeneous reaction takes place at the SiO_2–Si interface. Since the reaction is first-order, the use of Eq. (2.114) yields

$$N_{A_z} = k_1'' c_{A_\delta} \qquad \Rightarrow \qquad c_{A_\delta} = \frac{1}{k_1''} N_{A_z} \tag{5.146}$$

Addition of Eqs. (5.143), (5.145), and (5.146) results in

$$N_{A_z} = \frac{c_{A_b}^*}{\dfrac{1}{k_c^*} + \dfrac{\delta}{\mathcal{D}_{eff}} + \dfrac{1}{k_1''}}, \tag{5.147}$$

in which the terms in the denominator indicate that the resistances are in series. Considering SiO_2 (species B) as a system, the macroscopic mass balance is written as

$$\begin{pmatrix} \text{Rate of generation} \\ \text{of mass } B \end{pmatrix} = \begin{pmatrix} \text{Rate of accumulation} \\ \text{of mass } B \end{pmatrix} \tag{5.148}$$

According to the stoichiometry of the reaction, consumption of 1 mole of O_2 produces 1 mole of SiO_2. Thus, Eq. (5.148) is expressed in the form

$$N_{A_z} A M_B = \frac{d}{dt}(A \delta \rho_B), \tag{5.149}$$

where A is the surface area of the slab. Substitution of Eq. (5.147) into Eq. (5.149) and rearrangement lead to

$$\widetilde{V}_B c_{A_b}^* \int_0^t dt = \int_0^\delta \left(\frac{1}{k_c^*} + \frac{\delta}{\mathcal{D}_{Aeff}} + \frac{1}{k_1''} \right) d\delta, \tag{5.150}$$

where $\widetilde{V}_B = M_B/\rho_B$ is the molar volume of SiO_2. Integration of Eq. (5.150) gives

$$\delta^2 + \Omega\delta - \Phi t = 0, \qquad (5.151)$$

where

$$\Omega = 2\mathcal{D}_{eff}\left(\frac{1}{k_c^*} + \frac{1}{k_1''}\right) \qquad \text{and} \qquad \Phi = 2\mathcal{D}_{eff}\widetilde{V}_B c_{A_b}^* \qquad (5.152)$$

The solution of the quadratic equation given by Eq. (5.151) is

$$\boxed{\delta = \frac{\Omega}{2}\left(\sqrt{\frac{4\Phi t}{\Omega^2} + 1} - 1\right)} \qquad (5.153)$$

Now let us investigate the limiting cases of Eq. (5.153).

• Heterogeneous reaction controls the growth of the oxide layer

When the thickness of the oxide layer is small or the diffusion coefficient is large, the rate determining step is the heterogeneous reaction at the SiO_2–Si interface. In this case

$$\frac{1}{k_1''} \gg \frac{\delta}{\mathcal{D}_{eff}} \qquad \text{and} \qquad \frac{1}{k_1''} \gg \frac{1}{k_c^*} \qquad (5.154)$$

When δ is small, the δ^2 term in Eq. (5.151) may be neglected to obtain

$$\Omega\delta - \Phi t = 0 \qquad \Rightarrow \qquad \delta = \frac{\Phi}{\Omega}t = \left(\widetilde{V}_B c_{A_b}^* k_1''\right)t \qquad (5.155)$$

Therefore, the thickness of the oxide layer changes linearly with time.

• Diffusion of O_2 through the SiO_2 layer controls the growth of the oxide layer

When the thickness of the oxide layer is large or the oxidation time is long, the rate determining step is the diffusion of oxygen through the porous SiO_2 layer. In this case

$$\frac{\delta}{\mathcal{D}_{eff}} \gg \frac{1}{k_c^*} \qquad \text{and} \qquad \frac{\delta}{\mathcal{D}_{eff}} \gg \frac{1}{k_1''} \qquad (5.156)$$

Since Ω is small, Eq. (5.151) simplifies to

$$\delta^2 - \Phi t = 0 \qquad \Rightarrow \qquad \delta = \sqrt{\Phi t} = \sqrt{2\mathcal{D}_{eff}\widetilde{V}_B c_{A_b}^* t} \qquad (5.157)$$

Therefore, the thickness of the oxide layer changes with the square root of time.

5.9.2 SPHERICAL GEOMETRY

Consider a spherical solid particle (species B) of initial radius R_o undergoing a heterogeneous reaction with gas species A according to the reaction

$$A(g) + bB(s) \rightarrow C(s),$$

which can be modeled as a shrinking core model as shown in Figure 5.8.

   The molar flux of species A from the bulk gas to the surface of the product layer is given by

$$-N_{A_r} = k_c(c_{A_b} - c_{A_s}) \qquad (5.158)$$

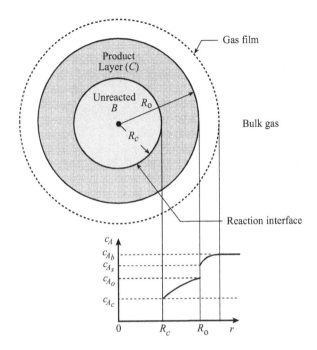

Figure 5.8 Shrinking core model.

The minus sign in Eq. (5.158) is due to the fact that species A diffuses in the negative r-direction, i.e., $(-N_{A_r})$ is a positive quantity. At $r = R_o$, the use of Eq. (2.223) gives the relationship between c_{A_s} and c_{A_o} as

$$c_{A_o} = \frac{1}{\mathcal{H}_A^*} \overline{P}_{A_s} = \frac{RT}{\mathcal{H}_A^*} c_{A_s} \tag{5.159}$$

Substitution of Eq. (5.159) into Eq. (5.158) gives

$$-N_{A_r} = k_c^* (c_{A_b}^* - c_{A_o}), \tag{5.160}$$

where

$$k_c^* = \frac{\mathcal{H}_A^*}{RT} k_c \qquad \text{and} \qquad c_{A_b}^* = \frac{RT}{\mathcal{H}_A^*} c_{A_b} \tag{5.161}$$

Thus, the molar flow rate of species A from the bulk gas to the outer surface of the product layer is

$$\mathcal{W}_A = 4\pi R_o^2 k_c^* (c_{A_b}^* - c_{A_o}) \qquad \Rightarrow \qquad c_{A_b}^* - c_{A_o} = \frac{1}{4\pi R_o^2 k_c^*} \mathcal{W}_A \tag{5.162}$$

A pseudosteady-state approximation is used for the molar flow rate of species A through the product layer. Under steady conditions, the molar flow rate of species A is given by Eq. (4.52) as

$$\mathcal{W}_A = 4\pi D_{eff} \left[\frac{c_{A_o} - c_{A_c}}{(1/R_c) - (1/R_o)} \right] \qquad \Rightarrow \qquad c_{A_o} - c_{A_c} = \left[\frac{(1/R_c) - (1/R_o)}{4\pi D_{eff}} \right] \mathcal{W}_A \tag{5.163}$$

On the surface of the unreacted solid particle, the heterogeneous reaction results in the following molar flow rate of species A:

$$\mathcal{W}_A = 4\pi R_c^2 k_1'' c_{A_c} \qquad \Rightarrow \qquad c_{A_c} = \frac{1}{4\pi R_c^2 k_1''} \mathcal{W}_A \tag{5.164}$$

Addition of Eqs. (5.162)–(5.164) results in

$$W_A = \frac{4\pi c_{A_b}^*}{\dfrac{1}{R_o^2 k_c^*} + \dfrac{(1/R_c) - (1/R_o)}{\mathcal{D}_{eff}} + \dfrac{1}{R_c^2 k_1''}},\qquad (5.165)$$

in which the terms in the denominator indicate that the resistances are in series. Considering species B as a system, the macroscopic mass balance is written as

$$-\,\text{Consumption rate of } B = \text{Accumulation rate of } B \qquad (5.166)$$

From the stoichiometry of the reaction, 1 mole of species A reacts with b moles of species B. Therefore, Eq. (5.166) is expressed as

$$-b\,W_A M_B = \frac{d}{dt}\left(\frac{4}{3}\pi R_c^3 \rho_B\right) = 4\pi R_c^2 \rho_B \frac{dR_c}{dt} \qquad (5.167)$$

Substitution of Eq. (5.165) into Eq. (5.167) and rearrangement give

$$b\widetilde{V}_B c_{A_b}^* \int_0^t dt = -\int_{R_o}^{R_c}\left[\frac{1}{R_o^2 k_c^*} + \frac{(1/R_c) - (1/R_o)}{\mathcal{D}_{eff}} + \frac{1}{R_c^2 k_1''}\right] R_c^2\, dR_c \qquad (5.168)$$

In terms of the dimensionless distance ξ, defined by

$$\xi = \frac{R_c}{R_o}, \qquad (5.169)$$

Eq. (5.169) takes the form

$$\begin{aligned}
\frac{b\widetilde{V}_B c_{A_b}^*}{R_o} t &= \frac{1}{k_c^*}\int_\xi^1 \xi^2\, d\xi + \frac{R_o}{\mathcal{D}_{eff}}\int_\xi^1 (\xi - \xi^2)\, d\xi + \frac{1}{k_1''}\int_\xi^1 d\xi \\
&= \frac{1 - \xi^3}{3k_c^*} + \frac{R_o(1 - 3\xi^2 + 2\xi^3)}{6\mathcal{D}_{eff}} + \frac{1 - \xi}{k_1''}
\end{aligned} \qquad (5.170)$$

The fractional conversion of species B, X_B, is defined by

$$X_B = 1 - \left(\frac{R_c}{R_o}\right)^3 \qquad \Rightarrow \qquad X_B = 1 - \xi^3 \qquad (5.171)$$

In terms of the fraction conversion, Eq. (5.170) is expressed as

$$\boxed{\frac{b\widetilde{V}_B c_{A_b}^*}{R_o} t = \frac{1}{3k_c^*} X_B + \frac{R_o}{6\mathcal{D}_{eff}}\left[1 - 3(1 - X_B)^{2/3} + 2(1 - X_B)\right] + \frac{1}{k_1''}\left[1 - (1 - X_B)^{1/3}\right]} \qquad (5.172)$$

The time, t^*, required for complete conversion, i.e., $X_B = 1$, is

$$t^* = \frac{R_o}{b\widetilde{V}_B c_{A_b}^*}\left(\frac{1}{3k_c^*} + \frac{R_o}{6\mathcal{D}_{eff}} + \frac{1}{k_1''}\right) \qquad (5.173)$$

In the analysis presented here, R_o is assumed constant throughout the process. When the densities of the reacting solid and the product layer are different from each other, volume does not remain constant. In general, volume increases as a result of the porous structure of the product layer. Now let us investigate the limiting cases of Eq. (5.172).

● **Diffusion through the film controls the mass transfer rate**

In this case

$$\frac{1}{R_o^2 k_c^*} \gg \frac{(1/R_c) - (1/R_o)}{\mathcal{D}_{eff}} \quad \text{and} \quad \frac{1}{R_o^2 k_c^*} \gg \frac{1}{R_c^2 k_1''} \tag{5.174}$$

As a result, Eqs. (5.172) and (5.173) simplify to

$$t = \left(\frac{R_o}{3b\widetilde{V}_B c_{A_b}^* k_c^*} \right) X_B \quad \text{and} \quad t^* = \frac{R_o}{3b\widetilde{V}_B c_{A_b}^* k_c^*} \tag{5.175}$$

Thus,

$$\boxed{\frac{t}{t^*} = X_B} \tag{5.176}$$

● **Diffusion through the product layer controls the mass transfer rate**

In this case,

$$\frac{(1/R_c) - (1/R_o)}{\mathcal{D}_{eff}} \gg \frac{1}{R_o^2 k_c^*} \quad \text{and} \quad \frac{(1/R_c) - (1/R_o)}{\mathcal{D}_{eff}} \gg \frac{1}{R_c^2 k_1''} \tag{5.177}$$

As a result, Eqs. (5.172) and (5.173) simplify to

$$t = \frac{R_o^2}{6b\widetilde{V}_B c_{A_b}^* \mathcal{D}_{eff}} \left[1 - 3(1 - X_B)^{2/3} + 2(1 - X_B) \right] \quad \text{and} \quad t^* = \frac{R_o^2}{6b\widetilde{V}_B c_{A_b}^* \mathcal{D}_{eff}} \tag{5.178}$$

Thus,

$$\boxed{\frac{t}{t^*} = 1 - 3(1 - X_B)^{2/3} + 2(1 - X_B)} \tag{5.179}$$

● **Heterogeneous reaction controls the mass transfer rate**

In this case,

$$\frac{1}{R_c^2 k_1''} \gg \frac{1}{R_o^2 k_c^*} \quad \text{and} \quad \frac{1}{R_c^2 k_1''} \gg \frac{(1/R_c) - (1/R_o)}{\mathcal{D}_{eff}} \tag{5.180}$$

As a result, Eqs. (5.172) and (5.173) simplify to

$$t = \frac{R_o}{b\widetilde{V}_B c_{A_b}^* k_1''} \left[1 - (1 - X_B)^{1/3} \right] \quad \text{and} \quad t^* = \frac{R_o}{b\widetilde{V}_B c_{A_b}^* k_1''} \tag{5.181}$$

Thus,

$$\boxed{\frac{t}{t^*} = 1 - (1 - X_B)^{1/3}} \tag{5.182}$$

The variation in the fractional conversion with time depending on the controlling resistance to mass transfer is shown in Figure 5.9.

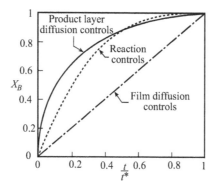

Figure 5.9 Effects of controlling mass transfer resistances on the variation in the fractional conversion with time.

Problems

5.1 A rectangular PVC box has dimensions $0.3 \times 0.4 \times 0.7$ m and has a wall thickness of 0.8 mm. The box initially contains carbon dioxide at 3 atm and 298 K. How long does it take for the pressure in the tank to decrease to 2.8 atm? For the CO_2–PVC system, the permeability is given by

$$P_M^* = 1 \times 10^{-13} \frac{\text{m}^3(\text{STP}).\text{m}}{\text{day}.\text{m}^2.\text{Pa}}$$

The partial pressure of CO in the atmosphere is about 3×10^{-4} atm.

(Answer: 344 days)

5.2 Consider reservoir-based drug delivery systems in three different geometries as shown in the figure below.

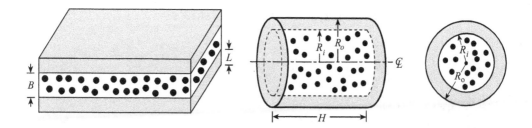

The number of moles of drug (species A) released at time t, $\mathbb{N}_A$, from such geometries are given by Siepmann and Siepmann (2012) in the following table. The term $\mathbb{N}_{A_\infty}$ stands for the number of moles of species A initially present in the reservoir. The term K_A is the partition coefficient. In case (i), the reservoir is assumed to contain a saturated solution with a large excess of undissolved species A. Therefore, the saturation concentration of species A, c_A^{eq}, remains constant during the diffusion process. In case (ii), however, the concentration of species A in the reservoir is below the saturation concentration and changes with time as the diffusion process takes place. Verify the formulas given in the table.

| Geometry | Number of moles of species A released in time t $(\mathbb{N}_A)$ | | | |
	Case (i)		Case (ii)	
Slab	$\mathbb{N}_A = \dfrac{A\mathcal{D}_{AB}K_A c_A^{eq}}{L}t$	(A)	$\dfrac{\mathbb{N}_A}{\mathbb{N}_{A\infty}} = 1 - \exp\left(-\dfrac{\mathcal{D}_{AB}K_A}{LB}t\right)$	(B)
Cylinder	$\mathbb{N}_A = \dfrac{2\pi H\mathcal{D}_{AB}K_A c_A^{eq}}{\ln(R_o/R_i)}t$	(C)	$\dfrac{\mathbb{N}_A}{\mathbb{N}_{A\infty}} = 1 - \exp\left[-\dfrac{2\mathcal{D}_{AB}K_A}{R_i^2 \ln(R_o/R_i)}t\right]$	(D)
Sphere	$\mathbb{N}_A = \dfrac{4\pi R_i R_o \mathcal{D}_{AB}K_A c_A^{eq}}{R_o - R_i}t$	(E)	$\dfrac{\mathbb{N}_A}{\mathbb{N}_{A\infty}} = 1 - \exp\left[-\dfrac{3R_o \mathcal{D}_{AB}K_A}{R_i^2(R_o - R_i)}t\right]$	(F)

5.3 In the original article by Siepmann and Siepmann (2012), Eq. (D) of the table given in Problem 5.2 is expressed in the form

$$\frac{\mathbb{N}_A}{\mathbb{N}_{A\infty}} = 1 - \exp\left\{-\frac{\left[(R_i + R_o)H + 2R_i R_o\right]\mathcal{D}_{AB}K_A}{R_i^2 H \ln(R_o/R_i)}t\right\}$$

Show that this equation is derived by approximating the logarithmic mean area in Eq. (4.36) to be equal to

$$A_{LM} \simeq \pi(R_i + R_o)H + 2\pi R_i R_o$$

Interested readers may refer to Paterson (1984) and Chen (1987) for expressing logarithmic mean in terms of arithmetic and geometric means.

5.4 A solid sphere of salicylic acid (species A) with an initial radius of R_o is dropped into a long cylindrical tank filled with pure water (species B). The initial acceleration period is negligible, and the sphere reaches its terminal velocity in the Stokes region instantaneously, i.e.,

$$v_t = \frac{2R^2 g(\rho_A - \rho_B)}{9\mu_B} \tag{1}$$

Let us further assume that the physical properties of water do not change as a result of mass transfer. It is required to calculate the time for the salicylic acid sphere to dissolve completely in water.

a) Choose the sphere as a system, and show that the macroscopic mass balance leads to

$$t = \frac{\rho_A R_o}{c_A^{eq} M_A}\int_0^1 \frac{du}{k_c}, \tag{2}$$

where c_A^{eq} is the saturation solubility of salicylic acid in water and u is the dimensionless parameter defined by

$$u = \frac{R}{R_o} \tag{3}$$

b) Both the terminal velocity and the Reynolds number change as the solid sphere dissolves in water. Use the Ranz–Marshall correlation, Eq. (5.41), to relate the mass transfer coefficient to the radius of the sphere and show that

$$k_c = \frac{\mathcal{D}_{AB}}{R_o}\left(\frac{1 + \alpha u^{3/2}}{u}\right), \tag{4}$$

where

$$\alpha = 0.3 \text{Re}_o^{1/2} \, \text{Sc}^{1/3}, \tag{5}$$

in which Re_o is the Reynolds number based on the initial radius and initial terminal velocity of the sphere.

c) Substitute Eq. (4) into Eq. (2) to obtain

$$t = \frac{\rho_A R_o^2}{c_{A_w} M_A \mathcal{D}_{AB}} \int_0^1 \frac{u}{1 + \alpha u^{3/2}} \, du \tag{6}$$

Integrate Eq. (6), and show that the time for complete dissolution of a salicylic acid sphere is given by

$$t = \frac{\rho_A R_o^2}{c_{A_w} M_A \mathcal{D}_{AB}} \left\{ \frac{2}{\alpha} - \frac{1}{3\alpha^{4/3}} \ln \left[\frac{(1 + \alpha^{1/3})^2}{1 + \alpha^{2/3} - \alpha^{1/3}} \right] - \frac{2}{\sqrt{3}\alpha^{4/3}} \left[\tan^{-1} \left(\frac{2\alpha^{1/3} - 1}{\sqrt{3}} \right) + \frac{\pi}{6} \right] \right\} \tag{7}$$

5.5 Formation of carbonaceous residues, known as coke deposition, on the surface of a catalyst over time leads to loss of catalyst activity and/or selectivity. Regeneration of such a catalyst is achieved by burning the coke in an oxygen atmosphere. Consider a spherical carbon particle of initial radius R_o surrounded by an atmosphere of oxygen.

a) For a very rapid heterogeneous reaction

$$C + O_2 \rightarrow CO_2$$

taking place on the outer surface of the carbon particle, show that the time it takes for the carbon particle to disappear completely is given by

$$t = \frac{\rho_C R_o^2}{24 c \mathcal{D}_{O_2 - CO_2}},$$

where ρ_C is the density of carbon.

b) For a very rapid heterogeneous reaction,

$$2C + O_2 \rightarrow 2CO$$

taking place on the outer surface of the carbon particle, show that the time it takes for the carbon particle to disappear completely is given by

$$t = \frac{\rho_C R_o^2}{33.271 \, c \mathcal{D}_{O_2 - CO}}$$

5.6 Repeat the analysis given in Section 5.8.2 for a cylindrical geometry shown in the figure below. Assuming radial diffusion only, show that

$$b \tilde{V}_B c_{A_b}^* t = \frac{R_o}{2k_c^*} X_B + \frac{R_o^2}{4 \mathcal{D}_{eff}} \left[X_B + (1 - X_B) \ln(1 - X_B) \right] + \frac{R_o}{k_1''} \left[1 - (1 - X_B)^{1/2} \right],$$

where the fractional conversion for species B is given by

$$X_B = 1 - \left(\frac{R_c}{R_o} \right)^2$$

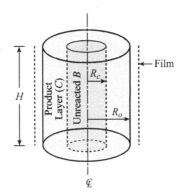

REFERENCES

Asai, S., Y. Konishi and Y. Sasaki. 1988. Mass transfer between fine particles and liquids in agitated vessels. *J. Chem. Eng. Japan* 21(2):107–12.

Bedingfield, C. H. and T. B. Drew. 1950. Analogy between heat transfer and mass transfer. A psychometric study. *Ind. Eng. Chem.* 42(6):1164–73.

Blausius, H. 1908. Grenzschichten in Flussigkeiten mit kleiner Reibung. *Z. Angew. Math. Phys.* 56:1-37; 60:397–398.

Chen, J. J. J. 1987. Comments on improvements on a replacement for the logarithmic mean. *Chem. Eng. Sci.* 42(10):2488–89.

Cussler, E. N. 1984. How we make mass transfer seem difficult. *Chem. Eng. Ed.* 18(3):124–7; 149–52.

Cussler, E. N., 2009. *Diffusion – Mass Transfer in Fluid Systems.* 3rd edn. Cambridge: Cambridge University Press.

Delgado, J. M. P. Q. 2007. Molecular diffusion coefficients of organic compounds in water at different temperatures. *J. Phase Equil. Diff.* 28(5):427–32.

Dwivedi, P. N. and S. N. Upadhyay. 1977. Particle-fluid mass transfer in fixed and fluidized beds. *Ind. Eng. Chem. Process Des. Dev.* 16(2):157–65.

Frossling, N. 1938. The evaporation of falling drops (in German), *Gerlands Beiträge zur Geophysik.* 52:170–216.

Gilliland, E. R. and T. K. Sherwood. 1934. Diffusion of vapors into air streams. *Ind. Eng. Chem.* 26(5):516–23.

Jessop, P. G., D. J. Heldebrant, X. Li, C. A. Eckert and C. L. Liotta. 2005. Reversible nonpolar-to-polar solvent. *Nature* 436(7054):1102.

Kulov, N. N., E. K. Nikolaishvili, V. M. Barabash, L. N. Braginski, V. A. Malyusov and N. M. Zhavoronkov. 1983. Dissolution of solid particles suspended in agitated vessels. *Chem. Eng. Commun.* 21:259–71.

Kwon, K. C., T. H. Ibrahim, Y. K. Park and C. M. Simmons. 2002. Inexpensive and simple binary molecular diffusion experiments. *Chem. Eng. Ed.* 36(1):68–73.

Lewis, W. K. 1916. Laboratory and plant: The principles of counter-current extraction. *Ind. Eng. Chem.* 8(9):825–33.

Linton, W. H. and T. K. Sherwood. 1950. Mass transfer from solid shapes to water in streamline and turbulent flow. *Chem. Eng. Prog.* 46:258–64.

Lozar, J., C. Laguerie and J. P. Couderc. 1975. Diffusivité de l'acide benzoïque dans l'eau: Influence de la température. *Can. J. Chem. Eng.* 53(2):200–3.

Miller, D. N. 1971. Scale-up of agitated tanks: Mass transfer from suspended solute particles. *Ind. Eng. Chem. Process Des. Develop.* 10(3):365–75.

Nanta, P., W. Skolpap, K. Kasemwong and Y. Shimoyama. 2018. Development of a diffusion-limited shrinking particle model of cellulose dissolution in a carbon dioxide switchable system. *Chem. Eng. Sci.* 179:214–20.

Pangarkar, V. G., A. A. Yawalkar, M. M. Sharma and A. A. C. M. Beenackers. 2002. Particle-liquid mass transfer coefficient in two-/three-phase stirred tank reactors. *Ind. Eng. Chem. Res.* 41(17):4141–67.

Paterson, W. R. 1984. A replacement for the logarithmic mean. *Chem. Eng. Sci.* 39(11):1635–36.

Ranz, W. E. and W. R. Marshall. 1952a. Evaporation from drops - Part I. *Chem. Eng. Prog.* 48(3):141–46.

Ranz, W. E. and W. R. Marshall. 1952b. Evaporation from drops - Part II. *Chem. Eng. Prog.* 48(4):173–180.

Siepmann, J. and F. Siepmann. 2012. Modeling of diffusion controlled drug delivery. *J. Control. Release* 161:351–62.

Steinberger, R. L. and R. E. Treybal. 1960. Mass transfer from a solid soluble sphere to a flowing liquid stream. *AIChE J.* 6(2):227–32.

Tosun, I. 2007. *Modeling in Transport Phenomena—A Conceptual Approach*, 2nd edn. Amsterdam: Elsevier.

Wang, G. Q., X. G. Yuan and K. T. Yu. 2005. Review of mass-transfer correlations for packed columns. *Ind. Eng. Chem. Res.* 44(23):8715–29.

Whitman, W. G. 1923. Preliminary experimental confirmation of the two-film theory of gas absorption. *Chem. Met. Eng.* 29(4):146–54.

Wickramasinghe, S. R., M. J. Semmens and E. L. Cussler. 1992. Mass transfer in various hollow fiber geometries. *J. Memb. Sci.* 69(3):235–50.

6 Mass Transfer in Binary Systems without Bulk Flow: Unsteady-State Examples

When concentration depends on time as well as position, the species continuity equation becomes a partial differential equation in at least one dimension. The solution method is dependent not only on the structure of the equation itself, i.e., homogeneous or nonhomogeneous, but also on the types of boundary conditions. This obviously leads to numerous possibilities. A mathematical treatise of diffusion and heat conduction problems is completely analogous. The comprehensive book by Carslaw and Jaeger (1959) provides analytical solutions to a variety of heat conduction problems. The counterpart of this book for diffusion is the one written by Crank (1975). In that respect, it is always advantageous to write the governing equation and its associated initial and boundary conditions in dimensionless form since they represent the solution to the entire class of geometrically similar problems when they are applied to a particular geometry. In this chapter, some representative examples of unsteady-state diffusion problems in the Cartesian, cylindrical, and spherical coordinate systems will be presented in detail.

6.1 GOVERNING EQUATIONS

In the absence of bulk flow, transfer of species into and/or out of the system takes place by diffusion. In this case, the equation of continuity for species A reduces to

$$\frac{\partial c_A}{\partial t} = \mathcal{D}_{AB} \nabla^2 c_A + \mathcal{R}_A, \tag{6.1}$$

which is presented in the different coordinate systems in Table 6.1.

Table 6.1

Equation of Continuity for Species A when Convection Is Negligible

Cartesian Coordinates

$$\frac{\partial c_A}{\partial t} = \mathcal{D}_{AB} \left(\frac{\partial^2 c_A}{\partial x^2} + \frac{\partial^2 c_A}{\partial y^2} + \frac{\partial^2 c_A}{\partial z^2} \right) + \mathcal{R}_A \tag{A}$$

Cylindrical Coordinates

$$\frac{\partial c_A}{\partial t} = \mathcal{D}_{AB} \left[\frac{1}{r} \frac{\partial}{\partial r} \left(r \frac{\partial c_A}{\partial r} \right) + \frac{1}{r^2} \frac{\partial^2 c_A}{\partial \theta^2} + \frac{\partial^2 c_A}{\partial z^2} \right] + \mathcal{R}_A \tag{B}$$

Spherical Coordinates

$$\frac{\partial c_A}{\partial t} = \mathcal{D}_{AB} \left[\frac{1}{r^2} \frac{\partial}{\partial r} \left(r^2 \frac{\partial c_A}{\partial r} \right) + \frac{1}{r^2 \sin \theta} \frac{\partial}{\partial \theta} \left(\sin \theta \frac{\partial c_A}{\partial \theta} \right) + \frac{1}{r^2 \sin^2 \theta} \frac{\partial^2 c_A}{\partial \phi^2} \right] + \mathcal{R}_A \tag{C}$$

6.2   DIFFUSION INTO A RECTANGULAR SLAB

Consider a rectangular solid slab (species B) of thickness $2L$ as shown in Figure 6.1. Initially the concentration of species A within the slab is uniform at a value of c_{A_o}. At $t = 0$, the surfaces at $z = \pm L$ are exposed to a fluid having a concentration of c_{A_∞}, with $c_{A_\infty} > c_{A_o}$. We are interested in the amount of species A transferred into the slab as a function of time. For this purpose, it is first necessary to determine the concentration distribution of species A within the slab as a function of position and time.

Let us assume $\mathrm{Bi}_H > 40$ so that the resistance to mass transfer in the fluid phase is negligible and the concentration of species A in the fluid phase at the solid–fluid interface is also c_{A_∞}. Under equilibrium conditions, a partition coefficient K_A relates the concentrations of species A on both sides of the interface as

$$c_A^{solid}\Big|_{z=\pm L} = K_A c_{A_\infty} \tag{6.2}$$

In the absence of a chemical reaction, Eq. (A) of Table 6.1 reduces to

$$\frac{\partial c_A}{\partial t} = \mathcal{D}_{AB} \left(\frac{\partial^2 c_A}{\partial x^2} + \frac{\partial^2 c_A}{\partial y^2} + \frac{\partial^2 c_A}{\partial z^2} \right) \tag{6.3}$$

The terms on the right side of Eq. (6.3) represent diffusion in the x-, y-, and z-directions, respectively. The order of magnitude estimates of these terms are

$$\frac{\partial^2 c_A}{\partial x^2} \sim O\left[\frac{(\Delta c_A)_{ch}}{H^2}\right] \qquad \frac{\partial^2 c_A}{\partial y^2} \sim O\left[\frac{(\Delta c_A)_{ch}}{W^2}\right] \qquad \frac{\partial^2 c_A}{\partial z^2} \sim O\left[\frac{(\Delta c_A)_{ch}}{L^2}\right], \tag{6.4}$$

where $(\Delta c_A)_{ch} = K_A c_{A_\infty} - c_{A_o}$. If $L/H \ll 1$ and $L/W \ll 1$, then

$$\frac{\partial^2 c_A/\partial x^2}{\partial^2 c_A/\partial z^2} \sim \left(\frac{L}{H}\right)^2 \ll 1 \qquad \text{and} \qquad \frac{\partial^2 c_A/\partial y^2}{\partial^2 c_A/\partial z^2} \sim \left(\frac{L}{W}\right)^2 \ll 1, \tag{6.5}$$

indicating that the dominant term is the diffusion in the z-direction, and Eq. (6.3) can be simplified to

$$\frac{\partial c_A}{\partial t} = \mathcal{D}_{AB} \frac{\partial^2 c_A}{\partial z^2} \tag{6.6}$$

The initial and boundary conditions associated with Eq. (6.6) are

$$\text{at} \quad t = 0 \qquad c_A = c_{A_o} \tag{6.7}$$

$$\text{at} \quad z = L \qquad c_A = K_A c_{A_\infty} \tag{6.8}$$

$$\text{at} \quad z = -L \qquad c_A = K_A c_{A_\infty} \tag{6.9}$$

Note that $z = 0$ represents a plane of symmetry across which there is no net flux, i.e., $\partial c_A/\partial z = 0$. Therefore, it is also possible to express the initial and boundary conditions as

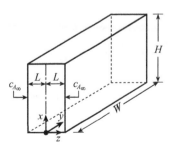

Figure 6.1   Mass transfer into a rectangular slab.

$$\text{at} \quad t = 0 \qquad c_A = c_{A_o} \tag{6.10}$$

$$\text{at} \quad z = 0 \qquad \frac{\partial c_A}{\partial z} = 0 \tag{6.11}$$

$$\text{at} \quad z = L \qquad c_A = K_A c_{A_\infty} \tag{6.12}$$

The boundary condition at $z = 0$ can also be interpreted as an impermeable surface, i.e., the concentration gradient is zero since there is no flux through the surface located at $z = 0$. As a result, the governing equation for concentration, Eq. (6.6), together with the initial and boundary conditions given by Eqs. (6.10)–(6.12), may also represent the following problem statement: *"Initially the concentration of species A within a slab of thickness L is uniform at a value of c_{A_o}. While one of the surfaces is impermeable to species A, the other is exposed to a fluid having constant concentration c_{A_∞}, with $c_{A_\infty} > c_{A_o}$ for $t > 0$."*

The order of magnitude of the term on the left side of Eq. (6.6) is

$$\frac{\partial c_A}{\partial t} \sim O\left[\frac{(\Delta c_A)_{ch}}{t}\right] \tag{6.13}$$

Thus, the ratio of the rate of diffusion to the rate of mass accumulation is given by

$$\frac{\text{Rate of diffusion}}{\text{Rate of mass accumulation}} = \frac{\mathcal{D}_{AB}(\Delta c_A)_{ch}/L^2}{(\Delta c_A)_{ch}/t} = \frac{\mathcal{D}_{AB} t}{L^2}, \tag{6.14}$$

which is known as the dimensionless *Fourier number*, τ.

Introduction of the dimensionless quantities

$$\theta = \frac{K_A c_{A_\infty} - c_A}{K_A c_{A_\infty} - c_{A_o}} \qquad \tau = \frac{\mathcal{D}_{AB} t}{L^2} \qquad \xi = \frac{z}{L} \tag{6.15}$$

reduces Eqs. (6.6) and (6.10)–(6.12) to

$$\frac{\partial \theta}{\partial \tau} = \frac{\partial^2 \theta}{\partial \xi^2} \tag{6.16}$$

$$\text{at} \quad \tau = 0 \qquad \theta = 1 \tag{6.17}$$

$$\text{at} \quad \xi = 0 \qquad \frac{\partial \theta}{\partial \xi} = 0 \tag{6.18}$$

$$\text{at} \quad \xi = 1 \qquad \theta = 0 \tag{6.19}$$

The solution of Eq. (6.16) by the Laplace transformation technique is presented in Example E.10 in Appendix E. The solution in the Laplace domain is

$$\overline{\theta} = \frac{1}{s} - \frac{\cosh(\xi \sqrt{s})}{s \cosh \sqrt{s}} \tag{6.20}$$

and the inverse Laplace transformation yields

$$\boxed{\theta = \frac{4}{\pi} \sum_{n=0}^{\infty} \frac{(-1)^n}{2n+1} e^{-\left(\frac{2n+1}{2}\right)^2 \pi^2 \tau} \cos\left[\left(\frac{2n+1}{2}\right) \pi \xi\right]} \tag{6.21}$$

The molar flux of species A at the surface of the slab is

$$N_{A_z}\big|_{z=L} = -\mathcal{D}_{AB} \frac{\partial c_A}{\partial z}\bigg|_{z=L} = \frac{\mathcal{D}_{AB}(K_A c_{A_\infty} - c_{A_o})}{L} \frac{\partial \theta}{\partial \xi}\bigg|_{\xi=1} \tag{6.22}$$

The use of Eq. (6.21) in Eq. (6.22) gives

$$N_{A_z}\big|_{z=L} = \frac{2\mathcal{D}_{AB}\left(K_A c_{A_\infty} - c_{A_o}\right)}{L} \sum_{n=0}^{\infty} \exp\left[-\left(\frac{2n+1}{2}\right)^2 \pi^2 \tau\right] \tag{6.23}$$

The molar rate of flow of species A entering the slab from both surfaces is

$$\mathcal{W}_A = \frac{4WH\mathcal{D}_{AB}\left(K_A c_{A_\infty} - c_{A_o}\right)}{L} \sum_{n=0}^{\infty} \exp\left[-\left(\frac{2n+1}{2}\right)^2 \pi^2 \tau\right] \tag{6.24}$$

The number of moles of species A transferred into the slab, $\mathbb{N}_A$, over time t is calculated from

$$\mathbb{N}_A = \int_0^t \mathcal{W}_A \, dt = \frac{L^2}{\mathcal{D}_{AB}} \int_0^\tau \mathcal{W}_A \, d\tau \tag{6.25}$$

Substitution of Eq. (6.24) into Eq. (6.25) and integration lead to

$$\frac{\mathbb{N}_A}{\mathbb{N}_{A_\infty}} = 1 - \frac{8}{\pi^2} \sum_{n=0}^{\infty} \frac{1}{(2n+1)^2} \exp\left[-\left(\frac{2n+1}{2}\right)^2 \pi^2 \tau\right], \tag{6.26}$$

where $\mathbb{N}_{A_\infty}$ represents the maximum number of moles of species A transferred into the slab, i.e.,

$$\mathbb{N}_{A_\infty} = 2LWH\left(K_A c_{A_\infty} - c_{A_o}\right) \tag{6.27}$$

6.2.1 CALCULATION OF THE MOLAR FLUX – AN ALTERNATIVE APPROACH

If the ultimate purpose is to obtain the molar flux of species A at the surface of the slab, there is no need to obtain the concentration distribution, Eq. (6.21), by taking the inverse Laplace transformation of Eq. (6.20). The Laplace transformed molar flux at the surface of the slab is

$$\overline{N}_{A_z}\big|_{z=L} = \frac{\mathcal{D}_{AB}\left(K_A c_{A_\infty} - c_{A_o}\right)}{L} \frac{d\overline{\theta}}{d\xi}\bigg|_{\xi=1} \tag{6.28}$$

The use of Eq. (6.20) in Eq. (6.28) yields

$$\overline{N}_{A_z}\big|_{z=L} = \frac{\mathcal{D}_{AB}\left(K_A c_{A_\infty} - c_{A_o}\right)}{L} \frac{\sinh\sqrt{s}}{\sqrt{s}\cosh\sqrt{s}} \tag{6.29}$$

Using Eq. (30) from Table E.6 in Appendix E, the inverse Laplace transform becomes

$$N_{A_z}\big|_{z=L} = \frac{2\mathcal{D}_{AB}\left(K_A c_{A_\infty} - c_{A_o}\right)}{L} \sum_{n=1}^{\infty} (-1)^{n-1} e^{-\left(\frac{2n+1}{2}\right)^2 \pi^2 \tau} \sin\left[\left(\frac{2n-1}{2}\right)\pi\right] \tag{6.30}$$

Using

$$m = n - 1 \tag{6.31}$$

Eq. (6.30) becomes

$$N_{A_z}\big|_{z=L} = \frac{2\mathcal{D}_{AB}\left(K_A c_{A_\infty} - c_{A_o}\right)}{L} \sum_{m=0}^{\infty} \exp\left[-\left(\frac{2m+1}{2}\right)^2 \pi^2 \tau\right] \tag{6.32}$$

which is identical with Eq. (6.23).

Example 6.1 A 2.5-mm-thick membrane (species B) in the form of a flat sheet is initially free of species A. It is immersed in a well-stirred 0.2 M solution of species A.

a) Estimate the concentration of species A at the center of the membrane after 10 min if $\mathcal{D}_{AB} = 4 \times 10^{-10}\,\text{m}^2/\text{s}$ and $K_A = 0.85$.

b) How long will it take for the system to reach steady-state?

Solution

a) Since $\xi = 0$ represents the center of the membrane and $c_{A_o} = 0$, Eq. (6.21) gives the concentration at this location as

$$\frac{K_A c_{A_\infty} - c_A|_{\xi=0}}{K_A c_{A_\infty}} = \frac{4}{\pi}\sum_{n=0}^{\infty}\frac{(-1)^n}{2n+1}\exp\left[-\left(\frac{2n+1}{2}\right)^2\pi^2\tau\right] \tag{1}$$

As can be seen from the Mathcad worksheet, $c_A|_{\xi=0} = 0.024$ M after 10 min.

b) If the time to reach steady-state, t_∞, is defined as the time for the center concentration to reach 99% of the surface concentration, i.e.,

$$c_A|_{\xi=0} = 0.99\,K_A c_{A_\infty},$$

then from the Mathcad worksheet $t_\infty = 2.131$ h.

$K := 0.85$ $cAinf := 0.2$ $t := 10$ $L := \dfrac{2.5 \cdot 10^{-3}}{2}$ $D := 4 \cdot 10^{-10}$

$$\tau := \frac{D \cdot t \cdot 60}{L^2}$$

Part (a)

$$cAcenter := K \cdot cAinf \cdot \left[1 - \frac{4}{\pi} \cdot \sum_{n=0}^{20}\left[\frac{(-1)^n}{2n+1} \cdot \exp\left[-\left(\frac{2n+1}{2}\right)^2 \cdot \pi^2 \cdot \tau\right]\right]\right] = 0.024$$

Part (b)

$$cAcenter := 0.99\,K \cdot cAinf$$

$$\tau := \frac{-4}{\pi^2} \cdot \ln\left[\frac{\pi}{4} \cdot \left(\frac{K \cdot cAinf - cAcenter}{K \cdot cAinf}\right)\right] = 1.964 \qquad \text{This is the initial guess value}$$

Given

$$\frac{K \cdot cAinf - cAcenter}{K \cdot cAinf} = \frac{4}{\pi} \cdot \sum_{n=0}^{20}\left[\frac{(-1)^n}{2n+1} \cdot \exp\left[-\left(\frac{2n+1}{2}\right)^2 \cdot \pi^2 \cdot \tau\right]\right]$$

$$\tau := \text{Find}(\tau) = 1.964$$

$$time := \frac{\tau \cdot L^2}{3600\,D} = 2.131$$

Mathcad worksheet of Example 6.1.

Comment: In Section 5.1, the time it takes for a given process to reach steady-state is defined as

$$t_{ch}^D = \frac{L_{ch}^2}{\mathcal{D}_{AB}},$$

where L is the half-thickness of the membrane. Substitution of the values into Eq. (2) gives

$$t_{ch}^D = \frac{(2.5 \times 10^{-3}/2)^2}{4 \times 10^{-10}} \frac{1}{3600} = 1.085h,$$

which is quite satisfactory as far as the orders of magnitude are concerned. Interested readers may refer to Carr (2017) for a more detailed analysis of the problem.

6.2.2 SOLUTION FOR SHORT TIMES

At small values of time, species A does not penetrate very far into the slab. Within this very thin region adjacent to the surface of the slab, called *penetration depth* (δ), concentration changes from Kc_{A_∞} to c_{A_o}. Since short-time solutions correspond to large values of s in the Laplace domain, the hyperbolic terms in Eq. (6.20) are approximated in terms of exponential functions as

$$\cosh(\xi \sqrt{s}) = \frac{e^{\xi \sqrt{s}} + e^{-\xi \sqrt{s}}}{2} \simeq \frac{e^{\xi \sqrt{s}}}{2} \qquad (6.33)$$

$$\cosh \sqrt{s} = \frac{e^{\sqrt{s}} + e^{-\sqrt{s}}}{2} \simeq \frac{e^{\sqrt{s}}}{2} \qquad (6.34)$$

Substitution of Eqs. (6.33) and (6.34) into Eq. (6.20) yields

$$\overline{\theta} = \frac{1}{s} - \frac{e^{-\sqrt{s}(1-\xi)}}{s} \qquad (6.35)$$

Using Eqs. (1) and (16) from Table E.6 in Appendix E, the inverse Laplace transform becomes

$$\boxed{\theta = 1 - \text{erfc}\left(\frac{1-\xi}{2\sqrt{\tau}}\right) = \text{erf}\left(\frac{1-\xi}{2\sqrt{\tau}}\right)} \qquad (6.36)$$

The use of Eq. (6.36) in Eq. (6.22) gives the molar flux at the surface as

$$\boxed{N_{A_z}\big|_{z=L} = (Kc_{A_\infty} - c_{A_o}) \sqrt{\frac{\mathcal{D}_{AB}}{\pi t}}} \qquad (6.37)$$

The molar rate of flow of species A entering the slab from both surfaces is

$$\boxed{\mathcal{W}_A = 2WH(K_A c_{A_\infty} - c_{A_o}) \sqrt{\frac{\mathcal{D}_{AB}}{\pi t}}} \qquad (6.38)$$

The number of moles of species A transferred into the slab, $\mathbb{N}_A$, over time t is calculated from

$$\boxed{\mathbb{N}_A = \int_0^t \mathcal{W}_A \, dt = 4WH(Kc_{A_\infty} - c_{A_o}) \sqrt{\frac{\mathcal{D}_{AB} t}{\pi}}} \qquad (6.39)$$

Thus,

$$\boxed{\frac{\mathbb{N}_A}{\mathbb{N}_{A_\infty}} = \frac{2}{L} \sqrt{\frac{\mathcal{D}_{AB} t}{\pi}}} \qquad \text{Short-time solution} \qquad (6.40)$$

One should be careful when interpreting the term L in Eq. (6.40). It is defined by

$$L = \begin{cases} \text{Total thickness} & \text{When mass transfer takes place from one surface} \\ \text{Half-thickness} & \text{When mass transfer takes place from both surfaces} \end{cases} \tag{6.41}$$

A representative plot of $\mathbb{N}_A/\mathbb{N}_{A\infty}$ versus $\sqrt{t}$ is shown in Figure 6.2.

In terms of dimensional quantities, Eq. (6.36) is expressed in the form

$$\frac{K_A c_{A\infty} - c_A}{K_A c_{A\infty} - c_{A_0}} = \text{erf}\left(\frac{L-z}{2\sqrt{\mathcal{D}_{AB}t}}\right) \tag{6.42}$$

Let s be the distance measured from the slab surface, i.e., $s = L - z$, so that Eq. (6.36) becomes

$$\frac{K_A c_{A\infty} - c_A}{K_A c_{A\infty} - c_{A_0}} = \text{erf}\left(\frac{s}{2\sqrt{\mathcal{D}_{AB}t}}\right) \tag{6.43}$$

Rearrangement of Eq. (6.43) gives

$$\frac{c_A - c_{A_0}}{K_A c_{A\infty} - c_{A_0}} = 1 - \text{erf}\left(\frac{s}{2\sqrt{\mathcal{D}_{AB}t}}\right) \tag{6.44}$$

The term on the left side of Eq. (6.44) is plotted versus the distance measured from the slab surface, s, with $2\sqrt{\mathcal{D}_{AB}t}$ being a parameter in Figure 6.3.

The penetration depth, δ, is the distance over which the concentration change takes place, i.e.,

$$c_A = c_{A_0} \qquad \text{when} \qquad s = \delta \tag{6.45}$$

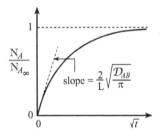

Figure 6.2 Fractional uptake versus $\sqrt{t}$.

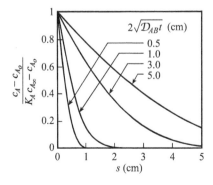

Figure 6.3 Variation in concentration as a function of s.

The use of Eq. (6.45) in Eq. (6.44) gives

$$\text{erf}\left(\frac{\delta}{2\sqrt{\mathcal{D}_{AB}t}}\right) = \underbrace{1}_{\text{erf}(2)} \qquad \Rightarrow \qquad \frac{\delta}{2\sqrt{\mathcal{D}_{AB}t}} = 2 \tag{6.46}$$

Thus, the penetration depth is given by

$$\boxed{\delta = 4\sqrt{\mathcal{D}_{AB}t}} \tag{6.47}$$

Note that the short-time solution, Eq. (6.44), is valid as long as the concentration at $s = L$ is less than or equal to c_{A_o}, i.e.,

$$\text{erf}\left(\frac{L}{2\sqrt{\mathcal{D}_{AB}t}}\right) \geq \underbrace{1}_{\text{erf}(2)} \tag{6.48}$$

or

$$\boxed{t \leq \frac{L^2}{16\mathcal{D}_{AB}}} \qquad \begin{array}{c} \text{Criterion for the validity of} \\ \text{short-time solution} \end{array} \tag{6.49}$$

6.2.3 DIFFUSION INTO A SEMI-INFINITE DOMAIN

Consider one-dimensional diffusion of species A into a semi-infinite slab of width W and height H. Initially the concentration of species A within the slab is uniform at a value of c_{A_o}. Let s be the distance measured from the surface of the slab. The surface of the slab is exposed to a fluid with a concentration of c_{A_∞}. The governing equation and its associated initial and boundary conditions are given as

$$\frac{\partial\theta}{\partial t} = \mathcal{D}_{AB}\frac{\partial^2\theta}{\partial s^2}$$

$$\begin{array}{lll} t = 0 & \theta = 0 \\ s = 0 & \theta = 1 \\ s = \infty & \theta = 0, \end{array} \tag{6.50}$$

where the dimensionless concentration θ is defined by

$$\theta = \frac{c_A - c_{A_o}}{K_A c_{A_\infty} - c_{A_o}} \tag{6.51}$$

The solution can be obtained from Example E.8 in Appendix E as

$$\theta = \frac{c_A - c_{A_o}}{K_A c_{A_\infty} - c_{A_o}} = 1 - \text{erf}\left(\frac{s}{2\sqrt{\mathcal{D}_{AB}t}}\right), \tag{6.52}$$

which is identical with Eq. (6.44). This implies that the short-time solution is another way of treating the diffusion domain as semi-infinite. Therefore, the semi-infinite medium assumption holds as long as the criterion given by Eq. (6.49) is satisfied.

The number of moles of species A transferred into the semi-infinite medium, $\mathbb{N}_A$, can be determined from

$$\begin{aligned} \mathbb{N}_A &= WH\int_0^\infty (c_A - c_{A_o})\,ds = WH\left(K_A c_{A_\infty} - c_{A_o}\right)\int_0^\infty\left[1 - \text{erf}\left(\frac{s}{2\sqrt{\mathcal{D}_{AB}t}}\right)\right]\,ds \\ &= 2WH\left(Kc_{A_\infty} - c_{A_o}\right)\sqrt{\frac{\mathcal{D}_{AB}t}{\pi}} \end{aligned} \tag{6.53}$$

Example 6.2   Segel et al. (1977) carried out the following experimental procedure to quantify the average motility of bacterial populations. A capillary tube of cross-sectional area A is filled with phosphate buffer. The open end of the tube is placed in a suspension of bacteria (species A) of known concentration c_{A_o}. The tube is removed after time t and the number of bacteria that it contains is counted. Postulating one-dimensional diffusion and a semi-infinite medium, the governing equation and its associated initial and boundary conditions are given as

$$\frac{\partial \theta}{\partial t} = \mathcal{D}_{AB} \frac{\partial^2 \theta}{\partial z^2}$$

$$
\begin{aligned}
t &= 0 & \theta &= 0 \\
z &= 0 & \theta &= 1 \\
z &= \infty & \theta &= 0,
\end{aligned}
\tag{1}
$$

where z is the axial distance measured from the open end of the tube and θ is the dimensionless concentration defined by

$$\theta = \frac{c_A}{c_{A_o}} \tag{2}$$

Since Eq. (1) is identical with Eq. (6.50), the solution is given by Eq. (6.52), i.e.,

$$\frac{c_A}{c_{A_o}} = 1 - \mathrm{erf}\left(\frac{z}{2\sqrt{\mathcal{D}_{AB}t}}\right) \tag{3}$$

The flux at the open end of the capillary tube is

$$N_{A_z}\big|_{z=0} = -\mathcal{D}_{AB} \frac{\partial c_A}{\partial z}\bigg|_{z=0} = c_{A_o}\sqrt{\frac{\mathcal{D}_{AB}}{\pi t}} \tag{4}$$

The flow rate of bacteria into the capillary is

$$\mathcal{W}_A = A\,N_{A_z}\big|_{z=0} = A c_{A_o}\sqrt{\frac{\mathcal{D}_{AB}}{\pi t}}, \tag{5}$$

where A is the cross-sectional area of the capillary tube. Thus, the number of bacteria entering the capillary, $\mathbb{N}_A$, can be calculated from

$$\mathbb{N}_A = \int_0^t \mathcal{W}_A\,dt = 2A c_{A_o}\sqrt{\frac{\mathcal{D}_{AB}t}{\pi}} \tag{6}$$

or

$$\mathbb{N}_A^2 = \left(\frac{4A^2 c_{A_o}^2 \mathcal{D}_{AB}}{\pi}\right)t \tag{7}$$

The diffusion coefficient (or motility of bacteria) can be determined from the slope of the $\mathbb{N}_A^2$ versus t plot, i.e.,

$$\mathcal{D}_{AB} = \frac{\pi(\mathrm{slope})}{4A^2 c_{A_o}^2} \tag{8}$$

Using a 1-μL capillary tube 32mm in length, Segel et al. (1977) reported the following data for $c_{A_o} = 7 \times 10^7$ bacteria/mL:

t (min)	2	5	10	12.5	15	20
$\mathbb{N}_A$	1,800	3,700	4,800	5,500	6,700	8,000

The plot of $\mathbb{N}_A^2$ versus time is shown below. The slope of the best straight line (correlation coefficient is 0.984) passing through the data points is 3.28×10^6.

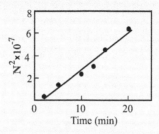

The cross-sectional area of the capillary is

$$A = \frac{V}{L} = \frac{10^{-3}}{3.2} = 3.125 \times 10^{-4} \text{cm}^2$$

Thus, the diffusion coefficient is calculated from Eq. (8) as

$$\mathcal{D}_{AB} = \frac{\pi(3.28 \times 10^6)}{4(3.125 \times 10^{-4})^2(7 \times 10^7)^2} = 5.38 \times 10^{-3} \text{cm}^2/\text{min} = 8.97 \times 10^{-5} \text{cm}^2/\text{s}$$

Comment: Is it logical to make a semi-infinite medium assumption for a tube of length 32 mm? This assumption is valid as long as the concentration at $z = 3.2$ cm is less than or equal to zero as stated by Eq. (6.49) or

$$t \leq \frac{(3.2)^2}{(16)(8.97 \times 10^{-5})} = 7135 \text{ s} = 119 \text{ min}$$

Since the maximum experimentation time is 20 min, it is plausible to assume a semi-infinite medium.

6.2.4 SOLUTION FOR LONG TIMES

When τ is large, only the first term of the series in Eq. (6.26) is important. Thus,

$$\boxed{\frac{\mathbb{N}_A}{\mathbb{N}_{A_\infty}} = 1 - \frac{8}{\pi^2} \exp\left(-\frac{\pi^2 \mathcal{D}_{AB} t}{4L^2}\right),} \qquad \begin{array}{l} \text{Long-time} \\ \text{solution} \end{array} \qquad (6.54)$$

in which the term L is defined by Eq. (6.41).

6.3 DRUG RELEASE FROM A SPHERICAL MATRIX

Consider a monolithic drug delivery system in which the drug (species A) is dispersed uniformly in a spherical polymeric matrix of radius R. The drug is surrounded by a fluid having a concentration of c_{A_∞}. We are interested in the amount of drug released as a function of time. If the effective diffusion coefficient, $\mathcal{D}_{eff}$, is independent of concentration, Eq. (C) of Table 6.1 gives the governing equation as

$$\frac{\partial c_A}{\partial t} = \frac{\mathcal{D}_{eff}}{r^2} \frac{\partial}{\partial r}\left(r^2 \frac{\partial c_A}{\partial r}\right) \qquad (6.55)$$

The initial and boundary conditions associated with Eq. (6.55) are

$$\text{at} \quad t = 0 \qquad c_A = c_{A_o} \tag{6.56}$$

$$\text{at} \quad r = 0 \qquad \frac{\partial c_A}{\partial r} = 0 \tag{6.57}$$

$$\text{at} \quad r = R \qquad c_A = K_A c_{A_\infty} \tag{6.58}$$

Introduction of the dimensionless quantities

$$\theta = \frac{c_A - K_A c_{A_\infty}}{c_{A_o} - K_A c_{A_\infty}} \qquad \tau = \frac{\mathcal{D}_{eff} t}{R^2} \qquad \xi = \frac{r}{R} \tag{6.59}$$

reduces Eqs. (6.55)–(6.58) to

$$\frac{\partial \theta}{\partial \tau} = \frac{1}{\xi^2} \frac{\partial}{\partial \xi} \left(\xi^2 \frac{\partial \theta}{\partial \xi} \right) \tag{6.60}$$

$$\text{at} \quad \tau = 0 \qquad \theta = 1 \tag{6.61}$$

$$\text{at} \quad \xi = 0 \qquad \frac{\partial \theta}{\partial \xi} = 0 \tag{6.62}$$

$$\text{at} \quad \xi = 1 \qquad \theta = 0 \tag{6.63}$$

The transformation

$$\theta(\tau, \xi) = \frac{u(\tau, \xi)}{\xi} \tag{6.64}$$

converts Eqs. (6.60)–(6.63) to

$$\frac{\partial u}{\partial \tau} = \frac{\partial^2 u}{\partial \xi^2} \tag{6.65}$$

$$\text{at} \quad \tau = 0 \qquad u = \xi \tag{6.66}$$
$$\text{at} \quad \xi = 0 \qquad u = 0 \tag{6.67}$$
$$\text{at} \quad \xi = 1 \qquad u = 0 \tag{6.68}$$

The Laplace transform of Eq. (6.65) gives the following ordinary differential equation (ODE):

$$\frac{d^2 \bar{u}}{d\xi^2} - s \bar{u} = -\xi, \tag{6.69}$$

where $\bar{u}$ is the Laplace transformed variable, defined by

$$\bar{u} = \int_0^\infty e^{-s\tau} u \, d\tau \tag{6.70}$$

The solution of Eq. (6.70) is given by

$$\bar{u} = C_1 \sinh(\xi \sqrt{s}) + C_2 \cosh(\xi \sqrt{s}) + \frac{\xi}{s} \tag{6.71}$$

Using the boundary conditions in the Laplace domain, i.e.,

$$\text{at} \quad \xi = 0 \qquad \bar{u} = 0 \tag{6.72}$$
$$\text{at} \quad \xi = 1 \qquad \bar{u} = 0 \tag{6.73}$$

the constants are evaluated as

$$C_1 = -\frac{1}{s \sinh \sqrt{s}} \qquad \text{and} \qquad C_2 = 0 \tag{6.74}$$

so that the solution in the Laplace domain is written as

$$\bar{u} = \frac{\xi}{s} - \frac{\sinh(\xi \sqrt{s})}{s \sinh \sqrt{s}} \tag{6.75}$$

Using Eqs. (1) and (32) from Table E.6 in Appendix E, the inverse Laplace transform becomes

$$u = \xi - \left[\xi + \frac{2}{\pi} \sum_{n=1}^{\infty} \frac{(-1)^n}{n} e^{-n^2\pi^2\tau} \sin(n\pi\xi) \right] = -\frac{2}{\pi} \sum_{n=1}^{\infty} \frac{(-1)^n}{n} e^{-n^2\pi^2\tau} \sin(n\pi\xi) \tag{6.76}$$

Substitution of Eq. (6.76) into Eq. (6.64) gives the dimensionless concentration distribution as

$$\boxed{\theta = -\frac{2}{\pi} \sum_{n=1}^{\infty} \frac{(-1)^n}{n} e^{-n^2\pi^2\tau} \frac{\sin(n\pi\xi)}{\xi}} \tag{6.77}$$

The molar flux of species A on the surface of the sphere is

$$N_{A_r}|_{r=R} = -\mathcal{D}_{AB} \left. \frac{\partial c_A}{\partial r} \right|_{r=R} = -\frac{\mathcal{D}_{AB}(c_{A_o} - K_A c_{A_\infty})}{R} \left. \frac{\partial \theta}{\partial \xi} \right|_{\xi=1} \tag{6.78}$$

The use of Eq. (6.77) in Eq. (6.78) yields

$$N_{A_r}|_{r=R} = \frac{2\mathcal{D}_{AB}(c_{A_o} - K_A c_{A_\infty})}{R} \sum_{n=1}^{\infty} \exp\left(-n^2\pi^2\tau\right) \tag{6.79}$$

The molar flow rate of species A leaving through the surface of the sphere is given by

$$\mathcal{W}_A = 4\pi R^2 N_{A_r}|_{r=R} = 8\pi R \mathcal{D}_{AB}(c_{A_o} - K_A c_{A_\infty}) \sum_{n=1}^{\infty} \exp\left(-n^2\pi^2\tau\right) \tag{6.80}$$

The number of moles of species A released from the sphere is given by

$$\mathbb{N}_A = \int_0^t \mathcal{W}_A \, dt = \frac{R^2}{\mathcal{D}_{AB}} \int_0^\tau \mathcal{W}_A \, d\tau \tag{6.81}$$

Substitution of Eq. (6.80) into Eq. (6.81) results in

$$\mathbb{N}_A = \frac{8R^3(c_{A_o} - K_A c_{A_\infty})}{\pi} \left[\sum_{n=1}^{\infty} \frac{1}{n^2} - \sum_{n=1}^{\infty} \frac{1}{n^2} \exp\left(-n^2\pi^2\tau\right) \right] \tag{6.82}$$

The maximum number of moles of species A released from the sphere is

$$\mathbb{N}_{A_\infty} = \frac{4}{3} \pi R^3 (c_{A_o} - K_A c_{A_\infty}) \tag{6.83}$$

Noting that

$$\sum_{n=1}^{\infty} \frac{1}{n^2} = \frac{\pi^2}{6} \tag{6.84}$$

and using Eqs. (6.83) and (6.84) in Eq. (6.82) lead to

$$\boxed{\frac{\mathbb{N}_A}{\mathbb{N}_{A_\infty}} = 1 - \frac{6}{\pi^2} \sum_{n=1}^{\infty} \frac{1}{n^2} \exp\left(-n^2\pi^2\tau\right)} \tag{6.85}$$

6.3.1 INVESTIGATION OF THE LIMITING CASES

• Short-time solution

Short-time solutions ($\tau \to 0$) correspond to large values of s in the Laplace domain, i.e., $s \to \infty$. Thus, the hyperbolic terms in Eq. (6.75) are approximated in terms of the exponential functions as

$$\sinh(\xi\sqrt{s}) = \frac{e^{\xi\sqrt{s}} - e^{-\xi\sqrt{s}}}{2} \simeq \frac{e^{\xi\sqrt{s}}}{2} \tag{6.86}$$

$$\sinh\sqrt{s} = \frac{e^{\sqrt{s}} - e^{-\sqrt{s}}}{2} \simeq \frac{e^{\sqrt{s}}}{2} \tag{6.87}$$

Substitution of Eqs. (6.86) and (6.87) into Eq. (6.75) leads to

$$\overline{u} = \frac{\xi}{s} - \frac{e^{-(1-\xi)\sqrt{s}}}{s} \tag{6.88}$$

Using Eqs. (1) and (17) from Table E.6 in Appendix E, the inverse Laplace transform becomes

$$u = \xi - \text{erfc}\left(\frac{1-\xi}{2\sqrt{\tau}}\right) = \xi - 1 + \text{erf}\left(\frac{1-\xi}{2\sqrt{\tau}}\right) \tag{6.89}$$

Substitution of Eq. (6.89) into Eq. (6.64) gives the solution as

$$\boxed{\theta = 1 - \frac{1}{\xi} + \frac{1}{\xi}\text{erf}\left(\frac{1-\xi}{2\sqrt{\tau}}\right)} \tag{6.90}$$

The use of Eq. (6.89) in Eq. (6.78) gives

$$N_{A_r}|_{r=R} = \frac{\mathcal{D}_{AB}\left(c_{A_o} - K_A c_{A_\infty}\right)}{R}\left(\frac{1}{\sqrt{\pi\tau}} - 1\right) \tag{6.91}$$

The molar flow rate of species A leaving through the surface of the sphere is given by

$$\mathcal{W}_A = 4\pi R^2 N_{A_r}|_{r=R} = 4\pi R \mathcal{D}_{AB}\left(c_{A_o} - K_A c_{A_\infty}\right)\left(\frac{1}{\sqrt{\pi\tau}} - 1\right) \tag{6.92}$$

The number of moles of species A released from the sphere is given by

$$\mathbb{N}_A = \int_0^t \mathcal{W}_A\, dt = \frac{R^2}{\mathcal{D}_{AB}}\int_0^\tau \mathcal{W}_A\, d\tau \tag{6.93}$$

Substitution of Eq. (6.92) into Eq. (6.93) and integration yield

$$\mathbb{N}_A = 4\pi R^3\left(c_{A_o} - K_A c_{A_\infty}\right)\left(2\sqrt{\frac{\tau}{\pi}} - \tau\right) \tag{6.94}$$

or

$$\boxed{\frac{\mathbb{N}_A}{\mathbb{N}_{A_\infty}} = 6\sqrt{\frac{\mathcal{D}_{AB}t}{\pi R^2}} - \frac{3\mathcal{D}_{AB}t}{R^2}} \quad \begin{matrix}\text{Short-time}\\ \text{solution}\end{matrix} \tag{6.95}$$

• Long-time solution

When τ is large, only the first term of the series in Eq. (6.85) is important. Thus,

$$\boxed{\frac{\mathbb{N}_A}{\mathbb{N}_{A_\infty}} = 1 - \frac{6}{\pi^2} \exp\left(-\frac{\pi^2 \mathcal{D}_{AB} t}{R^2}\right)} \quad \begin{array}{l} \text{Long-time} \\ \text{solution} \end{array} \tag{6.96}$$

Example 6.3 Calculate the time required to release half the initial mass contained in a spherical drug of 5mm diameter if the effective diffusion coefficient is $2.8 \times 10^{-6} \text{cm}^2/\text{s}$. Assume a perfect sink condition at the outer surface of the drug.

Solution

• Case (i): Analytical solution

The use of Eq. (6.85) gives

$$0.5 = 1 - \frac{6}{\pi^2} \sum_{n=1}^{\infty} \frac{1}{n^2} \exp\left(-n^2 \pi^2 \tau\right) \tag{1}$$

Considering the first 20 terms of the series, the solution by Mathcad gives $t = 681\,\text{s}\,(\sim 11\,\text{min})$ as shown in the worksheet below.

• Case (ii): Numerical solution

The dimensionless forms of the governing equation together with the initial and boundary conditions are given by Eqs. (6.60)–(6.63). The amount of species A within the sphere is calculated from

$$\mathbb{N}_A = \int_0^{2\pi} \int_0^{\pi} \int_0^R c_A\, r^2 \sin\theta\, dr d\theta d\phi = 4\pi R^3 c_{A_o} \int_0^1 \theta\, \xi^2\, d\xi \tag{2}$$

The initial amount is

$$\mathbb{N}_{A_\infty} = \frac{4}{3}\pi R^3 c_{A_o} \tag{3}$$

Thus

$$\frac{\mathbb{N}_A}{\mathbb{N}_{A_\infty}} = 3 \int_0^1 \theta\, \xi^2\, d\xi \tag{4}$$

Mathcad does not accept Greek letters as subscripts. As a result, in the Mathcad worksheet shown below, τ and ξ are replaced by t and r, respectively. The upper limit of the dimensionless time in the argument of "Pdesolve" affects the result. For example, if the upper limit of the dimensionless time is changed from 0.1 to 5, the time required changes from 681.07 to 674.274s.

6.4 DIFFUSION AND REACTION IN A POLYMER MICROSPHERE

Poly(D,L-lactic-co-glycolic acid) (PLGA) microspheres are biodegradable polymeric devices that are widely studied for controlled-release drug delivery (Versypt et al., 2015). Consider a PLGA microsphere of radius R. The chemical species of interest is the autocatalytic carboxylic acid end groups of the polymer chains or *autocatalyst* (species A). The initial concentration of species A within the microsphere is c_{A_o}. As species A diffuses from the sphere, it is generated by an irreversible first-order reaction, i.e., $\mathcal{R}_A = k_1''' c_A$. The autocatalyst concentration at the surface of the microsphere, c_{A_R}, is considered constant. If the effective diffusion coefficient, $\mathcal{D}_{eff}$, is independent of concentration, Eq. (C) of Table 6.1 gives the equation of continuity for the autocatalyst as

$R := 0.25 \qquad D := 2.8 \cdot 10^{-6}$

Case (i)

$\tau := 0.1 \qquad$ This is the initial guess value

Given

$$0.5 = 1 - \frac{6}{\pi^2} \cdot \sum_{n=1}^{200} \left(\frac{1}{n^2} \cdot \exp\left(-n^2 \cdot \pi^2 \cdot \tau\right) \right)$$

$\tau := \text{Find}(\tau) = 0.0305$

$$\text{time} := \frac{\tau \cdot R^2}{D} = 681.842$$

Case (ii)

Given

$$\theta_t(r,t) = \begin{vmatrix} \left(3\,\theta_{rr}(r,t)\right) & \text{if } r = 0 \\[2mm] \left(\theta_{rr}(r,t) + \frac{2}{r} \cdot \theta_r(r,t)\right) & \text{otherwise} \end{vmatrix}$$

$\theta(r,0) = 1 \qquad\qquad \theta_r(0,t) = 0 \qquad\qquad \theta(1,t) = 0$

$$\theta := \text{Pdesolve}\left[\theta, r, \begin{pmatrix} 0 \\ 1 \end{pmatrix}, t, \begin{pmatrix} 0 \\ 0.1 \end{pmatrix}\right]$$

$t := 0.1 \qquad$ This is the initial guess value

Given

$$0.5 = 3 \int_0^1 \theta(r,t) \cdot r^2 \; dr$$

$\tau := \text{Find}(t) = 0.031$

$$\text{Time} := \frac{\tau \cdot R^2}{D} = 681.07$$

Mathcad worksheet of Example 6.3.

$$\frac{\partial c_A}{\partial t} = \frac{\mathcal{D}_{eff}}{r^2} \frac{\partial}{\partial r} \left(r^2 \frac{\partial c_A}{\partial r} \right) + k_1''' c_A \tag{6.97}$$

The initial and boundary conditions are given by

$$\text{at} \quad t = 0 \qquad c_A = c_{A_o} \tag{6.98}$$

$$\text{at} \quad r = 0 \qquad \frac{\partial c_A}{\partial r} = 0 \tag{6.99}$$

$$\text{at} \quad r = R \qquad c_A = c_{A_R} \tag{6.100}$$

Introduction of the dimensionless quantities

$$\theta = \frac{c_A}{c_{A_R}} \qquad \tau = \frac{\mathcal{D}_{eff} t}{R^2} \qquad \xi = \frac{r}{R} \qquad \Lambda^2 = \frac{k_1''' R^2}{\mathcal{D}_{eff}} \qquad \beta = \frac{c_{A_o}}{c_{A_R}} \tag{6.101}$$

reduces Eqs. (6.97)–(6.100) to

$$\frac{\partial \theta}{\partial \tau} = \frac{1}{\xi^2} \frac{\partial}{\partial \xi} \left(\xi^2 \frac{\partial \theta}{\partial \xi} \right) + \Lambda^2 \theta \tag{6.102}$$

$$\text{at} \quad \tau = 0 \qquad \theta = \beta \tag{6.103}$$

$$\text{at} \quad \xi = 0 \qquad \frac{\partial \theta}{\partial \xi} = 0 \tag{6.104}$$

$$\text{at} \quad \xi = 1 \qquad \theta = 1 \tag{6.105}$$

The transformation

$$\theta(\tau, \xi) = \frac{u(\tau, \xi)}{\xi} \tag{6.106}$$

converts Eq. (6.102) to

$$\frac{\partial u}{\partial \tau} = \frac{\partial^2 u}{\partial \xi^2} + \Lambda^2 u \tag{6.107}$$

with the following initial and boundary conditions:

$$\text{at} \quad \tau = 0 \qquad u = \xi \beta \tag{6.108}$$
$$\text{at} \quad \xi = 0 \qquad u = 0 \tag{6.109}$$
$$\text{at} \quad \xi = 1 \qquad u = 1 \tag{6.110}$$

Since the boundary condition at $\xi = 1$ is not homogeneous, let us propose a solution in the form

$$u(\tau, \xi) = u_t(\tau, \xi) + u_\infty(\xi), \tag{6.111}$$

in which $u_\infty(\xi)$ is the solution to the steady-state problem given by

$$\frac{d^2 u_\infty}{d\xi^2} + \Lambda^2 u_\infty = 0 \tag{6.112}$$

with the following boundary conditions:

$$\text{at} \quad \xi = 0 \qquad u_\infty = 0 \tag{6.113}$$
$$\text{at} \quad \xi = 1 \qquad u_\infty = 1 \tag{6.114}$$

The steady-state solution is

$$u_\infty = \frac{\sin(\Lambda \xi)}{\sin \Lambda} \tag{6.115}$$

The use of Eq. (6.115) in (6.111) gives

$$u(\tau, \xi) = u_t(\tau, \xi) + \frac{\sin(\Lambda \xi)}{\sin \Lambda} \tag{6.116}$$

Substitution of Eq. (6.116) into Eqs. (6.107)–(6.110) leads to the following governing equation for the transient problem together with the initial and boundary conditions:

$$\frac{\partial u_t}{\partial \tau} = \frac{\partial^2 u_t}{\partial \xi^2} + \Lambda^2 u_t \tag{6.117}$$

$$\text{at} \quad \tau = 0 \quad u_t = \xi \beta - \frac{\sin(\Lambda \xi)}{\sin \Lambda} \tag{6.118}$$

$$\text{at} \quad \xi = 0 \quad u_t = 0 \tag{6.119}$$

$$\text{at} \quad \xi = 1 \quad u_t = 0 \tag{6.120}$$

Representing the solution as a product of two functions of the form

$$u_t(\tau, \xi) = F(\tau) G(\xi) \tag{6.121}$$

reduces Eq. (6.117) to

$$\frac{1}{F} \frac{dF}{d\tau} - \Lambda^2 = \frac{1}{G} \frac{d^2 G}{d\xi^2} = -\lambda^2, \tag{6.122}$$

which results in two ODEs:

$$\frac{dF}{d\tau} - (\Lambda^2 - \lambda^2)F = 0 \quad \Rightarrow \quad F(\tau) = C_1 e^{-(\lambda^2 - \Lambda^2)\tau} \tag{6.123}$$

$$\frac{d^2 G}{d\xi^2} + \lambda^2 G = 0 \quad \Rightarrow \quad G(\xi) = C_2 \sin(\lambda \xi) + C_3 \cos(\lambda \xi) \tag{6.124}$$

The boundary conditions for $G(\xi)$ are

$$\text{at} \quad \xi = 0 \quad G = 0 \tag{6.125}$$

$$\text{at} \quad \xi = 1 \quad G = 0 \tag{6.126}$$

Application of Eq. (6.125) gives $C_3 = 0$. The use of Eq. (6.126) leads to

$$C_2 \sin \lambda = 0 \tag{6.127}$$

For a nontrivial solution, the eigenvalues are given by

$$\sin \lambda = 0 \quad \Rightarrow \quad \lambda_n = n\pi \quad n = 1, 2, 3, \ldots \tag{6.128}$$

The corresponding eigenfunctions are

$$G_n(\xi) = \sin(n\pi \xi) \tag{6.129}$$

Thus, the transient solution is

$$u_t = \sum_{n=1}^\infty C_n e^{-(n^2 \pi^2 - \Lambda^2)\tau} \sin(n\pi \xi) \tag{6.130}$$

The unknown coefficients C_n can be determined by using the initial condition given by Eq. (6.118). The result is

$$\beta \underbrace{\int_0^1 \xi \sin(n\pi\xi)\,d\xi}_{-\frac{(-1)^n}{n\pi}} - \frac{1}{\sin\Lambda} \underbrace{\int_0^1 \sin(\Lambda\xi)\sin(n\pi\xi)\,d\xi}_{-\frac{(-1)^n n\pi}{n^2\pi^2-\Lambda^2}\sin\Lambda} = C_n \underbrace{\int_0^1 \sin^2(n\pi\xi)\,d\xi}_{\frac{1}{2}} \tag{6.131}$$

or

$$C_n = 2(-1)^n \left(\frac{n\pi}{n^2\pi^2-\Lambda^2} - \frac{\beta}{n\pi} \right) \tag{6.132}$$

Addition of Eqs. (6.115) and (6.132) and making use of the transformation given by Eq. (6.106) yield the concentration distribution as

$$\boxed{\frac{c_A}{c_{A_R}} = \frac{1}{\sin\Lambda}\frac{\sin(\Lambda\xi)}{\xi} + 2\sum_{n=1}^{\infty}(-1)^n \left(\frac{n\pi}{n^2\pi^2-\Lambda^2} - \frac{\beta}{n\pi} \right) e^{-(n^2\pi^2-\Lambda^2)\tau}\frac{\sin(n\pi\xi)}{\xi}} \tag{6.133}$$

The molar flux at the outer surface of the sphere is given by

$$N_{A_r}\big|_{r=R} = -D_{AB}\frac{\partial c_A}{\partial r}\bigg|_{r=R} = -\frac{D_{AB}}{R}\frac{\partial c_A}{\partial \xi}\bigg|_{\xi=1} \tag{6.134}$$

The use of Eq. (6.133) in Eq. (6.134) leads to

$$\boxed{N_{A_r}\big|_{r=R} = \frac{D_{AB}c_{A_R}}{R}\left[1 - \Lambda\cot\Lambda - 2\sum_{n=1}^{\infty}\left(\frac{n^2\pi^2}{n^2\pi^2-\Lambda^2} - \beta \right)\exp\left[-(n^2\pi^2-\Lambda^2)\tau \right] \right]} \tag{6.135}$$

The molar flow rate of species A through the outer surface is

$$\boxed{\mathcal{W}_A = 4\pi R D_{AB} c_{A_R}\left[1 - \Lambda\cot\Lambda - 2\sum_{n=1}^{\infty}\left(\frac{n^2\pi^2}{n^2\pi^2-\Lambda^2} - \beta \right)\exp\left[-(n^2\pi^2-\Lambda^2)\tau \right] \right]} \tag{6.136}$$

6.5 DRUG RELEASE FROM A CYLINDRICAL MATRIX

Consider a monolithic drug delivery system in which the drug (species A) is dispersed uniformly in a cylindrical polymeric matrix of radius R and height H. The drug is surrounded by a fluid having a concentration of c_{A_∞}. We are interested in the amount of drug released as a function of time. The effective diffusion coefficient, $\mathcal{D}_{eff}$, is assumed constant. If $O(R) \sim O(H)$, we have a two-dimensional unsteady-state problem at hand and Eq. (B) in Table 6.1 gives the governing equation as

$$\frac{\partial c_A}{\partial t} = \frac{\mathcal{D}_{eff}}{r}\frac{\partial}{\partial r}\left(r\frac{\partial c_A}{\partial r} \right) + \mathcal{D}_{eff}\frac{\partial^2 c_A}{\partial z^2} \tag{6.137}$$

The initial and boundary conditions associated with Eq. (6.137) are given by

$$\text{at} \quad t=0 \qquad c_A = c_{A_o} \tag{6.138}$$

$$\text{at} \quad r=0 \qquad \frac{\partial c_A}{\partial r} = 0 \quad \text{and} \quad \theta \text{ is finite} \tag{6.139}$$

$$\text{at} \quad r=R \qquad c_A = K_A c_{A_\infty} \tag{6.140}$$

$$\text{at} \quad z=0 \qquad c_A = K_A c_{A_\infty} \tag{6.141}$$

$$\text{at} \quad z=H \qquad c_A = K_A c_{A_\infty} \tag{6.142}$$

Introduction of the dimensionless quantities

$$\theta = \frac{c_A - K_A c_{A\infty}}{c_{A_o} - K_A c_{A\infty}} \qquad \tau = \frac{\mathcal{D}_{eff} t}{R^2} \qquad \xi = \frac{r}{R} \qquad \eta = \frac{z}{H} \qquad \Omega = \frac{R}{H} \qquad (6.143)$$

reduces Eqs. (6.137)–(6.142) to

$$\frac{\partial \theta}{\partial \tau} = \frac{1}{\xi} \frac{\partial}{\partial \xi} \left(\frac{\partial \theta}{\partial \xi} \right) + \Omega^2 \frac{\partial^2 \theta}{\partial \eta^2} \qquad (6.144)$$

$$\text{at} \quad \tau = 0 \qquad \theta = 1 \qquad (6.145)$$

$$\text{at} \quad \xi = 0 \qquad \frac{\partial \theta}{\partial \xi} = 0 \quad \text{and} \quad \theta \text{ is finite} \qquad (6.146)$$

$$\text{at} \quad \xi = 1 \qquad \theta = 0 \qquad (6.147)$$

$$\text{at} \quad z = 0 \qquad \theta = 0 \qquad (6.148)$$

$$\text{at} \quad z = H \qquad \theta = 0 \qquad (6.149)$$

The use of the method of separation of variables in which the solution is sought in the form

$$\theta(\tau, \xi, \eta) = E(\tau) F(\xi) G(\eta) \qquad (6.150)$$

reduces Eq. (6.144) to

$$\frac{1}{E} \frac{dE}{d\tau} = \frac{1}{\xi F} \frac{d}{d\xi} \left(\frac{dF}{d\xi} \right) + \frac{\Omega^2}{G} \frac{d^2 G}{d\eta^2} = -\lambda^2, \qquad (6.151)$$

where λ^2 is a separation constant. From Eq. (6.151), we can write

$$\frac{1}{E} \frac{dE}{d\tau} = -\lambda^2 \qquad \Rightarrow \qquad E = C_1 e^{-\lambda^2 \tau} \qquad (6.152)$$

and

$$\frac{1}{\xi F} \frac{d}{d\xi} \left(\frac{dF}{d\xi} \right) + \frac{\Omega^2}{G} \frac{d^2 G}{d\eta^2} = -\lambda^2 \qquad (6.153)$$

Equation (6.153) can be rearranged in the form

$$\frac{1}{\xi F} \frac{d}{d\xi} \left(\frac{dF}{d\xi} \right) = -\frac{\Omega^2}{G} \frac{d^2 G}{d\eta^2} - \lambda^2 = -\beta^2, \qquad (6.154)$$

where β^2 is another separation constant. Equation (6.154) results in two ODEs:

$$\frac{d}{d\xi} \left(\frac{dF}{d\xi} \right) + \beta^2 \xi F = 0 \qquad \Rightarrow \qquad F = C_2 J_o(\beta \xi) + C_3 Y_o(\beta \xi) \qquad (6.155)$$

$$\frac{d^2 G}{d\eta^2} + \left(\frac{\lambda^2 - \beta_n^2}{\Omega^2} \right) G = 0 \quad \Rightarrow \quad G = C_4 \sin \left(\sqrt{\frac{\lambda^2 - \beta_n^2}{\Omega^2}} \, \eta \right) + C_5 \cos \left(\sqrt{\frac{\lambda^2 - \beta_n^2}{\Omega^2}} \, \eta \right)$$

$$(6.156)$$

The boundary conditions for $F(\xi)$ are

$$\text{at} \quad \xi = 0 \qquad F \text{ is finite} \qquad (6.157)$$

$$\text{at} \quad \xi = 1 \qquad F = 0 \qquad (6.158)$$

Since $Y_o(0) = -\infty$, $C_3 = 0$. Application of Eq. (6.158) yields

$$C_2 J_o(\beta) = 0 \tag{6.159}$$

For a nontrivial solution, the eigenvalues, β_n, are the roots of the following transcendental equation:

$$\boxed{J_o(\beta_n) = 0} \qquad n = 1, 2, 3, \ldots \tag{6.160}$$

The corresponding eigenfunctions, $J_o(\beta_n \xi)$, are orthogonal to each other with respect to the weight function ξ. The boundary conditions for $G(\eta)$ are

$$\begin{array}{lll} \text{at} & \eta = 0 & G = 0 \end{array} \tag{6.161}$$
$$\begin{array}{lll} \text{at} & \eta = 1 & G = 0 \end{array} \tag{6.162}$$

Application of Eq. (6.161) gives $C_5 = 0$. Application of Eq. (6.162) leads to

$$C_4 \sin\left(\sqrt{\frac{\lambda^2 - \beta_n^2}{\Omega^2}}\right) = 0 \qquad \Rightarrow \qquad \sqrt{\frac{\lambda^2 - \beta_n^2}{\Omega^2}} = m\pi \qquad m = 1, 2, 3, \ldots \tag{6.163}$$

Thus

$$\boxed{\lambda_m^2 = m^2 \pi^2 \Omega^2 + \beta_n^2} \qquad m = 1, 2, 3, \ldots \tag{6.164}$$

The solution is the sum of all solutions

$$\theta = \sum_{n=1}^{\infty} \sum_{m=1}^{\infty} C_{nm} e^{-(m^2 \pi^2 \Omega^2 + \beta_n^2)\tau} J_o(\beta_n \xi) \sin(m\pi\eta) \tag{6.165}$$

The unknown coefficients C_{nm} can be determined by using the initial condition given by Eq. (6.145), i.e.,

$$1 = \sum_{n=1}^{\infty} \sum_{m=1}^{\infty} C_{nm} J_o(\beta_n \xi) \sin(m\pi\eta) \tag{6.166}$$

Multiplication of Eq. (6.166) by $\xi J_o(\beta_u \xi) \sin(v\pi\eta) \, d\xi \, d\eta$ and integration from $\xi = 0$ to $\xi = 1$ and $\eta = 0$ to $\eta = 1$ give

$$\underbrace{\left(\int_0^1 \xi J_o(\beta_n \xi) \, d\xi\right)}_{\frac{J_1(\beta_n)}{\beta_n}} \underbrace{\left(\int_0^1 \sin(m\pi\eta) \, d\eta\right)}_{\frac{1-(-1)^m}{m\pi}} = C_{nm} \underbrace{\left(\int_0^1 \xi J_o^2(\beta_n \xi) \, d\xi\right)}_{\frac{1}{2} J_1^2(\beta_n)} \underbrace{\left(\int_0^1 \sin^2(m\pi\eta) \, d\eta\right)}_{\frac{1}{2}}$$

$$\tag{6.167}$$

or

$$C_{nm} = \frac{4[1 - (-1)^m]}{m\pi \beta_n J_1(\beta_n)} \tag{6.168}$$

Therefore, the solution becomes

$$\theta = \frac{4}{\pi} \sum_{n=1}^{\infty} \frac{1}{\beta_n J_1(\beta_n)} e^{-\beta_n^2 \tau} J_o(\beta_n \xi) \sum_{m=1}^{\infty} \frac{[1 - (-1)^m]}{m} e^{-m^2 \pi^2 \Omega^2 \tau} \sin(m\pi\eta) \tag{6.169}$$

Note that

$$[1 - (-1)^m] = \begin{cases} 2 & m \text{ is odd} \\ 0 & m \text{ is even} \end{cases} \tag{6.170}$$

Thus, Eq. (6.169) is expressed as

$$\theta = \frac{8}{\pi} \sum_{n=1}^{\infty} \frac{1}{\beta_n J_1(\beta_n)} e^{-\beta_n^2 \tau} J_o(\beta_n \xi) \sum_{m=1,3,5...}^{\infty} \frac{1}{m} e^{-m^2 \pi^2 \Omega^2 \tau} \sin(m\pi\eta) \qquad (6.171)$$

Using

$$m = 2k+1 \qquad k = 0,1,2,\dots \qquad (6.172)$$

the solution takes the final form of

$$\boxed{\theta = \frac{8}{\pi} \sum_{n=1}^{\infty} \frac{1}{\beta_n J_1(\beta_n)} e^{-\beta_n^2 \tau} J_o(\beta_n \xi) \sum_{k=0}^{\infty} \frac{1}{2k+1} e^{-(2k+1)^2 \pi^2 \Omega^2 \tau} \sin\left[(2k+1)\pi\eta\right]} \qquad (6.173)$$

The average concentration, $\langle c_A \rangle$, is

$$\langle c_A \rangle = \frac{\int_0^H \int_0^R c_A r\,dr\,dz}{\int_0^H \int_0^R r\,dr\,dz} = 2 \int_0^1 \int_0^1 c_A \xi\,d\xi\,d\eta \qquad (6.174)$$

Thus, the average dimensionless concentration, $\langle \theta \rangle$, becomes

$$\langle \theta \rangle = \frac{\langle c_A \rangle - K_A c_{A_\infty}}{c_{A_o} - K_A c_{A_\infty}} = 2 \int_0^1 \int_0^1 \theta \xi\,d\xi\,d\eta \qquad (6.175)$$

The use of Eq. (6.173) in (6.175) leads to

$$\boxed{\langle \theta \rangle = \frac{32}{\pi^2} \sum_{n=1}^{\infty} \frac{1}{\beta_n^2} \exp\left(-\beta_n^2 \tau\right) \sum_{k=0}^{\infty} \frac{1}{(2k+1)^2} \exp\left[-(2k+1)^2 \pi^2 \Omega^2 \tau\right]} \qquad (6.176)$$

The fractional uptake is then expressed as

$$\boxed{\begin{aligned} \frac{\mathbb{N}_A}{\mathbb{N}_{A_\infty}} &= \frac{c_{A_o} - \langle c_A \rangle}{c_{A_o} - K_A c_{A_\infty}} = 1 - \langle \theta \rangle \\[2mm] &= 1 - \frac{32}{\pi^2} \sum_{n=1}^{\infty} \frac{1}{\beta_n^2} \exp\left(-\beta_n^2 \tau\right) \sum_{k=0}^{\infty} \frac{1}{(2k+1)^2} \exp\left[-(2k+1)^2 \pi^2 \Omega^2 \tau\right] \end{aligned}} \qquad (6.177)$$

6.6 DIFFUSION INTO A SLAB FROM A LIMITED VOLUME OF SOLUTION

A long slab of thickness $2L$ is suspended in a well-mixed fluid with a limited volume of V_s as shown in Figure 6.4. While the slab is initially solute-free, the solute concentration in the solution is c_{s_o}. It is required to obtain an expression relating solute uptake of the slab as a function of time.

Let c and c_s be the solute concentrations in the slab and the solution, respectively. When $L/H \ll 1$, the governing equations for the slab and the solution take the forms

$$\text{Slab} \qquad \frac{\partial c}{\partial t} = \mathcal{D} \frac{\partial^2 c}{\partial z^2} \qquad (6.178)$$

$$\text{Solution} \qquad -\left(\mathcal{D} \frac{\partial c}{\partial z}\bigg|_{z=L}\right) 2A = V_s \frac{dc_s}{dt}, \qquad (6.179)$$

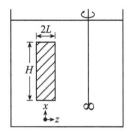

Figure 6.4 Diffusion into a thin slab from a limited volume.

where A is the cross-sectional area of the slab. The initial and boundary conditions are

$$\text{at} \quad t = 0 \quad\quad c = 0 \quad \text{and} \quad c_s = c_{s_o} \tag{6.180}$$

$$\text{at} \quad z = 0 \quad\quad \frac{\partial c}{\partial z} = 0 \tag{6.181}$$

$$\text{at} \quad z = L \quad\quad c = Kc_s, \tag{6.182}$$

where K is a partition coefficient. Introduction of the dimensionless variables

$$\theta = \frac{c}{Kc_{s_o}} \quad\quad \theta_s = \frac{c_s}{c_{s_o}} \quad\quad \xi = \frac{z}{L} \quad\quad \tau = \frac{Dt}{L^2} \quad\quad \Omega = \frac{V_s}{2ALK} \tag{6.183}$$

reduces Eqs. (6.178)–(6.182) to the forms

$$\text{Slab} \quad\quad \frac{\partial \theta}{\partial \tau} = \frac{\partial^2 \theta}{\partial \xi^2} \tag{6.184}$$

$$\text{Solution} \quad\quad -\frac{\partial \theta}{\partial \xi}\bigg|_{\xi=1} = \Omega \frac{d\theta_s}{d\tau} \tag{6.185}$$

$$\text{at} \quad \tau = 0 \quad\quad \theta = 0 \quad \text{and} \quad \theta_s = 1 \tag{6.186}$$

$$\text{at} \quad \xi = 0 \quad\quad \frac{\partial \theta}{\partial \xi} = 0 \tag{6.187}$$

$$\text{at} \quad \xi = 1 \quad\quad \theta = \theta_s \tag{6.188}$$

The Laplace transform of Eq. (6.184) is

$$s\bar{\theta} = \frac{d^2\bar{\theta}}{d\xi^2}, \tag{6.189}$$

which has the solution

$$\bar{\theta} = C_1 \sinh\left(\xi \sqrt{s}\right) + C_2 \cosh\left(\xi \sqrt{s}\right) \tag{6.190}$$

Application of the boundary condition given by Eq. (6.187) in the Laplace domain gives

$$\text{at} \quad \xi = 0 \quad\quad \frac{d\bar{\theta}}{d\xi} = 0 \quad\quad \Rightarrow \quad\quad C_1 = 0 \tag{6.191}$$

Thus, Eq. (6.190) becomes

$$\bar{\theta} = C_2 \cosh\left(\xi \sqrt{s}\right) \tag{6.192}$$

Taking the Laplace transform of Eq. (6.185), we obtain

$$-\left.\frac{d\overline{\theta}}{d\xi}\right|_{\xi=1} = \Omega\left(s\overline{\theta}_s - 1\right) \tag{6.193}$$

Substitution of Eq. (6.192) into Eq. (6.193) yields

$$\overline{\theta}_s = \frac{1}{s} - C_2\frac{\sinh(\sqrt{s})}{\Omega\sqrt{s}} \tag{6.194}$$

Using the boundary condition given by Eq. (6.188) in the Laplace domain, i.e., $\left.\overline{\theta}\right|_{\xi=1} = \left.\overline{\theta}_s\right|_{\xi=1}$, leads to

$$C_2 = \frac{\Omega}{\Omega s\cosh(\sqrt{s}) + \sqrt{s}\sinh(\sqrt{s})} \tag{6.195}$$

Substitution of Eq. (6.195) into Eq. (6.194) gives the Laplace domain solution for the concentration within the slab as

$$\overline{\theta} = \frac{\Omega\cosh(\xi\sqrt{s})}{\sqrt{s}\left[\Omega\sqrt{s}\cosh(\sqrt{s}) + \sinh(\sqrt{s})\right]} \tag{6.196}$$

To take the inverse Laplace transform of Eq. (6.196), note that it is in the form given by Eq. (E.46) in Appendix E with

$$P(s) = \cosh(\xi\sqrt{s}) \tag{6.197}$$

$$Q(s) = \sqrt{s}\left[\Omega\sqrt{s}\cosh(\sqrt{s}) + \sinh(\sqrt{s})\right] \tag{6.198}$$

The roots of $Q(s) = 0$ are

$$s = 0 \qquad \text{and} \qquad s = -\lambda_n^2 \tag{6.199}$$

According to Eq. (E.46), the solution is

$$\theta = \Omega\left[\frac{P(0)}{Q'(0)} + \sum_{n=1}^{\infty}\frac{P(-\lambda_n^2)}{Q'(-\lambda_n^2)}e^{-\lambda_n^2\tau}\right], \tag{6.200}$$

where $Q' = dQ/ds$. Substitution of $s = -\lambda_n^2$ into $Q(s) = 0$ gives the following transcendental equation for the eigenvalues:

$$\boxed{\tan\lambda_n = -\Omega\lambda_n} \quad n = 1,2,3,\ldots \tag{6.201}$$

The terms $P(0)$ and $Q'(0)$ are

$$P(0) = 1 \qquad Q'(0) = 1 + \Omega \tag{6.202}$$

On the other hand, the terms $P(-\lambda_n^2)$ and $Q'(-\lambda_n^2)$ are

$$P(-\lambda_n^2) = \cos(\lambda_n\xi) \tag{6.203}$$

$$Q'(-\lambda_n^2) = \frac{1}{2}\left(\Omega\cos\lambda_n - \Omega\lambda_n\sin\lambda_n + \cos\lambda_n\right) \tag{6.204}$$

The use of Eq. (6.201) in Eq. (6.204) gives

$$Q'(-\lambda_n^2) = -\frac{\sin\lambda_n}{2}\left(\frac{1 + \Omega + \Omega^2\lambda_n^2}{\Omega\lambda_n}\right) \tag{6.205}$$

Substitution of Eqs. (6.202), (6.203), and (6.205) into Eq. (6.200) gives the dimensionless solute distribution within the slab as

$$\theta = \frac{\Omega}{1+\Omega} - 2\Omega^2 \sum_{n=1}^{\infty} \left(\frac{\lambda_n}{1+\Omega+\Omega^2\lambda_n^2} \right) \frac{1}{\sin\lambda_n} e^{-\lambda_n^2\tau} \cos(\lambda_n\xi) \qquad (6.206)$$

The solute uptake of the slab is determined from

$$\mathbb{N}_A = 2A \int_0^L c\,dz = 2ALKc_{s_o} \int_0^1 \theta\,d\xi \qquad (6.207)$$

Substitution of Eq. (6.206) into Eq. (6.207) and integration lead to

$$\mathbb{N}_A = 2ALKc_{s_o} \left[\frac{\Omega}{1+\Omega} - 2\sum_{n=1}^{\infty} \frac{\Omega^2}{1+\Omega+\Omega^2\lambda_n^2} \exp\left(-\lambda_n^2\tau\right) \right] \qquad (6.208)$$

The solute concentration within the slab under steady conditions, c_∞, can be determined from a macroscopic balance as

$$V_s c_{s_o} = V_s c_\infty + 2ALKc_\infty \qquad (6.209)$$

or

$$c_\infty = \left(\frac{\Omega}{1+\Omega} \right) c_{s_o} \qquad (6.210)$$

Therefore, the maximum amount of solute transferred into the slab is

$$\mathbb{N}_{A_\infty} = 2ALKc_\infty = 2ALKc_{s_o} \left(\frac{\Omega}{1+\Omega} \right) \qquad (6.211)$$

Finally, the fractional uptake is expressed as

$$\frac{\mathbb{N}_A}{\mathbb{N}_{A_\infty}} = 1 - 2\sum_{n=1}^{\infty} \frac{\Omega(1+\Omega)}{1+\Omega+\Omega^2\lambda_n^2} \exp\left(-\lambda_n^2\tau\right) \qquad (6.212)$$

6.7 LOSCHMIDT DIFFUSION CELL

The Loschmidt[1] cell is used to determine the diffusion coefficients of binary gas mixtures. As shown in Figure 6.5, it consists of two equally sized vertical cylinders separated by a partition. Initially, the

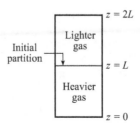

Figure 6.5 A schematic diagram of the Loschmidt cell.

---

[1] Josef Loschmidt (1821–1895), Austrian physicist and chemist.

cylinders are filled with pure gases, the heavier one being placed in the lower cylinder to minimize convection effects. The two gases are allowed to diffuse by removing the partition. Variation in the concentration change with time leads to the estimation of the diffusion coefficient.

The equation of continuity for species A is

$$\frac{\partial y_A}{\partial t} = \mathcal{D}_{AB} \frac{\partial^2 y_A}{\partial z^2} \tag{6.213}$$

The initial condition is given by

$$y_A = \begin{cases} 1 & 0 \leq z < L \\ 0 & L < z \leq 2L \end{cases} \tag{6.214}$$

Since the upper and lower boundaries of the cell are impermeable to gases

$$\text{at} \quad z = 0 \quad \text{and} \quad z = 2L \qquad \frac{\partial y_A}{\partial z} = 0 \tag{6.215}$$

Introduction of the dimensionless quantities

$$\tau = \frac{\mathcal{D}_{AB} t}{L^2} \qquad \xi = \frac{z}{L} \tag{6.216}$$

reduces Eq. (6.213) to

$$\frac{\partial y_A}{\partial \tau} = \frac{\partial^2 y_A}{\partial \xi^2} \tag{6.217}$$

Representing the solution as a product of two functions of the form

$$y_A(\tau, \xi) = F(\tau) G(\xi) \tag{6.218}$$

reduces Eq. (6.217) to

$$\frac{1}{F} \frac{dF}{d\tau} = \frac{1}{G} \frac{d^2 G}{d\xi^2} = -\lambda^2, \tag{6.219}$$

which results in two ODEs:

$$\frac{dF}{d\tau} + \lambda^2 F = 0 \qquad \Rightarrow \qquad F(\tau) = C_1 e^{-\lambda^2 \tau} \tag{6.220}$$

$$\frac{d^2 G}{d\xi^2} + \lambda^2 G = 0 \qquad \Rightarrow \qquad G(\xi) = C_2 \sin(\lambda \xi) + C_3 \cos(\lambda \xi) \tag{6.221}$$

The boundary conditions for $G(\xi)$ are

$$\text{at} \quad \xi = 0 \quad \text{and} \quad \xi = 2 \qquad \frac{dG}{d\xi} = 0 \tag{6.222}$$

The use of the boundary condition at $\xi = 0$ gives $C_2 = 0$. Application of the boundary condition at $\xi = 2$ gives

$$\sin 2\lambda = 0 \qquad \Rightarrow \qquad \boxed{\lambda_n = \frac{n\pi}{2}} \qquad n = 1, 2, 3, \ldots \tag{6.223}$$

The corresponding eigenfunctions are

$$G_n = \cos\left(\frac{n\pi\xi}{2}\right) \qquad n = 0, 1, 2, \ldots \tag{6.224}$$

Note that $n = 0$ is also included in Eq. (6.224) since the eigenfunction $G_o = 1$ corresponding to $\lambda_o = 0$ is nonzero. Therefore, the solution is

$$y_A = C_o + \sum_{n=1}^{\infty} C_n e^{-(n\pi/2)^2 \tau} \cos\left(\frac{n\pi\xi}{2}\right) \tag{6.225}$$

Since the mole fraction of species A over the entire cylinder will be $1/2$ as $\tau \to \infty$, $C_o = 1/2$. The coefficients C_n are calculated by the application of the initial condition, i.e.,

$$\int_0^1 \cos\left(\frac{n\pi\xi}{2}\right) d\xi = C_n \int_0^2 \cos^2\left(\frac{n\pi\xi}{2}\right) d\xi \quad \Rightarrow \quad C_n = \frac{2}{n\pi} \sin\left(\frac{n\pi}{2}\right) \tag{6.226}$$

Therefore, the mole fraction distribution is given by[2]

$$\boxed{y_A = \frac{1}{2} + \frac{2}{\pi} \sum_{n=1}^{\infty} \frac{1}{n} \sin\left(\frac{n\pi}{2}\right) e^{-(n\pi/2)^2 \tau} \cos\left(\frac{n\pi\xi}{2}\right)} \tag{6.227}$$

Variation in the mole fraction of species A as a function of the dimensionless distance at various values of the dimensionless time is shown in Figure 6.6. When $\tau \geq 2$, the mole fraction of species A is almost equal to 0.5 throughout the cylinder.

The average mole fraction of species A in the lower cylinder is

$$\langle y_A \rangle^L = \frac{1}{L} \int_0^L y_A \, dz = \int_0^1 y_A \, d\xi \tag{6.228}$$

Substitution of Eq. (6.227) into Eq. (6.228) and integration result in

$$\langle y_A \rangle^L = \frac{1}{2} + \frac{4}{\pi^2} \sum_{n=1}^{\infty} \frac{1}{n^2} \sin^2\left(\frac{n\pi}{2}\right) \exp\left[-\left(\frac{n\pi}{2}\right)^2 \tau\right] \tag{6.229}$$

Note that

$$\sin^2\left(\frac{n\pi}{2}\right) = \begin{cases} 1 & n = 1, 3, 5, \dots \\ 0 & n = 2, 4, 6, \dots \end{cases} \tag{6.230}$$

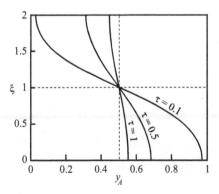

Figure 6.6   Variation in y_A as a function of ξ at various values of τ.

---

[2]Ravi (2007) pointed out the ambiguities and discrepancies in the analytical solutions of the Loschmidt problem reported in the literature.

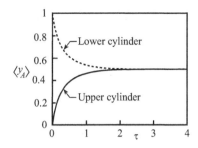

Figure 6.7 Variations in the average mole fractions as a function of dimensionless time.

Therefore, replacing n by $2k+1$ leads to

$$\langle y_A \rangle^L = \frac{1}{2} + \frac{4}{\pi^2} \sum_{k=0}^{\infty} \frac{1}{(2k+1)^2} \exp\left\{ -\left[\frac{(2k+1)\pi}{2} \right]^2 \tau \right\} \tag{6.231}$$

Similarly, the average mole fraction of species A in the upper cylinder is given by

$$\langle y_A \rangle^U = \frac{1}{2} - \frac{4}{\pi^2} \sum_{k=0}^{\infty} \frac{1}{(2k+1)^2} \exp\left\{ -\left[\frac{(2k+1)\pi}{2} \right]^2 \tau \right\} \tag{6.232}$$

Variations in the average mole fractions of species A in the lower and upper cylinders as a function of dimensionless time are shown in Figure 6.7. When $\tau \geq 2$, the average mole fractions of species A in the lower and upper cylinders are equal to 0.5.

6.8 DIFFUSION FROM INSTANTANEOUS SOURCES

In this section, diffusion of species released into a stagnant medium from instantaneous sources will be examined. In that respect, plane (or surface), line, and point sources will be considered.

6.8.1 DIFFUSION FROM A PLANE SOURCE

An infinitely long rectangular duct in the x-direction is filled with a stagnant liquid. At time $t = 0$, M_A amount of species A is injected uniformly across the y-z plane with an infinitesimally small width as shown in Figure 6.8. The governing equation for one-dimensional unsteady-state diffusion is expressed as

$$\frac{\partial c_A}{\partial t} = \mathcal{D}_x \frac{\partial^2 c_A}{\partial x^2}, \tag{6.233}$$

where $\mathcal{D}_x$ is the diffusion coefficient in the x-direction. The conservation of mass is expressed as

$$M_A = A \int_{-\infty}^{\infty} c_A(t,x)\, dx = A \int_{-\infty}^{\infty} c_A(0,x)\, dx = \text{constant}, \tag{6.234}$$

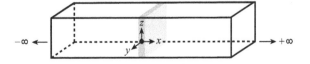

Figure 6.8 Diffusion from a plane source.

where A stands for the area of the y–z plane. Rearrangement of Eq. (6.234) in the form

$$\frac{M_A}{A} = \int_{-\infty}^{\infty} c_A(0,x)\, dx \tag{6.235}$$

shows that the plane source, M_A/A, has the unit of kg(or kmol)$/\text{m}^2$, depending on the unit of c_A (kg/m^3 or kmol/m^3). Mathematically, the initial condition is expressed in terms of the Dirac delta function as

$$\text{at} \quad t = 0 \qquad c_A = \frac{M_A}{A}\, \delta(x) \tag{6.236}$$

The boundary conditions are given by

$$\text{at} \quad x = \pm\infty \qquad c_A = 0 \tag{6.237}$$

This problem is solved in Example E.12 in Appendix E with the solution

$$\boxed{c_A = \frac{M_A/A}{2\sqrt{\pi \mathcal{D}_x t}}\, \exp\left(-\frac{x^2}{4\mathcal{D}_x t}\right)} \tag{6.238}$$

The factor 2 in the denominator comes from the fact that species A diffuses in the negative and positive x-directions. If the diffusion of species A in the negative x-direction is prevented, then the amount of species A diffusing in the positive x-direction is doubled and the factor 2 in the denominator of Eq. (6.238) should be eliminated.

The Gaussian distribution, also known as the "bell-shaped curve" or "normal distribution," is expressed by the density function $P(x)$, given by

$$P(x) = \frac{1}{\sqrt{2\pi\sigma^2}}\, \exp\left[-\frac{(x-\mu)^2}{2\sigma^2}\right], \tag{6.239}$$

where the parameters μ and σ stand for the mean and standard deviation of the distribution, respectively. The standard deviation, σ, is a measure of the distribution width. Comparison of Eqs. (6.238) and (6.239) indicates that $\mu = 0$ and $\sigma = \sqrt{2\mathcal{D}_x t}$. The plot of $c_A/(M_A/A)$ versus x with $\mathcal{D}_x t$ as a parameter is shown in Figure 6.9. The diffusing patch of species spreads as time progresses. The concentration reaches its maximum value at the center of mass, i.e., $x = 0$, and it is given by

$$c_{A\text{max}} = \frac{M_A/A}{2\sqrt{\pi \mathcal{D}_x t}} \tag{6.240}$$

The use of Eq. (6.240) in Eq. (6.238) leads to

$$c_A = c_{A\text{max}} \exp\left(-\frac{x^2}{4\mathcal{D}_x t}\right) \tag{6.241}$$

As shown in Figure 6.10, the standard deviation corresponds to the half-width of the peak at about 61% of the maximum concentration. In addition, 68% of the total mass falls within $\pm\sigma$. Similarly, 95% of the total mass falls within $\pm 2\sigma$. Therefore, once the mass M_A is introduced into a stagnant medium as the Dirac delta function, it spreads according to the Gaussian curve with the height proportional to $1/\left(2\sqrt{\pi \mathcal{D}_x t}\right)$ and the width proportional to $\sqrt{2\mathcal{D}_x t}$.

The width of a diffusing patch is generally defined as the length of the region that contains 95% of the species, i.e., $-2\sigma \leq x \leq 2\sigma$. Then, the concentration at the edges of the patch, i.e., $x = 2\sqrt{2\mathcal{D}_x t}$, is calculated from Eq. (6.241) as

$$c_A = c_{A\text{max}} \exp(-2) \simeq 0.14\, c_{A\text{max}} \tag{6.242}$$

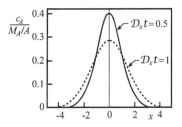

Figure 6.9 Variation in concentration as a function of position for an instantaneous plane source.

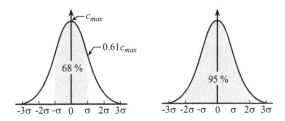

Figure 6.10 Gaussian probability distribution of concentration.

Example 6.4 Two kilograms of a chemical accidentally spills in a canal of 8 m width. The diffusion coefficient of the chemical in water is $0.065\,\text{m}^2/\text{s}$. We want to determine the time for the chemical spill to reach a house located 150 m away from where the incident occurred.

Note that we can use the equations developed in this section only if the water in the canal is stagnant and the chemical mixes rapidly across the width of the canal in order to consider it as a plane source. In its present form, the problem statement is vague. It should be stated as "what is the time for the edges of the chemical patch with two standard deviations to reach a house located 150 m away from where the incident occurred?" Thus,

$$x = 150 = 2\sigma = 2\sqrt{2\mathcal{D}_x t}$$

or

$$t = \frac{150^2}{(4)(2)(0.065)} = 43,269\,\text{s} = 12\,\text{h}$$

Let H be the depth of the canal. The maximum concentration at $t = 12\,\text{h}$ can be calculated from Eq. (6.240) as

$$c_{A_{max}}H = \frac{2/8}{2\sqrt{\pi(0.065)(43,269)}} = 1.33 \times 10^{-3}\,\text{kg/m}^2$$

Therefore, the concentration at the edge of the patch (or in front of the house) is calculated from Eq. (6.242) as

$$c_A H = (0.14)(1.33 \times 10^{-3}) = 1.86 \times 10^{-4}\,\text{kg/m}^2$$

The concentration in front of the house will change with time. To calculate the time when this concentration reaches its maximum value, we have to differentiate Eq. (6.238) with respect to time to obtain

$$t = \frac{x^2}{2\mathcal{D}_x} = \frac{150^2}{(2)(0.065)} = 173,076\,\text{s}$$

The value of concentration at this time is

$$c_A H = \frac{2/8}{2\sqrt{\pi(0.065)(173,076)}}\exp\left[-\frac{150^2}{(4)(0.065)(173,076)}\right] = 4 \times 10^{-4}\,\text{kg/m}^2$$

By definition, the variance is the square of the standard deviation. Thus, the variance of an instantaneous plane source is

$$\sigma^2 = 2\mathcal{D}_x t \tag{6.243}$$

Differentiation of Eq. (6.243) with respect to time gives

$$\mathcal{D}_x = \frac{1}{2}\frac{d\sigma^2}{dt} = \frac{1}{2}\left(\frac{\sigma_2^2 - \sigma_1^2}{t_2 - t_1}\right) \tag{6.244}$$

Hence, the diffusion coefficient can be estimated by measuring the change in variance with time.

6.8.2 DIFFUSION FROM A LINE SOURCE

A rectangular duct, infinitely long in the x- and y-directions, is filled with a stagnant liquid. At time $t = 0$, M_A amount of species A is injected uniformly in the z-direction. The governing equation for two-dimensional unsteady-state diffusion is expressed as

$$\frac{\partial c_A}{\partial t} = \mathcal{D}_x \frac{\partial^2 c_A}{\partial x^2} + \mathcal{D}_y \frac{\partial^2 c_A}{\partial y^2}, \tag{6.245}$$

where $\mathcal{D}_x$ and $\mathcal{D}_y$ are the diffusion coefficients in the x- and y-directions, respectively. The conservation of mass is expressed as

$$M_A = L \int_{-\infty}^{\infty} \int_{-\infty}^{\infty} c_A(t,x,y)\,dx\,dy = L \int_{-\infty}^{\infty} \int_{-\infty}^{\infty} c_A(0,x,y)\,dx\,dy = \text{constant}, \tag{6.246}$$

where L is the length in the z-direction. Rearrangement of Eq. (6.246) in the form

$$\frac{M_A}{L} = \int_{-\infty}^{\infty} \int_{-\infty}^{\infty} c_A(0,x,y)\,dx\,dy \tag{6.247}$$

shows that the line source, M_A/L, has the unit of kg(or kmol)/m, depending on the unit of c_A (kg/m^3 or kmol/m^3). Mathematically, the initial condition is expressed in terms of the Dirac delta function as

$$\text{at} \quad t = 0 \qquad c_A = \frac{M_A}{L}\delta(x)\delta(y) \tag{6.248}$$

The boundary conditions are given by

$$\text{at} \quad x = \pm\infty \qquad c_A = 0 \tag{6.249}$$
$$\text{at} \quad y = \pm\infty \qquad c_A = 0 \tag{6.250}$$

Proposing a solution in the form

$$c_A(t,x,y) = f(t,x)\,g(t,y) \tag{6.251}$$

reduces Eq. (6.245) to

$$g\left(\frac{\partial f}{\partial t} - \mathcal{D}_x \frac{\partial^2 f}{\partial x^2}\right) + f\left(\frac{\partial g}{\partial t} - \mathcal{D}_y \frac{\partial^2 g}{\partial x^2}\right) = 0 \tag{6.252}$$

For a nontrivial solution, the equations inside the parentheses must be zero, i.e.,

$$\frac{\partial f}{\partial t} - \mathcal{D}_x \frac{\partial^2 f}{\partial x^2} = 0 \quad \Rightarrow \quad f = \frac{K_1}{2\sqrt{\pi \mathcal{D}_x t}}\exp\left(-\frac{x^2}{4\mathcal{D}_x t}\right) \tag{6.253}$$

$$\frac{\partial g}{\partial t} - \mathcal{D}_y \frac{\partial^2 g}{\partial x^2} = 0 \quad \Rightarrow \quad g = \frac{K_2}{2\sqrt{\pi \mathcal{D}_y t}} \exp\left(-\frac{y^2}{4\mathcal{D}_y t}\right) \tag{6.254}$$

Substitution of Eqs. (6.253) and (6.254) into Eq. (6.251) yields

$$c_A = \frac{K_1 K_2}{4\pi t \sqrt{\mathcal{D}_x \mathcal{D}_y}} \exp\left(-\frac{x^2}{4\mathcal{D}_x t} - \frac{y^2}{4\mathcal{D}_y t}\right), \tag{6.255}$$

where K_1 and K_2 are constants. Application of Eq. (6.246) gives

$$\underbrace{\int_{-\infty}^{\infty} \int_{-\infty}^{\infty} c_A(t, x, y)\, dx\, dy}_{M_A/L} = \frac{K_1 K_2}{4\pi t \sqrt{\mathcal{D}_x \mathcal{D}_y}} \underbrace{\int_{-\infty}^{\infty} e^{-\frac{x^2}{4\mathcal{D}_x t}}\, dx}_{\sqrt{4\pi \mathcal{D}_x t}} \underbrace{\int_{-\infty}^{\infty} e^{-\frac{y^2}{4\mathcal{D}_y t}}\, dy}_{\sqrt{4\pi \mathcal{D}_y t}} \tag{6.256}$$

Thus, $K_1 K_2 = M_A/L$, and the solution takes the form

$$\boxed{c_A = \frac{M_A/L}{4\pi t \sqrt{\mathcal{D}_x \mathcal{D}_y}} \exp\left(-\frac{x^2}{4\mathcal{D}_x t} - \frac{y^2}{4\mathcal{D}_y t}\right)} \tag{6.257}$$

The concentration reaches its maximum value at the center of mass, i.e., $x = y = 0$, and it is given by

$$c_{A_{\max}} = \frac{M_A/L}{4\pi t \sqrt{\mathcal{D}_x \mathcal{D}_y}} \tag{6.258}$$

In this case, the length scales (or widths) of the diffusing cloud in the x- and y-directions are $-2\sigma_x \leq x \leq 2\sigma_x$ and $-2\sigma_y \leq y \leq 2\sigma_y$, respectively. When $\mathcal{D}_x = \mathcal{D}_y = \mathcal{D}$, Eq. (6.257) simplifies to

$$c_A = \frac{M_A/L}{4\pi \mathcal{D} t} \exp\left(-\frac{r^2}{4\mathcal{D} t}\right), \tag{6.259}$$

where $r = \sqrt{x^2 + y^2}$ stands for the radial distance in the cylindrical coordinate system.

6.8.3 DIFFUSION FROM A POINT SOURCE

A rectangular duct, infinitely long in the x-, y-, and z-directions, is filled with a stagnant liquid. At time $t = 0$, M_A amount of species A is released from a point source. The governing equation for three-dimensional unsteady-state diffusion is expressed as

$$\frac{\partial c_A}{\partial t} = \mathcal{D}_x \frac{\partial^2 c_A}{\partial x^2} + \mathcal{D}_y \frac{\partial^2 c_A}{\partial y^2} + \mathcal{D}_z \frac{\partial^2 c_A}{\partial z^2}, \tag{6.260}$$

The conservation of mass is expressed as

$$M_A = \int_{-\infty}^{\infty} \int_{-\infty}^{\infty} \int_{-\infty}^{\infty} c_A(t, x, y, z)\, dx\, dy\, dz = \int_{-\infty}^{\infty} \int_{-\infty}^{\infty} \int_{-\infty}^{\infty} c_A(0, x, y, z)\, dx\, dy\, dz = \text{constant} \tag{6.261}$$

Following the procedure given in Section 6.8.2, the solution is expressed in the form

$$\boxed{c_A = \frac{M_A}{8\left(\pi t\right)^{3/2} \sqrt{\mathcal{D}_x \mathcal{D}_y \mathcal{D}_z}} \exp\left(-\frac{x^2}{4\mathcal{D}_x t} - \frac{y^2}{4\mathcal{D}_y t} - \frac{z^2}{4\mathcal{D}_z t}\right)} \tag{6.262}$$

The concentration reaches its maximum value at the center of mass, i.e., $x = y = z = 0$, and it is given by

$$c_{A_{\max}} = \frac{M_A}{8\left(\pi t\right)^{3/2} \sqrt{\mathcal{D}_x \mathcal{D}_y \mathcal{D}_z}} \tag{6.263}$$

When $\mathcal{D}_x = \mathcal{D}_y = \mathcal{D}_z = \mathcal{D}$, Eq. (6.262) simplifies to

$$c_A = \frac{M_A}{8(\pi \mathcal{D}t)^{3/2}} \exp\left(-\frac{r^2}{4\mathcal{D}t}\right), \tag{6.264}$$

where $r = \sqrt{x^2 + y^2 + z^2}$ stands for the radial distance in the spherical coordinate system.

PROBLEMS

6.1 Consider mass transfer into a rectangular slab as described in Section 6.2. If the slab is initially free of species A, show that the time required for the center concentration to reach 99% of the final concentration is given by

$$t \simeq \frac{2L^2}{\mathcal{D}_{AB}}$$

6.2 Derive Eq. (6.53). It is different from Eq. (6.39) by a factor of 2. Why?

6.3 In the analysis given in Section 6.2, the external resistance to mass transfer is considered negligible. In the case of an appreciable resistance, the boundary condition at the fluid–solid interface becomes

$$z = L \qquad \mathcal{D}_{AB}\frac{\partial c_A}{\partial z} = k_c(c_{A_\infty} - c_A^f), \tag{1}$$

where k_c is the mass transfer coefficient, and c_A and c_A^f represent the concentrations of species A in the solid and fluid phases, respectively. Since these concentrations are related by the partition coefficient K_A, i.e., $c_A = K_A c_A^f$, Eq. (1) takes the form

$$z = L \qquad \mathcal{D}_{AB}\frac{\partial c_A}{\partial z} = \frac{k_c}{K_A}(K_A c_{A_\infty} - c_A) \tag{2}$$

a) Show that the governing equation and the initial and boundary conditions are given by

$$\frac{\partial \theta}{\partial \tau} = \frac{\partial^2 \theta}{\partial \xi^2} \tag{3}$$

$$\text{at} \quad \tau = 0 \qquad \theta = 1 \tag{4}$$

$$\text{at} \quad \xi = 0 \qquad \frac{\partial \theta}{\partial \xi} = 0 \tag{5}$$

$$\text{at} \quad \xi = 1 \qquad -\frac{\partial \theta}{\partial \xi} = \mathrm{Bi_M}\,\theta, \tag{6}$$

where the Biot number for mass transfer is defined by

$$\mathrm{Bi_M} = \frac{k_c L}{K_A \mathcal{D}_{AB}} \tag{7}$$

b) Show that the solution is expressed as

$$\theta = 4\sum_{n=1}^{\infty} \frac{\sin \lambda_n}{2\lambda_n + \sin 2\lambda_n}\, e^{-\lambda_n^2 \tau} \cos(\lambda_n \xi), \tag{8}$$

where the eigenvalues are the roots of the transcendental equation given by

$$\lambda_n \tan \lambda_n = \mathrm{Bi_M} \qquad n = 1, 2, 3, \ldots \tag{9}$$

c) Show that when $\mathrm{Bi_M} \to \infty$ Eq. (8) reduces to Eq. (6.21).

d) The dimensionless average concentration $\langle \theta \rangle$ can be defined as

$$\langle \theta \rangle = \frac{K_A c_{A_\infty} - \langle c_A \rangle}{K_A c_{A_\infty} - c_{A_o}} = \int_0^1 \theta \, d\xi \tag{10}$$

Show that the substitution of Eq. (8) into Eq. (10) and integration lead to

$$\langle \theta \rangle = 4 \sum_{n=1}^{\infty} \frac{\sin^2 \lambda_n}{\lambda_n (2\lambda_n + \sin 2\lambda_n)} \exp\left(-\lambda_n^2 \tau\right) \tag{11}$$

e) Show that the use of Eq. (9) in Eq. (10) results in

$$\langle \theta \rangle = 2 \sum_{n=1}^{\infty} \frac{\mathrm{Bi_M^2}}{\lambda_n^2 (\lambda_n^2 + \mathrm{Bi_M^2} + \mathrm{Bi_M})} \exp\left(-\lambda_n^2 \tau\right) \tag{12}$$

Thus, show that the fractional uptake is given by

$$\frac{\mathbb{N}_A}{\mathbb{N}_{A_\infty}} = 1 - 2 \sum_{n=1}^{\infty} \frac{\mathrm{Bi_M^2}}{\lambda_n^2 (\lambda_n^2 + \mathrm{Bi_M^2} + \mathrm{Bi_M})} \exp\left(-\lambda_n^2 \tau\right) \tag{13}$$

6.4 One of the techniques used for measuring the diffusion coefficient is the so-called "time-lag method." The apparatus consists of two large chambers separated by a membrane of thickness L and cross-sectional area A. Initially, a vacuum is applied to both chambers for some time to ensure that the membrane is free of the diffusing species A. At $t = 0$, one of the chambers is filled with gas A at a pressure of P_{A_o}, and the increase in the pressure of gas A in the low-pressure chamber is monitored continuously.

a) Show that the governing equation and its associated initial and boundary conditions are given as

$$\frac{\partial c_A}{\partial t} = \mathcal{D}_{AB} \frac{\partial^2 c_A}{\partial z^2}$$

$$\begin{array}{ll}
t = 0 & c_A = 0 \\
z = 0 & c_A = S_A P_{A_o} \\
z = L & c_A = 0,
\end{array} \tag{1}$$

where S_A is the solubility coefficient for the gas–membrane system. State your assumptions.

b) Write Eq. (1) in terms of the dimensionless quantities

$$\theta = \frac{c_A}{S_A P_{A_o}} \qquad \tau = \frac{\mathcal{D}_{AB} t}{L^2} \qquad \xi = \frac{z}{L} \tag{2}$$

and show that the solution is given by

$$\theta = 1 - \xi - \frac{2}{\pi} \sum_{n=1}^{\infty} \frac{1}{n} \exp\left(-n^2 \pi^2 \tau\right) \sin(n\pi\xi) \tag{3}$$

c) Show that the molar flux of species A at $z = L$ is

$$N_{A_z}\big|_{z=L} = \frac{\mathcal{D}_{AB} S_A P_{A_o}}{L}\left[1 + 2\sum_{n=1}^{\infty}(-1)^n \exp\left(-n^2\pi^2\tau\right)\right] \tag{4}$$

d) Show that the total number of moles of species A, $\mathbb{N}_A$, that entered the low-pressure side of the chamber over time t is given by

$$\frac{\mathbb{N}_A}{ALS_A P_{A_o}} = \tau - \frac{1}{6} - \frac{2}{\pi^2}\sum_{n=1}^{\infty}\frac{(-1)^n}{n^2}\exp\left(-n^2\pi^2\tau\right) \tag{5}$$

e) Express Eq. (5) in terms of the pressure in the low-pressure chamber, P_A, to obtain

$$\left(\frac{V}{RTALS_A P_{A_o}}\right)P_A = \left(\frac{\mathcal{D}_{AB}}{L^2}\right)t - \frac{1}{6} - \frac{2}{\pi^2}\sum_{n=1}^{\infty}\frac{(-1)^n}{n^2}\exp\left[-\left(\frac{n^2\pi^2\mathcal{D}_{AB}}{L^2}\right)t\right], \tag{6}$$

where V is the volume of the low-pressure side of the chamber.

f) Simplify Eq. (6) as $t \to \infty$ to show that

$$\left(\frac{V}{RTALS_A P_{A_o}}\right)P_A = \left(\frac{\mathcal{D}_{AB}}{L^2}\right)t - \frac{1}{6}, \tag{7}$$

which is a straight line with an intercept on the t axis, t^*, given by

$$t^* = \frac{L^2}{6\mathcal{D}_{AB}}$$

In the literature, t^* is called the *time lag*. Show that a representative plot of P_A versus t according to Eq. (6) looks like the following:

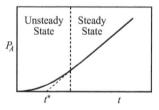

Thus, the diffusion coefficient is calculated from

$$\mathcal{D}_{AB} = \frac{L^2}{6t^*} \tag{8}$$

g) The increase in the pressure of the low-pressure chamber is reported as

$$P_A = 73(t - 2.3),$$

where P_A is in mmHg and t is in seconds. If the thickness of the membrane is 50μm, calculate the diffusion coefficient.

h) Is it possible to use this method to estimate the diffusion coefficient for liquid systems? If yes, how would you carry out the experiment?

(Answer: g) 1.81×10^{-6}cm^2/s)

6.5 Consider one-dimensional diffusion of a drug (species A) through a tissue (species B) of thickness L. The initial concentration of drug within the tissue is c_{A_o}. Let c_{A_1} and c_{A_2} be the drug concentrations at $z = 0$ and $z = L$, respectively ($c_{A_1} > c_{A_2}$). Drug concentrations at the edges remain constant.

a) Write down the governing equation and its associated initial and boundary conditions in terms of the following dimensionless quantities:

$$\theta = \frac{c_A - c_{A_o}}{c_{A_1} - c_{A_o}} \qquad \tau = \frac{\mathcal{D}_{AB}\,t}{L^2} \qquad \xi = \frac{z}{L}$$

b) Show that the concentration distribution is expressed in the form

$$\theta = 1 - (1 - \theta^*)\xi + \frac{2}{\pi}\sum_{n=1}^{\infty}\frac{1}{n}\left[(-1)^n\theta^* - 1\right]e^{-n^2\pi^2\tau}\sin(n\pi\xi),$$

where

$$\theta^* = \frac{c_{A_2} - c_{A_o}}{c_{A_1} - c_{A_o}}$$

c) Show that the molar transfer rate of the drug through the surface at $z = L$ is given by

$$W_A = \frac{\mathcal{D}_{AB}(c_{A_1} - c_{A_o})A}{L}\left\{1 - \theta^* - 2\sum_{n=1}^{\infty}\left[\theta^* - (-1)^n\right]\exp\left(-n^2\pi^2\tau\right)\right\},$$

where A is the surface area of the tissue.

d) Show that the total number of moles of the drug transferred through the surface at $z = L$ at time t is

$$\mathbb{N}_A = AL(c_{A_1} - c_{A_o})\left\{(1 - \theta^*)\tau - \frac{2}{\pi^2}\sum_{n=1}^{\infty}\frac{1}{n^2}\left[\theta^* - (-1)^n\right]\left[1 - \exp\left(-n^2\pi^2\tau\right)\right]\right\}$$

e) Calculate the time required for the transfer of 10 g of drug using the following data:

$$c_{A_o} = c_{A_2} = 0.6\,\text{kg/m}^3 \qquad c_{A_1} = 2.9\,\text{kg/m}^3 \qquad \mathcal{D}_{AB} = 3.4 \times 10^{-4}\,\text{m}^2/\text{s}$$

$$L = 2\,\text{mm} \qquad A = 0.15\,\text{cm}^2$$

(Answer: 1705s)

6.6 Consider sublimation of a circular disc of p-dichlorobenzene (species A) that is placed on an impermeable surface. Air (species B) surrounding the disc is stagnant at a temperature of T_∞. The initial thickness of the disc is H_o. Estimate the time required for the disc to disappear completely by the following analysis:

a) Show that the governing equation and its associated initial and boundary conditions representing the diffusion of p-dichlorobenzene in stagnant air are given as

$$\frac{\partial c_A}{\partial t} = \mathcal{D}_{AB}\frac{\partial^2 c_A}{\partial z^2} \tag{1}$$

$$\begin{array}{lll} t = 0 & c_A = 0 & \\ z = 0 & c_A = c_A^{eq} & \tag{2} \\ z = \infty & c_A = 0, & \end{array}$$

where z is the distance measured from the surface of the disc.

b) Show that the solution is

$$\frac{c_A}{c_A^{eq}} = 1 - \text{erf}\left(\frac{z}{2\sqrt{\mathcal{D}_{AB}t}}\right) \tag{3}$$

c) Show that the molar flux of p-dichlorobenzene at the surface is given by

$$N_{A_z}\big|_{z=0} = c_A^{eq}\sqrt{\frac{\mathcal{D}_{AB}}{\pi t}} \tag{4}$$

d) Taking the disc as a system show that the macroscopic mass balance leads to

$$-N_{A_z}\big|_{z=0} = \frac{1}{2\widetilde{V}_A}\frac{dH}{dt}, \tag{5}$$

where $\widetilde{V}_A$ is the molar volume of solid p-dichlorobenzene and H is the thickness of the disc.

e) Substitute Eq. (4) into Eq. (5) and integrate the resulting equation to show that the time for the disc to completely disappear is given by

$$t = \frac{\pi}{\mathcal{D}_{AB}}\left(\frac{H_o}{4\widetilde{V}_A c_A^{eq}}\right)^2 \tag{6}$$

6.7 The bottom of a vertical cylindrical tank of radius R is covered with a salt layer (species A) of thickness L_o. The tank is filled with pure water (species B) at $t = 0$. The height of the water layer H is such that $H \gg L_o$ and $H \ll R$.

a) Show that the governing equation and its associated initial and boundary conditions are given as

$$\frac{\partial c_A}{\partial t} = \mathcal{D}_{AB}\frac{\partial^2 c_A}{\partial z^2}$$

$$\begin{array}{ll} t = 0 & c_A = 0 \\ z = 0 & c_A = c_A^{eq} \\ z = \infty & c_A = 0, \end{array} \tag{1}$$

where z is the distance measured from the surface of the salt layer to the liquid phase.

b) Show that the concentration distribution is given by

$$\frac{c_A}{c_A^{eq}} = 1 - \text{erf}\left(\frac{z}{2\sqrt{\mathcal{D}_{AB}t}}\right) \tag{2}$$

c) Show that the change in the salt layer thickness, L, with time is expressed as

$$L(t) = L_o - \frac{2c_A^{eq}M_A}{\rho_A^S}\sqrt{\frac{\mathcal{D}_{AB}}{\pi t}}, \tag{3}$$

where M_A and ρ_A^S are the molecular weight of salt and density of solid salt, respectively.

d) Calculate the decrease in the thickness of the salt layer after 10 h using the following data:

$$c_A^{eq} = 7000\,\text{mol/m}^3 \qquad \mathcal{D}_{AB} = 1.3 \times 10^{-9}\,\text{m}^2/\text{s} \qquad M_A = 58\,\text{g/mol} \qquad \rho_A^S = 2100\,\text{kg/m}^3$$

(Answer: d) 1.49×10^{-3} m)

6.8 The bottom of a vertical cylindrical tank of radius R is coated with a catalyst. At $t = 0$, the cylinder is filled with a liquid containing dissolved species A with a concentration of c_{A_o}. An irreversible first-order reaction

$$A \rightarrow B$$

takes place on the catalyst surface.

a) Show that the governing equation and its associated initial and boundary conditions are given as

$$\frac{\partial c_A}{\partial t} = \mathcal{D}_{AB} \frac{\partial^2 c_A}{\partial z^2}$$

$$
\begin{array}{lll}
t = 0 & c_A = c_{A_o} & \quad (1) \\
z = 0 & \mathcal{D}_{AB} \dfrac{\partial c_A}{\partial z} = k_1'' c_A & \\
z = \infty & c_A = c_{A_o}, &
\end{array}
$$

where z is the distance measured from the bottom of the tank. State your assumptions.

b) Write Eq. (1) in terms of the dimensionless quantities

$$\theta = \frac{c_A}{c_{A_o}} \qquad \tau = \frac{(k_1'')^2 t}{\mathcal{D}_{AB}} \qquad \xi = \frac{k_1'' z}{\mathcal{D}_{AB}} \qquad (2)$$

and show that the solution is given by

$$\theta = 1 + e^{\tau + \xi} \operatorname{erfc}\left(\sqrt{\tau} + \frac{\xi}{2\sqrt{\tau}}\right) - \operatorname{erfc}\left(\frac{\xi}{2\sqrt{\tau}}\right) \qquad (3)$$

c) Show that the molar rate of consumption of species A on the catalyst surface, $\mathcal{W}_A$, is given by

$$\mathcal{W}_A = \pi R^2 k_1'' c_{A_o} e^{\tau} \operatorname{erfc}\left(\sqrt{\tau}\right) \qquad (4)$$

d) Using Table E.5 in Appendix E, show that the limiting values of Eq. (4) are given by

$$\mathcal{W}_A = \begin{cases} c_{A_o} R^2 \sqrt{\dfrac{\pi \mathcal{D}_{AB}}{t}} & \text{Fast reaction} \\[4mm] \pi R^2 k_1'' c_{A_o} \left(1 - 2k_1'' \sqrt{\dfrac{t}{\pi \mathcal{D}_{AB}}}\right) & \text{Short time} \end{cases} \qquad (5)$$

6.9 Carburization (or carburizing) is the process of introducing carbon into a metal by diffusion. For this purpose, the metal is exposed to carbon-rich gas at high temperature. Consider a 1-cm-thick steel sheet (species B) having a uniform carbon (species A) concentration of 0.20 wt %.

a) If the sheet is exposed to an atmosphere containing 1.3 wt % carbon at $1,200\,\text{K}$ for 2 h, estimate the concentration of carbon at a depth of 1 mm below the surface. Take $\mathcal{D}_{AB} = 1.8 \times 10^{-11}\,\text{m}^2/\text{s}$. State your assumptions.

b) Calculate the amount of carbon deposited in the steel sheet in 2 h. Express your result as a fraction of the maximum amount.

c) How long will it take to achieve a carbon concentration of 0.7 wt % at a depth of 0.5 mm below the surface?

(Answer: a) 0.254 wt %, b) 0.081, c) 3 h 27 min)

6.10 Decarburization is the reversal of the process of carburization, i.e., removal of carbon (species A) from a metal (species B) by diffusion. A thick steel plate having a uniform concentration of 0.8 wt % is decarburized in a vacuum at $1,200\,\text{K}$. How long will it take for the carbon concentration at a depth of 0.5 mm below the surface to decrease to 0.4 wt %? Take $\mathcal{D}_{AB} = 1.8 \times 10^{-11}\,\text{m}^2/\text{s}$.
(Answer: 3 h 15 min)

6.11 For estimation of the durability of structures, it is highly desirable to quantify the chloride diffusion process in concrete (Vedalakshmi et al., 2009). The initiation and propagation periods are the two distinct periods of deterioration caused by corrosion. The initiation period (t_i) is the time taken for Cl^- or CO_2 to diffuse to the steel–concrete interface and activate the corrosion. The time to initiation of corrosion is given by

$$t_i = \frac{L^2}{4\mathcal{D}_{eff}\left[\text{erf}^{-1}\left(1 - \dfrac{c_A^*}{c_{A_s}}\right)\right]^2},$$

where L is the cover of concrete, $\mathcal{D}_{eff}$ is the effective diffusion coefficient of chloride, c_{A_s} is the concentration of chloride at the surface, and c_A^* is the threshold concentration of chloride at which corrosion initiates. Derive this equation, and state the assumptions.

6.12 A dopant (or a doping agent) is an impurity added to a semiconductor in trace amounts to change its electrical conductivity, producing n-type (negative) or p-type (positive) semiconductors. Boron and phosphorus are the common dopants for producing p- and n-type semiconductors, respectively.

Consider doping of a 1-mm-thick silicon wafer by exposing one side of it to hot boron gas at $1,300\,\text{K}$ for 4 h. The surface concentration is constant at $4.3 \times 10^{20}\,\text{atoms/cm}^3$ and $\mathcal{D}_{AB} = 5 \times 10^{-19}\,\text{m}^2/\text{s}$.

a) Estimate the boron concentration at a depth of $0.25\,\mu\text{m}$ below the silicon surface.
b) Calculate the diffusion penetration depth.
(Answer: a) $1.6 \times 10^{19}\,\text{atoms/cm}^3$, b) $0.34\,\mu\text{m}$)

6.13 Consider one-dimensional diffusion of species A into a semi-infinite slab of width W and height H. Initially, the concentration of species A within the slab is uniform at a value of c_{A_o}.

a) If the surface of the slab at $z = 0$ is exposed to constant molar flux, i.e.,

$$\text{at} \quad z = 0 \qquad -\mathcal{D}_{AB}\frac{\partial c_A}{\partial z} = N_{A_s} = \text{constant},$$

show that the concentration distribution is given by

$$c_A - c_{A_o} = 2N_{A_s}\sqrt{\frac{t}{\pi\mathcal{D}_{AB}}}\exp\left(-\frac{z^2}{4\mathcal{D}_{AB}t}\right) - \frac{N_{A_s}z}{\mathcal{D}_{AB}}\text{erfc}\left(\frac{z}{2\sqrt{\mathcal{D}_{AB}t}}\right)$$

b) The surface of the slab at $z = 0$ is exposed to a constant concentration c_{A_∞}. If the external resistance to mass transfer cannot be neglected, then the boundary condition at the slab surface is given by

$$\text{at} \quad z = 0 \qquad -\mathcal{D}_{AB}\frac{\partial c_A}{\partial z} = k_c(c_{A_\infty} - c_A),$$

in which the partition coefficient is considered unity. First show that the concentration distribution is given by

$$\frac{c_A - c_{A_o}}{c_{A_\infty} - c_{A_o}} = \text{erfc}\left(\frac{z}{2\sqrt{\mathcal{D}_{AB}t}}\right) - \exp\left[\frac{k_c(z + k_c t)}{\mathcal{D}_{AB}}\right]\text{erfc}\left(\frac{z}{2\sqrt{\mathcal{D}_{AB}t}} + k_c\sqrt{\frac{t}{\mathcal{D}_{AB}}}\right)$$

and then show that the total number of moles of species A transferred into the slab over time t is given by

$$\mathbb{N}_A = WH(c_{A_\infty} - c_{A_o}) \left[\frac{\mathcal{D}_{AB}}{k_c} \exp\left(\frac{k_c^2 t}{\mathcal{D}_{AB}}\right) \operatorname{erfc}\left(k_c \sqrt{\frac{t}{\mathcal{D}_{AB}}}\right) - \frac{\mathcal{D}_{AB}}{k_c} + 2\sqrt{\frac{\mathcal{D}_{AB}t}{\pi}} \right]$$

6.14 Consider one-dimensional diffusion of species A into a semi-infinite slab. The initial concentration of species A in the slab is c_{A_o}. At $t = 0$, the surface of the slab is exposed to a concentration varying with time according to the relation

$$c_A = c_{A_o} + \frac{\beta}{\sqrt{t}},$$

where $\beta > 0$. Show that the concentration distribution is given by

$$c_A = c_{A_o} + \frac{\beta}{\sqrt{t}} \exp\left(-\frac{z^2}{4\mathcal{D}_{AB}t}\right)$$

6.15 Consider one-dimensional diffusion of species A into a semi-infinite slab of width W and height H. Initially, the slab is free of species A. At $t = 0$, the surface of the slab at $z = 0$ is exposed to a concentration that is a periodic function of time in the form

$$c_A = c_{A_o} \cos(\omega t - \phi)$$

Using Duhamel's theorem show that

$$\frac{c_A}{c_{A_o}} = \exp\left(-\sqrt{\frac{\omega}{2\mathcal{D}_{AB}}}\, z\right) \cos\left(\omega t - \sqrt{\frac{\omega}{2\mathcal{D}_{AB}}}\, z - \phi\right)$$
$$- \frac{2}{\sqrt{\pi}} \int_0^{z/2\sqrt{\mathcal{D}_{AB}t}} \exp\left(-\beta^2\right) \cos\left[\omega\left(t - \frac{z^2}{4\mathcal{D}_{AB}\beta^2}\right) - \phi\right] d\beta,$$

where β is a dummy variable.

6.16 Consider one-dimensional diffusion of species A into a semi-infinite slab of width W and height H. Initially, the slab is free of species A. Once the surface of the slab at $z = 0$ is exposed to a constant concentration c_{A_∞}, species A diffuses into the slab and also undergoes an irreversible first-order reaction, i.e., $\mathcal{R}_A = -k_1''' c_A$.

a) Show that the concentration distribution is given by

$$\frac{c_A}{K_A c_{A_\infty}} = \frac{1}{2} \exp\left(-\sqrt{\frac{k_1'''}{\mathcal{D}_{AB}}}\, z\right) \operatorname{erfc}\left(\frac{z}{2\sqrt{\mathcal{D}_{AB}t}} - \sqrt{k_1''' t}\right)$$
$$+ \frac{1}{2} \exp\left(\sqrt{\frac{k_1'''}{\mathcal{D}_{AB}}}\, z\right) \operatorname{erfc}\left(\frac{z}{2\sqrt{\mathcal{D}_{AB}t}} + \sqrt{k_1''' t}\right),$$

where K_A is the partition coefficient.

b) Show that the molar rate of flow of species A entering the slab is given by

$$\mathcal{W}_A = WHK_A c_{A_\infty} \left[\sqrt{k_1''' \mathcal{D}_{AB}} \operatorname{erf}\left(\sqrt{k_1''' t}\right) + \sqrt{\frac{\mathcal{D}_{AB}}{\pi t}} \exp\left(-k_1''' t\right) \right]$$

c) Show that the total number of moles of species A transferred into the slab over time t is given by

$$\mathbb{N}_A = WHK_A c_{A_\infty} \sqrt{\mathcal{D}_{AB} t} \left[\left(\sqrt{k_1''' t} + \frac{1}{2\sqrt{k_1''' t}} \right) \text{erf} \left(\sqrt{k_1''' t} \right) + \sqrt{\frac{1}{\pi}} \exp \left(-k_1''' t \right) \right]$$

Hint: Study Example E.14 in Appendix E.

6.17 Consider absorption of species A into a spherical liquid droplet (species B) of radius R. The liquid droplet is initially A-free. Assume that the total concentration within the droplet is constant and the convective flux is negligible compared to the diffusive flux.

a) Show that the concentration distribution is given by

$$\frac{c_A}{c_A^{eq}} = 1 + \frac{2}{\pi} \sum_{n=1}^{\infty} \frac{(-1)^n}{n} e^{-n^2 \pi^2 \tau} \frac{\sin(n\pi\xi)}{\xi},$$

where c_A^{eq} is the equilibrium solubility of species A in liquid B and τ and ξ are the dimensionless quantities defined by

$$\tau = \frac{\mathcal{D}_{AB} t}{R^2} \qquad \xi = \frac{r}{R}$$

b) Show that the time required for the center concentration to reach 99% of the final concentration is given by

$$t \simeq \frac{0.54 R^2}{\mathcal{D}_{AB}}$$

6.18 The hypertextbook *Biofilms*[3] indicates that the time required for a solute to reach 90% of the bulk fluid concentration at the base of a flat biofilm is given by

$$t_{90} = 1.03 \frac{L^2}{\mathcal{D}_{eff}}, \tag{1}$$

where $\mathcal{D}_{eff}$ is the effective diffusion coefficient of solute in the biofilm. On the other hand, the time required for a solute to reach 90% of the bulk fluid concentration at the center of a spherical biofilm of radius R is given by

$$t_{90} = 0.31 \frac{R^2}{\mathcal{D}_{eff}} \tag{2}$$

Derive these equations. What does L represent in Eq. (1)?

6.19 Consider a cylinder (species B) of radius R and height H with $R \ll H$. Initially, the concentration of species A within the cylinder is uniform at a value of c_{A_o}. At $t = 0$, the cylinder is exposed to a fluid with a constant concentration of c_{A_∞} ($c_{A_\infty} > c_{A_o}$). Let us assume $\text{Bi}_M > 40$ so that the resistance to mass transfer in the fluid phase is negligible.

a) Show that the governing differential equation is given by

$$\frac{\partial \theta}{\partial \tau} = \frac{1}{\xi} \frac{\partial}{\partial \xi} \left(\xi \frac{\partial \theta}{\partial \xi} \right) \tag{1}$$

---

[3]http://hypertextbookshop.com/biofilmbook/v005/r001/default.html

subject to the initial and boundary conditions

$$\text{at} \quad \tau = 0 \qquad \theta = 1 \tag{2}$$

$$\text{at} \quad \xi = 0 \qquad \frac{\partial \theta}{\partial \xi} = 0 \tag{3}$$

$$\text{at} \quad \xi = 1 \qquad \theta = 0, \tag{4}$$

where the dimensionless quantities are defined by

$$\theta = \frac{K_A c_{A_\infty} - c_A}{K_A c_{A_\infty} - c_{A_o}} \qquad \xi = \frac{r}{R} \qquad \tau = \frac{\mathcal{D}_{AB} t}{R^2}, \tag{5}$$

in which K_A is the partition coefficient.

b) Take the Laplace transform of Eq. (1) and show that the solution in the Laplace domain is given by

$$\overline{\theta} = \frac{1}{s} - \frac{I_o(\xi \sqrt{s})}{s I_o(\sqrt{s})} \tag{6}$$

c) Use the identity

$$I_n(x) = e^{-n\pi i/2} J_n(ix) \tag{7}$$

and show that the dimensionless concentration distribution is given by

$$\theta = 2 \sum_{n=1}^{\infty} \frac{1}{\lambda_n J_1(\lambda_n)} \exp\left(-\lambda_n^2 \tau\right) J_o(\lambda_n \xi), \tag{8}$$

where the eigenvalues are calculated from

$$J_o(\lambda_n) = 0 \qquad n = 1, 2, 3, \ldots \tag{9}$$

d) The dimensionless average concentration $\langle \theta \rangle$ can be defined as

$$\langle \theta \rangle = \frac{K_A c_{A_\infty} - \langle c_A \rangle}{K_A c_{A_\infty} - c_{A_o}} = 2 \int_0^1 \theta \xi \, d\xi \tag{10}$$

Show that the substitution of Eq. (8) into Eq. (10) and integration lead to

$$\langle \theta \rangle = 4 \sum_{n=1}^{\infty} \frac{1}{\lambda_n^2} \exp\left(-\lambda_n^2 \tau\right) \tag{11}$$

e) Show that the fractional uptake is given by

$$\frac{N_A}{N_{A_\infty}} = 1 - 4 \sum_{n=1}^{\infty} \frac{1}{\lambda_n^2} \exp\left(-\lambda_n^2 \tau\right) \tag{12}$$

6.20 Problem 4.12 is about the steady-state diffusion of a bleaching agent into the dentin layer of a tooth. Now let us consider the unsteady-state version of this problem.

a) Show that the concentration distribution is given by

$$\theta = \xi + 2 \sum_{n=1}^{\infty} \frac{(-1)^n}{n\pi} \left\{ \frac{\Lambda^2 + n^2 \pi^2 \exp\left[-(n^2 \pi^2 + \Lambda^2)\tau\right]}{n^2 \pi^2 + \Lambda^2} \right\} \sin(n\pi\xi),$$

where the dimensionless quantities are defined as follows:

$$\theta = \frac{c_A}{c_{A_o}} \qquad \tau = \frac{\mathcal{D}_{AB}t}{\delta^2} \qquad \xi = 1 - \frac{z}{\delta} \qquad \Lambda^2 = \frac{k_1''' \delta^2}{\mathcal{D}_{AB}}$$

b) Show that the molar flux of a bleaching agent entering the dentin layer is given by

$$N_{A_z}\big|_{z=0} = \frac{\mathcal{D}_{AB}c_{A_o}}{\delta} \left(1 + 2 \sum_{n=1}^{\infty} \left\{ \frac{\Lambda^2 + n^2\pi^2 \exp\left[-(n^2\pi^2 + \Lambda^2)\tau\right]}{n^2\pi^2 + \Lambda^2} \right\} \right)$$

c) Show that the number of moles of a bleaching agent entering the dentin layer is

$$\mathbb{N}_A = \delta c_{A_o} A \left\{ \tau + 2 \sum_{n=1}^{\infty} \frac{n^2\pi^2 \left[1 + \Lambda^2\tau - e^{-(n^2\pi^2 + \Lambda^2)\tau} \right] + \Lambda^4\tau}{(n^2\pi^2 + \Lambda^2)^2} \right\},$$

where A is the cross-sectional area of the dentin layer.

6.21 Steady-state diffusion of species A in a liquid with a homogeneous reaction is described in Section 4.8. Now consider the unsteady-state version of the same problem.

a) Using the dimensionless quantities

$$\theta = \frac{c_A}{c_{A_o}} \qquad \xi = \frac{z}{L} \qquad \tau = \frac{\mathcal{D}_{AB}t}{L^2} \qquad \Lambda^2 = \frac{k_1''' L^2}{\mathcal{D}_{AB}}$$

express the governing equation together with initial and boundary conditions in dimensionless form and show that the concentration distribution is given by

$$\theta = \frac{\cosh\left[\Lambda(1-\xi)\right]}{\cosh\Lambda} - 2\sum_{n=0}^{\infty} \frac{\lambda_n}{\lambda_n^2 + \Lambda^2} \exp\left[-(\lambda_n^2 + \Lambda^2)\tau\right] \sin(\lambda_n\xi),$$

where the eigenvalues are given as

$$\lambda_n = \left(\frac{2n+1}{2}\right)\pi \qquad n = 0,1,2,\ldots$$

b) Show that the molar flow rate of species A entering the liquid is

$$\mathcal{W}_A = \frac{A\mathcal{D}_{AB}c_{A_o}}{L} \left\{ \Lambda\tanh\Lambda + 2\sum_{n=0}^{\infty} \frac{\lambda_n^2}{\lambda_n^2 + \Lambda^2} \exp\left[-(\lambda_n^2 + \Lambda^2)\tau\right] \right\}$$

6.22 Raudino et al. (1999) studied the formation and diffusion of methyl methacrylate (MMA) monomer in a thin film of poly(methyl methacrylate) (PMMA) subjected to pulsed ion beam irradiation. For this purpose, $4\,\text{cm}^2$ square samples of PMMA (thickness $= L = 8600\,\text{Å}$) placed on a SiO$_2$ support were irradiated at different temperatures. The working pressure in the irradiation chamber was $\sim 10^{-7}$torr. If the formation of MMA (species A) follows the zeroth-order reaction, the governing equation is

$$\frac{\partial c_A}{\partial t} = D_{eff}\frac{\partial^2 c_A}{\partial z^2} + k_o''' f(t), \tag{1}$$

where $f(t)$ is a function of the irradiation time that describes the depolymerization reaction induced by the ion beam. The function $f(t)$ suddenly goes to zero when the beam is turned off at $t > t_o$, with t_o being the irradiation time, and is unity for $t < t_o$. Thus, it is expressed as

$$f(t) = 1 - H(t - t_o), \tag{2}$$

where $H(t - t_o)$ is the *Heaviside function* (or unit step function) defined by

$$H(t - t_o) = \begin{cases} 0 & t < t_o \\ 1 & t \geq t_o \end{cases} \tag{3}$$

The initial and boundary conditions associated with Eq. (1) are

$$\text{at} \quad t = 0 \qquad c_A = 0 \tag{4}$$

$$\text{at} \quad z = 0 \qquad \frac{\partial c_A}{\partial z} = 0 \tag{5}$$

$$\text{at} \quad z = L \qquad c_A = 0 \tag{6}$$

The boundary condition given by Eq. (5) indicates no mass transfer through the PMMA film–inert support (SiO_2) interface. Equation (6) implies complete evaporation of species A at the PMMA film–vacuum interface.

a) Rewrite Eqs. (1) and (4)–(6) in terms of the following dimensionless variables:

$$\tau = \frac{\mathcal{D}_{eff} t}{L^2} \qquad \xi = \frac{z}{L} \qquad \Omega^2 = \frac{k_o''' L^2}{\mathcal{D}_{eff}} \tag{7}$$

b) Show that the solution in the Laplace domain is given by

$$\bar{c}_A = -\frac{\Omega^2 (1 - e^{-st_o})}{s^2 \cosh \sqrt{s}} \cosh(\sqrt{s}\xi) + \frac{\Omega^2 (1 - e^{-st_o})}{s^2} \tag{8}$$

c) Since we are interested in the flux of monomer escaping from the PMMA film–vacuum interface, first show that the flux in the Laplace domain is given by

$$\bar{N}_{A_z}\big|_{z=L} = k_o''' L \left(\frac{1 - e^{-st_o}}{s} \right) \frac{\sinh \sqrt{s}}{\sqrt{s} \cosh \sqrt{s}} \tag{9}$$

and then take the inverse Laplace transformation to obtain

$$N_{A_z}\big|_{z=L} = k_o''' L \left\{ 1 - \frac{8}{\pi^2} \sum_{n=1}^{\infty} \frac{1}{(2n-1)^2} \exp\left[-\frac{(2n-1)^2 \pi^2 \mathcal{D}_{eff}}{4L^2} t \right] \right\} \qquad \text{when } t < t_o \tag{10}$$

$$N_{A_z}\big|_{z=L} = \frac{8 k_o''' L}{\pi^2} \sum_{n=1}^{\infty} \frac{1}{(2n-1)^2} \exp\left[-\frac{(2n-1)^2 \pi^2 \mathcal{D}_{eff}}{4L^2} t \right]$$
$$\times \left\{ \exp\left[-\frac{(2n-1)^2 \pi^2 \mathcal{D}_{eff} t_o}{4L^2} \right] - 1 \right\} \qquad \text{when } t \geq t_o \tag{11}$$

6.23 Repeat the analysis given in Section 6.6 for a spherical particle of radius R. First show that the governing equations are given as

$$\text{Sphere} \qquad \frac{\partial \theta}{\partial \tau} = \frac{1}{\xi^2} \frac{\partial}{\partial \xi}\left(\xi^2 \frac{\partial \theta}{\partial \xi} \right)$$

$$\text{Solution} \qquad -\frac{\partial \theta}{\partial \xi}\bigg|_{\xi=1} = \frac{\Omega}{3} \frac{d\theta_s}{d\tau},$$

where the dimensionless quantities are defined by

$$\theta = \frac{c}{Kc_{s_o}} \qquad \theta_s = \frac{c_s}{c_{s_o}} \qquad \xi = \frac{r}{R} \qquad \tau = \frac{Dt}{R^2} \qquad \Omega = \frac{V_s}{\frac{4}{3}\pi R^3 K}$$

Then, use the method of Laplace transform to show that

$$\frac{c_s}{c_{s_o}} = \frac{\Omega}{1+\Omega} + 6\Omega \sum_{n=1}^{\infty} \frac{1}{\Omega^2 \lambda_n^2 + 9(1+\Omega)} e^{-\lambda_n^2 \tau},$$

where λ_n are the roots of

$$\tan \lambda_n = \frac{3\lambda_n}{3 + \Omega \lambda_n^2} \qquad n = 1, 2, 3, \ldots$$

6.24 Consider the following governing equation together with the initial and boundary conditions in dimensionless form:

$$\frac{\partial \theta}{\partial \tau} = \frac{\partial^2 \theta}{\partial \xi^2} \tag{1}$$

$$\text{at} \quad \tau = 0 \qquad \theta = 0 \tag{2}$$

$$\text{at} \quad \xi = 0 \qquad \theta = 1 \tag{3}$$

$$\text{at} \quad \xi = 1 \qquad \frac{\partial \theta}{\partial \xi} = 0 \tag{4}$$

a) Show that the solution is

$$\theta = 1 - 2 \sum_{n=0}^{\infty} \frac{1}{\lambda_n} \exp\left(-\lambda_n^2 \tau\right) \sin(\lambda_n \xi), \tag{5}$$

where

$$\lambda_n = \frac{(2n+1)\pi}{2} \qquad n = 0, 1, 2, \ldots \tag{6}$$

b) Give examples of mass transfer problems in real life that will be modeled by Eqs. (1)–(4).

6.25 Consider the following governing equation together with the initial and boundary conditions in dimensionless form:

$$\frac{\partial \theta}{\partial \tau} = \frac{\partial^2 \theta}{\partial \xi^2} - \Lambda \tag{1}$$

$$\text{at} \quad \tau = 0 \qquad \theta = 0 \tag{2}$$

$$\text{at} \quad \xi = 0 \qquad \theta = 1 \tag{3}$$

$$\text{at} \quad \xi = 1 \qquad \frac{\partial \theta}{\partial \xi} = 0 \tag{4}$$

a) Show that the solution is

$$\theta = 1 - \Lambda \xi + \frac{\Lambda}{2} \xi^2 + 2 \sum_{n=0}^{\infty} \frac{1}{\lambda_n} \left(\frac{\Lambda}{\lambda_n^2} - 1\right) \exp\left(-\lambda_n^2 \tau\right) \sin(\lambda_n \xi), \tag{5}$$

where

$$\lambda_n = \frac{(2n+1)\pi}{2} \qquad n = 0, 1, 2, \ldots \tag{6}$$

b) Give examples of mass transfer problems in real life that will be modeled by Eqs. (1)–(4).

6.26 Consider the following governing equation together with the initial and boundary conditions in dimensionless form:

$$\frac{\partial\theta}{\partial\tau} = \frac{\partial^2\theta}{\partial\xi^2} \tag{1}$$

$$\text{at} \quad \tau = 0 \qquad \theta = \delta(\xi) \tag{2}$$

$$\text{at} \quad \xi = 0 \qquad \frac{\partial\theta}{\partial\xi} = 0 \tag{3}$$

$$\text{at} \quad \xi = 1 \qquad \theta = 0, \tag{4}$$

where $\delta(\xi)$ is the Dirac delta function.

a) Show that the solution is

$$\theta = 2\sum_{n=0}^{\infty} \exp\left(-\lambda_n^2\tau\right)\cos(\lambda_n\xi), \tag{5}$$

where

$$\lambda_n = \frac{(2n+1)\pi}{2} \qquad n = 0,1,2,\dots \tag{6}$$

b) Give examples of mass transfer problems in real life that will be modeled by Eqs. (1)–(4).

6.27 Transdermal drug delivery is the transfer of active ingredients by diffusion through the skin into the bloodstream. Transdermal patches, such as nicotine, EMSAM (antidepressant), fentanyl (pain), and clonidine (high blood pressure) find extensive use in our daily lives. Consider the diffusion of a drug (species A) from a transdermal patch to the skin as shown in the figure below.

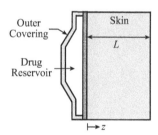

a) Considering the skin as a homogeneous layer of thickness L, show that the governing equation for species A is given by

$$\frac{\partial c_A}{\partial t} = \mathcal{D}_{\text{eff}}\frac{\partial^2 c_A}{\partial z^2}$$

subject to the following initial and boundary conditions:

$$
\begin{array}{ll}
t = 0 & c_A = 0 \\
z = 0 & c_A = c_{A_o} \\
z = L & c_A = 0
\end{array}
$$

What is the physical significance of the boundary condition at $z = L$?

b) Show that the concentration distribution is given by

$$\theta = 1 - \xi - \frac{2}{\pi}\sum_{n=1}^{\infty}\frac{1}{n}e^{-n^2\pi^2\tau}\sin(n\pi\xi),$$

where the dimensionless quantities are defined by

$$\theta = \frac{c_A}{c_{A_o}} \qquad \tau = \frac{\mathcal{D}_{eff} t}{L^2} \qquad \xi = \frac{z}{L}$$

c) Show that the number of moles of drug penetrating into the skin is given by

$$\mathbb{N}_{A_{in}} = A L c_{A_o} \left(\tau + \frac{1}{3} - \frac{2}{\pi^2} \sum_{n=1}^{\infty} \frac{1}{n^2} e^{-n^2 \pi^2 \tau} \right)$$

d) Show that the number of moles of drug carried out by the bloodstream is given by

$$\mathbb{N}_{A_{out}} = A L c_{A_o} \left(\tau - \frac{1}{6} - \frac{2}{\pi^2} \sum_{n=1}^{\infty} \frac{(-1)^n}{n^2} e^{-n^2 \pi^2 \tau} \right)$$

6.28 The nerve cells in the brain that are responsible for communication are called neurons. A neuron mainly consists of three parts: dendrites, an axon, and a cell body (soma). Neurons receive input from other cells via their dendrites. Neurons talk to each other by sending an electrical message, called an action potential, throughout the entire axon. The junction between an axon and a neighboring dendrite is called a synapse, and the tiny opening between neurons is called the synaptic cleft. The axon ends in an enlargement known as the presynaptic terminal, containing tiny vesicles filled with molecules, such as acetylcholine, dopamine, glutamate, and serotonin. These substances are known as neurotransmitters. When an electrical signal arrives at the presynaptic terminal, the neurotransmitters are released from the vesicles into the synaptic cleft, where they diffuse to the postsynaptic surface and bind to their specific receptors.

    If the diffusion of a neurotransmitter through the synaptic cleft is modeled as

$$\frac{\partial c_A}{\partial t} = \mathcal{D}_{AB} \frac{\partial^2 c_A}{\partial z^2} - k_1''' c_A$$

subject to the initial and boundary conditions

$$\text{at} \quad t = 0 \qquad c_A = \frac{M_A}{A} \delta(z)$$

$$\text{at} \quad z = 0 \qquad \frac{\partial c_A}{\partial z} = 0$$

$$\text{at} \quad z = L \qquad -\mathcal{D}_{AB} \frac{\partial c_A}{\partial z} = k_1'' c_A$$

obtain the concentration distribution.

6.29 Consider diffusion from a plane source and show that the concentration at one standard deviation from the center of mass is $0.61 c_{max}$.

6.30 Consider diffusion from a plane source as explained in Section 6.8.1.

a) If the mass M_A is released at $x = x_1$ instead of $x = 0$, show that the concentration distribution is given by

$$c_A = \frac{M_A / A}{2 \sqrt{\pi \mathcal{D}_x t}} \exp \left[-\frac{(x - x_1)^2}{4 \mathcal{D}_x t} \right]$$

b) If there are two plane sources, M_{A_1} / A and M_{A_2} / A located at $x = x_1$ and $x = x_2$, respectively, show that the concentration distribution is given by

$$c_A = \frac{M_{A_1} / A}{2 \sqrt{\pi \mathcal{D}_x t}} \exp \left[-\frac{(x - x_1)^2}{4 \mathcal{D}_x t} \right] + \frac{M_{A_2} / A}{2 \sqrt{\pi \mathcal{D}_x t}} \exp \left[-\frac{(x - x_2)^2}{4 \mathcal{D}_x t} \right]$$

6.31 The top and bottom of a vertical cylindrical column of height L are closed once it is filled with sand. At $t = 0$, M_A amount of species is injected into the column at $z = z^*$, where z is the distance measured from the bottom of the cylinder, uniformly across the cross-sectional area, A, of the cylinder. Show that the concentration distribution is given by

$$c_A = \frac{M_A}{AL}\left[1 + 2\sum_{n=1}^{\infty}\exp\left(-\frac{n^2\pi^2\mathcal{D}_{eff}t}{L^2}\right)\cos\left(\frac{n\pi z^*}{L}\right)\cos\left(\frac{n\pi z}{L}\right)\right]$$

6.32 Five kilograms of a chemical accidentally spills in a canal of 5 m width and 3 m deep. The diffusion coefficient of the chemical in water is $3.5 \times 10^{-9}\,\mathrm{m^2/s}$. Estimate the width and the maximum concentration of the diffusing patch after 24 h.

(Answer: 0.098 m, 5.41 kg/m^3)

6.33 Consider one-dimensional diffusion from a plane source. While diffusing, species A undergoes an irreversible first-order homogeneous reaction. If the rate of depletion of species A per unit volume is represented by

$$\mathcal{R}_A = -k_1''' c_A$$

show that the concentration distribution is given by

$$c_A = \frac{M_A/A}{2\sqrt{\pi\mathcal{D}_x t}}\exp\left(-\frac{x^2}{4\mathcal{D}_x t} - k_1''' t\right)$$

REFERENCES

Carr, E. J. 2017. Calculating how long it takes for a diffusion process to effectively reach steady state without computing the transient solution. *Phys. Rev. E.* 96:012116.

Carslaw, H. S. and J. C. Jaeger. 1959. *Conduction of Heat in Solids*, 2nd edn. London: Oxford University Press.

Crank, J. 1975. *The Mathematics of Diffusion*, 2nd edn. London: Oxford University Press.

Raudino, A., M. E. Fragala, G. Compagnini and O. Puglisi. 1999. Modeling of low-temperature depolymerization of poly(methyl methacrylate) promoted by ion-beam. *J. Chem. Phys.* 111(4):1721–31.

Ravi, R. 2007. Mathematical treatment of the Loschmidt tube experiment: Some clarifications. *Chem. Eng. Comm.* 194:170–76.

Segel, L. E., I. Chet and Y. Henis. 1977. A simple quantitative assay for bacterial motility. *J. Gen. Microbiol.* 98:329–37.

Vedalakshmi, R., V. Saraswathy, H. W. Song and N. Palaniswamy. 2009. Determination of diffusion coefficient of chloride in concrete using Warburg diffusion coefficient. *Corros. Sci.* 51(6):1299–307.

Versypt, A. N. F., P. D. Arendt, D. W. Pack and R. D. Braatz. 2015. Reaction-diffusion model for autocatalytic degradation and erosion in polymeric microspheres, *PLoS ONE* 10(8):e0135506.

7 Mass Transfer in Binary Systems with Bulk Flow

Chapters 4–6 dealt with mass transfer in binary systems without bulk flow. In the problems presented in those chapters, convection was either induced by the diffusion process itself or considered negligible. This chapter is devoted to mass transfer in moving fluids. The presence of the convective (or advective[1]) term in the equation of continuity for species A usually introduces nonlinearity into the governing equation. Since the choice of a characteristic velocity is arbitrary, it is more convenient to select a characteristic velocity that will make the convective term zero and thus yield a simpler problem. Most of the time, however, none of the characteristic velocities are zero. As a result, analytical solutions of the problems become rather difficult if not impossible to obtain. Examples are chosen from a wide range of topics to illustrate the effect of bulk flow in mass transfer problems.

7.1 GOVERNING EQUATIONS

The equation of continuity for species A is presented in different forms in Section 2.4.3. In the case of dilute liquid solutions, it takes the form

$$\frac{\partial c_A}{\partial t} + \underbrace{\mathbf{v} \cdot \nabla c_A}_{\text{Convection}} = \mathcal{D}_{AB} \nabla^2 c_A + \mathcal{R}_A \tag{7.1}$$

Table 2.4 shows this equation in the Cartesian, cylindrical, and spherical coordinate systems. When the bulk flow is appreciable, we have to consider all the terms appearing in Eq. (7.1). The order of magnitude estimates of the unsteady-state and convection terms are

$$\text{Unsteady-state term} \sim O\left[\frac{(\Delta c_A)_{ch}}{t_{ch}^C}\right] \qquad \text{Convection term} \sim O\left[v_{ch} \frac{(\Delta c_A)_{ch}}{L_{ch}}\right], \tag{7.2}$$

where $(\Delta c_A)_{ch}$, t_{ch}^C, v_{ch}, and L_{ch} represent the characteristic concentration difference of species A, characteristic time for convection, characteristic velocity, and characteristic convection length, respectively. The existence of these two terms in the continuity equation implies that they have the same order of magnitude, i.e.,

$$O\left[\frac{(\Delta c)_{ch}}{t_{ch}^C}\right] = O\left[v_{ch} \frac{(\Delta c_A)_{ch}}{L_{ch}}\right] \tag{7.3}$$

or

$$\boxed{t_{ch}^C = \frac{L_{ch}}{v_{ch}}} \tag{7.4}$$

The term t_{ch}^C, referred to as the *convective timescale,* represents the time it takes for species A to travel distance L_{ch} at velocity v_{ch}. It is important to keep in mind that the characteristic length used in the diffusion timescale, Eq. (5.4), may be different from the one used in the convective timescale.

---

[1] In general, there is a subtle difference between the terms "convection" and "advection." While convection includes mass transfer by both bulk flow and diffusion, advection only considers mass transfer by bulk flow.

7.2   FORCED CONVECTION MASS TRANSFER IN A PIPE

Consider the steady, laminar flow of an incompressible Newtonian liquid (species B) in a circular pipe of radius R under the action of a pressure gradient. The fully developed velocity profile[2] is given by

$$v_z = 2 \langle v_z \rangle \left[1 - \left(\frac{r}{R} \right)^2 \right], \tag{7.5}$$

where $\langle v_z \rangle$ is the average velocity. For $z < 0$, the liquid has a uniform species A concentration of c_{A_o}. The inner surface of the pipe is coated with species A for $z \geq 0$. As a result of the mass transfer from the pipe wall to the flowing liquid, species A concentration starts to change in the radial and axial directions. Since the analogous heat transfer problem was first solved by Graetz (1883), problems of this type are known as *"Graetz problems"* in the literature.

Postulating $c_A = c_A(r,z)$, Eq. (B) of Table 2.4 reduces to

$$\underbrace{v_z \frac{\partial c_A}{\partial z}}_{\substack{\text{Convection in} \\ z\text{-direction}}} = \underbrace{\frac{\mathcal{D}_{AB}}{r} \frac{\partial}{\partial r} \left(r \frac{\partial c_A}{\partial r} \right)}_{\text{Diffusion in } r\text{-direction}} + \underbrace{\mathcal{D}_{AB} \frac{\partial^2 c_A}{\partial z^2}}_{\substack{\text{Diffusion in} \\ z\text{-direction}}} \tag{7.6}$$

In the axial direction, mass of species A is transported by both convection and diffusion. The order of magnitude estimates of these terms are

$$\text{Convection in } z\text{-direction} \quad \sim \quad O \left[\langle v_z \rangle \frac{(\Delta c_A)_{ch}}{L} \right] \tag{7.7}$$

$$\text{Diffusion in } z\text{-direction} \quad \sim \quad O \left[\mathcal{D}_{AB} \frac{(\Delta c_A)_{ch}}{L^2} \right] \tag{7.8}$$

In the z-direction, diffusion may be considered negligible with respect to convection when

$$O \left[\langle v_z \rangle \frac{(\Delta c_A)_{ch}}{L} \right] \gg O \left[\mathcal{D}_{AB} \frac{(\Delta c_A)_{ch}}{L^2} \right] \tag{7.9}$$

Thus, the criterion is

$$\frac{\langle v_z \rangle L}{\mathcal{D}_{AB}} \gg 1 \tag{7.10}$$

Equation (7.10) can be rearranged in the form

$$\underbrace{\frac{\rho \langle v_z \rangle D}{\mu}}_{\text{Re}} \underbrace{\frac{\mu}{\rho \mathcal{D}_{AB}}}_{\text{Sc}} \frac{L}{D} \gg 1 \tag{7.11}$$

Since the product of the Reynolds and Schmidt numbers gives the Peclet number for mass transfer, Eq. (7.11) is expressed as

$$\boxed{\text{Pe}_\text{M} \frac{L}{D} \gg 1} \tag{7.12}$$

In the literature, axial diffusion is generally neglected compared to convection on the basis of large Peclet numbers without considering the L/D term.

---

[2]*Fully developed flow* implies there is no variation in velocity in the axial direction. In this way, the flow development regions near the entrance and exit are not taken into consideration. In other words, "end effects" are neglected.

If the constraint given by Eq. (7.12) is satisfied, then Eq. (7.6) reduces to

$$v_z \frac{\partial c_A}{\partial z} = \frac{\mathcal{D}_{AB}}{r} \frac{\partial}{\partial r} \left(r \frac{\partial c_A}{\partial r} \right) \tag{7.13}$$

Substitution of the velocity distribution, Eq. (7.5), into Eq. (7.13) gives

$$2 \langle v_z \rangle \left[1 - \left(\frac{r}{R} \right)^2 \right] \frac{\partial c_A}{\partial z} = \frac{\mathcal{D}_{AB}}{r} \frac{\partial}{\partial r} \left(r \frac{\partial c_A}{\partial r} \right) \tag{7.14}$$

The boundary conditions associated with Eq. (7.14) are

$$\text{at} \quad z = 0 \qquad c_A = c_{A_o} \tag{7.15}$$

$$\text{at} \quad r = 0 \qquad \frac{\partial c_A}{\partial r} = 0 \tag{7.16}$$

$$\text{at} \quad r = R \qquad c_A = c_A^{eq}, \tag{7.17}$$

where the concentration at the wall surface, c_A^{eq}, is constant and equals the saturation solubility of species A in the liquid. Introduction of the dimensionless quantities

$$\theta = \frac{c_A - c_A^{eq}}{c_{A_o} - c_A^{eq}} \qquad \xi = \frac{r}{R} \qquad \eta = \frac{\mathcal{D}_{AB} z}{2R^2 \langle v_z \rangle} \tag{7.18}$$

reduces Eqs. (7.14)–(7.17) to

$$(1 - \xi^2) \frac{\partial \theta}{\partial \eta} = \frac{1}{\xi} \frac{\partial}{\partial \xi} \left(\xi \frac{\partial \theta}{\partial \xi} \right) \tag{7.19}$$

$$\text{at} \quad \eta = 0 \qquad \theta = 1 \tag{7.20}$$

$$\text{at} \quad \xi = 0 \qquad \frac{\partial \theta}{\partial \xi} = 0 \tag{7.21}$$

$$\text{at} \quad \xi = 1 \qquad \theta = 0 \tag{7.22}$$

Representing the solution as a product of two functions of the form

$$\theta(\eta, \xi) = F(\eta) G(\xi) \tag{7.23}$$

reduces Eq. (7.19) to

$$\frac{1}{F} \frac{dF}{d\eta} = \frac{1}{\xi(1 - \xi^2)} \frac{1}{G} \frac{d}{d\xi} \left(\xi \frac{dG}{d\xi} \right) = -\lambda^2, \tag{7.24}$$

which results in two ordinary differential equations (ODEs):

$$\frac{dF}{d\eta} + \lambda^2 F = 0 \qquad \Longrightarrow \qquad F(\eta) = C_1 e^{-\lambda^2 \eta} \tag{7.25}$$

$$\frac{d}{d\xi} \left(\xi \frac{dG}{d\xi} \right) + \lambda^2 \xi(1 - \xi^2) G = 0 \tag{7.26}$$

Note that the choice of a negative constant, $-\lambda^2$, in Eq. (7.24) is due to the fact that the solution will decay to zero, i.e., $\theta \to 0$ ($c_A \to c_A^{eq}$), as $z \to \infty$.

Equation (7.26) is a Sturm–Liouville equation with a weight function of $\xi(1 - \xi^2)$, and the boundary conditions associated with it are

$$\text{at} \quad \xi = 0 \qquad \frac{dG}{d\xi} = 0 \tag{7.27}$$

$$\text{at} \quad \xi = 1 \qquad G = 0 \tag{7.28}$$

Let us introduce the transformations in the form

$$Z = \lambda \xi^2 \quad \text{and} \quad W = e^{Z/2} G \tag{7.29}$$

The chain rule of differentiation leads to

$$\frac{dG}{d\xi} = \frac{dG}{dZ}\frac{dZ}{d\xi} \quad \text{and} \quad \frac{d^2G}{d\xi^2} = \frac{d^2G}{dZ^2}\left(\frac{dZ}{d\xi}\right)^2 + \frac{dG}{dZ}\frac{d^2Z}{d\xi^2} \tag{7.30}$$

Noting that

$$\frac{dG}{dZ} = e^{-Z/2}\left(\frac{dW}{dZ} - \frac{1}{2}W\right) \qquad \frac{d^2G}{dZ^2} = e^{-Z/2}\left(\frac{d^2W}{dZ^2} - \frac{dW}{dZ} + \frac{1}{4}W\right) \tag{7.31}$$

$$\frac{dZ}{d\xi} = 2\frac{Z}{\xi} \qquad \frac{d^2Z}{d\xi^2} = 2\frac{Z}{\xi^2} \tag{7.32}$$

Eq. (7.26) is expressed in the form

$$Z\frac{d^2W}{dZ^2} + (1-Z)\frac{dW}{dZ} - \left(\frac{1}{2} - \frac{\lambda}{4}\right)W = 0 \tag{7.33}$$

The solution of Eq. (7.33) is given by

$$W = C_2 M\left(\frac{1}{2} - \frac{\lambda}{4}, 1, Z\right) + C_3 U\left(\frac{1}{2} - \frac{\lambda}{4}, 1, Z\right), \tag{7.34}$$

where M and U are known as *Kummer's function of the first kind* and *Kummer's function of the second kind*, respectively (Abramowitz and Stegun, 1972), defined by

$$M(a,b,Z) = 1 + \frac{a}{b}Z + \frac{a(a+1)}{b(b+1)}\frac{Z^2}{2!} + \cdots + \frac{a(a+1)\cdots(a+n-1)}{b(b+1)\cdots(b+n-1)}\frac{Z^n}{n!} + \cdots \tag{7.35}$$

and

$$U(a,b,Z) = \frac{\Gamma(1-b)}{\Gamma(a-b+1)}M(a,b,Z) + \frac{\Gamma(b-1)}{\Gamma(a)}Z^{1-b}M(a-b+1,2-b,Z), \tag{7.36}$$

where $\Gamma(u)$ is the *gamma function* defined by

$$\Gamma(u) = \int_0^\infty t^{u-1}e^{-t}\,dt \tag{7.37}$$

Using Eq. (7.36), the term $U\left(\frac{1}{2} - \frac{\lambda}{4}, 1, Z\right)$ is expressed as

$$U\left(\frac{1}{2} - \frac{\lambda}{4}, 1, Z\right) = \frac{\Gamma(0)}{\Gamma\left(\frac{1}{2} - \frac{\lambda}{4}\right)}\left[M\left(\frac{1}{2} - \frac{\lambda}{4}, 1, Z\right) + M\left(-\frac{1}{2} - \frac{\lambda}{4}, 1, Z\right)\right] \tag{7.38}$$

Since $\Gamma(0)$ is unbounded, $C_3 = 0$ and Eq. (7.34) reduces to

$$W = C_2 M\left(\frac{1}{2} - \frac{\lambda}{4}, 1, Z\right) \tag{7.39}$$

Application of the boundary condition given by Eq. (7.28), i.e.,

$$\text{at} \quad Z = \lambda \quad W = 0, \tag{7.40}$$

gives the following transcendental equation for the eigenvalues:

$$M\left(\frac{1}{2} - \frac{\lambda_n}{4}, 1, \lambda_n\right) = 0 \qquad n = 1, 2, 3, \dots \tag{7.41}$$

The first ten eigenvalues are given in Table 7.1. Thus, the solution is expressed in the form

$$\theta = \sum_{n=1}^{\infty} C_n \underbrace{e^{-\lambda_n^2 \eta}}_{F_n(\eta)} \underbrace{e^{-\lambda_n \xi^2/2} M\left(\frac{1}{2} - \frac{\lambda_n}{4}, 1, \lambda_n \xi^2\right)}_{G_n(\xi)} \tag{7.42}$$

Application of Eq. (7.20) gives the constants C_n as

$$C_n = \frac{\displaystyle\int_0^1 \xi(1-\xi^2) G_n(\xi) d\xi}{\displaystyle\int_0^1 \xi(1-\xi^2) G_n^2(\xi) d\xi} = -\frac{2}{\lambda_n \, (dG_n/d\lambda_n)|_{\xi=1}} \tag{7.43}$$

The values of $(dG_n/d\lambda_n)|_{\xi=1}$ are also given in Table 7.1.

As shown in Section 5.3, mass transfer correlations are expressed in terms of the Sherwood number. The solution given by Eq. (7.42) can be related to the Sherwood number by the following analysis.

The molar flux of species A on the pipe surface can be represented by

$$\mathcal{D}_{AB} \frac{\partial c_A}{\partial r}\bigg|_{r=R} = k_c (c_A^{eq} - c_{A_b}), \tag{7.44}$$

where c_{A_b} is the bulk concentration, defined by

$$c_{A_b} = \frac{\displaystyle\int_0^{2\pi} \int_0^R v_z c_A \, r \, dr \, d\theta}{\displaystyle\int_0^{2\pi} \int_0^R v_z \, r \, dr \, d\theta} = \frac{\displaystyle\int_0^R v_z c_A \, r \, dr}{\displaystyle\int_0^R v_z \, r \, dr} \tag{7.45}$$

Table 7.1
The Values of λ_n, $(dG_n/d\lambda_n)|_{\xi=1}$, and $(dG_n/d\xi)|_{\xi=1}$

n	λ_n	$(dG_n/d\lambda_n)|_{\xi=1}$	$(dG_n/d\xi)|_{\xi=1}$
1	2.7044	-0.5009	-1.0143
2	6.6790	0.3715	1.3492
3	10.6734	-0.3183	-1.5723
4	14.6711	0.2865	1.7460
5	18.6699	-0.2645	-1.8909
6	22.6691	0.2480	2.0165
7	26.6687	-0.2350	-2.1282
8	30.6683	0.2243	2.2293
9	34.6681	-0.2153	-2.3219
10	38.6679	0.2077	2.4078

Therefore, the Sherwood number is expressed as

$$\text{Sh} = \frac{k_c D}{\mathcal{D}_{AB}} = \frac{2R \, (\partial c_A/\partial r)|_{r=R}}{c_A^{eq} - c_{A_b}} \tag{7.46}$$

In dimensionless form, Eq. (7.46) becomes

$$\text{Sh} = -2 \frac{(\partial \theta/\partial \xi)|_{\xi=1}}{\theta_b}, \tag{7.47}$$

where the dimensionless bulk concentration is defined by

$$\theta_b = \frac{c_{A_b} - c_A^{eq}}{c_{A_o} - c_A^{eq}} = \frac{\int_0^1 \xi(1-\xi^2)\,\theta\,d\xi}{\int_0^1 \xi(1-\xi^2)\,d\xi} = 4\int_0^1 \xi(1-\xi^2)\,\theta\,d\xi \tag{7.48}$$

Substitution of Eq. (7.42) into Eq. (7.48) yields

$$\theta_b = 4\sum_{n=1}^{\infty} C_n e^{-\lambda_n^2 \eta} \int_0^1 \xi(1-\xi^2)\,G_n\,d\xi \tag{7.49}$$

From Eq. (7.26)

$$\xi(1-\xi^2)\,G_n = -\frac{1}{\lambda_n^2}\frac{d}{d\xi}\left(\xi\frac{dG_n}{d\xi}\right) \tag{7.50}$$

Substitution of Eq. (7.50) into Eq. (7.49) and integration lead to

$$\theta_b = -4\sum_{n=1}^{\infty}\left(\frac{C_n}{\lambda_n^2}\right)e^{-\lambda_n^2 \eta}\frac{dG_n}{d\xi}\bigg|_{\xi=1} \tag{7.51}$$

On the other hand, the expression $\partial \theta/\partial \xi|_{\xi=1}$ becomes

$$\frac{\partial \theta}{\partial \xi}\bigg|_{\xi=1} = \sum_{n=1}^{\infty} C_n e^{-\lambda_n^2 \eta}\frac{dG_n}{d\xi}\bigg|_{\xi=1} \tag{7.52}$$

Substitution of Eqs. (7.51) and (7.52) into Eq. (7.47) gives the Sherwood number as

$$\boxed{\text{Sh} = \frac{1}{2}\frac{\displaystyle\sum_{n=1}^{\infty} C_n e^{-\lambda_n^2 \eta}\frac{dG_n}{d\xi}\bigg|_{\xi=1}}{\displaystyle\sum_{n=1}^{\infty}\left(\frac{C_n}{\lambda_n^2}\right)e^{-\lambda_n^2 \eta}\frac{dG_n}{d\xi}\bigg|_{\xi=1}}} \tag{7.53}$$

The values of $(dG_n/d\xi)|_{\xi=1}$ are given in Table 7.1.

7.2.1 ASYMPTOTIC SOLUTION FOR LARGE VALUES OF z

For large values of z (or η), only the first term in each sum in Eq. (7.53) is needed. Thus, Eq. (7.53) simplifies to

$$\lim_{\eta\to\infty}\text{Sh} = \frac{\lambda_1^2}{2} \tag{7.54}$$

Since $\lambda_1 = 2.7044$ from Table 7.1, the Sherwood number at large η is

$$\boxed{\text{Sh} = \frac{(2.7044)^2}{2} = 3.657} \tag{7.55}$$

7.2.2 ASYMPTOTIC SOLUTION FOR SMALL VALUES OF z

In the entrance region of the pipe, the concentration change from c_A^{eq} to c_{A_o} occurs in a very thin region adjacent to the pipe wall, called the *concentration boundary layer*, as shown in Figure 7.1. The thickness of the concentration boundary layer, $\delta_c(z)$, is very small compared to the radius of the pipe, R.

The governing equation, Eq. (7.13), can be simplified with the help of the following assumptions:

- Let s be the distance measured from the pipe wall, i.e.,

$$s = R - r \tag{7.56}$$

- The velocity profile, Eq. (7.5), becomes

$$v_z = 2\langle v_z \rangle \left[1 - \left(\frac{R-s}{R} \right)^2 \right] = 2\langle v_z \rangle \left[\frac{2s}{R} - \left(\frac{s}{R} \right)^2 \right] \tag{7.57}$$

Since $s/R \ll 1$, Eq. (7.57) simplifies to

$$v_z = 4\langle v_z \rangle \frac{s}{R} \tag{7.58}$$

In other words, the velocity profile is regarded as linear within the concentration boundary layer.

- The term on the right side of Eq. (7.13) is expressed in terms of s as

$$\frac{\mathcal{D}_{AB}}{(R-s)} \frac{\partial}{\partial s} \left[(R-s) \frac{\partial c_A}{\partial s} \right] = \underbrace{\mathcal{D}_{AB} \frac{\partial^2 c_A}{\partial s^2}}_{\text{I}} - \underbrace{\frac{\mathcal{D}_{AB}}{(R-s)} \frac{\partial c_A}{\partial s}}_{\text{II}}, \tag{7.59}$$

in which the terms I and II represent the diffusion in the s-direction and the change in flux due to area change in cylindrical coordinates, respectively. In a very thin region adjacent to the pipe wall, curvature effects may be ignored, and the problem is treated as though the wall were flat. Consequently, the term II is neglected.

Substitution of Eqs. (7.58) and (7.59) into Eq. (7.13) gives

$$4\langle v_z \rangle \frac{s}{R} \frac{\partial c_A}{\partial z} = \mathcal{D}_{AB} \frac{\partial^2 c_A}{\partial s^2} \tag{7.60}$$

The boundary conditions associated with Eq. (7.60) are as follows:

$$\text{at} \quad z = 0 \qquad c_A = c_{A_o} \tag{7.61}$$

$$\text{at} \quad s = 0 \qquad c_A = c_A^{eq} \tag{7.62}$$

$$\text{at} \quad s = \infty \qquad c_A = c_{A_o} \tag{7.63}$$

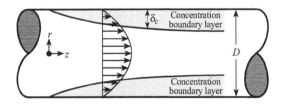

Figure 7.1 Development of the concentration boundary layer in the entrance region of a pipe.

Since $c_A = c_{A_o}$ outside the concentration boundary layer, we may consider the s-direction as semi-infinite and use Eq. (7.63) as the boundary condition instead of the boundary condition at the center of the pipe, Eq. (7.16). Introduction of the dimensionless quantities

$$\theta = \frac{c_A - c_A^{eq}}{c_{A_o} - c_A^{eq}} \qquad \xi = \frac{s}{R} \qquad \eta = \frac{\mathcal{D}_{AB}z}{4R^2 \langle v_z \rangle} \tag{7.64}$$

reduces Eqs. (7.60)–(7.63) to

$$\xi \frac{\partial \theta}{\partial \eta} = \frac{\partial^2 \theta}{\partial \xi^2} \tag{7.65}$$

$$\text{at} \quad \eta = 0 \qquad \theta = 1 \tag{7.66}$$
$$\text{at} \quad \xi = 0 \qquad \theta = 0 \tag{7.67}$$
$$\text{at} \quad \xi = \infty \qquad \theta = 1 \tag{7.68}$$

The solution is sought in the form

$$\theta = \theta(\chi), \tag{7.69}$$

where the dimensionless similarity variable χ combines the independent variables, η and ξ, in the form

$$\chi = \frac{\xi}{\sqrt[3]{9\eta}} \tag{7.70}$$

Therefore, Eq. (7.65) transforms into the following second-order ODE:

$$\frac{d^2\theta}{d\chi^2} + 3\chi^2 \frac{d\theta}{d\chi} = 0 \tag{7.71}$$

The boundary conditions associated with Eq. (7.71) are

$$\text{at} \quad \chi = 0 \qquad \theta = 0 \tag{7.72}$$
$$\text{at} \quad \chi = \infty \qquad \theta = 1 \tag{7.73}$$

The solution of Eq. (7.71) is

$$\boxed{\theta = \frac{1}{\Gamma(4/3)} \int_0^\chi e^{-u^3} du} \tag{7.74}$$

When the concentration boundary layer is thin, the bulk concentration can be approximated by the concentration of the fluid entering the pipe. Thus, Eq. (7.44) is expressed as

$$\mathcal{D}_{AB} \frac{\partial c_A}{\partial r} \bigg|_{r=R} = -\mathcal{D}_{AB} \frac{\partial c_A}{\partial s} \bigg|_{s=0} = k_c (c_A^{eq} - c_{A_o}) \tag{7.75}$$

and the Sherwood number takes the form

$$\text{Sh} = \frac{k_c D}{\mathcal{D}_{AB}} = -\frac{2R \, (\partial c_A / \partial s)|_{s=0}}{c_A^{eq} - c_{A_o}} \tag{7.76}$$

In dimensionless form, Eq. (7.76) becomes

$$\text{Sh} = 2 \left. \frac{\partial \theta}{\partial \xi} \right|_{\xi=0} = \frac{2}{\sqrt[3]{9\eta}} \left. \frac{d\theta}{d\chi} \right|_{\chi=0} = \frac{2}{9^{1/3}\Gamma(4/3)} \left(\frac{1}{\eta} \right)^{1/3} \tag{7.77}$$

or

$$\boxed{\text{Sh} = 1.357 \, \text{Pe}_{\text{M}}^{1/3} \left(\frac{R}{z} \right)^{1/3}} \tag{7.78}$$

In the literature, this problem is known as the *Lévêque problem.*

7.3 MORE ON THE FORCED CONVECTION MASS TRANSFER IN A PIPE

When the concentration profile is "fully developed," rather than dealing with the complicated mathematics leading to Eq. (7.53), the expression for the Sherwood number can be easily obtained by the averaging technique. For this purpose, Eq. (7.6) is integrated over the cross-sectional area of the pipe to obtain the governing equation for the bulk concentration of species A defined by Eq. (7.45). Note that Eq. (7.45) can also be expressed as

$$c_{A_b} = \frac{2}{\langle v_z \rangle R^2} \int_0^R v_z c_A \, r \, dr \tag{7.79}$$

Before proceeding any further, the definition of the "fully developed concentration profile" should be understood. While the local concentration changes in both the radial and axial directions, the bulk and wall concentrations change only in the z-direction. When the ratio

$$\frac{c_A - c_{A_b}}{c_A^{eq} - c_{A_b}} \tag{7.80}$$

does not vary along the axial direction, the concentration profile is said to be *fully developed*. In other words[3]

$$\frac{\partial}{\partial z} \left(\frac{c_A - c_{A_b}}{c_A^{eq} - c_{A_b}} \right) = 0 \tag{7.81}$$

Equation (7.81) indicates that

$$\frac{\partial c_A}{\partial z} = \left(\frac{c_A^{eq} - c_A}{c_A^{eq} - c_{A_b}} \right) \frac{dc_{A_b}}{dz} + \left(\frac{c_A - c_{A_b}}{c_A^{eq} - c_{A_b}} \right) \frac{dc_A^{eq}}{dz} \tag{7.82}$$

The following conclusions can be drawn when the concentration profile is fully developed:

- For a fluid with constant physical properties, the mass transfer coefficient is constant.
- For a constant wall mass flux, the concentration gradient in the axial direction, $\partial c_A / \partial z$, remains constant.

---

[3] In the literature, the condition for *the fully developed concentration profile* is also given in the form

$$\frac{\partial}{\partial z} \left(\frac{c_A^{eq} - c_A}{c_A^{eq} - c_{A_b}} \right) = 0$$

Note that

$$\frac{c_A^{eq} - c_A}{c_A^{eq} - c_{A_b}} = 1 - \frac{c_A - c_{A_b}}{c_A^{eq} - c_{A_b}}$$

Integration of Eq. (7.6) over the cross-sectional area of the tube leads to

$$\int_0^{2\pi} \int_0^R v_z \frac{\partial c_A}{\partial z} \, r \, dr \, d\theta = \mathcal{D}_{AB} \int_0^{2\pi} \int_0^R \frac{1}{r} \frac{\partial}{\partial r} \left(r \frac{\partial c_A}{\partial r} \right) r \, dr \, d\theta \tag{7.83}$$

Since v_z and c_A are independent of θ, Eq. (7.83) simplifies to

$$\int_0^R v_z \frac{\partial c_A}{\partial z} \, r \, dr = \mathcal{D}_{AB} \int_0^R \frac{\partial}{\partial r} \left(r \frac{\partial c_A}{\partial r} \right) dr \tag{7.84}$$

The term on the left side of Eq. (7.84) can be rearranged as

$$\int_0^R v_z \frac{\partial c_A}{\partial z} \, r \, dr = \int_0^R \frac{\partial (v_z c_A)}{\partial z} \, r \, dr = \frac{d}{dz} \int_0^R v_z c_A \, r \, dr \tag{7.85}$$

The use of Eq. (7.79) in Eq. (7.85) yields

$$\int_0^R v_z \frac{\partial c_A}{\partial z} \, r \, dr = \frac{\langle v_z \rangle R^2}{2} \frac{dc_{A_b}}{dz} \tag{7.86}$$

On the other hand, since $\partial c_A / \partial r = 0$ as a result of the symmetry condition at the center of the tube, the term on the right side of Eq. (7.84) takes the form

$$\mathcal{D}_{AB} \int_0^R \frac{\partial}{\partial r} \left(r \frac{\partial c_A}{\partial r} \right) dr = \mathcal{D}_{AB} R \left. \frac{\partial c_A}{\partial r} \right|_{r=R} \tag{7.87}$$

Substitution of Eqs. (7.86) and (7.87) into Eq. (7.84) gives the governing equation for the bulk concentration in the form

$$\boxed{\frac{dc_{A_b}}{dz} = \frac{2}{\langle v_z \rangle R} \mathcal{D}_{AB} \left. \frac{\partial c_A}{\partial r} \right|_{r=R},} \tag{7.88}$$

which is in a much simpler form than the governing equation for the local concentration, Eq. (7.6).

7.3.1 SHERWOOD NUMBER FOR CONSTANT WALL CONCENTRATION

The molar flux of species A at the pipe surface, N_{A_w}, is

$$N_{A_w} = \mathcal{D}_{AB} \left. \frac{\partial c_A}{\partial r} \right|_{r=R} = k_c (c_A^{eq} - c_{A_b}) \tag{7.89}$$

Substitution of Eq. (7.89) into Eq. (7.88) gives

$$\frac{dc_{A_b}}{dz} = \frac{2 k_c (c_A^{eq} - c_{A_b})}{\langle v_z \rangle R} \tag{7.90}$$

Since c_A^{eq} is constant, Eq. (7.82) simplifies to

$$\frac{\partial c_A}{\partial z} = \left(\frac{c_A^{eq} - c_A}{c_A^{eq} - c_{A_b}} \right) \frac{dc_{A_b}}{dz} \tag{7.91}$$

The use of Eq. (7.90) in Eq. (7.91) yields

$$\frac{\partial c_A}{\partial z} = \frac{2 k_c (c_A^{eq} - c_A)}{\langle v_z \rangle R} \tag{7.92}$$

Substitution of Eqs. (7.5) and (7.92) into Eq. (7.6) gives the governing equation as

$$\frac{2}{R^2} \left(\frac{2 k_c R}{\mathcal{D}_{AB}} \right) \left[1 - \left(\frac{r}{R} \right)^2 \right] (c_A^{eq} - c_A) = \frac{1}{r} \frac{\partial}{\partial r} \left(r \frac{\partial c_A}{\partial r} \right) \tag{7.93}$$

In terms of the dimensionless variables

$$\theta = \frac{c_A^{eq} - c_A}{c_A^{eq} - c_{A_b}} \qquad \xi = \frac{r}{R} \qquad Sh = \frac{k_c D}{\mathcal{D}_{AB}} \tag{7.94}$$

Eq. (7.93) takes the form

$$-2 \, Sh \, (1 - \xi^2) \, \theta = \frac{1}{\xi} \frac{d}{d\xi} \left(\xi \frac{d\theta}{d\xi} \right) \tag{7.95}$$

The boundary conditions associated with Eq. (7.95) are

$$\text{at} \quad \xi = 0 \qquad \frac{d\theta}{d\xi} = 0 \tag{7.96}$$

$$\text{at} \quad \xi = 1 \qquad \theta = 0 \tag{7.97}$$

Equation (7.95) can be solved for Sh by the method of Stodola and Vianello as explained in Section E.1.4 in Appendix E as follows[4]:

- A reasonable first guess for θ that satisfies the boundary conditions is

$$\theta_1(\xi) = 1 - \xi^2 \tag{7.98}$$

- Substitution of Eq. (7.98) into the left side of Eq. (7.95) gives

$$\frac{d}{d\xi} \left(\xi \frac{d\theta}{d\xi} \right) = -2 \, Sh \, (\xi - 2\xi^3 + \xi^5) \tag{7.99}$$

- The solution of Eq. (7.99) is

$$\theta = Sh \underbrace{\left(\frac{11 - 18\xi^2 + 9\xi^4 - 2\xi^6}{36} \right)}_{f_1(\xi)} \tag{7.100}$$

- Therefore, the first approximation to the Sherwood number is

$$Sh^{(1)} = \frac{\displaystyle\int_0^1 \xi \, (1 - \xi^2) f_1(\xi) \, \theta_1(\xi) \, d\xi}{\displaystyle\int_0^1 \xi \, (1 - \xi^2) f_1^2(\xi) \, d\xi} \tag{7.101}$$

Substitution of $f_1(\xi)$ and $\theta_1(\xi)$ from Eqs. (7.100) and (7.98), respectively, into Eq. (7.101) and evaluation of the integrals give

$$Sh = 3.663 \tag{7.102}$$

---

[4]Tosun (2007) applied this approach to calculate the Nusselt number for forced convection heat transfer in circular pipes with constant wall temperature.

- The trial function for the second approximation is

$$\theta_2(\xi) = \frac{11 - 18\xi^2 + 9\xi^4 - 2\xi^6}{36} \tag{7.103}$$

- Substitution of Eq. (7.103) into the left side of Eq. (7.95) gives

$$\frac{d}{d\xi}\left(\xi\frac{d\theta}{d\xi}\right) = -\frac{Sh}{18}\left(11\xi - 29\xi^3 + 27\xi^5 - 11\xi^7 + 2\xi^9\right) \tag{7.104}$$

- The solution of Eq. (7.104) is

$$\theta = Sh\underbrace{\left(\frac{2{,}457 - 4{,}400\xi^2 + 2{,}900\xi^4 - 1{,}200\xi^6 + 275\xi^8 - 32\xi^{10}}{28{,}800}\right)}_{f_2(\xi)} \tag{7.105}$$

- Therefore, the second approximation to the Sherwood number is given by

$$Sh^{(2)} = \frac{\displaystyle\int_0^1 \xi\,(1-\xi^2)f_2(\xi)\,\theta_2(\xi)\,d\xi}{\displaystyle\int_0^1 \xi\,(1-\xi^2)f_2^2(\xi)\,d\xi} \tag{7.106}$$

Substitution of $f_2(\xi)$ and $\theta_2(\xi)$ from Eqs. (7.105) and (7.103), respectively, into Eq. (7.106) and evaluation of the integrals give

$$\boxed{Sh = 3.657,} \tag{7.107}$$

which is exactly equal to the Sherwood number for large values of z as calculated in Section 7.2, i.e., Eq. (7.55). This is an expected result since the concentration profile becomes "fully developed" for large values of z.

7.3.2   SHERWOOD NUMBER FOR CONSTANT WALL MASS FLUX

The molar flux of species A at the pipe surface is

$$N_{A_w} = \mathcal{D}_{AB}\left.\frac{\partial c_A}{\partial r}\right|_{r=R} = k_c\left(c_A^{eq} - c_{A_b}\right) = \text{constant} \implies \frac{dc_A^{eq}}{dz} = \frac{dc_{A_b}}{dz} \tag{7.108}$$

Thus, Eq. (7.82) simplifies to

$$\frac{\partial c_A}{\partial z} = \frac{dc_{A_b}}{dz} = \frac{dc_A^{eq}}{dz} \tag{7.109}$$

Replacing dc_{A_b}/dz by $\partial c_A/\partial z$ on the left side of Eq. (7.88) yields

$$\frac{\partial c_A}{\partial z} = \frac{2N_{A_w}}{\langle v_z\rangle R} = \text{constant} \tag{7.110}$$

or

$$\frac{\partial c_A}{\partial z} = \frac{2k_c(c_A^{eq} - c_{A_b})}{\langle v_z\rangle R} \tag{7.111}$$

Since we are interested in the determination of the Sherwood number, it is appropriate to express $\partial c_A / \partial z$ in terms of the Sherwood number. Note that the Sherwood number is given by

$$\text{Sh} = \frac{k_c D}{\mathcal{D}_{AB}} \quad \Rightarrow \quad k_c = \frac{\text{Sh}\,\mathcal{D}_{AB}}{2R} \tag{7.112}$$

Substitution of Eq. (7.112) into Eq. (7.111) results in

$$\frac{\partial c_A}{\partial z} = \frac{\text{Sh}\,(c_A^{eq} - c_{A_b})\,\mathcal{D}_{AB}}{\langle v_z \rangle R^2} \tag{7.113}$$

Substitution of Eqs. (7.5) and (7.113) into Eq. (7.6) gives the governing equation as

$$\frac{2}{R^2}\left[1 - \left(\frac{r}{R}\right)^2\right]\text{Sh}\,(c_A^{eq} - c_{A_b}) = \frac{1}{r}\frac{\partial}{\partial r}\left(r\frac{\partial c_A}{\partial r}\right) \tag{7.114}$$

In terms of the dimensionless variables

$$\theta = \frac{c_A - c_{A_b}}{c_A^{eq} - c_{A_b}} \qquad \xi = \frac{r}{R} \tag{7.115}$$

Eq. (7.114) takes the form

$$2\,\text{Sh}\,(1 - \xi^2) = \frac{1}{\xi}\frac{d}{d\xi}\left(\xi\frac{d\theta}{d\xi}\right) \tag{7.116}$$

The boundary conditions associated with Eq. (7.116) are

$$\text{at} \quad \xi = 0 \qquad \frac{d\theta}{d\xi} = 0 \tag{7.117}$$

$$\text{at} \quad \xi = 1 \qquad \theta = 1 \tag{7.118}$$

The solution of Eq. (7.116) is

$$\theta = 1 - \frac{\text{Sh}}{8}\left(3 - 4\xi^2 + \xi^4\right) \tag{7.119}$$

The bulk concentration in dimensionless form can be expressed as

$$\theta_b = \frac{c_{A_b} - c_{A_b}}{c_A^{eq} - c_{A_b}} = 0 = \frac{\displaystyle\int_0^1 (1 - \xi^2)\,\theta\,\xi\,d\xi}{\displaystyle\int_0^1 (1 - \xi^2)\,\xi\,d\xi} \tag{7.120}$$

Substitution of Eq. (7.119) into Eq. (7.120) and carrying out the integrations give the Sherwood number as

$$\boxed{\text{Sh} = \frac{48}{11}} \tag{7.121}$$

How realistic is the "fully developed concentration profile" assumption? For water flowing in a circular pipe of diameter D at a Reynolds number of 100 and at a temperature of 293K, Skelland (1974) calculated the length of the tube, L, required for the velocity, temperature, and concentration distributions to reach a fully developed profile as follows:

$$\frac{L}{D} = \begin{cases} 5 & \text{fully developed velocity profile} \\ 35 & \text{fully developed temperature profile} \\ 6,000 & \text{fully developed concentration profile} \end{cases} \tag{7.122}$$

Therefore, a fully developed concentration profile is generally not attained for fluids with high Schmidt number[5], and the use of Eqs. (7.102) and (7.121) may lead to erroneous results.

When the velocity profile is fully developed, it is recommended to use the following semi-empirical correlations suggested by Hausen (1943):

$$\text{Sh} = 3.66 + \frac{0.668\left[(D/L)\,\text{Re}\,\text{Sc}\right]}{1 + 0.04\left[(D/L)\,\text{Re}\,\text{Sc}\right]^{2/3}} \qquad c_A^{eq} = \text{constant} \qquad (7.123)$$

$$\text{Sh} = 4.36 + \frac{0.023\left[(D/L)\,\text{Re}\,\text{Sc}\right]}{1 + 0.0012\left[(D/L)\,\text{Re}\,\text{Sc}\right]} \qquad N_{A_w} = \text{constant} \qquad (7.124)$$

7.4 CONVECTIVE MASS TRANSPORT WITH A WALL REACTION IN A PIPE

Consider the steady, laminar flow of an incompressible Newtonian liquid (species B) in a circular pipe of radius R under the action of a pressure gradient. The fully developed velocity distribution is given by

$$v_z = 2\langle v_z\rangle\left[1 - \left(\frac{r}{R}\right)^2\right] \qquad (7.125)$$

For $z < 0$, the wall is inert, and the liquid has a uniform species A concentration of c_{A_o}. For $z \geq 0$, the wall is coated with a catalyst on which a first-order irreversible chemical reaction takes place. The system is isothermal, the fluid mixture has constant physical properties, and it behaves as a Newtonian fluid. It is required to find the bulk concentration as a function of the axial direction.

Postulating $c_A = c_A(r,z)$, Eq. (B) in Table 2.4 reduces to

$$2\langle v_z\rangle\left[1 - \left(\frac{r}{R}\right)^2\right]\frac{\partial c_A}{\partial z} = \frac{\mathcal{D}_{AB}}{r}\frac{\partial}{\partial r}\left(r\frac{\partial c_A}{\partial r}\right), \qquad (7.126)$$

in which the convective term is assumed dominant over the diffusive one in the z-direction. The boundary conditions associated with Eq. (7.126) are

$$\text{at} \quad z = 0 \qquad c = c_{A_o} \qquad (7.127)$$

$$\text{at} \quad r = 0 \qquad \frac{\partial c_A}{\partial r} = 0 \qquad (7.128)$$

$$\text{at} \quad r = R \qquad -\mathcal{D}_{AB}\frac{\partial c_A}{\partial r} = k_1'' c_A \qquad (7.129)$$

Introduction of the dimensionless variables

$$\theta = \frac{c_A}{c_{A_o}} \qquad \xi = \frac{r}{R} \qquad \eta = \frac{\mathcal{D}_{AB}\,z}{2R^2\langle v_z\rangle} \qquad \Lambda = \frac{k_1''R}{\mathcal{D}_{AB}} \qquad (7.130)$$

reduces Eqs. (7.126)–(7.129) to

$$(1 - \xi^2)\frac{\partial\theta}{\partial\eta} = \frac{1}{\xi}\frac{\partial}{\partial\xi}\left(\xi\frac{\partial\theta}{\partial\xi}\right) \qquad (7.131)$$

---

[5]For various substances in water, a typical value for the Schmidt number is $1,200$.

$$\text{at} \quad \eta = 0 \qquad \theta = 1 \tag{7.132}$$

$$\text{at} \quad \xi = 0 \qquad \frac{\partial \theta}{\partial \xi} = 0 \tag{7.133}$$

$$\text{at} \quad \xi = 1 \qquad -\frac{\partial \theta}{\partial \xi} = \Lambda \theta \tag{7.134}$$

Representing the solution as a product of two functions of the form

$$\theta(\eta, \xi) = F(\eta) G(\xi) \tag{7.135}$$

reduces Eq. (7.131) to

$$\frac{1}{F} \frac{dF}{d\eta} = \frac{1}{\xi(1-\xi^2)G} \frac{d}{d\xi}\left(\xi \frac{dG}{d\xi}\right) = -\lambda^2, \tag{7.136}$$

which results in two ODEs:

$$\frac{dF}{d\eta} + \lambda^2 F = 0 \qquad \Rightarrow \qquad F(\eta) = C_1 e^{-\lambda^2 \eta} \tag{7.137}$$

$$\frac{d}{d\xi}\left(\xi \frac{dG}{d\xi}\right) + \lambda^2 \xi (1-\xi^2) G = 0 \tag{7.138}$$

The transformations in the forms

$$X = \lambda \xi^2 \qquad \text{and} \qquad W = e^{X/2} G \tag{7.139}$$

reduce Eq. (7.138) to

$$X \frac{d^2 W}{dX^2} + (1-X) \frac{dW}{dX} - \left(\frac{1}{2} - \frac{\lambda}{4}\right) W = 0, \tag{7.140}$$

which is Kummer's equation with the solution

$$W = C_2 M\left(\frac{1}{2} - \frac{\lambda}{4}, 1, X\right) + C_3 U\left(\frac{1}{2} - \frac{\lambda}{4}, 1, X\right) \tag{7.141}$$

Since U is unbounded, $C_3 = 0$ and Eq. (7.141) simplifies to

$$W = C_2 M\left(\frac{1}{2} - \frac{\lambda}{4}, 1, X\right) \tag{7.142}$$

Application of the boundary condition given by Eq. (7.129), i.e.,

$$\text{at} \quad X = \lambda \qquad -\frac{dW}{dX} = \left(\frac{1}{2} - \frac{\Lambda}{2\lambda}\right) W, \tag{7.143}$$

gives the following transcendental equation for the eigenvalues:

$$\boxed{\left(\frac{1}{2} - \frac{\Lambda}{2\lambda_n}\right) M\left(\frac{1}{2} - \frac{\lambda_n}{4}, 1, \lambda_n\right) = \left(\frac{1}{2} - \frac{\lambda_n}{4}\right) M\left(\frac{3}{2} - \frac{\lambda_n}{4}, 2, \lambda_n\right)} \quad n = 1, 2, 3, \ldots \tag{7.144}$$

The first ten eigenvalues for various values of Λ are given in Table 7.2.

Therefore, the solution is given by

$$\theta = \sum_{n=1}^{\infty} C_n \underbrace{e^{-\lambda_n^2 \eta}}_{F_n(\eta)} \underbrace{e^{-\lambda_n \xi^2/2} M\left(\frac{1}{2} - \frac{\lambda_n}{4}, 1, \lambda_n \xi^2\right)}_{G_n(\xi)} \tag{7.145}$$

Application of Eq. (7.132) gives the constants C_n as

$$C_n = \frac{\displaystyle\int_0^1 \xi \left(1 - \xi^2\right) G_n(\xi)\, d\xi}{\displaystyle\int_0^1 \xi \left(1 - \xi^2\right) G_n^2(\xi)\, d\xi} \tag{7.146}$$

The bulk concentration, c_{A_b}, is defined by

$$c_{A_b} = \frac{\displaystyle\int_0^{2\pi}\int_0^R c_A v_z\, r\, dr\, d\theta}{\displaystyle\int_0^{2\pi}\int_0^R v_z\, r\, dr\, d\theta} \tag{7.147}$$

In terms of the dimensionless quantities, Eq. (7.147) takes the form

$$\theta_b = \frac{c_{A_b}}{c_{A_o}} = \frac{\displaystyle\int_0^1 \xi \left(1 - \xi^2\right) \theta\, d\xi}{\displaystyle\int_0^1 \xi \left(1 - \xi^2\right) d\xi} = 4\int_0^1 \xi \left(1 - \xi^2\right) \theta\, d\xi \tag{7.148}$$

The use of Eq. (7.145) in Eq. (7.148) gives the dimensionless bulk concentration as

$$\theta_b = -4\sum_{n=1}^{\infty} \left(\frac{C_n}{\lambda_n^2}\right) e^{-\lambda_n^2 \eta} \frac{dG_n}{d\xi}\bigg|_{\xi=1} \tag{7.149}$$

Table 7.2

The Roots of Eq. (7.144) as a Function of Λ

	λ_n			
n	$\Lambda = 0.1$	$\Lambda = 0.5$	$\Lambda = 1.0$	$\Lambda = 2.0$
1	0.6183	1.2716	1.6413	2.0000
2	5.1169	5.2951	5.4783	5.7439
3	9.1889	9.3063	9.4360	9.6451
4	13.2211	13.3119	13.4152	13.5903
5	17.2399	17.3153	17.4026	17.5548
6	21.2524	21.3177	21.3939	21.5295
7	25.2615	25.3194	25.3875	25.5105
8	29.2684	29.3207	29.3826	29.4955
9	33.2738	33.3217	33.3787	33.4834
10	37.2783	37.3225	37.3755	37.4733

7.5 DIFFUSION INTO A FALLING LIQUID FILM

Consider gas absorption in a wetted-wall column as shown in Figure 7.2. An incompressible New-tonian liquid (species B) flows in laminar flow over a flat plate of width W and length L as a thin film of thickness δ under the action of gravity. The liquid has a uniform concentration of c_{A_o} for $z < 0$. Gas A flows in a countercurrent direction to the liquid, and it is required to determine the amount of species A absorbed by the liquid under steady conditions. Liquid viscosity is assumed to be unaffected by mass transfer. The fully developed velocity distribution is given by

$$v_z = v_{\max}\left[1 - \left(\frac{x}{\delta}\right)^2\right],\tag{7.150}$$

where

$$v_{\max} = \frac{\rho g \delta^2}{2\mu}\tag{7.151}$$

Postulating $c_A = c_A(x,z)$, Eq. (A) of Table 2.4 reduces to

$$\underbrace{v_z \frac{\partial c_A}{\partial z}}_{\substack{\text{Convection in}\\ \text{z-direction}}} = \underbrace{\mathcal{D}_{AB}\frac{\partial^2 c_A}{\partial x^2}}_{\substack{\text{Diffusion in}\\ \text{x-direction}}} + \underbrace{\mathcal{D}_{AB}\frac{\partial^2 c_A}{\partial z^2}}_{\substack{\text{Diffusion in}\\ \text{z-direction}}}\tag{7.152}$$

In the z-direction, the mass of species A is transported by both convection and diffusion. Neglecting the diffusion term compared to convection reduces Eq. (7.152) to

$$v_{\max}\left[1 - \left(\frac{x}{\delta}\right)^2\right]\frac{\partial c_A}{\partial z} = \mathcal{D}_{AB}\frac{\partial^2 c_A}{\partial x^2}\tag{7.153}$$

The boundary conditions associated with Eq. (7.153) are

$$\text{at}\quad z = 0 \qquad c_A = c_{A_o}\tag{7.154}$$

$$\text{at}\quad x = 0 \qquad c_A = c_A^{eq}\tag{7.155}$$

$$\text{at}\quad x = \delta \qquad \frac{\partial c_A}{\partial x} = 0\tag{7.156}$$

At the liquid–gas interface, the value of c_A^{eq} is determined from the solubility data, i.e., Henry's law. Equation (7.156) indicates that species A cannot diffuse through the wall.

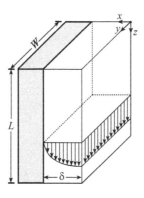

Figure 7.2 Diffusion into a falling liquid film.

Introduction of the dimensionless quantities

$$\theta = \frac{c_A^{eq} - c_A}{c_A^{eq} - c_{A_o}} \qquad \xi = \frac{x}{\delta} \qquad \eta = \frac{\mathcal{D}_{AB} z}{v_{max} \delta^2} \qquad (7.157)$$

reduces Eqs. (7.153)–(7.156) to

$$(1 - \xi^2) \frac{\partial \theta}{\partial \eta} = \frac{\partial^2 \theta}{\partial \xi^2} \qquad (7.158)$$

$$\text{at} \quad \eta = 0 \qquad \theta = 1 \qquad (7.159)$$

$$\text{at} \quad \xi = 0 \qquad \theta = 0 \qquad (7.160)$$

$$\text{at} \quad \xi = 1 \qquad \frac{\partial \theta}{\partial \xi} = 0 \qquad (7.161)$$

Representing the solution as a product of two functions of the form

$$\theta(\eta, \xi) = F(\eta) G(\xi) \qquad (7.162)$$

reduces Eq. (7.158) to

$$\frac{1}{F} \frac{dF}{d\eta} = \frac{1}{G(1 - \xi^2)} \frac{d^2 G}{d\xi^2} = -\lambda^2, \qquad (7.163)$$

which results in two ODEs:

$$\frac{dF}{d\eta} + \lambda^2 F = 0 \qquad \Rightarrow \qquad F = C_1 e^{-\lambda^2 \tau} \qquad (7.164)$$

$$\frac{d^2 G}{d\xi^2} + (1 - \xi^2) \lambda^2 G = 0 \qquad (7.165)$$

The complete solution is a linear combination of products of the form

$$\boxed{\theta = \sum_{n=1}^{\infty} C_n e^{-\lambda_n^2 \eta} G_n(\xi)} \qquad (7.166)$$

Application of Eq. (7.159) gives the constants C_n as

$$C_n = \frac{\displaystyle\int_0^1 (1 - \xi^2) G_n \, d\xi}{\displaystyle\int_0^1 (1 - \xi^2) G_n^2 \, d\xi} \qquad (7.167)$$

7.5.1   EXPRESSION FOR THE SHERWOOD NUMBER

The molar flux of species A at the gas–liquid interface is given by

$$-\mathcal{D}_{AB} \left. \frac{\partial c_A}{\partial x} \right|_{x=0} = k_c (c_A^{eq} - c_{A_b}), \qquad (7.168)$$

where c_{A_b} is the bulk concentration defined by

$$c_{A_b} = \frac{\displaystyle\int_0^W \int_0^\delta c_A v_z \, dx \, dy}{\displaystyle\int_0^W \int_0^\delta v_z \, dx \, dy} = \frac{\displaystyle\int_0^\delta c_A v_z \, dx}{\displaystyle\int_0^\delta v_z \, dx} \qquad (7.169)$$

Therefore, the Sherwood number is expressed as

$$\mathrm{Sh} = \frac{k_c \delta}{\mathcal{D}_{AB}} = -\frac{\delta (\partial c_A/\partial x)|_{x=0}}{\mathcal{D}_{AB}} \tag{7.170}$$

In dimensionless form, Eq. (7.170) becomes

$$\mathrm{Sh} = \frac{(\partial \theta/\partial \xi)|_{\xi=0}}{\theta_b}, \tag{7.171}$$

where the dimensionless bulk concentration is defined by

$$\theta_b = \frac{c_A^{eq} - c_{A_b}}{c_A^{eq} - c_{A_o}} = \frac{\int_0^1 (1-\xi^2)\,\theta\,d\xi}{\int_0^1 (1-\xi^2)\,d\xi} = \frac{3}{2} \int_0^1 (1-\xi^2)\,\theta\,d\xi \tag{7.172}$$

Substitution of Eq. (7.166) into Eq. (7.172) yields

$$\theta_b = \frac{3}{2} \sum_{n=1}^{\infty} \left(\frac{C_n}{\lambda_n^2}\right) e^{-\lambda_n^2 \eta} \left. \frac{dG_n}{d\xi} \right|_{\xi=0} \tag{7.173}$$

On the other hand, the expression $(\partial \theta/\partial \xi)|_{\xi=0}$ becomes

$$\left. \frac{\partial \theta}{\partial \xi} \right|_{\xi=0} = \sum_{n=1}^{\infty} C_n e^{-\lambda_n^2 \eta} \left. \frac{dG_n}{d\xi} \right|_{\xi=0} \tag{7.174}$$

Substitution of Eqs. (7.173) and (7.174) into Eq. (7.171) gives the Sherwood number as

$$\boxed{\mathrm{Sh} = \frac{2}{3} \frac{\displaystyle\sum_{n=1}^{\infty} C_n e^{-\lambda_n^2 \eta} \left. \frac{dG_n}{d\xi} \right|_{\xi=0}}{\displaystyle\sum_{n=1}^{\infty} \left(\frac{C_n}{\lambda_n^2}\right) e^{-\lambda_n^2 \eta} \left. \frac{dG_n}{d\xi} \right|_{\xi=0}}} \tag{7.175}$$

7.5.2 LONG CONTACT TIMES

For large values of η, only the first term in each sum in Eq. (7.175) is needed. Thus, Eq. (7.175) simplifies to

$$\lim_{\eta \to \infty} \mathrm{Sh} = \frac{2}{3} \lambda_1^2 \tag{7.176}$$

The first eigenvalue of Eq. (7.165), rearranged in the form

$$\frac{d^2 G}{d\xi^2} = -(1-\xi^2)\lambda^2 G, \tag{7.177}$$

can be obtained by the method of Stodola and Vianello as explained in Section E.1.4 in Appendix E as follows:

- A reasonable first guess for θ that satisfies the boundary conditions is

$$\theta_1(\xi) = \xi(\xi - 2) \tag{7.178}$$

- Substitution of Eq. (7.178) into the left side of Eq. (7.177) gives

$$\frac{d^2G}{d\xi^2} = -\lambda_1^2(1-\xi^2)\xi(\xi-2) \tag{7.179}$$

- The solution of Eq. (7.179) is

$$G = \lambda_1^2 \underbrace{\left(\frac{\xi^3}{3} - \frac{\xi^4}{12} - \frac{\xi^5}{10} + \frac{\xi^6}{30} - \frac{11\xi}{30}\right)}_{f_1(\xi)} \tag{7.180}$$

- Therefore, the first approximation to λ_1^2 is

$$[\lambda_1^2]^{(1)} = \frac{\displaystyle\int_0^1 (1-\xi^2)f_1(\xi)\,\theta_1(\xi)\,d\xi}{\displaystyle\int_0^1 (1-\xi^2)f_1^2(\xi)\,d\xi} \tag{7.181}$$

Substitution of $f_1(\xi)$ and $\theta_1(\xi)$ from Eqs. (7.180) and (7.178), respectively, into Eq. (7.181) and evaluation of the integrals give $\lambda_1^2 = 5.122$. Therefore, the Sherwood number is

$$\boxed{\text{Sh} = \left(\frac{2}{3}\right)(5.122) = 3.41} \tag{7.182}$$

7.5.3 SHORT CONTACT TIMES

If the solubility of species A in the liquid B is low, species A penetrates only a short distance into the falling liquid film for short contact times. Under these circumstances, species A, for the most part, has the impression that the film is moving throughout at a velocity equal to v_{max}. Furthermore, species A does not feel the presence of the solid wall at $x = \delta$. In other words, if the film were of infinite thickness moving at the velocity v_{max}, species A would not know the difference.

In the light of the above discussion, Eqs. (7.152)–(7.156) take the following form:

$$v_{max}\frac{\partial\phi}{\partial z} = \mathcal{D}_{AB}\frac{\partial^2\phi}{\partial x^2} \tag{7.183}$$

$$\text{at}\quad z=0 \qquad \phi=0 \tag{7.184}$$
$$\text{at}\quad x=0 \qquad \phi=1 \tag{7.185}$$
$$\text{at}\quad x=\infty \qquad \phi=0, \tag{7.186}$$

where ϕ is the dimensionless concentration, defined by

$$\phi = 1-\theta = \frac{c_A - c_{A_o}}{c_A^{eq} - c_{A_o}} \tag{7.187}$$

With the help of Example E.10 in Appendix E, the solution is expressed as

$$\boxed{\frac{c_A - c_{A_o}}{c_A^{eq} - c_{A_o}} = 1 - \text{erf}\left(\frac{x}{2\sqrt{\mathcal{D}_{AB}z/v_{max}}}\right)} \tag{7.188}$$

The molar transfer rate of species A at the gas–liquid interface is

$$\mathcal{W}_A = W\int_0^L N_{A_x}|_{x=0}\,dz = -W\mathcal{D}_{AB}\int_0^L \frac{\partial c_A}{\partial x}\bigg|_{x=0}\,dz \tag{7.189}$$

The use of Eq. (7.188) in Eq. (7.189) leads to

$$\mathcal{W}_A = 2WL(c_A^{eq} - c_{A_o}) \sqrt{\frac{v_{max}\mathcal{D}_{AB}}{\pi L}} \tag{7.190}$$

The molar transfer rate of species A in terms of the mass transfer coefficient is expressed as

$$\mathcal{W}_A = (WL)k_c\,(c_A^{eq} - c_{A_o}) \tag{7.191}$$

Comparison of Eqs. (7.190) and (7.191) indicates that

$$k_c = 2\sqrt{\frac{v_{max}\mathcal{D}_{AB}}{\pi L}} \tag{7.192}$$

Therefore, the Sherwood number is expressed in the form

$$\text{Sh} = \frac{k_c\,\delta}{\mathcal{D}_{AB}} = 2\sqrt{\frac{v_{max}\,\delta^2}{\pi \mathcal{D}_{AB}L}} = \sqrt{\left(\frac{1}{\pi}\right)\left(\frac{v_{max}}{\langle v_z \rangle}\right)\left(\frac{4\rho\langle v_z\rangle\delta}{\mu}\right)\left(\frac{\mu}{\rho\mathcal{D}_{AB}}\right)\left(\frac{\delta}{L}\right)} \tag{7.193}$$

The Reynolds[6] and Schmidt numbers are defined by

$$\text{Re} = \frac{4\delta\langle v_z\rangle\rho}{\mu} \qquad \text{and} \qquad \text{Sc} = \frac{\mu}{\rho\mathcal{D}_{AB}} \tag{7.194}$$

Noting that $v_{max}/\langle v_z \rangle = 3/2$, Eq. (7.193) is expressed as

$$\text{Sh} = 0.691\,\text{Re}^{1/2}\,\text{Sc}^{1/2}\left(\frac{\delta}{L}\right)^{1/2} \tag{7.195}$$

Equation (7.195) is recommended when $100 < \text{Re} < 1,200$. It should be kept in mind that the use of Eq. (7.191) underestimates $\mathcal{W}_A$ values due to ripple formation even at very small values of Re.

In the literature, Eq. (7.192) is also expressed in the form

$$k_c = 2\sqrt{\frac{\mathcal{D}_{AB}}{\pi t_{\text{exp}}}}, \tag{7.196}$$

where the exposure time, or gas–liquid contact time, is defined by

$$t_{\text{exp}} = \frac{L}{v_{max}} \tag{7.197}$$

Equation (7.196) is also applicable to gas absorption to laminar liquid jets and mass transfer from ascending bubbles, if the penetration distance of the solute is small.

Is it possible to have an estimate of the axial distance, z, over which "short contact time" approximation is valid? Keep in mind that we are interested in a very thin region in the liquid phase adjacent to the interface in which $v_z \simeq v_{max}$ and the concentration changes from c_A^{eq} to c_{A_o}. Over this region, let us assume that

$$\frac{v_z}{v_{max}} = 0.95 \qquad \text{and} \qquad \frac{c_A - c_{A_o}}{c_A^{eq} - c_{A_o}} = 0.05 \tag{7.198}$$

---

[6]The term 4δ represents the hydraulic equivalent diameter.

The use of Eq. (7.150) gives $x/\delta = 0.224$. Substitution of the numerical values into Eq. (7.188) leads to

$$0.05 = 1 - \text{erf}\left[\left(\frac{1}{2}\right)(0.224)\frac{\delta}{\sqrt{\mathcal{D}_{AB}z/v_{max}}}\right] \quad \Rightarrow \quad z = 6.53 \times 10^{-3}\frac{v_{max}\,\delta^2}{\mathcal{D}_{AB}} \quad (7.199)$$

Consider a dilute water film of thickness 0.05 cm with the following physical properties:

$$\frac{\mu}{\rho} = 8.9 \times 10^{-3}\,\text{cm}^2/\text{s} \qquad \mathcal{D}_{AB} = 1 \times 10^{-5}\,\text{cm}^2/\text{s}$$

From Eq. (7.151),

$$v_{max} = \frac{(980)(0.05)^2}{(2)(8.9 \times 10^{-3})} = 137.6\,\text{cm/s}$$

Substitution of the numerical values into Eq. (7.199) results in

$$z = \frac{(6.53 \times 10^{-3})(137.6)(0.05)^2}{1 \times 10^{-5}} = 225\,\text{cm}$$

7.6 STEFAN DIFFUSION PROBLEM REVISITED: UNSTEADY-STATE CASE

The steady-state and pseudosteady-state cases of the Stefan diffusion problem were analyzed in Sections 4.3 and 5.5, respectively. Now let us consider the unsteady-state evaporation of pure liquid A into a gas mixture of A and B in a tube of infinite length. The solution of this problem for a stationary liquid–vapor interface is attributed to Arnold (1944). As stated by Mitrovic (2012), this problem actually was first solved by Stefan in 1889.[7] However, the existence of such a solution was not known in scientific circles. The analysis presented here for a moving liquid–vapor interface is taken from Slattery and Mhetar (1997). The problem will be analyzed with the following assumptions:

- The pressure and temperature throughout the system are uniform.
- Species A and B form an ideal gas mixture. Thus, the total molar concentration of the gas mixture, c, is constant.
- Species B is insoluble in liquid A.
- There is no homogeneous reaction.
- The diffusion coefficient is constant.

The equation of continuity for the mixture, Eq. (2.103), reduces to

$$\frac{\partial v_z^*}{\partial z} = 0 \quad \Rightarrow \quad v_z^* = v_z^*(t) \quad (7.200)$$

The equation of continuity for species A, Eq. (2.170), simplifies to

$$\frac{\partial y_A}{\partial t} + v_z^* \frac{\partial y_A}{\partial z} = \mathcal{D}_{AB}\frac{\partial^2 y_A}{\partial z^2} \quad (7.201)$$

The initial and boundary conditions associated with Eq. (7.201) are

$$\text{at} \quad t = 0 \qquad y_A = y_{A_o} \quad (7.202)$$

$$\text{at} \quad z = h(t) \qquad y_A = y_A^{eq} = P_A^{vap}/P \quad (7.203)$$

$$\text{at} \quad z = \infty \qquad y_A = y_{A_o}, \quad (7.204)$$

where $z = h(t)$ represents the location of the liquid–vapor interphase.

---

[7] Stefan's original solution for a moving phase interface is presented by Mitrovic (2012).

To proceed further, we have to relate v_z^* to y_A with the help of overall jump mass balance, Eq. (2.240), and jump mass balance for species A, Eq. (2.239). Let α-phase be the pure liquid A and β-phase be the gaseous mixture of A and B. Therefore, the unit normal vector pointing from the α-phase to the β-phase is given by

$$\lambda_{\alpha\beta} = -\lambda_{\beta\alpha} = \mathbf{e}_z \tag{7.205}$$

Since the α-phase is stagnant, we have

$$(\mathbf{v}^*)^\alpha = 0 \quad\text{and}\quad \mathbf{v}_A^\alpha = 0 \tag{7.206}$$

The concentrations are given as

$$c^\alpha = c_A^\alpha = c^L \quad\text{and}\quad c^\beta = c_A + c_B = c = \frac{P}{RT} \tag{7.207}$$

The molar flux of species A is expressed as

$$N_{A_z} = c_A^\beta \mathbf{v}_A^\beta \cdot \mathbf{e}_z \tag{7.208}$$

As a result, the overall and the species A jump mass balances at $z = h(t)$ simplify to

$$-c^L w - c(v_z^* - w) = 0 \quad\Rightarrow\quad w = \left(\frac{c}{c - c^L}\right) v_z^* \tag{7.209}$$

and

$$-c^L w - N_{A_z}\big|_{z=h} + c_A^{eq} w = 0 \quad\Rightarrow\quad N_{A_z}\big|_{z=h} = (c y_A^{eq} - c^L) w \tag{7.210}$$

Elimination of w between Eqs. (7.209) and (7.210) gives

$$N_{A_z}\big|_{z=h} = \frac{c(c y_A^{eq} - c^L)}{c - c^L} v_z^* \tag{7.211}$$

From Eq. (2.145), the total molar flux of species A is expressed as

$$N_{A_z} = -c\mathcal{D}_{AB} \frac{\partial y_A}{\partial z} + c y_A v_z^* \tag{7.212}$$

Evaluation of Eq. (7.212) at $z = h(t)$ gives

$$N_{A_z}\big|_{z=h} = -c\mathcal{D}_{AB} \frac{\partial y_A}{\partial z}\bigg|_{z=h} + c y_A^{eq} v_z^* \tag{7.213}$$

An expression for the molar average velocity can be obtained from Eqs. (7.211) and (7.213) as

$$v_z^* = -\left(\frac{c^L - c}{c^L}\right)\left(\frac{1}{1 - y_A^{eq}}\right) \mathcal{D}_{AB} \frac{\partial y_A}{\partial z}\bigg|_{z=h} \tag{7.214}$$

Substitution of Eq. (7.214) into Eq. (7.201) leads to

$$\frac{\partial y_A}{\partial t} - \left[\left(\frac{c^L - c}{c^L}\right)\left(\frac{1}{1 - y_A^{eq}}\right) \mathcal{D}_{AB} \frac{\partial y_A}{\partial z}\bigg|_{z=h}\right] \frac{\partial y_A}{\partial z} = \mathcal{D}_{AB} \frac{\partial^2 y_A}{\partial z^2} \tag{7.215}$$

In terms of the dimensionless concentration defined by

$$\theta = \frac{y_A - y_{A_o}}{y_A^{eq} - y_{A_o}} \tag{7.216}$$

Eq. (7.215) is expressed as

$$\frac{\partial \theta}{\partial t} - \left[\left(\frac{c^L - c}{c^L} \right) \left(\frac{y_A^{eq} - y_{A_o}}{1 - y_A^{eq}} \right) \mathcal{D}_{AB} \frac{\partial \theta}{\partial z} \bigg|_{z=h} \right] \frac{\partial \theta}{\partial z} = \mathcal{D}_{AB} \frac{\partial^2 \theta}{\partial z^2} \tag{7.217}$$

The solution is sought in the form

$$\theta = \theta(\eta), \tag{7.218}$$

where the dimensionless similarity variable η combines the independent variables, t and z, in the form

$$\eta = \frac{z}{2 \sqrt{\mathcal{D}_{AB} t}} \tag{7.219}$$

The chain rule of differentiation gives

$$\frac{\partial \theta}{\partial t} = \frac{d\theta}{d\eta} \frac{\partial \eta}{\partial t} = -\frac{1}{2} \frac{\eta}{t} \frac{d\theta}{d\eta} \tag{7.220}$$

$$\frac{\partial \theta}{\partial z} = \frac{d\theta}{d\eta} \frac{\partial \eta}{\partial z} = \frac{1}{2 \sqrt{\mathcal{D}_{AB} t}} \frac{d\theta}{d\eta} \tag{7.221}$$

$$\frac{\partial^2 \theta}{\partial z^2} = \frac{d^2 \theta}{d\eta^2} \left(\frac{\partial \eta}{\partial z} \right)^2 + \frac{d\theta}{d\eta} \frac{\partial^2 \eta}{\partial z^2} = \frac{1}{4 \mathcal{D}_{AB} t} \frac{d^2 \theta}{d\eta^2} \tag{7.222}$$

Substitution of Eqs. (7.220)–(7.222) into Eq. (7.217) results in the following second-order ODE:

$$\frac{d^2 \theta}{d\eta^2} + 2 (\eta - \varphi) \frac{d\theta}{d\eta} = 0, \tag{7.223}$$

where

$$\varphi = -\frac{1}{2} \left(\frac{c^L - c}{c^L} \right) \left(\frac{y_A^{eq} - y_{A_o}}{1 - y_A^{eq}} \right) \frac{d\theta}{d\eta} \bigg|_{\eta=\lambda} \tag{7.224}$$

and

$$\lambda = \frac{h}{2 \sqrt{\mathcal{D}_{AB} t}} \tag{7.225}$$

The boundary conditions associated with Eq. (7.223) are

$$\text{at} \quad \eta = \lambda \qquad \theta = 1 \tag{7.226}$$

$$\text{at} \quad \eta = \infty \qquad \theta = 0 \tag{7.227}$$

The solution is given by

$$\theta = 1 - \frac{\displaystyle\int_\lambda^\eta \exp\left[-(u - \varphi)^2 \right] du}{\displaystyle\int_\lambda^\infty \exp\left[-(u - \varphi)^2 \right] du} \tag{7.228}$$

The substitution

$$\beta = u - \varphi \tag{7.229}$$

transforms Eq. (7.228) into

$$
\begin{aligned}
\theta &= 1 - \frac{\int_{\lambda-\varphi}^{\eta-\varphi} \exp\left(-\beta^2\right) d\beta}{\int_{\lambda-\varphi}^{\infty} \exp\left(-\beta^2\right) d\beta} = 1 - \frac{\int_{0}^{\eta-\varphi} \exp\left(-\beta^2\right) d\beta - \int_{0}^{\lambda-\varphi} \exp\left(-\beta^2\right) d\beta}{\int_{0}^{\infty} \exp\left(-\beta^2\right) d\beta - \int_{0}^{\lambda-\varphi} \exp\left(-\beta^2\right) d\beta} \\[2mm]
&= 1 - \frac{\operatorname{erf}(\eta-\varphi) - \operatorname{erf}(\lambda-\varphi)}{\operatorname{erf}(\infty) - \operatorname{erf}(\lambda-\varphi)}
\end{aligned}
\tag{7.230}
$$

Simplification of Eq. (7.230) gives the concentration distribution as

$$
\boxed{\theta = \frac{1 - \operatorname{erf}(\eta-\varphi)}{1 - \operatorname{erf}(\lambda-\varphi)}}
\tag{7.231}
$$

The use of Eq. (7.231) in Eq. (7.226) gives

$$
\boxed{\varphi = \frac{1}{\sqrt{\pi}} \left(\frac{c^L - c}{c^L}\right) \left(\frac{y_A^{eq} - y_{A_o}}{1 - y_A^{eq}}\right) \frac{\exp\left[-(\lambda-\varphi)^2\right]}{1 - \operatorname{erf}(\lambda-\varphi)}}
\tag{7.232}
$$

To characterize the rate of evaporation by the position of the interface, first let us express Eq. (7.214) in terms of the dimensionless quantities as

$$
v_z^* = \underbrace{-\frac{1}{2} \left(\frac{c^L - c}{c^L}\right) \left(\frac{y_A^{eq} - y_{A_o}}{1 - y_A^{eq}}\right) \mathcal{D}_{AB} \left.\frac{d\eta}{dz}\right|_{\eta=\lambda} \sqrt{\frac{\mathcal{D}_{AB}}{t}}}_{\varphi\,[\text{Eq. (7.224)}]}
\tag{7.233}
$$

The speed of the interface is given by

$$
w = \frac{dh}{dt} = \frac{d}{dt}\left(2\sqrt{\mathcal{D}_{AB}t}\right) = \lambda\sqrt{\frac{\mathcal{D}_{AB}}{t}}
\tag{7.234}
$$

Elimination of w between Eqs. (7.209) and (7.234) results in

$$
v_z^* = \left(\frac{c - c^L}{c}\right) \lambda \sqrt{\frac{\mathcal{D}_{AB}}{t}}
\tag{7.235}
$$

Equations (7.233) and (7.235) indicate that

$$
\boxed{\varphi = \left(\frac{c - c^L}{c}\right) \lambda}
\tag{7.236}
$$

Slattery and Mhetar (1997) provided the following physical properties for the evaporation of methanol (species A) into air (species B) at 298.6 K and 1.006×10^5 Pa:

$$
y_A^{eq} = 0.172 \quad y_{A_o} = 0 \quad c^L = 24.6\,\text{kmol/m}^3 \quad c = 0.0411\,\text{kmol/m}^3 \quad \mathcal{D}_{AB} = 1.558 \times 10^{-5}\,\text{m}^2/\text{s}
$$

As shown in the Mathcad worksheet given below, simultaneous solution of Eqs. (7.232) and (7.236) gives

$$
\varphi = 0.104 \quad\text{and}\quad \lambda = -1.735 \times 10^{-4}
$$

yeq := 0.172   y0 := 0 $D := 1.558\,10^{-5}$ cL := 24.6   c := 0.0411

$\varphi := 0.1$ $\lambda := 0.1$ These are the initial guess values

Given

$$\varphi = \frac{1}{\sqrt{\pi}} \cdot \left(\frac{cL - c}{cL}\right) \cdot \left(\frac{yeq - y0}{1 - yeq}\right) \cdot \frac{\exp\left[-(\lambda - \varphi)^2\right]}{1 - \mathrm{erf}(\lambda - \varphi)}$$

$$\varphi = \left(\frac{c - cL}{c}\right) \cdot \lambda$$

$$\mathrm{Find}(\varphi, \lambda) = \begin{pmatrix} 0.104 \\ -1.735 \times 10^{-4} \end{pmatrix}$$

Mathcad worksheet for Section 7.6.

7.7 STEFAN TUBE AT SUPERCRITICAL CONDITIONS

Ozguler et al. (2003) studied the applicability of the Stefan tube in the diffusion coefficient measurements of nonvolatile solids in supercritical fluids. For this purpose, they considered the carbon dioxide (B)–naphthalene (A) system as shown in Figure 7.3. Solid naphthalene diffuses from the bottom of the tube into the supercritical carbon dioxide that fills the rest of the tube and is swept away by the pure carbon dioxide that is flowing from the top of the tube.

The equation of continuity for species A, Eq. (2.170), simplifies to

$$\frac{\partial y_A}{\partial t} + v_z^* \frac{\partial y_A}{\partial z} = \mathcal{D}_{AB} \frac{\partial^2 y_A}{\partial z^2}, \tag{7.237}$$

in which the molar average velocity, v_z^*, is considered constant on the basis of negligible natural convection. The initial and boundary conditions associated with Eq. (7.237) are

$$\text{at} \quad t = 0 \quad y_A = 0 \tag{7.238}$$

$$\text{at} \quad z = 0 \quad y_A = y_A^{eq} \tag{7.239}$$

$$\text{at} \quad z = L \quad y_A = 0, \tag{7.240}$$

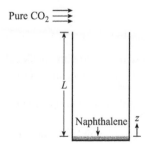

Figure 7.3 Diffusion of naphthalene into carbon dioxide.

where y_A^{eq} is the saturation mole fraction of naphthalene in carbon dioxide. In terms of the dimensionless variables,

$$\theta = \frac{y_A}{y_A^{eq}} \qquad \tau = \frac{\mathcal{D}_{AB}t}{L^2} \qquad \xi = \frac{z}{L} \qquad \Omega = \frac{Lv_z^*}{\mathcal{D}_{AB}} \tag{7.241}$$

Eqs. (7.237)–(7.240) are expressed as

$$\frac{\partial \theta}{\partial \tau} + \Omega \frac{\partial \theta}{\partial \xi} = \frac{\partial^2 \theta}{\partial \xi^2} \tag{7.242}$$

$$\text{at} \quad \tau = 0 \qquad \theta = 0 \tag{7.243}$$
$$\text{at} \quad \xi = 0 \qquad \theta = 1 \tag{7.244}$$
$$\text{at} \quad \xi = 1 \qquad \theta = 0 \tag{7.245}$$

Since the boundary condition at $\xi = 0$ is nonhomogeneous, let us propose a solution in the form

$$\theta(\tau, \xi) = \theta_\infty(\xi) + \theta_t(\tau, \xi), \tag{7.246}$$

in which $\theta_\infty(\xi)$ is the solution to the steady-state problem, i.e.,

$$\frac{d^2 \theta_\infty}{d\xi^2} - \Omega \frac{d\theta_\infty}{d\xi} = 0 \tag{7.247}$$

$$\text{at} \quad \xi = 0 \qquad \theta_\infty = 1 \tag{7.248}$$
$$\text{at} \quad \xi = 1 \qquad \theta_\infty = 0 \tag{7.249}$$

The steady-state solution is given by

$$\theta_\infty = \frac{\exp(\Omega\xi) - \exp(\Omega)}{1 - \exp(\Omega)} \tag{7.250}$$

The use of Eq. (7.250) in Eq. (7.246) gives

$$\theta(\tau, \xi) = \frac{\exp(\Omega\xi) - \exp(\Omega)}{1 - \exp(\Omega)} + \theta_t(\tau, \xi) \tag{7.251}$$

Substitution of Eq. (7.251) into Eqs. (7.242)–(7.245) leads to the following governing equation for the transient problem together with the initial and boundary conditions:

$$\frac{\partial \theta_t}{\partial \tau} + \Omega \frac{\partial \theta_t}{\partial \xi} = \frac{\partial^2 \theta_t}{\partial \xi^2} \tag{7.252}$$

$$\text{at} \quad \tau = 0 \qquad \theta_t = -\frac{\exp(\Omega\xi) - \exp(\Omega)}{1 - \exp(\Omega)} \tag{7.253}$$
$$\text{at} \quad \xi = 0 \qquad \theta_t = 0 \tag{7.254}$$
$$\text{at} \quad \xi = 1 \qquad \theta_t = 0 \tag{7.255}$$

Representing the solution as a product of two functions of the form

$$\theta_t(\tau, \xi) = F(\tau) G(\xi) \tag{7.256}$$

reduces Eq. (7.252) to

$$\frac{1}{F}\frac{dF}{d\tau} = \frac{1}{G}\frac{d^2G}{d\xi^2} - \Omega\frac{dG}{d\xi} = -\lambda^2, \tag{7.257}$$

which results in two ODEs:

$$\frac{dF}{d\tau} + \lambda^2 F = 0 \quad\Rightarrow\quad F(\tau) = C_1 e^{-\lambda^2\tau} \tag{7.258}$$

$$\frac{d^2G}{d\xi^2} - \Omega\frac{dG}{d\xi} + \lambda^2 G = 0 \tag{7.259}$$

The boundary conditions for $G(\xi)$ are

$$\text{at}\quad \xi = 0 \qquad G = 0 \tag{7.260}$$
$$\text{at}\quad \xi = 1 \qquad G = 0 \tag{7.261}$$

Proposing a solution of the form

$$G = e^{m\xi} \tag{7.262}$$

leads to the following characteristic equation:

$$m^2 - \Omega m + \lambda^2 = 0, \tag{7.263}$$

which has the roots

$$m = \frac{\Omega}{2} \pm \sqrt{\frac{\Omega^2}{4} - \lambda^2} \tag{7.264}$$

If we let

$$-\omega^2 - \frac{\Omega^2}{4} \quad \lambda^2 \tag{7.265}$$

Eq. (7.264) becomes

$$m = \frac{\Omega}{2} \pm i\omega \tag{7.266}$$

According to Eq. (D.24) given in Appendix D, the solution is given by

$$G = e^{\frac{\Omega\xi}{2}}\left[C_2\cos(\omega\xi) + C_3\sin(\omega\xi)\right] \tag{7.267}$$

Application of the boundary condition at $\xi = 0$ gives $C_2 = 0$. The boundary condition at $\xi = 1$ leads to

$$\sin\omega = 0 \quad\Rightarrow\quad \boxed{\omega = n\pi} \quad n = 1,2,3,\ldots \tag{7.268}$$

Substitution of Eq. (7.268) into Eq. (7.265) results in

$$\boxed{\lambda_n^2 = n^2\pi^2 + \frac{\Omega^2}{4}} \tag{7.269}$$

Therefore, the transient solution is expressed as

$$\theta_t = \exp\left(\frac{\Omega\xi}{2}\right)\sum_{n=1}^{\infty} C_n \exp\left[-(n^2\pi^2 + \frac{\Omega^2}{4})\tau\right]\sin(n\pi\xi) \tag{7.270}$$

Application of Eq. (7.253) yields

$$-\frac{\exp(\Omega\xi)-\exp(\Omega)}{1-\exp(\Omega)}=\exp\left(\frac{\Omega\xi}{2}\right)\sum_{n=1}^{\infty}C_n\sin(n\pi\xi) \tag{7.271}$$

Multiplication of Eq. (7.271) by $\exp(-\Omega\xi/2)\sin(m\pi\xi)d\xi$ and integration from $\xi=0$ to $\xi=1$ give

$$\frac{\exp(\Omega)}{1-\exp(\Omega)}\int_0^1\exp\left(-\frac{\Omega\xi}{2}\right)\sin(n\pi\xi)d\xi-\frac{1}{1-\exp(\Omega)}\int_0^1\exp\left(\frac{\Omega\xi}{2}\right)\sin(n\pi\xi)d\xi$$
$$=C_n\int_0^1\sin^2(n\pi\xi)d\xi \tag{7.272}$$

Evaluation of the integrals results in

$$C_n=-\frac{8n\pi}{4n^2\pi^2+\Omega^2} \tag{7.273}$$

The transient solution then becomes

$$\theta_t=-8\pi\exp\left(\frac{\Omega\xi}{2}\right)\sum_{n=1}^{\infty}\frac{n}{4n^2\pi^2+\Omega^2}\exp\left[-\left(n^2\pi^2+\frac{\Omega^2}{4}\right)\tau\right]\sin(n\pi\xi) \tag{7.274}$$

Substitution of Eqs. (7.250), (7.270), and (7.273) into Eq. (7.246) gives the solution[8] as

$$\boxed{\theta=\frac{\exp(\Omega\xi)-\exp(\Omega)}{1-\exp(\Omega)}-8\pi\exp\left(\frac{\Omega\xi}{2}\right)\sum_{n=1}^{\infty}\frac{n}{4n^2\pi^2+\Omega^2}\exp\left[-\left(n^2\pi^2+\frac{\Omega^2}{4}\right)\tau\right]\sin(n\pi\xi)}$$
$$\tag{7.275}$$

The molar flux of naphthalene at the interphase is given by

$$N_{A_z}\big|_{z=0}=-\frac{c\mathcal{D}_{AB}}{1-y_{A_o}}\frac{\partial y_A}{\partial z}\bigg|_{z=0}=-\frac{c\mathcal{D}_{AB}}{L}\frac{y_{A_o}}{1-y_{A_o}}\frac{\partial\theta}{\partial\xi}\bigg|_{\xi=0} \tag{7.276}$$

The use of Eq. (7.275) in Eq. (7.276) leads to

$$\boxed{N_{A_z}\big|_{z=0}=-\frac{c\mathcal{D}_{AB}}{L}\frac{y_{A_o}}{1-y_{A_o}}\left[\frac{\Omega}{1-\exp(\Omega)}-8\pi^2\sum_{n=1}^{\infty}\frac{n^2}{4n^2\pi^2+\Omega^2}\exp\left[-\left(n^2\pi^2+\frac{\Omega^2}{4}\right)\tau\right]\right]}$$
$$\tag{7.277}$$

Choosing the solid naphthalene as a system, the macroscopic mass balance is expressed as

$$-\left(\begin{array}{c}\text{Rate of}\\\text{mass }A\text{ out}\end{array}\right)=\left(\begin{array}{c}\text{Rate of accumulation}\\\text{of mass }A\end{array}\right) \tag{7.278}$$

or

$$-N_{A_z}\big|_{z=0}A=\frac{d\mathbb{N}_A}{dt}=\frac{\mathcal{D}_{AB}}{L^2}\frac{d\mathbb{N}_A}{d\tau}, \tag{7.279}$$

---

[8] The solution given by Ozguler et al., Eq. (15) in their paper, is in error.

where A is the cross-sectional area of the tube and $\mathbb{N}_A$ is the number of moles of naphthalene. Substitution of Eq. (7.277) into Eq. (7.279) and rearrangement give

$$
\int_{\mathbb{N}_{A_o}}^{\mathbb{N}_A} d\mathbb{N}_A = cAL\left(\frac{y_{A_o}}{1-y_{A_o}}\right)
$$

$$
\times \int_0^\tau \left\{ \frac{\Omega}{1-\exp(\Omega)} - 8\pi^2 \sum_{n=1}^\infty \frac{n^2}{4n^2\pi^2+\Omega^2} \exp\left[-\left(n^2\pi^2+\frac{\Omega^2}{4}\right)\tau\right]\right\} d\tau \quad (7.280)
$$

Therefore, the mass of naphthalene loss as a result of sublimation, i.e.,

$$
\text{Loss} = (\mathbb{N}_{A_o} - \mathbb{N}_A)M_A, \quad (7.281)
$$

where M_A is the molecular weight of naphthalene, is given by[9]

$$
\boxed{
\begin{aligned}
\text{Loss} = cAM_AL&\left(\frac{y_{A_o}}{1-y_{A_o}}\right)\left(\frac{\Omega\tau}{\exp(\Omega)-1}\right. \\
&\left. + 32\pi^2 \sum_{n=1}^\infty \left(\frac{n}{4n^2\pi^2+\Omega^2}\right)^2 \left\{1-\exp\left[-\left(n^2\pi^2+\frac{\Omega^2}{4}\right)\tau\right]\right\}\right)
\end{aligned}
}
\quad (7.282)
$$

7.7.1 LIMITING CASE WHEN $\Omega = 0$

When the molar-average velocity is negligible, the term Ω approaches zero. Application of L'Hôpital's rule, i.e., differentiation of the numerator and the denominator separately, to the first term on the right side of Eq. (7.275) yields

$$
\lim_{\Omega \to 0}\left[\frac{\exp(\Omega\xi)-\exp(\Omega)}{1-\exp(\Omega)}\right] = \lim_{\Omega \to 0}\left[\frac{\xi\exp(\Omega\xi)-\exp(\Omega)}{-\exp(\Omega)}\right] = 1-\xi \quad (7.283)
$$

Hence, Eq. (7.275) simplifies to

$$
\boxed{\theta = 1-\xi - \frac{2}{\pi}\sum_{n=1}^\infty \frac{1}{n}\exp\left(-n^2\pi^2\tau\right)\sin(n\pi\xi)} \quad (7.284)
$$

On the other hand, noting that

$$
\lim_{\Omega \to 0}\left[\frac{\Omega}{\exp(\Omega)-1}\right] = \lim_{\Omega \to 0}\left[\frac{1}{\exp(\Omega)}\right] = 1 \quad (7.285)
$$

Eq. (7.282) simplifies to

$$
\text{Loss} = cAM_AL\left(\frac{y_{A_o}}{1-y_{A_o}}\right)\left\{\tau + \frac{2}{\pi^2}\sum_{n=1}^\infty \frac{1}{n^2}\left[1-\exp\left(-n^2\pi^2\tau\right)\right]\right\} \quad (7.286)
$$

Making use of the identity

$$
\sum_{n=1}^\infty \frac{1}{n^2} = \frac{\pi^2}{6} \quad (7.287)
$$

---

[9] As a result of the flaw in concentration distribution, the equation given by Ozguler et al., Eq. (22) in their paper, is not correct.

Eq. (7.286) takes the final form of

$$\boxed{\text{Loss} = cAM_AL\left(\frac{y_{A_o}}{1-y_{A_o}}\right)\left[\tau + \frac{1}{3} - \frac{2}{\pi^2}\sum_{n=1}^{\infty}\frac{1}{n^2}\exp\left(-n^2\pi^2\tau\right)\right]} \tag{7.288}$$

7.8 DIFFUSION FROM INSTANTANEOUS SOURCES

Section 6.8 was about the diffusion of species released from instantaneous sources into a stagnant medium. Now, the same problem will be considered for a nonstationary medium.

7.8.1 DIFFUSION FROM A PLANE SOURCE

Fluid flows through an infinitely long rectangular duct in the x-direction. At $t = 0$, M_A amount of species A is injected uniformly across the y–z plane. The governing equation is

$$\frac{\partial c_A}{\partial t} + v_x\frac{\partial c_A}{\partial x} = \mathcal{D}_x\frac{\partial^2 c_A}{\partial x^2} \tag{7.289}$$

The initial and boundary conditions associated with Eq. (7.289) are

$$\text{at} \quad t = 0 \qquad c_A = \frac{M_A}{A}\delta(x) \tag{7.290}$$

$$\text{at} \quad x = \pm\infty \qquad c_A = 0 \tag{7.291}$$

The presence of the convection term obviously complicates the solution of the problem. If the velocity term remains more or less constant across the cross section of the duct, then it is possible to eliminate the convection term by the coordinate transformation in the form

$$\boxed{\bar{x} = x - v_x t} \tag{7.292}$$

Using the chain rule of differentiation,

$$\left(\frac{\partial c_A}{\partial t}\right)_x = \left(\frac{\partial c_A}{\partial t}\right)_{\bar{x}} + \left(\frac{\partial c_A}{\partial \bar{x}}\right)_t\left(\frac{\partial \bar{x}}{\partial t}\right)_x = \left(\frac{\partial c_A}{\partial t}\right)_{\bar{x}} - v_z\left(\frac{\partial c_A}{\partial \bar{x}}\right)_t \tag{7.293}$$

$$\left(\frac{\partial c_A}{\partial x}\right)_t = \left(\frac{\partial c_A}{\partial \bar{x}}\right)_t\left(\frac{\partial \bar{x}}{\partial x}\right)_t = \left(\frac{\partial c_A}{\partial \bar{x}}\right)_t \tag{7.294}$$

$$\left(\frac{\partial^2 c_A}{\partial x^2}\right)_t = \left(\frac{\partial^2 c_A}{\partial \bar{x}^2}\right)_t \tag{7.295}$$

Substitution of Eqs. (7.293)–(7.295) into Eq. (7.289) leads to

$$\left(\frac{\partial c_A}{\partial t}\right)_{\bar{x}} = \mathcal{D}_{AB}\left(\frac{\partial^2 c_A}{\partial \bar{x}^2}\right)_t \tag{7.296}$$

One can think of $(\partial c_A/\partial t)_{\bar{x}}$ as the time rate of change of c_A as reviewed by an observer moving at velocity v_x. Note that Eq. (7.296) is similar to Eq. (6.233). Thus, the solution is given by Eq. (6.238) as

$$c_A = \frac{M_A/A}{2\sqrt{\pi\mathcal{D}_x t}}\exp\left(-\frac{\bar{x}^2}{4\mathcal{D}_x t}\right) \tag{7.297}$$

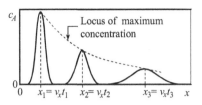

Figure 7.4 Evolution of concentration distribution.

Substitution of Eq. (7.292) into Eq. (7.297) gives the solution in the form

$$c_A = \frac{M_A/A}{2\sqrt{\pi \mathcal{D}_x t}} \exp\left[-\frac{(x - v_x t)^2}{4\mathcal{D}_x t}\right] \tag{7.298}$$

The standard deviation, i.e.,

$$\sigma = \sqrt{\pi \mathcal{D}_x t} \tag{7.299}$$

is again the measure of the width of the diffusing patch (or cloud) of species. The concentration reaches its maximum value at the center of mass, i.e., $x = v_x t$, and it is given by

$$c_{A_{\max}} = \frac{M_A/A}{2\sqrt{\pi \mathcal{D}_x t}} = \frac{M_A/A}{2\sqrt{\pi \mathcal{D}_x x / v_x}} \tag{7.300}$$

Figure 7.4 shows the evolution of concentration distribution and the locus of maximum concentration. Note that the maximum concentration is proportional to $x^{-1/2}$.

If the mass is released at $x = x_1$ instead of $x = 0$, the solution is shifted by the distance x_1 [10] and Eq. (7.298) becomes

$$c_A = \frac{M_A/A}{2\sqrt{\pi \mathcal{D}_x t}} \exp\left\{-\frac{\left[(x - x_1) - v_x t\right]^2}{4\mathcal{D}_x t}\right\} \tag{7.301}$$

7.8.2 DIFFUSION FROM A LINE SOURCE

The governing equation for two-dimensional unsteady-state diffusion from a line source into a non-stationary medium is

$$\frac{\partial c_A}{\partial t} + v_x \frac{\partial c_A}{\partial x} + v_y \frac{\partial c_A}{\partial y} = \mathcal{D}_x \frac{\partial^2 c_A}{\partial x^2} + \mathcal{D}_y \frac{\partial^2 c_A}{\partial y^2} \tag{7.302}$$

The coordinate transformations in the form

$$\bar{x} = x - v_x t \qquad \text{and} \qquad \bar{y} = y - v_y t \tag{7.303}$$

reduce Eq. (7.302) to

$$\frac{\partial c_A}{\partial t} = \mathcal{D}_x \frac{\partial^2 c_A}{\partial \bar{x}^2} + \mathcal{D}_y \frac{\partial^2 c_A}{\partial \bar{y}^2}, \tag{7.304}$$

which is identical with Eq. (6.245). Thus, the solution is given by Eq. (6.257) as

$$c_A = \frac{M_A/L}{4\pi t \sqrt{\mathcal{D}_x \mathcal{D}_y}} \exp\left(-\frac{\bar{x}^2}{4\mathcal{D}_x t} - \frac{\bar{y}^2}{4\mathcal{D}_y t}\right) \tag{7.305}$$

---

[10]See Problem 6.30.

Substitution of Eq. (7.303) into Eq. (7.305) gives the concentration distribution in the form

$$c_A = \frac{M_A/L}{4\pi t \sqrt{\mathcal{D}_x \mathcal{D}_y}} \exp\left[-\frac{(x - v_x t)^2}{4\mathcal{D}_x t} - \frac{(y - v_y t)^2}{4\mathcal{D}_y t}\right] \tag{7.306}$$

7.8.3 DIFFUSION FROM A POINT SOURCE

For three-dimensional diffusion, the procedure for obtaining the concentration distribution is similar to that for one- and two-dimensional cases and is left as an exercise for students. The result is

$$c_A = \frac{M_A}{8(\pi t)^{3/2}\sqrt{\mathcal{D}_x \mathcal{D}_y \mathcal{D}_z}} \exp\left[-\frac{(x - v_x t)^2}{4\mathcal{D}_x t} - \frac{(y - v_y t)^2}{4\mathcal{D}_y t} - \frac{(z - v_z t)^2}{4\mathcal{D}_z t}\right] \tag{7.307}$$

Example 7.1 Consider two-dimensional diffusion from a line source. The amount of mass released at $x = y = 0$ is $3\,\text{kg}$. The velocity field is given by

$$v_x = 1.5\,\text{cm/s} \quad\text{and}\quad v_y = 0,$$

and $\mathcal{D}_x = \mathcal{D}_y = 2.8\,\text{cm}^2/\text{s}$.

a) How long does it take for the maximum concentration to reach the probe located at $x = 200\,\text{cm}$ and $y = 0\,\text{cm}$?
b) What will be the width of the diffusion cloud when the maximum concentration reaches the probe?

Solution

a) Since $\mathcal{D}_x = \mathcal{D}_y = \mathcal{D}$ and $v_y = 0$, Eq. (7.306) becomes

$$c_A = \frac{M_A/L}{4\pi \mathcal{D} t} \exp\left[-\frac{(x - v_x t)^2}{4\mathcal{D} t} - \frac{y^2}{4\mathcal{D} t}\right]$$

The concentration will be maximum when

$$x - v_x t = 0 \quad\Rightarrow\quad t = \frac{x}{v_x} = \frac{200}{1.5} = 133.3\,\text{s}$$

b) The width, W, of the cloud in the x and y directions is the same and equals

$$W = 4\sigma = 4\sqrt{\pi \mathcal{D} t} = 4\sqrt{\pi(2.8)(133.3)} = 137\,\text{cm}$$

7.9 CONVECTION AND DIFFUSION IN A SEMI-INFINITE MEDIUM

Let us consider diffusion in an initially solute-free semi-infinite homogeneous medium with a continuous uniform input point source c_{A_o}. The governing equation and the initial and boundary conditions are

$$\frac{\partial c_A}{\partial t} + v_z \frac{\partial c_A}{\partial z} = \mathcal{D}_{eff} \frac{\partial^2 c_A}{\partial z^2} \tag{7.308}$$

$$\text{at} \quad t = 0 \qquad c_A = 0 \tag{7.309}$$

$$\text{at} \quad z = 0 \qquad c_A = c_{A_o} \tag{7.310}$$

$$\text{at} \quad z = \infty \qquad c_A = 0 \tag{7.311}$$

Ogata and Banks (1961) solved this problem to study dispersion phenomena in uniform flow through porous media. This equation is also useful in the analysis of dispersion and diffusion in environmental turbulent flows. In this case, the term $\mathcal{D}_{eff}$ is replaced by turbulent dispersivity.

Introduction of the new function $X(t,z)$ such that

$$c_A(t,z) = X(t,z) \exp\left(\frac{v_z z}{2\mathcal{D}_{eff}} - \frac{v_z^2 t}{4\mathcal{D}_{eff}}\right) \tag{7.312}$$

reduces Eq. (7.308) to

$$\frac{\partial X}{\partial t} = \mathcal{D}_{eff}\frac{\partial^2 X}{\partial z^2} \tag{7.313}$$

On the other hand, the initial and boundary conditions take the form

$$\text{at} \quad t = 0 \qquad X = 0 \tag{7.314}$$

$$\text{at} \quad z = 0 \qquad X = c_{A_o}\exp(\beta t) \tag{7.315}$$

$$\text{at} \quad z = \infty \qquad X = 0, \tag{7.316}$$

where

$$\beta = \frac{v_z^2}{4\mathcal{D}_{eff}} \tag{7.317}$$

Since the initial condition is zero and the boundary condition at $z = 0$ is time-dependent, Eq. (7.313) can be solved by the use of Duhamel's theorem as explained in Section E.3 in Appendix E.

The auxiliary problem is

$$\frac{\partial \varphi}{\partial t} = \mathcal{D}_{eff}\frac{\partial^2 \varphi}{\partial z^2} \tag{7.318}$$

$$\text{at} \quad t = 0 \qquad \varphi = 0 \tag{7.319}$$

$$\text{at} \quad z = 0 \qquad \varphi = 1 \tag{7.320}$$

$$\text{at} \quad z = \infty \qquad \varphi = 0 \tag{7.321}$$

The solution of the auxiliary problem can be obtained from Example E.10 in Appendix E as

$$\varphi = \frac{2}{\sqrt{\pi}}\int_{z/2\sqrt{\mathcal{D}_{eff}t}}^{\infty} e^{-\eta^2}\,d\eta \tag{7.322}$$

According to Eq. (E.69), the solution is given by

$$X = \frac{2c_{A_o}}{\sqrt{\pi}}\int_0^t e^{\beta u}\frac{\partial}{\partial t}\left[\int_{z/2\sqrt{\mathcal{D}_{eff}(t-u)}}^{\infty} e^{-\eta^2}\,d\eta\right]du \tag{7.323}$$

or

$$X = \frac{c_{A_o}z}{2\sqrt{\pi\mathcal{D}_{eff}}}\int_0^t e^{\beta u}e^{-z^2/4\mathcal{D}_{eff}(t-u)}\frac{1}{(t-u)^{3/2}}du \tag{7.324}$$

Making use of the substitution

$$\lambda = \frac{z}{2\sqrt{\mathcal{D}_{eff}(t-u)}} \tag{7.325}$$

Eq. (7.324) takes the form

$$X = \frac{2c_{A_o}}{\sqrt{\pi}} e^{\beta t} \int_{z/2\sqrt{\mathcal{D}_{eff}t}}^{\infty} \exp\left(-\frac{\beta z^2}{4\mathcal{D}_{eff}\lambda^2} - \lambda^2\right) d\lambda \tag{7.326}$$

Rearrangement of Eq. (7.326) gives

$$X = \frac{2c_{A_o}}{\sqrt{\pi}} \exp\left(\frac{v_z^2 t}{4\mathcal{D}_{eff}}\right) \left[\int_0^{\infty} \exp\left(-\frac{\Lambda^2}{\lambda^2} - \lambda^2\right) d\lambda - \int_0^{z/2\sqrt{\mathcal{D}_{eff}t}} \exp\left(-\frac{\Lambda^2}{\lambda^2} - \lambda^2\right) d\lambda\right], \tag{7.327}$$

where

$$\Lambda = \frac{v_z z}{4\mathcal{D}_{eff}} \tag{7.328}$$

The integrals in Eq. (7.327) are evaluated as

$$\int_0^{\infty} \exp\left(-\frac{\Lambda^2}{\lambda^2} - \lambda^2\right) d\lambda = \frac{\sqrt{\pi}}{2} e^{-2\Lambda} \tag{7.329}$$

$$\int_0^{z/2\sqrt{\mathcal{D}_{eff}t}} \exp\left(-\frac{\Lambda^2}{\lambda^2} - \lambda^2\right) d\lambda = \frac{1}{2}\left[e^{-2\Lambda} \int_{\Delta_1}^{\infty} e^{-u^2} du - e^{2\Lambda} \int_{\Delta_2}^{\infty} e^{-u^2} du\right], \tag{7.330}$$

where

$$\Delta_1 = \frac{v_z t - z}{2\sqrt{\mathcal{D}_{eff}t}} \quad \text{and} \quad \Delta_1 = \frac{v_z t + z}{2\sqrt{\mathcal{D}_{eff}t}} \tag{7.331}$$

Substitution of Eqs. (7.329) and (7.330) into Eq. (7.327) and expressing the integrals in terms of the error function lead to

$$X = \frac{c_{A_o}}{2} \exp\left(\frac{v_z^2 t}{4\mathcal{D}_{eff}}\right) \left[\exp\left(-\frac{v_z z}{2\mathcal{D}_{eff}}\right) \text{erfc}\left(\frac{z - v_z t}{2\sqrt{\mathcal{D}_{eff}t}}\right) + \exp\left(\frac{v_z z}{2\mathcal{D}_{eff}}\right) \text{erfc}\left(\frac{z + v_z t}{2\sqrt{\mathcal{D}_{eff}t}}\right)\right] \tag{7.332}$$

Substitution of Eq. (7.332) into Eq. (7.312) gives the final solution as

$$\boxed{\frac{c_A}{c_{A_o}} = \frac{1}{2}\left[\text{erfc}\left(\frac{z - v_z t}{2\sqrt{\mathcal{D}_{eff}t}}\right) + \exp\left(\frac{v_z z}{\mathcal{D}_{eff}}\right) \text{erfc}\left(\frac{z + v_z t}{2\sqrt{\mathcal{D}_{eff}t}}\right)\right]} \tag{7.333}$$

7.10 DEVELOPMENT OF TAYLOR–ARIS THEORY

Taylor (1953) studied the dispersion of a soluble salt when injected into a stream of solvent in laminar flow through a long capillary. Later, Aris (1956) generalized the development by removing some of the restrictions imposed by Taylor. In this section, the development of the so-called Taylor–Aris theory will be presented based on the averaging technique.

Consider a long capillary tube of radius R in which a solvent (species B) flows in laminar flow. When a pulse of solute (species A) is injected into the solvent, dispersion of the solute takes place by the combined action of the molecular diffusion and parabolic velocity distribution while the pulse travels through the capillary tube. Finally, the concentration distribution is represented by a bell-shaped curve as shown in Figure 7.5.

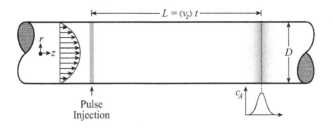

Figure 7.5   Dispersion of a pulse in a capillary tube.

The governing equation is expressed as

$$\frac{\partial c_A}{\partial t} + v_z \frac{\partial c_A}{\partial z} = \frac{\mathcal{D}_{AB}}{r} \frac{\partial}{\partial r}\left(r \frac{\partial c_A}{\partial r}\right) + \mathcal{D}_{AB} \frac{\partial^2 c_A}{\partial z^2}, \tag{7.334}$$

where the fully developed velocity distribution is given by

$$v_z = 2\langle v_z \rangle \left[1 - \left(\frac{r}{R}\right)^2\right] \tag{7.335}$$

The initial and boundary conditions associated with Eq. (7.334) are

$$\text{at}\quad t = 0 \qquad\qquad c_A = \frac{M_A}{\pi R^2}\,\delta(z) \tag{7.336}$$

$$\text{at}\quad r = 0 \ \& \ r = R \qquad \frac{\partial c_A}{\partial r} = 0 \tag{7.337}$$

$$\text{at}\quad z = \pm\infty \qquad\qquad c_A = 0 \tag{7.338}$$

For any quantity φ, the area-averaged form, $\langle\varphi\rangle$, is defined by

$$\langle\varphi\rangle = \frac{\displaystyle\int_0^{2\pi}\int_0^R \varphi\, r\,dr\,d\theta}{\displaystyle\int_0^{2\pi}\int_0^R r\,dr\,d\theta} = \frac{2}{R^2}\int_0^R \varphi\, r\,dr \tag{7.339}$$

Integration of Eq. (7.334) over the cross-sectional area of the capillary tube gives

$$\int_0^{2\pi}\int_0^R \frac{\partial c_A}{\partial t} r\,dr\,d\theta + \int_0^{2\pi}\int_0^R v_z \frac{\partial c_A}{\partial z} r\,dr\,d\theta =$$
$$\mathcal{D}_{AB}\int_0^{2\pi}\int_0^R \frac{1}{r}\frac{\partial}{\partial r}\left(r \frac{\partial c_A}{\partial r}\right) r\,dr\,d\theta + \mathcal{D}_{AB}\int_0^{2\pi}\int_0^R \frac{\partial^2 c_A}{\partial z^2} r\,dr\,d\theta \tag{7.340}$$

Simplification of Eq. (7.340) gives

$$\frac{\partial}{\partial t}\int_0^R c_A\, r\,dr + \frac{\partial}{\partial z}\int_0^R v_z c_A\, r\,dr = \mathcal{D}_{AB}\left(r \frac{\partial c_A}{\partial r}\right)\Bigg|_{r=0}^{r=R} + \frac{\partial^2}{\partial z^2}\int_0^R c_A\, r\,dr \tag{7.341}$$

The use of Eq. (7.339) in Eq. (7.341) leads to

$$\frac{\partial\langle c_A \rangle}{\partial t} + \frac{\partial\langle v_z c_A \rangle}{\partial z} = \mathcal{D}_{AB}\frac{\partial^2\langle c_A \rangle}{\partial z^2} \tag{7.342}$$

In order to express the average of a product in terms of the product of averages, spatial deviations are defined by

$$v_z = \langle v_z \rangle + \widetilde{v}_z \tag{7.343}$$

$$c_A = \langle c_A \rangle + \widetilde{c}_A \tag{7.344}$$

with the constraint that

$$\langle \widetilde{v}_z \rangle = \langle \widetilde{c}_A \rangle = 0 \qquad \text{and} \qquad \langle \langle v_z \rangle \rangle = \langle v_z \rangle \, \& \, \langle \langle c_A \rangle \rangle = \langle c_A \rangle \tag{7.345}$$

The term $\langle v_z c_A \rangle$ is expressed in the form

$$\langle v_z c_A \rangle = \langle (\langle v_z \rangle + \widetilde{v}_z)(\langle c_A \rangle + \widetilde{c}_A) \rangle = \langle \langle v_z \rangle \langle c_A \rangle + \langle v_z \rangle \widetilde{c}_A + \widetilde{v}_z \langle c_A \rangle + \widetilde{v}_z \widetilde{c}_A \rangle$$

$$= \langle v_z \rangle \langle c_A \rangle + \langle v_z \rangle \underbrace{\langle \widetilde{c}_A \rangle}_{0} + \underbrace{\langle \widetilde{v}_z \rangle}_{0} \langle c_A \rangle + \langle \widetilde{v}_z \widetilde{c}_A \rangle \tag{7.346}$$

Substitution of Eq. (7.346) into Eq. (7.342) gives

$$\frac{\partial \langle c_A \rangle}{\partial t} + \langle v_z \rangle \frac{\partial \langle c_A \rangle}{\partial z} = \mathcal{D}_{AB} \frac{\partial^2 \langle c_A \rangle}{\partial z^2} - \frac{\partial \langle \widetilde{v}_z \widetilde{c}_A \rangle}{\partial z} \tag{7.347}$$

The second term on the right side of Eq. (7.347) represents the dispersive transport. To proceed further, $\widetilde{v}_z$ and $\widetilde{c}_A$ must be expressed in terms of the area-averaged variables.

Substitution of Eq. (7.335) into Eq. (7.343) yields the deviation field for the velocity as

$$\widetilde{v}_z = \langle v_z \rangle \left[1 - 2 \left(\frac{r}{R} \right)^2 \right] \tag{7.348}$$

To obtain the governing equation for $\widetilde{c}_A$, first substitute Eqs. (7.343) and (7.344) into Eq. (7.334) to obtain

$$\frac{\partial \langle c_A \rangle}{\partial t} + \frac{\partial \widetilde{c}_A}{\partial t} + v_z \frac{\partial \langle c_A \rangle}{\partial z} + v_z \frac{\partial \widetilde{c}_A}{\partial z} = \mathcal{D}_{AB} \frac{1}{r} \frac{\partial}{\partial r} \left(r \frac{\partial \widetilde{c}_A}{\partial r} \right) + \mathcal{D}_{AB} \frac{\partial^2 \langle c_A \rangle}{\partial z^2} + \mathcal{D}_{AB} \frac{\partial^2 \widetilde{c}_A}{\partial z^2} \tag{7.349}$$

Subtraction of Eq. (7.334) from Eq. (7.348) yields the governing equation for the spatial deviation of concentration. The result is

$$\frac{\partial \widetilde{c}_A}{\partial t} + v_z \frac{\partial \widetilde{c}_A}{\partial z} + \widetilde{v}_z \frac{\partial \langle c_A \rangle}{\partial z} = \mathcal{D}_{AB} \left[\frac{1}{r} \frac{\partial}{\partial r} \left(r \frac{\partial \widetilde{c}_A}{\partial r} \right) + \frac{\partial^2 \widetilde{c}_A}{\partial z^2} \right] + \frac{\partial \langle \widetilde{v}_z \widetilde{c}_A \rangle}{\partial z} \tag{7.350}$$

The boundary conditions for $\widetilde{c}_A$ are

$$\text{at} \quad t = 0 \qquad \widetilde{c}_A = 0 \tag{7.351}$$

$$\text{at} \quad r = 0 \ \& \ r = R \qquad \frac{\partial \widetilde{c}_A}{\partial r} = 0 \tag{7.352}$$

$$\text{at} \quad z = \pm\infty \qquad \widetilde{c}_A = 0 \tag{7.353}$$

Comparison of Eq. (7.350) with Eq. (7.334) indicates that the governing equation for $\widetilde{c}_A$ is much more complicated than the equation for c_A. Since an approximate expression for $\widetilde{c}_A$ is required, Eq. (7.350) needs to be simplified. Examination of Eq. (7.350) indicates that the only source term is $\widetilde{v}_z \partial \langle c_A \rangle / \partial z$. Thus, we expect that $\widetilde{c}_A$ depends strongly on $\widetilde{v}_z$ and the gradient of the average concentration, $\partial \langle c_A \rangle / \partial z$.

Diffusion in the axial direction can be neglected relative to convective transport when

$$O \left(v_z \frac{\partial \widetilde{c}_A}{\partial z} \right) \gg O \left(\mathcal{D}_{AB} \frac{\partial^2 \widetilde{c}_A}{\partial z^2} \right) \tag{7.354}$$

or

$$\frac{\langle v_z \rangle L}{\mathcal{D}_{AB}} = \text{Pe}_M \frac{L}{D} \gg 1 \tag{3.355}$$

Thus, Eq. (7.350) simplifies to

$$\frac{\partial \tilde{c}_A}{\partial t} + v_z \frac{\partial \tilde{c}_A}{\partial z} + \tilde{v}_z \frac{\partial \langle c_A \rangle}{\partial z} = \mathcal{D}_{AB} \frac{1}{r} \frac{\partial}{\partial r} \left(r \frac{\partial \tilde{c}_A}{\partial r} \right) + \frac{\partial \langle \tilde{v}_z \tilde{c}_A \rangle}{\partial z} \tag{7.356}$$

The coordinate transformation in the form

$$\bar{z} = z - \langle v_z \rangle t \tag{7.357}$$

reduces Eq. (7.356) to

$$\left(\frac{\partial \tilde{c}_A}{\partial t} \right)_{\bar{z}} + \tilde{v}_z \frac{\partial \tilde{c}_A}{\partial z} + \tilde{v}_z \frac{\partial \langle c_A \rangle}{\partial z} = \mathcal{D}_{AB} \frac{1}{r} \frac{\partial}{\partial r} \left(r \frac{\partial \tilde{c}_A}{\partial r} \right) + \frac{\partial \langle \tilde{v}_z \tilde{c}_A \rangle}{\partial z} \tag{7.358}$$

One can claim that

$$O\left[\mathcal{D}_{AB} \frac{1}{r} \frac{\partial}{\partial r} \left(r \frac{\partial \tilde{c}_A}{\partial r} \right) \right] \gg O\left[\left(\frac{\partial \tilde{c}_A}{\partial t} \right)_{\bar{z}} \right] \tag{7.359}$$

if the following constraint is satisfied,

$$\frac{\mathcal{D}_{AB} t}{R^2} \gg 1 \tag{7.360}$$

It is also plausible to assume that

$$\frac{\partial \langle c_A \rangle}{\partial z} \gg \frac{\partial \tilde{c}_A}{\partial z} \tag{7.361}$$

With these simplifications, Eq. (7.358) takes the form

$$\tilde{v}_z \frac{\partial \langle c_A \rangle}{\partial z} = \mathcal{D}_{AB} \frac{1}{r} \frac{\partial}{\partial r} \left(r \frac{\partial \tilde{c}_A}{\partial r} \right) \tag{7.362}$$

or

$$\langle v_z \rangle \left[1 - 2 \left(\frac{r}{R} \right)^2 \right] \frac{\partial \langle c_A \rangle}{\partial z} = \mathcal{D}_{AB} \frac{1}{r} \frac{\partial}{\partial r} \left(r \frac{\partial \tilde{c}_A}{\partial r} \right) \tag{7.363}$$

Integration of Eq. (7.363) with respect to r twice gives $\tilde{c}_A$:

$$\tilde{c}_A = \frac{\langle v_z \rangle R^2}{4 \mathcal{D}_{AB}} \left[\left(\frac{r}{R} \right)^2 - \frac{1}{2} \left(\frac{r}{R} \right)^4 - \frac{1}{3} \right] \frac{\partial \langle c_A \rangle}{\partial z} \tag{7.364}$$

Once $\tilde{v}_z$ and $\tilde{c}_A$ are expressed in terms of the averaged quantities, the dispersive term becomes

$$\begin{aligned}
\frac{\partial \langle \tilde{v}_z \tilde{c}_A \rangle}{\partial z} &= \langle \tilde{v}_z \frac{\partial \tilde{c}_A}{\partial z} \rangle \\
&= \frac{2}{R^2} \int_0^R \langle v_z \rangle \left[1 - 2 \left(\frac{r}{R} \right)^2 \right] \frac{\langle v_z \rangle R^2}{4 \mathcal{D}_{AB}} \left[\left(\frac{r}{R} \right)^2 - \frac{1}{2} \left(\frac{r}{R} \right)^4 - \frac{1}{3} \right] \frac{\partial^2 \langle c_A \rangle}{\partial z^2} r \, dr
\end{aligned} \tag{7.365}$$

Carrying out the integration gives

$$\frac{\partial \langle \tilde{v}_z \tilde{c}_A \rangle}{\partial z} = -\frac{\langle v_z \rangle^2 R^2}{48 \mathcal{D}_{AB}} \frac{\partial^2 \langle c_A \rangle}{\partial z^2} \tag{7.366}$$

Substitution of Eq. (7.366) into Eq. (7.347) gives the final form of the equation as

$$\boxed{\frac{\partial \langle c_A \rangle}{\partial t} + \langle v_z \rangle \frac{\partial \langle c_A \rangle}{\partial z} = K \frac{\partial^2 \langle c_A \rangle}{\partial z^2},} \tag{7.367}$$

where K is the *dispersion coefficient*, defined by

$$K = \mathcal{D}_{AB} + \frac{\langle v_z \rangle^2 R^2}{48 \mathcal{D}_{AB}} \simeq \frac{\langle v_z \rangle^2 R^2}{48 \mathcal{D}_{AB}} \tag{7.368}$$

With the help of Eq. (7.298), the concentration distribution is expressed as

$$c_A = \frac{M_A / \pi R^2}{2 \sqrt{\pi K t}} \exp\left[-\frac{(z - \langle v_z \rangle t)^2}{4Kt} \right] \tag{7.369}$$

with the variance

$$\sigma^2 = 2Kt \tag{7.370}$$

The variance given in Eq. (7.370) is in the length unit. The mean residence time, t_R, and the variance, σ_t^2, with respect to time are defined by (van der Laan, 1958)

$$t_R = \frac{L}{\langle v_z \rangle} \left(1 + \frac{\sigma^2}{\langle v_z \rangle L t} \right) \tag{7.371}$$

$$\sigma_t^2 = \left(\frac{L}{\langle v_z \rangle} \right)^2 \left[\frac{\sigma^2}{\langle v_z \rangle L t} + 2 \left(\frac{\sigma^2}{\langle v_z \rangle L t} \right)^2 \right] \tag{7.372}$$

The deviation of the concentration distribution from a Gaussian curve becomes negligible when the following constraint is satisfied (Baldauf and Knapp, 1983):

$$0.1 \left(\frac{L}{R} \right)^2 > \text{Pe}_M \tag{7.373}$$

Under these circumstances, Eqs. (7.371) and (7.372) simplify to

$$t_R = \frac{L}{\langle v_z \rangle} \tag{7.374}$$

$$\sigma_t^2 = \frac{\sigma^2 t_R^2}{L^2} = \frac{2Kt_R}{\langle v_z \rangle^2} \tag{7.375}$$

Substitution of Eq. (7.368) into Eq. (7.375) leads to

$$\mathcal{D}_{AB} = \frac{t_R R^2}{24 \sigma_t^2} \tag{7.376}$$

For a Gaussian distribution, Baldauf and Knapp (1983) showed that

$$\sigma_t^2 = \frac{W_{1/2}^2}{8 \ln 2}, \tag{7.377}$$

where $W_{1/2}$ is the width of the peak at half height. The use of Eq. (7.377) in Eq. (7.376) gives

$$\boxed{\mathcal{D}_{AB} = \frac{\ln 2}{3} \frac{t_R R^2}{W_{1/2}^2}} \tag{7.378}$$

Later, Callendar and Leist (2006) generalized Eq. (7.378) as

$$(\mathcal{D}_{AB})_h = -\frac{\ln h}{3} \frac{t_R R^2}{W_h^2}, \tag{7.379}$$

where W_h is the peak width at arbitrary fractional peak height h.

PROBLEMS

7.1 Consider the flow of a fluid with constant physical properties. Show that the mass transfer coefficient is constant when the concentration profile is fully developed.

7.2 When the concentration profile is fully developed, show that the concentration gradient in the axial direction, $\partial c_A / \partial z$, remains constant for a constant wall mass flux.

7.3 Prove Eq. (7.43).

7.4 Consider two large parallel plates separated by a distance B as shown in the figure below. There is no pressure gradient in the system, and the plate at $x = 0$ is stationary. Fluid flow is due to the movement of the plate at $x = B$ in the positive z-direction with a constant velocity V. The system is isothermal, and it is continuously fed at $z = 0$ with a dilute solution of chemical species A with a uniform concentration c_{A_0}. While species A undergoes a first-order irreversible chemical reaction at the upper plate, the lower plate is impermeable to the mass transfer. The fluid mixture has constant physical properties and behaves as a Newtonian fluid. This problem is analyzed by Chen et al. (1996).

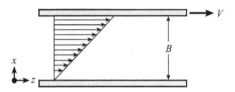

The fully developed velocity profile is given by

$$\frac{v_z}{V} = \frac{x}{B} \tag{1}$$

a) In terms of the dimensionless quantities,

$$\theta = \frac{c_A}{c_{A_o}} \qquad \xi = \frac{x}{B} \qquad \eta = \frac{\mathcal{D}_{AB}\, z}{V B^2} \qquad \Lambda = \frac{k_1'' B}{\mathcal{D}_{AB}} \tag{2}$$

show that the conservation of chemical species under steady conditions is expressed as

$$\xi \frac{\partial \theta}{\partial \eta} = \frac{\partial^2 \theta}{\partial \xi^2} \tag{3}$$

subject to the following dimensionless boundary conditions:

$$\text{at} \quad \eta = 0 \qquad \theta = 1 \tag{4}$$

$$\text{at} \quad \xi = 0 \qquad \frac{\partial \theta}{\partial \xi} = 0 \tag{5}$$

$$\text{at} \quad \xi = 1 \qquad -\frac{\partial \theta}{\partial \xi} = \Lambda \theta \tag{6}$$

b) Using the method of separation of variables, propose a solution in the form

$$\theta(\eta, \xi) = F(\xi) G(\eta) \tag{7}$$

and show that Eq. (3) yields the following ODEs:

$$\frac{dF}{d\eta} + \lambda F = 0 \tag{8}$$

$$\frac{d^2 G}{d\xi^2} + \lambda \xi G = 0, \tag{9}$$

where λ is a separation constant.

c) Show that the transformation

$$Z = -\lambda^{1/3}\xi \tag{10}$$

converts Eq. (9) to the form

$$\frac{d^2G}{dZ^2} - ZG = 0, \tag{11}$$

which is known as the *Airy equation*.

d) Show that the solution is given by

$$\theta = \sum_{n=1}^{\infty} C_n e^{-\lambda_n \eta} \left[\sqrt{3}\,\text{Ai}\left(-\lambda_n^{1/3}\xi\right) + \text{Bi}\left(-\lambda_n^{1/3}\xi\right) \right], \tag{12}$$

where Ai and Bi are the Airy functions of the first and second kinds, respectively, and the eigenvalues λ_n are the roots of the following transcendental equation:

$$\sqrt{3}\left[\text{Ai}'\left(-\lambda_n^{1/3}\right) - \Lambda\lambda_n^{1/3}\,\text{Ai}\left(-\lambda_n^{1/3}\right)\right] + \text{Bi}'\left(-\lambda_n^{1/3}\right) - \Lambda\lambda_n^{1/3}\,\text{Bi}\left(-\lambda_n^{1/3}\right) = 0 \tag{13}$$

The prime on the Airy functions represents differentiation.

e) Show that the coefficients C_n are given by

$$C_n = \frac{3\left[\sqrt{3}\,\text{Ai}'\left(-\lambda_n^{1/3}\right) + \text{Bi}'\left(-\lambda_n^{1/3}\right)\right]}{X + Y + Z}, \tag{14}$$

where

$$X = 3\left[\lambda_n^{2/3}\,\text{Ai}\left(-\lambda_n^{1/3}\right)^2 + \lambda_n^{1/3}\,\text{Ai}'\left(-\lambda_n^{1/3}\right)^2\right] + \lambda_n^{2/3}\,\text{Bi}\left(-\lambda_n^{1/3}\right)^2$$
$$+ \text{Bi}\left(-\lambda_n^{1/3}\right)\text{Bi}'\left(-\lambda_n^{1/3}\right) + \lambda_n^{1/3}\,\text{Bi}'\left(-\lambda_n^{1/3}\right)^2 \tag{15}$$

$$Y = \sqrt{3}\,\text{Ai}'\left(-\lambda_n^{1/3}\right)\left[\text{Bi}\left(-\lambda_n^{1/3}\right) + 2\lambda_n^{1/3}\,\text{Bi}'\left(-\lambda_n^{1/3}\right)\right] \tag{16}$$

$$Z = \text{Ai}\left(-\lambda_n^{1/3}\right)\left\{3\,\text{Ai}'\left(-\lambda_n^{1/3}\right) + \sqrt{3}\left[2\lambda_n^{2/3}\,\text{Bi}\left(-\lambda_n^{1/3}\right) + \text{Bi}'\left(-\lambda_n^{1/3}\right)\right]\right\} \tag{17}$$

f) Show that the dimensionless bulk concentration is defined by

$$\theta_b = \frac{c_{A_b}}{c_{A_o}} = 2\int_0^1 \theta\xi\,d\xi \tag{18}$$

g) Show that the substitution of Eq. (12) into Eq. (18) and integration lead to

$$\theta_b = 2\sum_{n=1}^{\infty} \frac{C_n}{\lambda_n^{2/3}}\, e^{-\lambda_n \eta}\left[\sqrt{3}\,\text{Ai}'\left(-\lambda_n^{1/3}\right) + \text{Bi}'\left(-\lambda_n^{1/3}\right)\right] \tag{19}$$

7.5 Consider the steady-state diffusion into a semi-infinite medium near a wall with a linear velocity profile as shown in the figure below. The surface of the wall is coated with species A for $z \geq 0$.

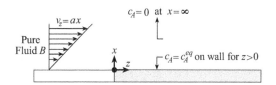

a) Postulate a solution in the form

$$\frac{c_A}{c_A^{eq}} = f(\eta),$$

where

$$\eta = x \sqrt[3]{\frac{a}{9\mathcal{D}_{AB}z}}$$

and show that the solution is given by

$$\frac{c_A}{c_A^{eq}} = 1 - \frac{\int_0^{\eta} e^{-u^3} du}{\int_0^{\infty} e^{-u^3} du} = \frac{1}{\Gamma(4/3)} \int_{\eta}^{\infty} e^{-u^3} du,$$

where $\Gamma(4/3)$ is the gamma function.

b) Show that the molar flux at the wall surface is given by

$$N_{A_x}\big|_{x=0} = \frac{c_A^{eq} \mathcal{D}_{AB}}{\Gamma(4/3)} \sqrt[3]{\frac{a}{9z}}$$

7.6 Consider the problem analyzed in Section 7.4. Using the dimensionless quantities defined by

$$\theta = \frac{c_A}{c_{A_o}} \qquad \xi = \frac{r}{R} \qquad \eta = \frac{\langle v_z \rangle z}{\mathcal{D}_{AB}} \qquad \mathrm{Pe_M} = \frac{\langle v_z \rangle R}{\mathcal{D}_{AB}} \qquad \Lambda = \frac{k_1'' R}{\mathcal{D}_{AB}}$$

and assuming plug flow, i.e.,

$$v_z = \langle v_z \rangle = \text{constant},$$

show that the concentration distribution is given by

$$\theta = 2 \sum_{n=1}^{\infty} \frac{\Lambda}{(\Lambda^2 + \lambda_n^2) J_0(\lambda_n)} \exp\left[-\left(\frac{\lambda_n}{\mathrm{Pe_M}}\right)^2 \eta\right] J_0(\lambda_n \xi),$$

where the eigenvalues are the roots of the following transcendental equation:

$$\lambda_n J_1(\lambda_n) = \Lambda J_0(\lambda_n) \qquad n = 1, 2, 3, \ldots$$

7.7 The solution of Eq. (7.152) subject to the boundary conditions given by Eqs. (7.154)–(7.156) was first obtained by Johnstone and Pigford (1942). Their series solution expresses the bulk concentration of species A at $z = L$ as

$$\frac{c_A^{eq} - (c_{A_b})_L}{c_A^{eq} - c_{A_o}} = 0.7857 \exp(-5.1213\eta) + 0.1001 \exp(-39.318\eta) + 0.03599 \exp(-105.64\eta) + \cdots,$$
$$(1)$$

where

$$\eta = \frac{\mathcal{D}_{AB}L}{\delta^2 v_{\max}} = \frac{2\mathcal{D}_{AB}L}{3\delta^2 \langle v_z \rangle} \tag{2}$$

a) Show that

$$\langle k_c \rangle = \frac{\dot{Q}}{WL} \ln\left[\frac{c_A^{eq} - c_{A_o}}{c_A^{eq} - (c_{A_b})_L}\right], \tag{3}$$

where the average mass transfer coefficient, $\langle k_c \rangle$, is defined by

$$\langle k_c \rangle = \frac{1}{L} \int_0^L k_c \, dz \tag{4}$$

and $\dot{Q}$ is the volumetric flow rate given by

$$\dot{Q} = \langle v_z \rangle W \delta \tag{5}$$

b) When $\eta > 0.1$, all the terms in Eq. (1), excluding the first, become almost zero. Substitute Eq. (1) into Eq. (3) to obtain

$$\langle k_c \rangle = \frac{\dot{Q}}{WL} (5.1213\eta + 0.241) \tag{6}$$

c) For large values of η, show that $Sh = 3.41$, which is identical with Eq. (7.182).

7.8 Consider the problem analyzed in Section 7.7.

a) Show that the introduction of the transformation in the form

$$\theta(\tau, \xi) = X(\tau, \xi) \exp\left(\frac{\Omega \xi}{2} - \frac{\Omega^2 \tau}{4}\right) \tag{1}$$

reduces Eqs. (7.242)–(7.245) to

$$\frac{\partial X}{\partial \tau} = \frac{\partial^2 X}{\partial \xi^2} \tag{2}$$

$$\text{at} \quad \tau = 0 \quad X = 0 \tag{3}$$

$$\text{at} \quad \xi = 0 \quad X = \exp\left(\frac{\Omega^2 \tau}{4}\right) \tag{4}$$

$$\text{at} \quad \xi = 1 \quad X = 0 \tag{5}$$

b) Using the method of Laplace transformation, show that the solution in the Laplace domain is given by

$$\overline{X} = \frac{\sinh\left[\sqrt{s}(1 - \xi)\right]}{\left(s - \dfrac{\Omega^2}{4}\right)\sinh \sqrt{s}}, \tag{6}$$

where

$$\overline{X} = \int_0^\infty e^{-s\tau} X \, d\tau \tag{7}$$

c) Take the inverse Laplace transformation of Eq. (6) by using the convolution integral to obtain Eq. (7.275).

Hint: Note that

$$1 - \xi = \frac{2}{\pi} \sum_{n=1}^{\infty} \frac{\sin(n\pi\xi)}{n} \tag{8}$$

7.9 For the Lévêque problem explained in Section 7.2.2, consider the case where the molar flux at the tube wall is constant, i.e.,

$$N_{A_s}\big|_{s=0} = -\mathcal{D}_{AB} \frac{\partial c_A}{\partial s}\bigg|_{s=0} = N_w = \text{constant} \tag{1}$$

a) Differentiate Eq. (7.60) with respect to s to obtain

$$\frac{4\langle v_z \rangle}{R\mathcal{D}_{AB}} \frac{\partial N_{A_s}}{\partial z} = \frac{\partial}{\partial s}\left(\frac{1}{s} \frac{\partial N_{A_s}}{\partial s}\right) \tag{2}$$

b) Using the dimensionless quantities,

$$\theta = \frac{N_{A_s}}{N_w} \qquad \eta = \frac{\mathcal{D}_{AB}\,z}{4R^2\langle v_z\rangle} \qquad \xi = \frac{s}{R} \tag{3}$$

express Eq. (2) and its associate boundary conditions in dimensionless form.

c) If the solution is sought in the form,

$$\theta = \theta(\chi), \qquad \text{where} \qquad \chi = \frac{\xi}{\sqrt[3]{9\eta}}, \tag{4}$$

obtain the solution as

$$\theta = \frac{3}{\Gamma(2/3)}\int_\chi^\infty u\,e^{-u^3}\,du \tag{5}$$

d) Note that

$$N_{A_s} = \theta\,N_w = -\mathcal{D}_{AB}\frac{\partial c_A}{\partial s} \tag{6}$$

Substitute Eq. (5) into Eq. (6) to obtain

$$c_A = \frac{3N_w R}{\mathcal{D}_{AB}\,\Gamma(2/3)}\int_\chi^\infty\left(\int_\varphi^\infty u\,e^{-u^3}\,du\right)d\varphi \tag{7}$$

e) Integrate the double integral in Eq. (7) by parts, and show that the concentration distribution is given by

$$c_A = \frac{3N_w R}{\mathcal{D}_{AB}\Gamma(2/3)}\left(\frac{e^{-\chi^3}}{3} - \chi\int_\chi^\infty u\,e^{-u^3}\,du\right) \tag{8}$$

Express the integral in Eq. (8) in terms of the incomplete gamma function as

$$\int_\chi^\infty u\,e^{-u^3}\,du = \frac{1}{3}\Gamma(2/3,\chi^3) \tag{9}$$

so that the solution becomes

$$c_A = \frac{N_w R}{\mathcal{D}_{AB}\,\Gamma(2/3)}\left[e^{-\chi^3} - \chi\Gamma(2/3,\chi^3)\right] \tag{10}$$

7.10 Two large parallel plates are separated by a distance H as shown in the figure below. Inner surfaces of both plates are coated with species A in order to maintain constant mass fractions of ω_{A_o} and ω_{A_H} at $x=0$ and $x=H$, respectively. Air (species B) is blown in the x-direction with a velocity of V. Assume that the total density is constant.

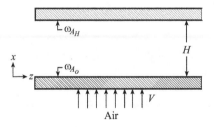

a) Show that the governing differential equation is given by

$$\frac{d^2\theta}{d\xi^2} - \beta\frac{d\theta}{d\xi} = 0,$$

where the dimensionless quantities are defined by

$$\theta = \frac{\omega_A - \omega_{A_o}}{\omega_{A_H} - \omega_{A_o}} \qquad \xi = \frac{x}{H} \qquad \beta = \frac{VH}{\mathcal{D}_{AB}}$$

b) Show that the solution is given by

$$\theta = \frac{1 - \exp(\beta\xi)}{1 - \exp\beta}$$

c) Show that the total mass flux at the lower plate is given by

$$n_{A_x}\big|_{x=0} = \rho V \left[\omega_{A_o} + \frac{\omega_{A_H} - \omega_{A_o}}{1 - \exp(VH/\mathcal{D}_{AB})} \right]$$

7.11 Repeat the analysis given in Example 4.11 if the medium moves at a constant velocity v_z.

a) Show that the solution of the governing equation

$$v_z \frac{dc_A}{dz} = \mathcal{D}_{AB} \frac{d^2 c_A}{dz^2} - k_1''' c_A$$

is given by

$$c_A^R = C_1 \exp\left[\frac{1}{2} \frac{v_z z}{\mathcal{D}_{AB}} \left(1 - \sqrt{1 + \frac{4k_1''' \mathcal{D}_{AB}}{v_z^2}} \right) \right] \qquad 0 < z < \infty$$

$$c_A^L = C_2 \exp\left[\frac{1}{2} \frac{v_z z}{\mathcal{D}_{AB}} \left(1 + \sqrt{1 + \frac{4k_1''' \mathcal{D}_{AB}}{v_z^2}} \right) \right] \qquad -\infty < z < 0,$$

where C_1 and C_2 are constants.

b) Using the equality of concentrations at the location of the source, show that $C_1 = C_2$.

c) Using the material balance in the form

$$\left(-\mathcal{D}_{AB} \frac{d^2 c_A^L}{dz^2} + v_z c_A^L \right)\bigg|_{z=0} + Q = \left(-\mathcal{D}_{AB} \frac{d^2 c_A^R}{dz^2} + v_z c_A^R \right)\bigg|_{z=0}$$

show that the concentration distribution is given as

$$c_A = \begin{cases} \dfrac{Q}{\sqrt{v_z^2 + 4k_1''' \mathcal{D}_{AB}}} \exp\left[\dfrac{1}{2} \dfrac{v_z z}{\mathcal{D}_{AB}} \left(1 - \sqrt{1 + \dfrac{4k_1''' \mathcal{D}_{AB}}{v_z^2}} \right) \right] & 0 < z < \infty \\[4mm] \dfrac{Q}{\sqrt{v_z^2 + 4k_1''' \mathcal{D}_{AB}}} C_2 \exp\left[\dfrac{1}{2} \dfrac{v_z z}{\mathcal{D}_{AB}} \left(1 + \sqrt{1 + \dfrac{4k_1''' \mathcal{D}_{AB}}{v_z^2}} \right) \right] & -\infty < z < 0 \end{cases}$$

7.12 To study the role of oxygen in modulating cellular functions, Allen and Bhatia (2003) modeled convective and diffusion transport of oxygen in the flat-plate bioreactor shown below. The inlet liquid has a constant oxygen concentration of $c_{A_{in}}$. While the top of the bioreactor is impermeable to oxygen, the cell monolayer placed at the bottom of the bioreactor consumes oxygen at a constant rate.

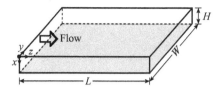

a) Assuming steady-state transport in a uniform flow field in the z-direction, show that the governing equation and the boundary conditions are written as

$$\langle v_z \rangle \frac{\partial c_A}{\partial z} = \mathcal{D}_{AB} \frac{\partial^2 c_A}{\partial x^2} \tag{1}$$

$$\text{at} \quad z = 0 \qquad c_A = c_{A_{in}} \tag{2}$$

$$\text{at} \quad x = 0 \qquad \frac{\partial c_A}{\partial x} = 0 \tag{3}$$

$$\text{at} \quad x = H \qquad -\mathcal{D}_{AB} \frac{\partial c_A}{\partial x} = N_{A_H} = \text{const.} \tag{4}$$

b) In terms of the dimensionless quantities

$$\theta = \frac{c_A}{c_{A_{in}}} \qquad \eta = \frac{z}{L} \qquad \xi = \frac{x}{H} \qquad \Lambda = \frac{\mathcal{D}_{AB} L}{\langle v_z \rangle H^2} \qquad \beta = \frac{N_{A_H} H}{\mathcal{D}_{AB} c_{A_{in}}} \tag{5}$$

show that Eqs. (1)–(4) take the form

$$\frac{\partial \theta}{\partial \eta} = \Lambda \frac{\partial^2 \theta}{\partial \xi^2} \tag{6}$$

$$\text{at} \quad \eta = 0 \qquad \theta = 1 \tag{7}$$

$$\text{at} \quad \xi = 0 \qquad \frac{\partial \theta}{\partial \xi} = 0 \tag{8}$$

$$\text{at} \quad \xi = 1 \qquad \frac{\partial \theta}{\partial \xi} = -\beta \tag{9}$$

c) To make the boundary condition at $\xi = 1$ homogeneous, use the transformation of the dependent variable in the form

$$\theta(\xi, \eta) = X(\xi, \eta) - \beta \left(\frac{\xi^2}{2} + \Lambda \eta \right) \tag{10}$$

and obtain the concentration distribution as

$$\theta = 1 + \beta \left[\frac{1}{6} - \frac{\xi^2}{2} - \Lambda \eta + \frac{2}{\pi^2} \sum_{n=1}^{\infty} \frac{(-1)^n}{n^2} \exp\left(-n^2 \pi^2 \Lambda \eta\right) \cos(n \pi \xi) \right] \tag{11}$$

REFERENCES

Abramowitz, M. and I. A. Stegun. 1972. *Handbook of Mathematical Functions with Formulas, Graphs, and Mathematical Tables*. New York: Dover Publications, Inc.

Allen, J. W. and S. N. Bhatia. 2003. Formation of steady-state oxygen gradients in vitro – Application to liver zonation. *Biotechnol. Bioeng.* 82:253–62.

Aris, R. 1956. On the dispersion of a solute in a fluid flowing through a tube. *Proc. Roy. Soc. Lond. A.* 235:67–77.

Arnold, J. H. 1944. Studies in diffusion: III. Unsteady-state vaporization and adsorption. *Trans. AIChE.* 40:361–78.

Baldauf, W. and H. Knapp. 1983. Measurements of diffusivities in liquids by the dispersion method. *Chem. Eng. Sci.* 38(7):1031–37.

Callendar, R. and D. G. Leaist. 2006. Diffusion coefficients for binary, ternary, and polydisperse solutions from peak-width analysis of Taylor dispersion profile. *J. Solution Chem.* 35(3):353–79.

Chen, Z., P. Arce and B. R. Locke. 1996. Convective-diffusive transport with a wall reaction in Couette flows. *Chem. Eng. J.* 61(2):63–71.

Graetz, L. 1883. Über die Wärmeleitfähigkeit von Flüssigkeiten (on the conduction of heat in liquids). *Annalen der Physik (N.F.).* 18:79–94.

Hausen, L. 1943. Darstellug des Wärmeiiberganges in Rohren durch verallgemeinerte Potenzbeziehungen. *Z. Ver. deutsch, Ing. Beih. Verfahrenstechnik* 4:91–5.

Johnstone, H. F. and R. L. Pigford. 1942. Distillation in a wetted-wall column. *Trans. AIChE.* 38:25–51.

Mitrovic, J. 2012. Josef Stefan and his evaporation-diffusion tube – the Stefan diffusion problem. *Chem. Eng. Sci.* 75:279–81.

Ogata, K. and R. B. Banks. 1961. A solution of the differential equation of longitudinal dispersion in porous media. *US Geol. Survey Professional Pap.* 411-A:A1–7.

Ozguler, E. I., S. G. Sunol and A. K. Sunol. 2003. Analysis of the Stefan tube at supercritical conditions and diffusion coefficient measurements. *Ind. Eng. Chem. Res.* 42:4389–97.

Skelland, A. H. P. 1974. *Diffusional Mass Transfer*. New York: Wiley.

Slattery, J. C. and V. R. Mhetar. 1997. Unsteady-state evaporation and the measurement of a binary diffusion coefficient. *Chem. Eng. Sci.* 52(9):1511–15.

Taylor, G. 1953. Dispersion of soluble matter in solvent flowing slowly through a tube. *Proc. Roy. Soc. Lond. A.* 219:186–203.

Tosun, I. 2007. Forced convection heat transfer in circular pipes. *Chem. Eng. Ed.* 41(1):39–42.

van der Laan, E. T. 1958. Notes on the diffusion type model for the longitudinal mixing in flow (O. Levenspiel and W. K. Smith). *Chem. Eng. Sci.* 7:187–91.

8 Mass Transfer in Multicomponent Mixtures

The governing equations for diffusion in multicomponent mixtures were developed in Chapter 3. This chapter is devoted to the applications of these equations to various problems involving ternary systems. For one-dimensional diffusion of a ternary mixture under steady conditions, the Maxwell–Stefan (MS) equations provide two independent equations in which the mole fraction of each component and the corresponding flux of each appear as variables. Since the existing solution procedures are quite lengthy, two Mathcad subroutines are developed for the "shooting method," which is necessary to solve the MS equations. Application of this numerical scheme is very simple, and the initial guess values do not affect the results. The MS equations in the case of coupled driving forces are also briefly covered.

8.1 TWO-BULB DIFFUSION EXPERIMENT BY DUNCAN AND TOOR

While investigating diffusion in three-component gas mixtures, Toor (1957) realized that the diffusive flux of a specific species is affected not only by its own mole fraction gradient but also the mole fraction gradients of other species present in the mixture and postulated the following three types of diffusion phenomena:

1. Diffusion barrier: The flux of a species is zero even though its concentration gradient is nonzero.
2. Osmotic diffusion: The flux of a species is nonzero even though its concentration gradient is zero.
3. Reverse (or uphill) diffusion: A species diffuses in the direction opposite to its concentration driving force.

Five years later, to test these hypotheses, Duncan and Toor (1962) carried out one of the most celebrated experiments on diffusion: a two-bulb diffusion experiment. As shown in Figure 8.1, the experimental setup consisted of bulbs A and B having almost equal volumes. The bulbs are connected by a 8.59-cm-long capillary tube, 2.08 mm in internal diameter. While the bulb A is initially filled with an equimolar mixture of hydrogen (1) and nitrogen (2), bulb B is filled with an equimolar mixture of nitrogen and carbon dioxide (3). These gas mixtures are separated from each other by keeping the stopcock closed. When the bulbs reach thermal and mechanical equilibrium, the stopcock is opened and diffusion is allowed to take place for a preset time period. At the end of the run, the stopcock is closed, and the contents of the bulbs are analyzed by gas chromatography. Experiments with the same initial bulb concentrations are repeated by varying the diffusion time.

Since bulb A initially contains no carbon dioxide and bulb B contains no hydrogen, once the stopcock is opened, one can easily predict that carbon dioxide will diffuse from bulb B to bulb A and hydrogen will diffuse from bulb A to bulb B. The experimental data shown in Figure 8.2 show

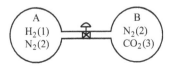

Figure 8.1 A two-bulb diffusion cell.

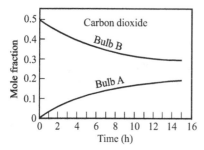
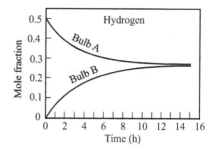

Figure 8.2 Variations in mole fractions of CO_2 and H_2 with time.

this is indeed the case. As the mole fraction of CO_2 in bulb B decreases, the mole fraction of CO_2 in bulb A increases. The mole fractions approach each other as time progresses. The same trend is observed for hydrogen but much more rapidly with respect to carbon dioxide.

When the system reaches equilibrium, the equilibrium mole fraction of species i, y_i^{eq}, would be

$$y_i^{eq} = \frac{y_{i_o}^A V_A + y_{i_o}^B V_B}{V_A + V_B}, \tag{8.1}$$

where $y_{i_o}^A$ and $y_{i_o}^B$ are the initial mole fractions of species i in bulbs A and B, respectively, and V_A and V_B are the volumes of bulbs A and B, respectively. Since $V_A \simeq V_B$, $y_1^{eq} = y_3^{eq} = 0.25$ and $y_2^{eq} = 0.5$.

When it comes to nitrogen, prediction of the direction of its flux is rather difficult since the initial mole fractions in both bulbs are the same. The experimental data shown in Figure 8.3 point out an unusual phenomenon in the diffusion of nitrogen. Although the initial mole fraction gradient of nitrogen is zero, nitrogen moves from bulb B to bulb A, i.e., osmotic diffusion. As a result, while the mole fraction of nitrogen in bulb A increases, the mole fraction of nitrogen in bulb B decreases. This is an example of reverse (or uphill) diffusion. This phenomenon continues until the mole fraction profiles reach a plateau at time t^*. At this point although the mole fraction gradient is large, the flux of nitrogen is zero, i.e., a diffusion barrier. For $t > t^*$, nitrogen diffuses from a region of high concentration (bulb A) to a region of low concentration (bulb B) as expected.

These anomalies in the diffusion behavior of nitrogen can be explained by using the MS equations. First of all, note that equimolar counterdiffusion takes place within the two-bulb system, i.e., $\sum_i N_i = 0$. Thus, the diffusive flux of species is equal to its total flux. The values of the MS diffusion coefficients are given as (Duncan and Toor, 1962)

$$Đ_{12} = 0.833 \, cm^2/s \qquad Đ_{13} = 0.680 \, cm^2/s \qquad Đ_{23} = 0.168 \, cm^2/s$$

For a ternary system, diffusive fluxes are given by Eq. (3.3), i.e.,

$$\mathbf{J}_1^* = -c\mathcal{D}_{11}^* \nabla y_1 - c\mathcal{D}_{12}^* \nabla y_2 \tag{8.2}$$

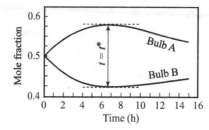

Figure 8.3 Variation in nitrogen mole fraction with time.

$$\mathbf{J}_2^* = -c\mathcal{D}_{21}^* \nabla y_1 - c\mathcal{D}_{22}^* \nabla y_2 \tag{8.3}$$

Osmotic diffusion implies that even though $\nabla y_2 = 0$, $\mathbf{J}_2^*$ may be nonzero due to ∇y_1. A diffusion barrier, on the other hand, implies that the two terms on the right side of Eq. (8.3) are equal in magnitude but have different signs.

Using Eqs. (3.131) and (3.132), the Fick diffusion coefficient matrix is given as

$$\begin{pmatrix} \mathcal{D}_{11}^* & \mathcal{D}_{12}^* \\ \mathcal{D}_{21}^* & \mathcal{D}_{22}^* \end{pmatrix} = \frac{\begin{pmatrix} Ð_{13}\left[y_1 Ð_{23} + (1-y_1)Ð_{12}\right] & y_1 Ð_{23}\left(Ð_{13} - Ð_{12}\right) \\ y_2 Ð_{13}\left(Ð_{23} - Ð_{12}\right) & Ð_{23}\left[y_2 Ð_{13} + (1-y_2)Ð_{12}\right] \end{pmatrix}}{y_1 Ð_{23} + y_2 Ð_{13} + y_3 Ð_{12}} \tag{8.4}$$

Figure 8.4 shows the results of the calculations at the equilibrium composition. Therefore, the one-dimensional form of Eq. (8.3) becomes

$$J_{2_z}^* = c\left(0.383\frac{dy_1}{dz} - 0.215\frac{dy_2}{dz}\right) \tag{8.5}$$

The gradients can be approximated as

$$\frac{dy_i}{dz} \simeq \frac{y_i^{eq} - y_i^A}{\delta} = \frac{\Delta y_i}{\delta}, \tag{8.6}$$

where δ is the length of the capillary tube. Equation (8.6) implies that the positive z-direction is directed from bulb A to bulb B. The use of Eq. (8.6) in Eq. (8.5) results in

$$J_{2_z}^* = \frac{c}{\delta}\left(0.383\Delta y_1 - 0.215\Delta y_2\right) \tag{8.7}$$

Initially $\Delta y_2 = 0$ and $\Delta y_1 = -0.25$. As a result, a large negative driving force causes nitrogen to diffuse from bulb B to bulb A. The reverse diffusion of nitrogen can also be explained by examining the magnitudes of the MS diffusion coefficients. As stated in Section 3.2, the MS diffusion coefficient may be interpreted as the reciprocal drag (or friction) coefficient between the species. Thus, the values of the MS diffusion coefficients imply that the drag coefficient between nitrogen

ORIGIN := 1

$$\text{Dms} := \begin{pmatrix} 0.833 \\ 0.680 \\ 0.168 \end{pmatrix} \qquad y := \begin{pmatrix} 0.25 \\ 0.50 \\ 0.25 \end{pmatrix}$$

$$D := \frac{\begin{bmatrix} \text{Dms}_2 \cdot \left[y_1 \cdot \text{Dms}_3 + \left(1 - y_1\right) \cdot \text{Dms}_1\right] & y_1 \cdot \text{Dms}_3 \cdot \left(\text{Dms}_2 - \text{Dms}_1\right) \\ y_2 \cdot \text{Dms}_2 \cdot \left(\text{Dms}_3 - \text{Dms}_1\right) & \text{Dms}_3 \cdot \left[y_2 \cdot \text{Dms}_2 + \left(1 - y_2\right) \cdot \text{Dms}_1\right] \end{bmatrix}}{y_1 \cdot \text{Dms}_3 + y_2 \cdot \text{Dms}_2 + y_3 \cdot \text{Dms}_1}$$

$$D = \begin{pmatrix} 0.768 & -0.011 \\ -0.383 & 0.215 \end{pmatrix}$$

Figure 8.4 Mathcad worksheet for the calculation of the Fick diffusion matrix.

and carbon dioxide is much larger than that between nitrogen and hydrogen. As the carbon dioxide stream moves from bulb B to bulb A, it drags nitrogen to bulb A as well. The condition

$$0.383\,\Delta y_1 - 0.215\,\Delta y_2 = 0$$

implies a diffusion barrier. In other words, although Δy_2 is nonzero, $J_{2_z}^* = 0$.

Example 8.1 This is an instructive example on reverse diffusion given by Krishna (2016) based on the experimental data published by Arnold and Toor (1967), who studied the unsteady-state diffusion of a ternary gas mixture of methane (1), argon (2), and hydrogen (3) in a Loschmidt cell at 307 K and 1 atm. The Loschmidt tubes are 12.7 mm in diameter and have a length of 0.406 m. The initial compositions in the upper and lower compartments are given as

$$y_1^U = 0 \qquad y_2^U = 0.509 \qquad y_3^U = 0.491$$

$$y_1^L = 0.515 \qquad y_2^L = 0.485 \qquad y_3^L = 0$$

The MS diffusion coefficients are reported as

$$Ð_{12} = 2.16 \times 10^{-5} \mathrm{m^2/s} \qquad Ð_{13} = 7.72 \times 10^{-5} \mathrm{m^2/s} \qquad Ð_{23} = 8.33 \times 10^{-5} \mathrm{m^2/s}$$

From the given data, we expect methane to move from the lower to the upper chamber while argon and hydrogen move from the upper to the lower chamber. The MS diffusion coefficients indicate that the drag coefficient between argon and methane is much larger than that between argon and hydrogen. Therefore, as methane diffuses from the lower to the upper chamber, it may drag argon with it, resulting in the reverse diffusion of argon. Let us quantify this conclusion by numerical calculations. The equilibrium mole fractions will be

$$y_1^{eq} = \frac{0.515}{2} = 0.2575 \qquad y_2^{eq} = \frac{0.509 + 0.485}{2} = 0.497 \qquad y_3^{eq} = \frac{0.491}{2} = 0.2455$$

At the equilibrium composition, the Fick diffusion coefficient matrix is calculated by using Eq. (8.4) as shown in the Mathcad worksheet. Diffusive fluxes at $t = 0$ can be calculated from

$$[J_i^*] = -c\,[D^*]\left[\frac{dy_i}{dz}\right] \tag{1}$$

Let us define the initial mole fraction gradient as

$$\frac{dy_i}{dz} = \frac{y_i^U - y_i^L}{\delta}, \tag{2}$$

implying the positive z-direction directing from the lower to the upper chamber. From the Mathcad worksheet, we see that the fluxes of methane and argon are positive, indicating movement from the lower to the upper chamber. On the other hand, the flux of hydrogen is negative as expected. The flux expression for argon is

$$J_{2_z}^* = -c\mathcal{D}_{21}^* \frac{dy_1}{dz} - c\mathcal{D}_{22}^* \frac{dy_2}{dz} \tag{3}$$

The magnitudes of the terms on the right side of Eq. (3) are

$$-c\mathcal{D}_{21}^* \frac{dy_1}{dz} = -(39.699)(3.635 \times 10^{-5})\left(\frac{0 - 0.515}{0.406}\right) = 1.83 \times 10^{-3} \mathrm{mol/m^2.s}$$

$$-c\mathcal{D}_{22}^* \frac{dy_2}{dz} = -(39.699)(6.298 \times 10^{-5})\left(\frac{0.509 - 0.485}{0.406}\right) = -1.48 \times 10^{-4} \mathrm{mol/m^2.s}$$

Since $J_{2_z}^* > 0$, argon is dragged by methane from the lower to the upper chamber.

$$\text{ORIGIN} := 1$$

$$\text{Dms} := \begin{pmatrix} 2.16 \\ 7.72 \\ 8.33 \end{pmatrix} \cdot 10^{-5} \qquad y := \begin{pmatrix} 0.2575 \\ 0.497 \\ 0.2455 \end{pmatrix} \qquad T := 307 \qquad P := 1 \qquad R := 82.05\ 10^{-6}$$

$$D := \frac{\begin{bmatrix} \text{Dms}_2 \cdot \left[y_1 \cdot \text{Dms}_3 + \left(1 - y_1 \right) \cdot \text{Dms}_1 \right] & y_1 \cdot \text{Dms}_3 \cdot \left(\text{Dms}_2 - \text{Dms}_1 \right) \\ y_2 \cdot \text{Dms}_2 \cdot \left(\text{Dms}_3 - \text{Dms}_1 \right) & \text{Dms}_3 \cdot \left[y_2 \cdot \text{Dms}_2 + \left(1 - y_2 \right) \cdot \text{Dms}_1 \right] \end{bmatrix}}{y_1 \cdot \text{Dms}_3 + y_2 \cdot \text{Dms}_2 + y_3 \cdot \text{Dms}_1}$$

$$D = \begin{pmatrix} 4.444 \times 10^{-5} & 1.831 \times 10^{-5} \\ 3.635 \times 10^{-5} & 6.298 \times 10^{-5} \end{pmatrix} \qquad c := \frac{P}{R \cdot T} = 39.699$$

$$J := -c \cdot D \cdot \begin{pmatrix} \dfrac{0 - 0.515}{0.406} \\ \dfrac{0.509 - 0.485}{0.406} \end{pmatrix} = \begin{pmatrix} 2.195 \times 10^{-3} \\ 1.683 \times 10^{-3} \end{pmatrix}$$

$$J_3 := -\left(J_1 + J_2 \right) = -3.878 \times 10^{-3}$$

Mathcad worksheet of Example 8.1.

8.2 MS EQUATIONS

For an ideal mixture, the MS equations in terms of total molar fluxes were given in Chapter 3:

$$\nabla x_i = \sum_{\substack{k=1 \\ k \neq i}}^{\mathcal{N}} \frac{x_i N_k - x_k N_i}{c Ð_{ik}}$$

$$= x_i \sum_{\substack{k=1 \\ k \neq i}}^{\mathcal{N}} \frac{N_k}{c Ð_{ik}} - N_i \sum_{\substack{k=1 \\ k \neq i}}^{\mathcal{N}-1} \frac{x_k}{c Ð_{ik}} - N_i \frac{x_{\mathcal{N}}}{c Ð_{i\mathcal{N}}} \tag{8.8}$$

Since mole fractions sum to unity, the mole fraction of species $\mathcal{N}$ is expressed as

$$x_{\mathcal{N}} = 1 - x_i - \sum_{\substack{k=1 \\ k \neq i}}^{\mathcal{N}-1} x_k \tag{8.9}$$

Substitution of Eq. (8.9) into Eq. (8.8) and rearrangement give

$$\nabla x_i = x_i \left(\frac{N_i}{c Ð_{i\mathcal{N}}} + \sum_{\substack{k=1 \\ k \neq i}}^{\mathcal{N}} \frac{N_k}{c Ð_{ik}} \right) + \sum_{\substack{k=1 \\ k \neq i}}^{\mathcal{N}-1} \left(\frac{N_i}{c Ð_{i\mathcal{N}}} - \frac{N_i}{c Ð_{ik}} \right) x_k - \frac{N_i}{c Ð_{i\mathcal{N}}} \tag{8.10}$$

For a ternary system, Eq. (8.10) is expressed for species 1 and 2 in the forms

$$\frac{dx_1}{dz} = \left(\frac{N_{1_z}}{c\mathcal{D}_{13}} + \frac{N_{2_z}}{c\mathcal{D}_{12}} + \frac{N_{3_z}}{c\mathcal{D}_{13}} \right) y_1 + \left(\frac{N_{1_z}}{c\mathcal{D}_{13}} - \frac{N_{1_z}}{c\mathcal{D}_{12}} \right) y_2 - \frac{N_{1_z}}{c\mathcal{D}_{13}} \tag{8.11}$$

$$\frac{dx_2}{dz} = \left(\frac{N_{2_z}}{c\mathcal{D}_{23}} - \frac{N_{2_z}}{c\mathcal{D}_{12}} \right) y_1 + \left(\frac{N_{1_z}}{c\mathcal{D}_{12}} + \frac{N_{2_z}}{c\mathcal{D}_{23}} + \frac{N_{3_z}}{c\mathcal{D}_{23}} \right) y_2 - \frac{N_{2_z}}{c\mathcal{D}_{23}} \tag{8.12}$$

8.2.1 STEADY-STATE MASS TRANSFER IN TERNARY GAS MIXTURES

The equation of continuity for species i is given by Eq. (2.99) as

$$\frac{\partial c_i}{\partial t} + \nabla \cdot \mathbf{N}_i = \mathcal{R}_i \tag{8.13}$$

Considering one-dimensional mass transfer under steady conditions with no homogeneous chemical reaction, Eq. (8.13) simplifies to

$$\frac{dN_{i_z}}{dz} = 0 \quad\Rightarrow\quad N_{i_z} = \text{constant} = N_i \tag{8.14}$$

Thus, Eqs. (8.11) and (8.12) are expressed in the forms

$$\frac{dy_1}{dz} = \left(\frac{N_1}{c\mathcal{D}_{13}} + \frac{N_2}{c\mathcal{D}_{12}} + \frac{N_3}{c\mathcal{D}_{13}} \right) y_1 + \left(\frac{N_1}{c\mathcal{D}_{13}} - \frac{N_1}{c\mathcal{D}_{12}} \right) y_2 - \frac{N_1}{c\mathcal{D}_{13}} \tag{8.15}$$

$$\frac{dy_2}{dz} = \left(\frac{N_2}{c\mathcal{D}_{23}} - \frac{N_2}{c\mathcal{D}_{12}} \right) y_1 + \left(\frac{N_1}{c\mathcal{D}_{12}} + \frac{N_2}{c\mathcal{D}_{23}} + \frac{N_3}{c\mathcal{D}_{23}} \right) y_2 - \frac{N_2}{c\mathcal{D}_{23}} \tag{8.16}$$

Introduction of the dimensionless quantities

$$\xi = \frac{z}{\delta} \qquad \Lambda_1 = \frac{N_1 \delta}{c\mathcal{D}_{12}} \qquad \Lambda_2 = \frac{N_2 \delta}{c\mathcal{D}_{12}} \qquad \Lambda_3 = \frac{N_3 \delta}{c\mathcal{D}_{12}} \qquad \beta_1 = \frac{\mathcal{D}_{12}}{\mathcal{D}_{13}} \qquad \beta_2 = \frac{\mathcal{D}_{12}}{\mathcal{D}_{23}} \tag{8.17}$$

transforms Eqs. (8.15) and (8.16) into

$$\boxed{\frac{dy_1}{d\xi} = (\Lambda_1 \beta_1 + \Lambda_2 + \Lambda_3 \beta_1)\, y_1 + \Lambda_1 (\beta_1 - 1)\, y_2 - \Lambda_1 \beta_1} \tag{8.18}$$

$$\boxed{\frac{dy_2}{d\xi} = \Lambda_2 (\beta_2 - 1)\, y_1 + (\Lambda_1 + \Lambda_2 \beta_2 + \Lambda_3 \beta_2)\, y_2 - \Lambda_2 \beta_2} \tag{8.19}$$

Example 8.2 At first glance, the problems shown in the figure below may look different from each other. However, they are completely analogous, and the same solution procedure is used for both cases.

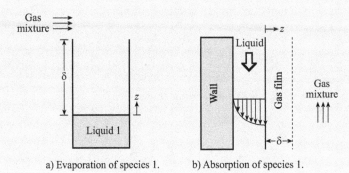

a) Evaporation of species 1.   b) Absorption of species 1.

In Problem (a), pure liquid 1 evaporates into a gas mixture consisting of species 1, 2, and 3 in a vertical tube. The distance from the liquid surface to the top of the tube is δ. In Problem (b), a gas mixture consisting of species 1, 2, and 3 flows in a wetted-wall column, and species 1 is absorbed by a nonvolatile liquid. Mass transfer takes place across the gas film of thickness δ. In both cases, the gas composition at $z = \delta$, i.e., y_{1_δ}, y_{2_δ}, y_{3_δ}, is known. In Problem (a), the mole fraction of species 1 at $z = 0$ can be calculated from $y_{1_o} = P_i^{vap}/P$. In Problem (b), y_{1_o} is given. Temperature, pressure, and the value of δ are also known quantities. To calculate the rate of evaporation or rate of absorption, we have to calculate the molar flux of species 1 at $z = 0$.

To simplify the problem, let us assume that the solubility of species 2 and 3 in the liquid is negligible, i.e., $N_2|_{z=0} = N_3|_{z=0} = 0$. Since N_2 and N_3 are constants, this implies that $N_2 = N_3 = 0$. Under these circumstances, Eqs. (8.18) and (8.19) simplify to

$$\frac{dy_1}{d\xi} = \Lambda_1 \beta_1 y_1 + \Lambda_1 (\beta_1 - 1) y_2 - \Lambda_1 \beta_1 \tag{1}$$

$$\frac{dy_2}{d\xi} = \Lambda_1 y_2 \tag{2}$$

Integration of Eq. (2) from $\xi = \xi$ to $\xi = 1$ yields

$$\int_{y_2}^{y_{2_\delta}} \frac{dy_2}{y_2} = \Lambda_1 \int_\xi^1 d\xi \quad \Rightarrow \quad y_2 = y_{2_\delta} e^{-\Lambda_1 (1-\xi)} \tag{3}$$

Substitution of Eq. (3) into Eq. (1) gives

$$\frac{dy_1}{d\xi} - \Lambda_1 \beta_1 y_1 = y_{2_\delta} \Lambda_1 (\beta_1 - 1) e^{-\Lambda_1 (1-\xi)} - \Lambda_1 \beta_1, \tag{4}$$

which is a first-order linear equation with the integrating factor, μ, of

$$\mu = e^{-\Lambda_1 \beta_1 \xi} \tag{5}$$

Multiplication of Eq. (4) by the integrating factor and rearrangement yield

$$\frac{d}{d\xi} \left(e^{-\Lambda_1 \beta_1 \xi} y_1 \right) = y_{2_\delta} \Lambda_1 (\beta_1 - 1) e^{-\Lambda_1 - \Lambda_1 (\beta_1 - 1)\xi} - \Lambda_1 \beta_1 e^{-\Lambda_1 \beta_1 \xi} \tag{6}$$

Integration of Eq. (6) leads to

$$y_1 = 1 - y_{2_\delta} e^{-\Lambda_1 (1-\xi)} + C e^{\Lambda_1 \beta_1 \xi}, \tag{7}$$

where C is an integration constant. The use of the boundary condition at $\xi = 1$ gives the concentration profile as

$$y_1 = 1 - y_{2_\delta} e^{-\Lambda_1 (1-\xi)} - y_{3_\delta} e^{-\Lambda_1 \beta_1 (1-\xi)} \tag{8}$$

By using the boundary condition at $\xi = 0$, the unknown quantity Λ_1 can be calculated from the following transcendental equation:

$$y_{1_o} = 1 - y_{2_\delta} e^{-\Lambda_1} - y_{3_\delta} e^{-\Lambda_1 \beta_1} \tag{9}$$

Now let us carry out a numerical calculation for Problem (a) using the following data:

$$P = 1\,\text{atm} \quad T = 325\,\text{K} \quad Đ_{12} = 0.41\,\text{cm}^2/\text{s} \quad Đ_{13} = 0.35\,\text{cm}^2/\text{s} \quad \delta = 9.5\,\text{cm}$$

$$y_{1_o} = 0.38 \quad y_{1_\delta} = 0.08 \quad y_{2_\delta} = 0.32 \quad y_{3_\delta} = 0.60$$

From the Mathcad worksheet shown below, $N_1 = 5.751 \times 10^{-7}\,\text{mol/cm}^2.\text{s}$.

$P := 1$ $T := 325$ $R := 82.05$ $\delta := 9.5$ $D12 := 0.41$ $D13 := 0.35$

$y10 := 0.38$ $y1\delta := 0.08$ $y2\delta := 0.32$ $y3\delta := 0.6$ $\beta1 := \dfrac{D12}{D13}$

$\Lambda1 := 0.4$

Given

$y10 = 1 - y2\delta \exp(-\Lambda1) - y3\delta \exp(-\Lambda1 \cdot \beta1)$

$\Lambda1 := \text{Find}(\Lambda1) = 0.3553$

$c := \dfrac{P}{R \cdot T} = 3.75 \times 10^{-5}$

$N1 := \dfrac{\Lambda1 \cdot c \cdot D12}{\delta} = 5.751 \times 10^{-7}$

Mathcad worksheet of Example 8.2.

Comment: In the case of gas absorption, the use of Eq. (9) will yield negative values for the flux of species 1 since it diffuses in the negative z-direction (see Problem 8.1).

Example 8.3 In Example 8.2, species 2 and 3 are considered insoluble in a liquid. Now suppose that only component 3 is insoluble in a liquid, i.e., $N_3 = 0$. In this case, Eqs. (8.18) and (8.19) become

$$\frac{dy_1}{d\xi} = (\Lambda_1 \beta_1 + \Lambda_2) y_1 + \Lambda_1 (\beta_1 - 1) y_2 - \Lambda_1 \beta_1 \tag{8.1}$$

$$\frac{dy_2}{d\xi} = \Lambda_2 (\beta_2 - 1) y_1 + (\Lambda_1 + \Lambda_2 \beta_2) y_2 - \Lambda_2 \beta_2 \tag{8.2}$$

Addition of Eqs. (1) and (2) and the use of the relationship

$$y_3 = 1 - y_1 - y_2 \tag{3}$$

lead to a simpler equation in terms of y_3 as

$$\frac{dy_3}{d\xi} = (\Lambda_1 \beta_1 + \Lambda_2 \beta_2) y_3 \tag{4}$$

Integration of Eq. (4) from $\xi = 0$ to $\xi = \xi$ yields

$$\int_{y_{3_o}}^{y_3} \frac{dy_3}{y_3} = (\Lambda_1 \beta_1 + \Lambda_2 \beta_2) \int_0^\xi d\xi \quad \Rightarrow \quad y_3 = y_{3_o} e^{(\Lambda_1 \beta_1 + \Lambda_2 \beta_2)\xi} \tag{5}$$

Substitution of $y_2 = 1 - y_1 - y_3$ into Eq. (1) gives

$$\frac{dy_1}{d\xi} = (\Lambda_1 + \Lambda_2) y_1 + \Lambda_1 (1 - \beta_1) y_3 - \Lambda_1 \tag{6}$$

Substitution of Eq. (5) into Eq. (6) gives

$$\frac{dy_1}{d\xi} - (\Lambda_1 + \Lambda_2) y_1 = \Lambda_1 (1 - \beta_1) y_{3_o} e^{(\Lambda_1 \beta_1 + \Lambda_2 \beta_2)\xi} - \Lambda_1, \tag{7}$$

which is a first-order linear equation with the integrating factor, μ, of

$$\mu = e^{-(\Lambda_1 + \Lambda_2)\xi} \tag{8}$$

Multiplication of Eq. (7) by the integrating factor and rearrangement yield

$$\frac{d}{d\xi}\left[e^{-(\Lambda_1+\Lambda_2)\xi}\,y_1\right] = \Lambda_1(1-\beta_1)y_{3_o}\,e^{[\Lambda_1(\beta_1-1)+\Lambda_2(\beta_2-1)]\xi} - \Lambda_1\,e^{-(\Lambda_1+\Lambda_2)\xi} \tag{9}$$

Integration of Eq. (9) leads to

$$y_1 = \frac{1}{1+(\Lambda_2/\Lambda_1)} - \frac{y_{3_o}}{1+(\Lambda_2/\Lambda_1)\Phi}\,e^{(\Lambda_1\beta_1+\Lambda_2\beta_2)\xi} + C\,e^{(\Lambda_1+\Lambda_2)\xi}, \tag{10}$$

where C is an integration constant and Φ is defined by

$$\Phi = \frac{\beta_2 - 1}{\beta_1 - 1} \tag{11}$$

The use of the boundary condition at $\xi = 0$ gives the concentration profile as

$$y_1 = \frac{1}{1+(\Lambda_2/\Lambda_1)} - \frac{y_{3_o}\,e^{(\Lambda_1\beta_1+\Lambda_2\beta_2)\xi}}{1+(\Lambda_2/\Lambda_1)\Phi} + \left[y_{1_o} - \frac{1}{1+(\Lambda_2/\Lambda_1)} + \frac{y_{3_o}}{1+(\Lambda_2/\Lambda_1)\Phi}\right]e^{(\Lambda_1+\Lambda_2)\xi} \tag{12}$$

To determine Λ_1 and Λ_2, Eqs. (5) and (12) have to be evaluated at $\xi = 1$:

$$\boxed{y_{3_\delta} = y_{3_o}\,e^{(\Lambda_1\beta_1+\Lambda_2\beta_2)}} \tag{13}$$

$$\boxed{y_{1_\delta} = \frac{1}{1+(\Lambda_2/\Lambda_1)} - \frac{y_{3_o}\,e^{(\Lambda_1\beta_1+\Lambda_2\beta_2)}}{1+(\Lambda_2/\Lambda_1)\Phi} + \left[y_{1_o} - \frac{1}{1+(\Lambda_2/\Lambda_1)} + \frac{y_{3_o}}{1+(\Lambda_2/\Lambda_1)\Phi}\right]e^{(\Lambda_1+\Lambda_2)}} \tag{14}$$

The values of Λ_1 and Λ_2 are determined from the simultaneous solution of Eqs. (13) and (14).

Carty and Schrodt (1975) studied evaporation of acetone (1) and methanol (2) into stagnant air (3) and provided the following data:

$$P = 0.981\,\text{atm} \qquad T = 328.5\,\text{K} \qquad \delta = 23.8\,\text{cm}$$

$$Ð_{12} = 0.0848\,\text{cm}^2/\text{s} \qquad Ð_{13} = 0.1372\,\text{cm}^2/\text{s} \qquad Ð_{23} = 0.1991\,\text{cm}^2/\text{s}$$

$$y_{1_o} = 0.319 \qquad y_{2_o} = 0.528 \qquad y_{3_o} = 0.153 \qquad y_{1_\delta} = y_{2_\delta} = 0 \qquad y_{3_\delta} = 1$$

From the Mathcad worksheet, the molar fluxes are calculated as

$$N_1 = 1.783 \times 10^{-7}\,\text{mol/cm}^2.\text{s} \qquad N_2 = 3.128 \times 10^{-7}\,\text{mol/cm}^2.\text{s}$$

Concentration profiles based on these molar flux values are determined from Eqs. (5) and (12) and plotted in the figure below.

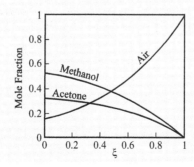

$T := 328.5$ $P := 0.981$ $R := 82.05$ $\delta := 23.8$

$y10 := 0.319$ $y20 := 0.528$ $y30 := 0.153$ $y1\delta := 0$ $y2\delta := 0$ $y3\delta := 1$

$D12 := 0.0848$ $D13 := 0.1372$ $D23 := 0.1991$

$\beta1 := \dfrac{D12}{D13}$ $\beta2 := \dfrac{D12}{D23}$ $c := \dfrac{P}{R \cdot T}$

$\Phi := \dfrac{\beta2 - 1}{\beta1 - 1}$

$\Lambda1 := 0.1$ $\Lambda2 := 0.2$

Given

$y3\delta = y30 \cdot \exp(\Lambda1 \cdot \beta1 + \Lambda2 \cdot \beta2)$

$y1\delta = \dfrac{1}{1 + \dfrac{\Lambda2}{\Lambda1}} - \dfrac{y30}{1 + \dfrac{\Lambda2}{\Lambda1} \cdot \Phi} \cdot \exp(\Lambda1 \cdot \beta1 + \Lambda2 \cdot \beta2) + \left(y10 - \dfrac{1}{1 + \dfrac{\Lambda2}{\Lambda1}} + \dfrac{y30}{1 + \dfrac{\Lambda2}{\Lambda1} \cdot \Phi} \right) \cdot \exp(\Lambda1 + \Lambda2)$

$\begin{pmatrix} \Lambda1 \\ \Lambda2 \end{pmatrix} := \text{Find}(\Lambda1, \Lambda2) = \begin{pmatrix} 1.375 \\ 2.412 \end{pmatrix}$

$N1 := \dfrac{\Lambda1 \cdot c \cdot D12}{\delta} = 1.783 \times 10^{-7}$ $N2 := \dfrac{\Lambda2 \cdot c \cdot D12}{\delta} = 3.128 \times 10^{-7}$

Mathcad worksheet of Example 8.3.

Example 8.4   Let us resolve Example 8.3 by using Mathcad's built-in function "rkfixed."[1] It is expressed in the form

$$\text{rkfixed(init,x1,x2,npoints,D)}$$

and uses a fixed step fourth-order Runge–Kutta method to solve a system of first-order ordinary differential equations (ODEs). The terms in the argument of "rkfixed" are defined as follows:

- "init" is a vector of initial values of the dependent variables.
- "x1" is the initial value of the independent variable.
- "x2" is the final value of the independent variable.
- "npoints" is the number of points beyond the initial point $\times 1$ at which the solution is to be evaluated. Thus, the number of solution points is (npoints + 1).
- "D" is a vector-valued function containing first derivatives of the dependent variables.

An iterative "shooting method" yields the solution as a matrix containing the values of the independent variable in the first column and the successive values of the dependent variables in vector D in the remaining columns.

The MS equations in dimensionless form are given by Eqs. (1) and (2) in Example 8.2:

$$\frac{dy_1}{d\xi} = (\Lambda_1 \beta_1 + \Lambda_2)\, y_1 + \Lambda_1\, (\beta_1 - 1)\, y_2 - \Lambda_1 \beta_1 \tag{1}$$

$$\frac{dy_2}{d\xi} = \Lambda_2\, (\beta_2 - 1)\, y_1 + (\Lambda_1 + \Lambda_2 \beta_2)\, y_2 - \Lambda_2 \beta_2 \tag{2}$$

---

[1] A similar procedure is also used by Benítez (2009).

ORIGIN := 1

$T := 328.5$ $P := 0.981$ $R := 82.05$ $\delta := 23.8$ npoints $:= 100$

$D12 := 0.0848$ $D13 := 0.1372$ $D23 := 0.1991$

$\beta 1 := \dfrac{D12}{D13}$ $\beta 2 := \dfrac{D12}{D23}$ $c := \dfrac{P}{R \cdot T}$

$$D(\xi, Y) := \begin{bmatrix} \left(Y_3 \cdot \beta 1 + Y_4\right) \cdot Y_1 + Y_3 \cdot (\beta 1 - 1) \cdot Y_2 - Y_3 \cdot \beta 1 \\ Y_4 \cdot (\beta 2 - 1) \cdot Y_1 + \left(Y_3 + Y_4 \cdot \beta 2\right) \cdot Y_2 - Y_4 \cdot \beta 2 \\ 0 \\ 0 \end{bmatrix}$$

$$\text{Sol}(\Lambda 1, \Lambda 2) := \text{rkfixed}\left[\begin{pmatrix} 0.319 \\ 0.528 \\ \Lambda 1 \\ \Lambda 2 \end{pmatrix}, 0, 1, \text{npoints}, D\right]$$

$\text{y1}(\Lambda 1, \Lambda 2) := \text{Sol}(\Lambda 1, \Lambda 2)^{\langle 2 \rangle}$ $\text{y2}(\Lambda 1, \Lambda 2) := \text{Sol}(\Lambda 1, \Lambda 2)^{\langle 3 \rangle}$

These are the initial guess values

$\Lambda 1 := 1$ $\Lambda 2 := 1$

Given

The following equations specify the values of y1 and y2 at z = 23.8 cm

$\text{y1}(\Lambda 1, \Lambda 2)_{\text{npoints}+1} = 0$ $\text{y2}(\Lambda 1, \Lambda 2)_{\text{npoints}+1} = 0$

$$\begin{pmatrix} \Lambda 1 \\ \Lambda 2 \end{pmatrix} := \text{Find}(\Lambda 1, \Lambda 2) = \begin{pmatrix} 1.375 \\ 2.412 \end{pmatrix}$$

$N1 := \dfrac{\Lambda 1 \cdot c \cdot D12}{\delta} = 1.783 \times 10^{-7}$ $N2 := \dfrac{\Lambda 2 \cdot c \cdot D12}{\delta} = 3.128 \times 10^{-7}$

Mathcad worksheet of Example 8.4.

Since there are four unknowns $[y_1, y_2, \Lambda_1 (\text{or } N_1), \Lambda_2 (\text{or } N_2)]$, we need two more equations. From the species continuity equation, we showed that N_1 and N_2 are constants. Thus,

$$\frac{dN_1}{dz} = 0 \quad \Rightarrow \quad \frac{d\Lambda_1}{d\xi} = 0 \tag{3}$$

$$\frac{dN_2}{dz} = 0 \quad \Rightarrow \quad \frac{d\Lambda_2}{d\xi} = 0 \tag{4}$$

If we let

$$y_1 = Y_1 \qquad y_2 = Y_2 \qquad \Lambda_1 = Y_3 \qquad \Lambda_2 = Y_4 \tag{5}$$

Eqs. (1)–(4) take the forms

$$\frac{dY_1}{d\xi} = (Y_3\beta_1 + Y_4)\,Y_1 + Y_3\,(\beta_1 - 1)\,Y_2 - Y_3\beta_1 \tag{6}$$

$$\frac{dY_2}{d\xi} = Y_4\,(\beta_2 - 1)\,Y_1 + (Y_3 + Y_4\beta_2)\,Y_2 - Y_4\beta_2 \tag{7}$$

$$\frac{dY_3}{d\xi} = 0 \qquad \frac{dY_4}{d\xi} = 0 \tag{8}$$

The Mathcad worksheet for Example 8.4 is shown above.

Alternative program: Equations (8.18) and (8.19) are solved by second-order[2] Runge–Kutta method, the subroutine of which is shown below. The terms in the argument of "rk2" are defined as follows:

$$
\begin{aligned}
&\text{rk2(yinit, npoints, F, } \Lambda) := \\
&\quad \xi \leftarrow 0 \\
&\quad j \leftarrow 1 \\
&\quad A_{j,1} \leftarrow \xi \\
&\quad A_{j,2} \leftarrow \text{yinit}_1 \\
&\quad A_{j,3} \leftarrow \text{yinit}_2 \\
&\quad \text{for } i \in 1..\text{npoints} \\
&\qquad h \leftarrow \frac{1}{\text{npoints}} \\
&\qquad k1 \leftarrow F(\xi, \text{yinit}, \Lambda) \\
&\qquad k2 \leftarrow F(\xi + h, \text{yinit} + h \cdot k1, \Lambda) \\
&\qquad \text{yinit} \leftarrow \text{yinit} + \frac{h}{2} \cdot (k1 + k2) \\
&\qquad \xi \leftarrow \xi + h \\
&\qquad A_{i+j,1} \leftarrow \xi \\
&\qquad A_{i+j,2} \leftarrow \text{yinit}_1 \\
&\qquad A_{i+j,3} \leftarrow \text{yinit}_2 \\
&\quad A
\end{aligned}
$$

Subroutine "rk2."

---

[2] Fourth-order is also possible.

- "yinit" is a vector of initial values of y_1 and y_2.
- "npoints" is the number of points beyond the initial point ($\xi = 0$) at which the solution is to be evaluated. Thus, the number of solution points is (npoints+1).
- "F" is a vector-valued function containing first derivatives of y_1 and y_2.
- "Λ" are the dimensionless flux values.

ORIGIN:= 1

$T := 328.5$ $\qquad$ $P := 0.981$ $\qquad$ $R := 82.05$ $\qquad$ npoints $:= 100$ $\qquad$ $\delta := 23.8$

$D12 := 0.0848$ $\qquad$ $D13 := 0.1372$ $\qquad$ $D23 := 0.1991$

$\beta1 := \dfrac{D12}{D13}$ $\qquad$ $\beta2 := \dfrac{D12}{D23}$ $\qquad$ $c := \dfrac{P}{R \cdot T}$

$$F(\xi, y, \Lambda) := \begin{bmatrix} \left(\Lambda_1 \cdot \beta1 + \Lambda_2 + \Lambda_3 \cdot \beta1\right) \cdot y_1 + \Lambda_1 \cdot (\beta1 - 1) \cdot y_2 - \Lambda_1 \cdot \beta1 \\ \Lambda_2 \cdot (\beta2 - 1) \cdot y_1 + \left(\Lambda_1 + \Lambda_2 \cdot \beta2 + \Lambda_3 \cdot \beta2\right) \cdot y_2 - \Lambda_2 \cdot \beta2 \end{bmatrix}$$

⯈ Reference:C:\Users\tosun\Desktop\Subroutines\rk2.xmcd

$yinit := \begin{pmatrix} 0.319 \\ 0.528 \end{pmatrix}$

$\Lambda := \begin{pmatrix} 1 \\ 1 \\ 0 \end{pmatrix}$ $\qquad$ **These are the initial guess values**

$Sol(\Lambda) := rk2(yinit, npoints, F, \Lambda)$

$y1(\Lambda) := Sol(\Lambda)^{\langle 2 \rangle}$ $\qquad\qquad$ $y2(\Lambda) := Sol(\Lambda)^{\langle 3 \rangle}$

Given

$y1(\Lambda)_{npoints+1} = 0.0$ $\qquad$ $y2(\Lambda)_{npoints+1} = 0$ $\qquad$ $\Lambda_3 = 0$

$\Lambda := Find(\Lambda) = \begin{pmatrix} 1.375 \\ 2.412 \\ 0 \end{pmatrix}$

$N1 := \dfrac{\Lambda_1 \cdot c \cdot D12}{\delta} = 1.783 \times 10^{-7}$ $\qquad$ $N2 := \dfrac{\Lambda_2 \cdot c \cdot D12}{\delta} = 3.128 \times 10^{-7}$

An alternative Mathcad worksheet of Example 8.4.

An alternative iterative "shooting method" yields the solution as a matrix containing the values of ξ, y_1, and y_2 in the first, second, and third columns, respectively. Subroutine "rk2" and the Mathcad worksheet for the alternative approach are shown on the previous pages.

In Example 8.2, two of the molar fluxes were zero. In Example 8.3, one of the molar fluxes was zero. The obvious question is, what happens if none of the molar fluxes are zero? Since the MS equations provide two independent equations, an additional equation, a so-called *bootstrap relation*, is needed. Some of the bootstrap relations are given below:

- In the absence of no net molar flow, i.e., equimolar counterdiffusion,

$$\sum_{i=1}^{\mathcal{N}} \mathbf{N}_i = 0 \tag{8.20}$$

- Taylor and Krishna (1993) stated that the equimolar counterdiffusion assumption is generally not valid in multicomponent distillation calculations. Instead, they recommended the use of the following relation:

$$\sum_{i=1}^{\mathcal{N}} \mathbf{N}_i \Delta \widetilde{H}_i^{vap} = 0, \tag{8.21}$$

where $\Delta \widetilde{H}_i^{vap}$ is the molar latent heat of vaporization of species i.
- When the mass-average velocity of the mixture is zero,

$$\sum_{i=1}^{\mathcal{N}} \mathbf{N}_i M_i = 0, \tag{8.22}$$

where M_i is the molecular weight of species i. Tai and Chang (1979) recommended the use of Eq. (8.22) for molecular diffusion in free space. For molecular diffusion in pores, they suggested the use of the following relation:

$$\sum_{i=1}^{\mathcal{N}} \mathbf{N}_i \sqrt{M_i} = 0 \tag{8.23}$$

- If one of the components does not diffuse through the interface, such as in filtration and gas absorption, then the flux of this component is zero:

$$\mathbf{N}_i\big|_{\text{interface}} = 0 \tag{8.24}$$

- When diffusion and the heterogeneous reaction take place simultaneously,

$$\sum_{i=1}^{\mathcal{N}} \frac{\mathbf{N}_i}{\alpha_i} = 0 \tag{8.25}$$

Example 8.5 Using Example 4.2.4 from Taylor and Krishna (1993), Amundson et al. (2003) studied the effect of changes in the boundary conditions on the concentration profiles of a ternary mixture of hydrogen (1), nitrogen (2), and carbon dichloride difluoride (3). The MS diffusion coefficients at 298 K and 1 atm are given as

$$Đ_{12} = 0.77\,\text{cm}^2/\text{s} \qquad Đ_{13} = 0.331\,\text{cm}^2/\text{s} \qquad Đ_{23} = 0.081\,\text{cm}^2/\text{s}$$

For equimolar counterdiffusion under steady conditions, the following three cases are considered:

Species	Case (a) y_o	Case (a) y_δ	Case (b) y_o	Case (b) y_δ	Case (c) y_o	Case (c) y_δ
1	0.55	0.01	0.55	0.10	0.55	0.01
2	0.05	0.45	0.05	0.72	0.05	0.98
3	0.40	0.54	0.40	0.18	0.40	0.01

The MS equations in dimensionless form are given by Eqs. (8.18) and (8.19), i.e.,

$$\frac{dy_1}{d\xi} = (\Lambda_1 \beta_1 + \Lambda_2 + \Lambda_3 \beta_1)\, y_1 + \Lambda_1 (\beta_1 - 1)\, y_2 - \Lambda_1 \beta_1 \tag{1}$$

$$\frac{dy_2}{d\xi} = \Lambda_2 (\beta_2 - 1)\, y_1 + (\Lambda_1 + \Lambda_2 \beta_2 + \Lambda_3 \beta_2)\, y_2 - \Lambda_2 \beta_2 \tag{2}$$

In addition, we have the following bootstrap relation:

$$\Lambda_1 + \Lambda_2 + \Lambda_3 = 0 \tag{3}$$

The Mathcad worksheet for Case (b) is shown below.

ORIGIN:= 1

D12 := 0.77   D13 := 0.331   D23 := 0.081   npoints := 100

$\beta 1 := \dfrac{D12}{D13}$ $\beta 2 := \dfrac{D12}{D23}$

$$F(\xi, y, \Lambda) := \begin{bmatrix} \left(\Lambda_1 \cdot \beta 1 + \Lambda_2 + \Lambda_3 \cdot \beta 1\right) \cdot y_1 + \Lambda_1 \cdot (\beta 1 - 1) \cdot y_2 - \Lambda_1 \cdot \beta 1 \\ \Lambda_2 \cdot (\beta 2 - 1) \cdot y_1 + \left(\Lambda_1 + \Lambda_2 \cdot \beta 2 + \Lambda_3 \cdot \beta 2\right) \cdot y_2 - \Lambda_2 \cdot \beta 2 \end{bmatrix}$$

→ Reference:C:\Users\tosun\Desktop\Subroutines\rk2.xmcd

$yinit := \begin{pmatrix} 0.55 \\ 0.05 \end{pmatrix}$

$\Lambda := \begin{pmatrix} 1 \\ 1 \\ 1 \end{pmatrix}$ **These are the initial guess values**

$Sol(\Lambda) := rk2(yinit, npoints, F, \Lambda)$

$y1(\Lambda) := Sol(\Lambda)^{\langle 2 \rangle}$ $y2(\Lambda) := Sol(\Lambda)^{\langle 3 \rangle}$

Given

$y1(\Lambda)_{npoints+1} = 0.1$ $y2(\Lambda)_{npoints+1} = 0.72$ $\Lambda_1 + \Lambda_2 + \Lambda_3 = 0$

Mathcad worksheet of Example 8.5 – Case (b).

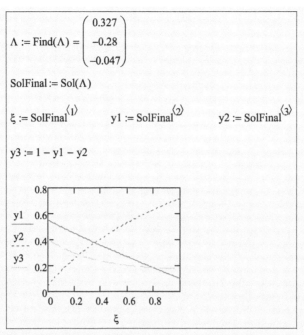

$$\Lambda := \text{Find}(\Lambda) = \begin{pmatrix} 0.327 \\ -0.28 \\ -0.047 \end{pmatrix}$$

$$\text{SolFinal} := \text{Sol}(\Lambda)$$

$$\xi := \text{SolFinal}^{\langle 1 \rangle} \qquad y1 := \text{SolFinal}^{\langle 2 \rangle} \qquad y2 := \text{SolFinal}^{\langle 3 \rangle}$$

$$y3 := 1 - y1 - y2$$

Mathcad worksheet of Example 8.5 – Case (b) (*continued*).

The calculated values of Λ_1, Λ_2, and Λ_3 and mole fraction profiles are given in Tables 8.1 and 8.2, respectively.

Table 8.1
Values of the Dimensionless Flux (Λ_1, Λ_2, Λ_3)

Case	Λ_1	Λ_2	Λ_3
(a)	0.304	−0.155	−0.149
(b)	0.327	−0.280	−0.047
(c)	0.471	−0.472	1.494×10^{-3}

Table 8.2
Variation in Mole Fraction as a Function of Dimensionless Distance

	Case (a)			Case (b)			Case (c)		
ξ	y_1	y_2	y_3	y_1	y_2	y_3	y_1	y_2	y_3
0.0	0.550	0.050	0.400	0.550	0.050	0.400	0.550	0.050	0.400
0.1	0.493	0.108	0.399	0.498	0.161	0.341	0.482	0.233	0.285
0.2	0.438	0.159	0.403	0.449	0.256	0.295	0.420	0.378	0.202
0.3	0.382	0.206	0.412	0.402	0.338	0.260	0.362	0.495	0.143
0.4	0.328	0.248	0.424	0.356	0.410	0.234	0.308	0.591	0.101
0.5	0.274	0.286	0.440	0.311	0.474	0.215	0.255	0.674	0.071
0.6	0.221	0.322	0.457	0.268	0.531	0.201	0.204	0.746	0.050
0.7	0.168	0.356	0.476	0.225	0.583	0.192	0.155	0.811	0.035
0.8	0.115	0.389	0.496	0.183	0.632	0.185	0.106	0.870	0.024
0.9	0.062	0.420	0.518	0.141	0.677	0.182	0.058	0.926	0.016
1.0	0.010	0.450	0.540	0.100	0.720	0.180	0.010	0.980	0.010

Concentration profiles for the three cases are shown in the figure below. In case (a), the fluxes are in the direction of decreasing mole fractions, as expected. In case (b), the flux of species 3 is in the direction of increasing concentration. Among the MS diffusion coefficients, $Đ_{23}$ has the smallest value, implying a large friction force between species 2 and 3. As a result, species 2 drags species 3 as it diffuses. In case (c), although species 3 has an appreciable concentration gradient, its flux is very close to zero.

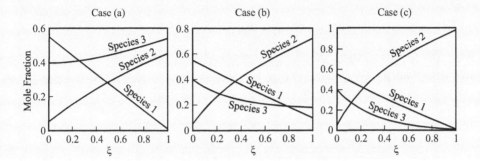

Example 8.6 Species A diffuses through a stagnant gas film of thickness δ as shown in the figure below. At the catalyst surface, A undergoes a first-order irreversible cracking reaction:

$$A \rightarrow B + C$$

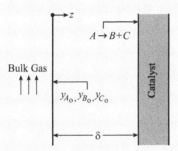

Let 1, 2, and 3 stand for A, B, and C, respectively. The following data are provided:

$$T = 1150\,\text{K} \qquad P = 1\,\text{atm} \qquad \delta = 1\,\text{mm}$$

$$Đ_{12} = 25\,\text{cm}^2/\text{s} \qquad Đ_{13} = 8\,\text{cm}^2/\text{s} \qquad Đ_{23} = 13\,\text{cm}^2/\text{s}$$

$$y_{1_o} = 0.75 \qquad y_{2_o} = 0.25$$

From the stoichiometry of the reaction, the molar fluxes are related as

$$N_1 = -N_2 = -N_3 \qquad \Rightarrow \qquad \Lambda_A = -\Lambda_B = -\Lambda_C \tag{1}$$

The mole fraction of species at the catalyst surface is not known. The boundary condition at the catalyst surface is expressed in the form

$$N_1 = k_1'' c_1 \qquad \text{at } z = \delta \tag{2}$$

In dimensionless form, Eq. (2) becomes

$$\Lambda_1 = \left(\frac{k_1'' \delta}{Đ_{12}}\right) y_{1_\delta}, \tag{3}$$

where the term $k_1'' \delta / Đ_{12}$ can be interpreted as the Thiele modulus (Θ). The Mathcad worksheet for $\Theta = 25$ is given below. Calculations are repeated for $\Theta = 0.05$ as well. The molar fluxes are calculated as

$$\Theta = 25 \qquad N_1 = -N_2 = -N_3 = 7.06\,\text{mol/m}^2.\text{s}$$
$$\Theta = 0.05 \qquad N_1 = -N_2 = -N_3 = 0.854\,\text{mol/m}^2.\text{s}$$

Concentration profiles for different values of the Thiele modulus are shown in the figure below. When the Thiele modulus is large, mass transfer is controlled by the diffusional resistance within the film. When the Thiele modulus is small, the reaction at the catalyst surface controls the mass transfer. As a result, the concentration profiles of species are almost flat.

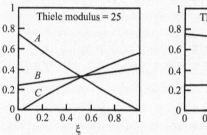
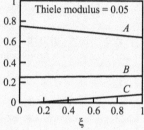

ORIGIN:= 1

$T := 1150$ $P := 1$ $R := 82.05 \cdot 10^{-6}$ npoints $:= 100$

$D12 := 25 \cdot 10^{-4}$ $D13 := 8 \cdot 10^{-4}$ $D23 := 13 \cdot 10^{-4}$ $\delta := 1 \cdot 10^{-3}$

$\beta 1 := \dfrac{D12}{D13}$ $\beta 2 := \dfrac{D12}{D23}$ $c := \dfrac{P}{R \cdot T}$

$$F(\xi, y, \Lambda) := \begin{bmatrix} (\Lambda_1 \cdot \beta 1 + \Lambda_2 + \Lambda_3 \cdot \beta 1) \cdot y_1 + \Lambda_1 \cdot (\beta 1 - 1) \cdot y_2 - \Lambda_1 \cdot \beta 1 \\ \Lambda_2 \cdot (\beta 2 - 1) \cdot y_1 + (\Lambda_1 + \Lambda_2 \cdot \beta 2 + \Lambda_3 \cdot \beta 2) \cdot y_2 - \Lambda_2 \cdot \beta 2 \end{bmatrix}$$

→ Reference:C:\Users\tosun\Desktop\Subroutines\rk2.xmcd

$\text{yinit} := \begin{pmatrix} 0.75 \\ 0.25 \end{pmatrix}$ $\Theta := 25$

$\Lambda := \begin{pmatrix} 1 \\ -1 \\ -1 \end{pmatrix}$ **These are the initial guess values**

$\text{Sol}(\Lambda) := \text{rk2}(\text{yinit}, \text{npoints}, F, \Lambda)$

$y1(\Lambda) := \text{Sol}(\Lambda)^{\langle 2 \rangle}$ $y2(\Lambda) := \text{Sol}(\Lambda)^{\langle 3 \rangle}$

Mathcad worksheet of Example 8.6.

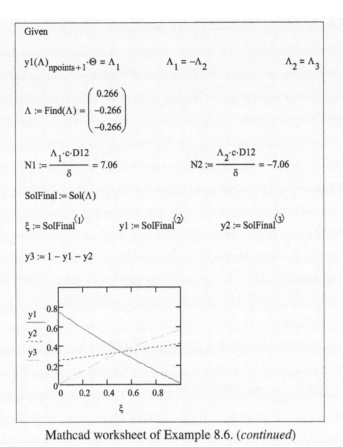

Given

$$y1(\Lambda)_{\text{npoints}+1} \cdot \Theta = \Lambda_1 \qquad \Lambda_1 = -\Lambda_2 \qquad \Lambda_2 = \Lambda_3$$

$$\Lambda := \text{Find}(\Lambda) = \begin{pmatrix} 0.266 \\ -0.266 \\ -0.266 \end{pmatrix}$$

$$N1 := \frac{\Lambda_1 \cdot c \cdot D12}{\delta} = 7.06 \qquad N2 := \frac{\Lambda_2 \cdot c \cdot D12}{\delta} = -7.06$$

$$\text{SolFinal} := \text{Sol}(\Lambda)$$

$$\xi := \text{SolFinal}^{\langle 1 \rangle} \qquad y1 := \text{SolFinal}^{\langle 2 \rangle} \qquad y2 := \text{SolFinal}^{\langle 3 \rangle}$$

$$y3 := 1 - y1 - y2$$

Mathcad worksheet of Example 8.6. (*continued*)

Example 8.7   Consider the reduction of zinc oxide by carbon monoxide gas at $1,400\,\text{K}$ and $1\,\text{atm}$:

$$\text{ZnO}\,(s) + \text{CO}\,(g) \rightleftharpoons \text{Zn}\,(g) + \text{CO}_2\,(g)$$

Let 1, 2, and 3 stand for CO, Zn, and CO_2, respectively. The bulk gas consists essentially of pure CO. Carbon monoxide diffuses through a stagnant gas film of thickness $0.1\,\text{cm}$ and, unlike the case given in Example 8.6, it undergoes a **reversible** reaction at the surface of zinc oxide. The Thiele modulus is large so that the mass transfer is controlled by diffusion and the mole fractions of species at the surface of the solid are very nearly the same as the equilibrium mole fractions. The equilibrium gas composition and the diffusion coefficients are given by

$$y_1^{eq} = 0.4734 \qquad y_2^{eq} = y_3^{eq} = 0.2633$$

$$Đ_{12} = 2.065\,\text{cm}^2/\text{s} \qquad Đ_{13} = 2.190\,\text{cm}^2/\text{s} \qquad Đ_{23} = 1.510\,\text{cm}^2/\text{s}$$

The MS equations in dimensionless form are given by Eqs. (8.18) and (8.19), i.e.,

$$\frac{dy_1}{d\xi} = (\Lambda_1\beta_1 + \Lambda_2 + \Lambda_3\beta_1)\,y_1 + \Lambda_1\,(\beta_1 - 1)\,y_2 - \Lambda_1\beta_1 \tag{1}$$

$$\frac{dy_2}{d\xi} = \Lambda_2\,(\beta_2 - 1)\,y_1 + (\Lambda_1 + \Lambda_2\beta_2 + \Lambda_3\beta_2)\,y_2 - \Lambda_2\beta_2 \tag{2}$$

From the stoichiometry of the reaction, the molar fluxes are related by

$$N_1 = -N_2 = -N_3 \quad \Rightarrow \quad \Lambda_1 = -\Lambda_2 = -\Lambda_3 \tag{3}$$

The analytical solution[3] of Eqs. (1)–(3) is given by Rao (1979). From the Mathcad worksheet, the flux values are calculated as

$$N_1 = -N_2 = -N_3 = 5.654 \times 10^{-5}\,\mathrm{mol/cm^2.s}$$

Approximate solution: The MS equation for species A, Eq. (8.11), is written as

$$c\frac{dy_A}{dz} = \left(\frac{N_A}{\text{\DJ}_{AC}} + \frac{N_B}{\text{\DJ}_{AB}} + \frac{N_C}{\text{\DJ}_{AC}}\right)y_A + \left(\frac{N_A}{\text{\DJ}_{AC}} - \frac{N_A}{\text{\DJ}_{AB}}\right)y_B - \frac{N_A}{\text{\DJ}_{AC}} \tag{4}$$

Eliminating N_B and N_C in favor of N_A with the help of Eq. (3) reduces Eq. (4) to

$$N_A = -c\left[\frac{y_A}{\text{\DJ}_{AB}} + \left(\frac{1}{\text{\DJ}_{AB}} - \frac{1}{\text{\DJ}_{AC}}\right)y_B + \frac{1}{\text{\DJ}_{AC}}\right]^{-1}\frac{dy_A}{dz} \tag{5}$$

Let us define an effective diffusion coefficient, $\text{\DJ}_{eff}$, as

$$N_A = -c\text{\DJ}_{eff}\frac{dy_A}{dz} + y_A(N_A + N_B + N_C) \tag{6}$$

The use of Eq. (3) simplifies Eq. (6) to

$$N_A = -\frac{c\text{\DJ}_{eff}}{(1+y_A)}\frac{dy_A}{dz} \tag{7}$$

Comparison of Eqs. (5) and (7) indicates that

$$\text{\DJ}_{eff} = (1+y_A)\left(\frac{y_A + y_B}{\text{\DJ}_{AB}} + \frac{1-y_B}{\text{\DJ}_{AC}}\right)^{-1} \tag{8}$$

The effective diffusivity will be considered constant and is evaluated by using the average values of the mole fractions, i.e.,

$$y_A = \frac{1+0.4734}{2} = 0.7367 \qquad y_B = \frac{0+0.2633}{2} = 0.13165$$

---

[3]Readers interested in the analytical solutions of multicomponent diffusion problems involving a heterogeneous reaction may refer to Hsu and Bird (1960).

ORIGIN:= 1

T := 1400   P := 1   R := 82.05   npoints := 100

D12 := 2.19   D13 := 2.065   D23 := 1.51 δ := 0.1

$$\beta1 := \frac{D12}{D13} \qquad \beta2 := \frac{D12}{D23} \qquad c := \frac{P}{R \cdot T}$$

$$F(\xi, y, \Lambda) := \begin{bmatrix} \left(\Lambda_1 \cdot \beta1 + \Lambda_2 + \Lambda_3 \cdot \beta1\right) \cdot y_1 + \Lambda_1 \cdot (\beta1 - 1) \cdot y_2 - \Lambda_1 \cdot \beta1 \\ \Lambda_2 \cdot (\beta2 - 1) \cdot y_1 + \left(\Lambda_1 + \Lambda_2 \cdot \beta2 + \Lambda_3 \cdot \beta2\right) \cdot y_2 - \Lambda_2 \cdot \beta2 \end{bmatrix}$$

➡ Reference:C:\Users\tosun\Desktop\Subroutines\rk2.xmcd

$$yinit := \begin{pmatrix} 1 \\ 0 \end{pmatrix}$$

$$\Lambda := \begin{pmatrix} 1 \\ -1 \\ -1 \end{pmatrix} \qquad \textbf{These are the initial guess values}$$

Sol(Λ) := rk2(yinit, npoints, F, Λ)

$$y1(\Lambda) := Sol(\Lambda)^{\langle 2 \rangle} \qquad\qquad y2(\Lambda) := Sol(\Lambda)^{\langle 3 \rangle}$$

Given

$$y1(\Lambda)_{npoints+1} = 0.4734 \qquad \Lambda_1 = -\Lambda_2 \qquad \Lambda_2 = \Lambda_3$$

$$\Lambda := Find(\Lambda) = \begin{pmatrix} 0.297 \\ -0.297 \\ -0.297 \end{pmatrix}$$

$$N1 := \frac{\Lambda_1 \cdot c \cdot D12}{\delta} = 5.654 \times 10^{-5} \qquad N2 := \frac{\Lambda_2 \cdot c \cdot D12}{\delta} = -5.654 \times 10^{-5}$$

Mathcad worksheet of Example 8.7.

Thus,

$$\mathcal{D}_{eff} = (1 + 0.7367) \left(\frac{0.7367 + 0.13165}{2.065} + \frac{1 - 0.13165}{2.19} \right)^{-1} = 2.126 \, \text{cm}^2/\text{s}$$

Integration of Eq. (7) yields

$$N_A \int_0^\delta dz = -c\mathcal{D}_{eff} \int_{y_{A_o}}^{y_{A\delta}} \frac{dy_A}{1+y_A} \tag{9}$$

or

$$N_A = \frac{c\mathcal{D}_{eff}}{\delta} \ln\left(\frac{1+y_{A_o}}{1+y_{A_\delta}}\right) \tag{10}$$

Substitution of the numerical values leads to

$$N_A = \frac{(8.705 \times 10^{-6})(2.126)}{0.1} \ln\left(\frac{1+1}{1+0.4734}\right) = 5.655 \times 10^{-5} \text{mol/cm}^2.\text{s},$$

which is almost equal to the result obtained from the numerical solution.

Example 8.8 Krishna (1981) considered nonequimolar distillation of a ternary mixture of pentane (1), ethanol (2), and water (3). We are interested in the molar fluxes of species at a point in a distillation column under the conditions of vapor-phase diffusion-controlled transfer. The following data are provided:

$$P = 1 \text{ bar} \qquad T = 346 \text{ K} \qquad \delta = 10 \,\mu\text{m}$$

$$\mathcal{D}_{12} = 7.27 \,\text{mm}^2/\text{s} \qquad \mathcal{D}_{13} = 14.4 \,\text{mm}^2/\text{s} \qquad \mathcal{D}_{23} = 20.9 \,\text{mm}^2/\text{s}$$

$$y_{1_o} = 0.630 \qquad y_{2_o} = 0.165 \qquad y_{1_\delta} = 0.590 \qquad y_{2_\delta} = 0.095$$

Partial molar enthalpies (in MJ/kmol) in the vapor and liquid phases are given as

$$\overline{H}_1^V = 38 \qquad \overline{H}_2^V = 50.6 \qquad \overline{H}_3^V = 47 \qquad \overline{H}_1^L = 15.5 \qquad \overline{H}_2^L = 10.1 \qquad \overline{H}_3^L = 5$$

In this case, we have to use Eq. (8.21) as the bootstrap relation. From the Mathcad worksheet, the molar flux values are calculated as

$$N_1 = 4.596 \,\text{mol/m}^2.\text{s} \qquad N_2 = -3.035 \,\text{mol/m}^2.\text{s} \qquad N_3 = -5.388 \text{mol/m}^2.\text{s}$$

ORIGIN:= 1

T := 346   P := 1   R := $8.314 \cdot 10^{-5}$ npoints := 100

D12 := $7.27 \cdot 10^{-6}$ D13 := $14.4 \cdot 10^{-6}$ D23 := $20.9 \cdot 10^{-6}$ δ := $10 \cdot 10^{-6}$

$$HV := \begin{pmatrix} 38 \\ 50.6 \\ 47 \end{pmatrix} \qquad HL := \begin{pmatrix} 15.5 \\ 10.1 \\ 5 \end{pmatrix}$$

$$\lambda := \overrightarrow{(HV - HL)} = \begin{pmatrix} 22.5 \\ 40.5 \\ 42 \end{pmatrix}$$

$$\beta 1 := \frac{D12}{D13} \qquad \beta 2 := \frac{D12}{D23} \qquad c := \frac{P}{R \cdot T}$$

$$F(\xi, y, \Lambda) := \begin{bmatrix} \left(\Lambda_1 \cdot \beta 1 + \Lambda_2 + \Lambda_3 \cdot \beta 1\right) \cdot y_1 + \Lambda_1 \cdot (\beta 1 - 1) \cdot y_2 - \Lambda_1 \cdot \beta 1 \\ \Lambda_2 \cdot (\beta 2 - 1) \cdot y_1 + \left(\Lambda_1 + \Lambda_2 \cdot \beta 2 + \Lambda_3 \cdot \beta 2\right) \cdot y_2 - \Lambda_2 \cdot \beta 2 \end{bmatrix}$$

Mathcad worksheet of Example 8.8.

➡ Reference:C:\Users\tosun\Desktop\Subroutines\rk2.xmcd

$$\text{yinit} := \begin{pmatrix} 0.63 \\ 0.165 \end{pmatrix}$$

$$\Lambda := \begin{pmatrix} 1 \\ 1 \\ -1 \end{pmatrix} \quad \textbf{These are the initial guess values}$$

$$\text{Sol}(\Lambda) := \text{rk2}(\text{yinit}, \text{npoints}, F, \Lambda)$$

$$y1(\Lambda) := \text{Sol}(\Lambda)^{\langle 2 \rangle} \qquad\qquad y2(\Lambda) := \text{Sol}(\Lambda)^{\langle 3 \rangle}$$

Given

$$y1(\Lambda)_{\text{npoints}+1} = 0.59 \qquad y2(\Lambda)_{\text{npoints}+1} = 0.095 \qquad \Lambda_1 \cdot \lambda_1 + \Lambda_2 \cdot \lambda_2 + \Lambda_3 \cdot \lambda_3 = 0$$

$$\Lambda := \text{Find}(\Lambda) = \begin{pmatrix} 0.182 \\ 0.12 \\ -0.213 \end{pmatrix}$$

$$N1 := \frac{\Lambda_1 \cdot c \cdot D12}{\delta} = 4.596 \qquad N2 := \frac{\Lambda_2 \cdot c \cdot D12}{\delta} = 3.035 \qquad N23 := \frac{\Lambda_3 \cdot c \cdot D12}{\delta} = -5.388$$

Mathcad worksheet of Example 8.8. (*continued*)

8.2.2 TWO-BULB DIFFUSION EXPERIMENT REVISITED: UNSTEADY-STATE CASE

In Section 8.1, the reason for nitrogen to move from a region of lower concentration to one of higher concentration is explained. Now let us generate Figures 8.1–8.3, i.e., variations in species mole fractions in the bulbs as a function of time, by numerical calculations. The analysis presented below is based on a pseudosteady-state approximation.

For an ideal gas mixture, the thermodynamic factor matrix is equal to an identity matrix, i.e., $[\Gamma] = [\mathbf{I}]$, and Eq. (3.124) simplifies to

$$-c\,[\nabla x] = [\mathbf{B}]\,[\mathbf{J}^*] \tag{8.26}$$

For a ternary gas mixture involved in the two-bulb experiment, using $\mathbf{N}_i = \mathbf{J}_i^*$ Eq. (8.26) is expressed in one-dimensional form as

$$-c\frac{d}{dz}\begin{pmatrix} y_1 \\ y_2 \end{pmatrix} = \begin{pmatrix} B_{11} & B_{12} \\ B_{21} & B_{22} \end{pmatrix}\begin{pmatrix} N_1 \\ N_2 \end{pmatrix} \tag{8.27}$$

Note that the components of $[\mathbf{B}]$, defined by Eq. (3.130), are dependent on composition. To simplify the calculations, the components of $[\mathbf{B}]$ will be evaluated at the average mole fraction of species. Since $[\mathbf{B}]$ is a constant, integration of Eq. (8.27) leads to

$$-c\begin{pmatrix} y_1 \\ y_2 \end{pmatrix} = \begin{pmatrix} B_{11} & B_{12} \\ B_{21} & B_{22} \end{pmatrix}\begin{pmatrix} N_1 \\ N_2 \end{pmatrix}\begin{pmatrix} z \\ z \end{pmatrix} + \begin{pmatrix} C_1 \\ C_2 \end{pmatrix}, \tag{8.28}$$

where C_1 and C_2 are dependent on time. The use of the boundary conditions

$$\text{at} \quad z = 0 \qquad y_1 = y_1^A \quad \& \quad y_2 = y_2^A \tag{8.29}$$

$$\text{at} \quad z = \delta \qquad y_1 = y_1^B \quad \& \quad y_2 = y_2^B \tag{8.30}$$

yields the solution as

$$\frac{c}{\delta}\begin{pmatrix} y_1^A - y_1^B \\ y_2^A - y_2^B \end{pmatrix} = \begin{pmatrix} B_{11} & B_{12} \\ B_{21} & B_{22} \end{pmatrix}\begin{pmatrix} N_1 \\ N_2 \end{pmatrix}$$ (8.31)

Multiplication of Eq. (8.31) by $[\mathbf{B}]^{-1}$ from the left side gives

$$\begin{pmatrix} N_1 \\ N_2 \end{pmatrix} = \frac{c}{\delta}\begin{pmatrix} B_{11} & B_{12} \\ B_{21} & B_{22} \end{pmatrix}^{-1}\begin{pmatrix} y_1^A - y_1^B \\ y_2^A - y_2^B \end{pmatrix}$$ (8.32)

Considering bulb A as the system, the macroscopic mass balance is written as

$$V_A \frac{dc_i^A}{dt} = -A N_i \qquad i = 1, 2,$$ (8.33)

where A is the cross-sectional area of the capillary tube. Noting that $c_i^A = c y_i^A$, Eq. (8.33) is written in matrix notation as

$$c V_A \frac{d}{dt}\begin{pmatrix} y_1^A \\ y_2^A \end{pmatrix} = -A\begin{pmatrix} N_1 \\ N_2 \end{pmatrix}$$ (8.34)

Combination of Eqs. (8.32) and (8.34) yields

$$\frac{d}{dt}\begin{pmatrix} y_1^A \\ y_2^A \end{pmatrix} = -\frac{A}{V_A \delta}\begin{pmatrix} B_{11} & B_{12} \\ B_{21} & B_{22} \end{pmatrix}^{-1}\begin{pmatrix} y_1^A - y_1^B \\ y_2^A - y_2^B \end{pmatrix}$$ (8.35)

Now let us eliminate y_i^B in favor of y_i^A by using the overall mass balance in the form

$$y_i^B V_B = y_i^{eq}(V_A + V_B) - y_i^A V_A$$ (8.36)

The result is

$$\frac{d}{dt}\begin{pmatrix} y_1^A \\ y_2^A \end{pmatrix} = -\phi\begin{pmatrix} B_{11} & B_{12} \\ B_{21} & B_{22} \end{pmatrix}^{-1}\begin{pmatrix} y_1^A - y_1^{eq} \\ y_2^A - y_2^{eq} \end{pmatrix},$$ (8.37)

where

$$\phi = \frac{A(V_A + V_B)}{\delta V_A V_B}$$ (8.38)

The substitution

$$u_i^A = y_i^A - y_i^{eq}$$ (8.39)

transforms Eq. (8.37) into a set of homogeneous linear first-order ODEs:

$$\frac{d}{dt}\begin{pmatrix} u_1^A \\ u_2^A \end{pmatrix} = F\begin{pmatrix} u_1^A \\ u_2^A \end{pmatrix},$$ (8.40)

where

$$F = -\phi\begin{pmatrix} B_{11} & B_{12} \\ B_{21} & B_{22} \end{pmatrix}^{-1}$$ (8.41)

Note that the inverse matrix in Eq. (8.41) is given by Eq. (3.132) as

$$
\begin{pmatrix} B_{11} & B_{12} \\ B_{21} & B_{22} \end{pmatrix}^{-1} = \frac{1}{\Delta} \begin{pmatrix} Đ_{13}\left[x_1 Đ_{23} + (1-x_1)Đ_{12}\right] & x_1 Đ_{23}(Đ_{13} - Đ_{12}) \\ x_2 Đ_{13}(Đ_{23} - Đ_{12}) & Đ_{23}\left[x_2 Đ_{13} + (1-x_2)Đ_{12}\right] \end{pmatrix}, \quad (8.42)
$$

where

$$
\Delta = x_1 Đ_{23} + x_2 Đ_{13} + x_3 Đ_{12} \tag{8.43}
$$

The solution of Eq. (8.40) is given as

$$
\begin{pmatrix} u_1^A \\ u_2^A \end{pmatrix} = K_1 \underbrace{\begin{pmatrix} G_1 \\ G_2 \end{pmatrix}}_{[G]} e^{\lambda_1 t} + K_1 \underbrace{\begin{pmatrix} H_1 \\ H_2 \end{pmatrix}}_{[H]} e^{\lambda_2 t}, \tag{8.44}
$$

where K_1 and K_2 are constants, λ_1 and λ_2 are the eigenvalues of F, and $[G]$ and $[H]$ are the eigenvectors of F corresponding to the eigenvalues λ_1 and λ_2, respectively. The Mathcad worksheet given in Figure 8.5 shows the calculations. The variations in concentrations of species in bulbs A and B as a function of time are also tabulated below.

t	Bulb A			Bulb B		
(h)	y_1	y_2	y_3	y_1	y_2	y_3
1	0.4404	0.5280	0.0316	0.0613	0.4714	0.4673
2	0.3946	0.5479	0.0575	0.1075	0.4513	0.4412
3	0.3599	0.5610	0.0791	0.1425	0.4381	0.4194
4	0.3338	0.5690	0.0972	0.1689	0.4300	0.4011
5	0.3140	0.5734	0.1126	0.1888	0.4256	0.3856
6	0.2990	0.5752	0.1258	0.2038	0.4239	0.3723
7	0.2877	0.5751	0.1372	0.2152	0.4240	0.3608
8	0.2792	0.5736	0.1472	0.2238	0.4254	0.3508
9	0.2727	0.5713	0.1560	0.2303	0.4278	0.3419
10	0.2678	0.5684	0.1638	0.2353	0.4307	0.3340
11	0.2641	0.5651	0.1708	0.2390	0.4340	0.3270
12	0.2613	0.5617	0.1770	0.2419	0.4375	0.3206
13	0.2591	0.5582	0.1827	0.2441	0.4410	0.3149
14	0.2575	0.5546	0.1879	0.2457	0.4445	0.3098
15	0.2563	0.5512	0.1925	0.2470	0.4480	0.3050

8.3 MS EQUATIONS FOR COUPLED DRIVING FORCES

As a result of multiple driving forces existing in multicomponent systems, coupled effects come into play in expressing mass and energy fluxes. As stated by Chapman and Cowling (1970), the "... elementary theories seem to be at least as troublesome mathematically and numerically as the exact theory," and the only way to understand the mechanism of coupled effects in mass and heat transfer is through study of the rigorous kinetic theory of gases. The rigorous kinetic theory of gases is, however, beyond the scope of this textbook. Thus, the mathematical description of these coupled effects is taken directly from the literature, and the derivations of these equations are omitted.

In Chapter 3, the generalized diffusional driving forces, $\mathbf{d}_i$, are given by Eq. (3.55) in the form

$$
cRT\mathbf{d}_i = c_i \nabla_{T,P} \overline{G}_i + (c_i \overline{V}_i - \omega_i)\nabla P - \rho_i \left(\widehat{\mathbf{F}}_i - \sum_{k=1}^{N} \omega_k \widehat{\mathbf{F}}_k \right) \tag{8.45}
$$

ORIGIN:= 1

$VA := 78.63 \qquad VB := 77.99 \qquad \delta := 8.59 \qquad D := 2.08 \cdot 10^{-1}$

$$Dms := \begin{pmatrix} 0.833 \\ 0.680 \\ 0.168 \end{pmatrix} \qquad yA := \begin{pmatrix} 0.50121 \\ 0.49879 \\ 0 \end{pmatrix} \qquad yB := \begin{pmatrix} 0 \\ 0.50086 \\ 0.49914 \end{pmatrix}$$

$$A := \frac{\pi\, D^2}{4} \qquad yav := \overrightarrow{\frac{(yA + yB)}{2}} = \begin{pmatrix} 0.251 \\ 0.5 \\ 0.25 \end{pmatrix} \qquad T := 308.3 \qquad P := 1 \qquad R := 82.05$$

$$Binv := \frac{\begin{bmatrix} Dms_2 \cdot \left[yav_1 \cdot Dms_3 + \left(1 - yav_1\right) \cdot Dms_1 \right] & yav_1 \cdot Dms_3 \cdot \left(Dms_2 - Dms_1 \right) \\ yav_2 \cdot Dms_2 \cdot \left(Dms_3 - Dms_1 \right) & Dms_3 \cdot \left[yav_2 \cdot Dms_2 + \left(1 - yav_2\right) \cdot Dms_1 \right] \end{bmatrix}}{yav_1 \cdot Dms_3 + yav_2 \cdot Dms_2 + yav_3 \cdot Dms_1} = \begin{pmatrix} 0.768 & -0.011 \\ -0.383 & 0.215 \end{pmatrix}$$

$$\phi := \frac{A \cdot (VA + VB)}{\delta \cdot VA \cdot VB} = 1.01 \times 10^{-4} \qquad c := \frac{P}{R \cdot T} = 3.953 \times 10^{-5}$$

$$F := -\phi \cdot Binv = \begin{pmatrix} -7.761 \times 10^{-5} & 1.103 \times 10^{-6} \\ 3.871 \times 10^{-5} & -2.177 \times 10^{-5} \end{pmatrix}$$

$$\lambda := eigenvals\,(F) = \begin{pmatrix} -7.836 \times 10^{-5} \\ -2.101 \times 10^{-5} \end{pmatrix}$$

$$G := eigenvec\left(F, \lambda_1\right) = \begin{pmatrix} -0.825 \\ 0.565 \end{pmatrix} \qquad H := eigenvec\left(F, \lambda_2\right) = \begin{pmatrix} 0.019 \\ 1 \end{pmatrix}$$

$$yeq := \overrightarrow{\frac{VA \cdot yA + VB \cdot yB}{VA \quad VB}} = \begin{pmatrix} 0.252 \\ 0.5 \\ 0.249 \end{pmatrix}$$

$$uA := \overrightarrow{(yA - yeq)} = \begin{pmatrix} 0.25 \\ -1.031 \times 10^{-3} \\ -0.249 \end{pmatrix}$$

Given

$$uA_1 = K1 \cdot G_1 + K2 \cdot H_1$$

$$uA_2 = K1 \cdot G_2 + K2 \cdot H_2$$

$$\begin{pmatrix} K1 \\ K2 \end{pmatrix} := Find(K1, K2) \rightarrow \begin{pmatrix} -0.2984288926424931133 \\ 0.16748849076714306263 \end{pmatrix}$$

Figure 8.5 Mathcad worksheet for unsteady-state calculations of two-bulb experiment.

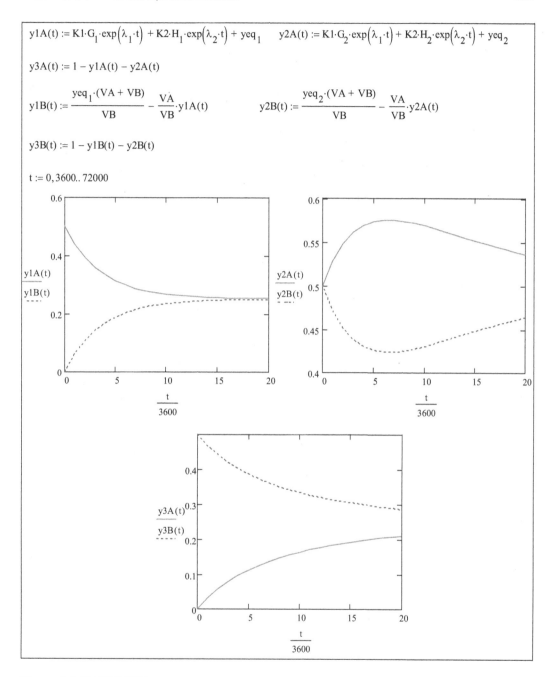

$$y1A(t) := K1 \cdot G_1 \cdot \exp(\lambda_1 \cdot t) + K2 \cdot H_1 \cdot \exp(\lambda_2 \cdot t) + yeq_1 \qquad y2A(t) := K1 \cdot G_2 \cdot \exp(\lambda_1 \cdot t) + K2 \cdot H_2 \cdot \exp(\lambda_2 \cdot t) + yeq_2$$

$$y3A(t) := 1 - y1A(t) - y2A(t)$$

$$y1B(t) := \frac{yeq_1 \cdot (VA + VB)}{VB} - \frac{VA}{VB} \cdot y1A(t) \qquad y2B(t) := \frac{yeq_2 \cdot (VA + VB)}{VB} - \frac{VA}{VB} \cdot y2A(t)$$

$$y3B(t) := 1 - y1B(t) - y2B(t)$$

$$t := 0, 3600 .. 72000$$

Figure 8.5 (CONTINUED)   Mathcad worksheet for unsteady-state calculations of two-bulb experiment.

From the development given in Section 3.2.1, the first term on the right side of Eq. (8.45) is expressed as

$$c_i \nabla_{T,P} \overline{G}_i = cRT \sum_{k=1}^{\mathcal{N}-1} \Gamma_{ik} \nabla x_k, \tag{8.46}$$

where

$$\Gamma_{ik} = \delta_{ik} + x_i \left(\frac{\partial \ln \gamma_i}{\partial x_k} \right)_{T,P,x_{j \neq k}} \tag{8.47}$$

The term $\widehat{\mathbf{F}}_i$ is the body force per unit mass acting on species i. In the case of a gravitational force, i.e., $\widehat{\mathbf{F}}_i = \mathbf{g}$, the third term on the right side of Eq. (8.45) becomes

$$\rho_i \left(\widehat{\mathbf{F}}_i - \sum_{k=1}^{\mathcal{N}} \omega_k \widehat{\mathbf{F}}_k \right) = \rho_i \left(\mathbf{g} - \mathbf{g} \sum_{k=1}^{\mathcal{N}} \omega_k \right) = 0 \tag{8.48}$$

Therefore, there is no effect of gravity on the diffusional force.

For nonisothermal systems, the diffusive mass flux with reference to mass-average velocity is given by Bird et al. (2007) as

$$\mathbf{j}_i = -D_i^T \nabla \ln T + \rho_i \sum_{k=1}^{\mathcal{N}} \mathfrak{D}_{ik} \mathbf{d}_k, \tag{8.49}$$

where D_i^T are *multicomponent thermal diffusion coefficients* in mass/(length)(time) and $\mathfrak{D}_{ik}$ are *multicomponent Fick diffusion coefficients*. The inversion of the mass flux expression is expressed in the form

$$\mathbf{d}_i = -\sum_{\substack{k=1 \\ k \neq i}}^{\mathcal{N}} \frac{x_i x_k}{\text{\DH}_{ik}} \left(\frac{D_i^T}{\rho_i} - \frac{D_k^T}{\rho_k} \right) \nabla \ln T - \sum_{\substack{k=1 \\ k \neq i}}^{\mathcal{N}} \frac{x_i x_k}{\text{\DH}_{ik}} \underbrace{\left(\frac{\mathbf{j}_i}{\rho_i} - \frac{\mathbf{j}_k}{\rho_k} \right)}_{\mathbf{v}_i - \mathbf{v}_k} \tag{8.50}$$

$\text{\DH}_{ik}$ are called *multicomponent MS diffusion coefficients*, and their relationship to the $\mathfrak{D}_{ik}$ is given by Curtiss and Bird (1999) and Bird et al. (2007). Combining Eqs. (8.45) and (8.50) yields

$$\sum_{\substack{k=1 \\ k \neq i}}^{\mathcal{N}} \frac{x_i x_k}{\text{\DH}_{ik}} (\mathbf{v}_i - \mathbf{v}_k) = -\sum_{k=1}^{\mathcal{N}-1} \Gamma_{ik} \nabla x_k - \sum_{\substack{k=1 \\ k \neq i}}^{\mathcal{N}} \frac{x_i x_k}{\text{\DH}_{ik}} \left(\frac{D_i^T}{\rho_i} - \frac{D_k^T}{\rho_k} \right) \nabla \ln T$$

$$- \frac{1}{cRT} \left[(c_i \overline{V}_i - \omega_i) \nabla P - \rho_i \left(\widehat{\mathbf{F}}_i - \sum_{k=1}^{\mathcal{N}} \omega_k \widehat{\mathbf{F}}_k \right) \right] \tag{8.51}$$

For binary diffusion in gases and liquids, Eq. (8.51) reduces to (Bird et al., 2007)

$$\mathbf{J}_A^* = -c\text{\DH}_{AB} \left\{ \left(1 + \frac{\partial \ln \gamma_A}{\partial \ln x_A} \right) \nabla x_A + k_T \nabla \ln T \right.$$

$$\left. + \frac{1}{cRT} \left[(c_A \overline{V}_A - \omega_A) \nabla P - \rho \omega_A \omega_B \left(\widehat{\mathbf{F}}_A - \widehat{\mathbf{F}}_B \right) \right] \right\}, \tag{8.52}$$

where k_T is the *thermal diffusion ratio*, defined by

$$k_T = \left(\frac{D_A^T}{\rho \text{\DH}_{AB}} \right) \left(\frac{x_A x_B}{\omega_A \omega_B} \right) \tag{8.53}$$

It is dimensionless and may be positive or negative.

8.3.1 DIFFUSION INDUCED BY A TEMPERATURE GRADIENT (THERMAL DIFFUSION)

Let us consider two bulbs connected by an insulated tube of small diameter and filled with an ideal gas mixture of A and B. The bulbs are maintained at constant temperatures of T_1 and T_2 ($T_2 > T_1$), respectively. We are interested in the composition of gases in the two bulbs when the system reaches equilibrium. At equilibrium, $\mathbf{J}_A^* = 0$ and Eq. (8.52) reduces to

$$\nabla y_A + k_T \nabla \ln T = 0 \tag{8.54}$$

For a one-dimensional case with the positive z-direction directing from the bulb at T_2 to the bulb at T_1, i.e., $dT/dz < 0$, Eq. (8.54) is written as

$$\frac{dy_A}{dz} = -\frac{k_T}{T}\frac{dT}{dz} \tag{8.55}$$

Depending on whether k_T is positive or negative, the movement of species A will be as follows:

$$
\begin{array}{llll}
k_T > 0 & dy_A/dz > 0 & \text{Species } A \text{ moves to the colder bulb} \\
k_T < 0 & dy_A/dz < 0 & \text{Species } A \text{ moves to the warmer bulb}
\end{array} \tag{8.56}
$$

It is customary to neglect the variation in k_T with temperature when it is evaluated at a mean temperature T_m, defined by

$$T_m = \frac{T_1 T_2}{T_2 - T_1}\ln\left(\frac{T_2}{T_1}\right) \tag{8.57}$$

Hence, integration of Eq. (8.55) yields

$$\boxed{y_{A_2} - y_{A_1} = -k_T(T_m)\ln\left(\frac{T_2}{T_1}\right)} \tag{8.58}$$

Example 8.9 A gas mixture consisting of 15 mol% deuterium (A) and 85% hydrogen (B) is charged into the two-bulb apparatus. The bulbs are kept at temperatures of 200 and 650K. The thermal diffusion ratio at the mean temperature is 0.017. Substitution of the numerical values into Eq. (8.58) gives

$$y_{A_2} - y_{A_1} = -(0.017)\ln\left(\frac{650}{200}\right) = -0.02$$

Thus, the mole fraction of deuterium in the colder bulb is greater than that in the warmer bulb by 0.02.

Comment: The existence of a temperature gradient causes a concentration gradient to build up in an initially uniform mixture. This phenomenon is called *thermal diffusion* or the *Soret effect*.

8.3.2 DIFFUSION INDUCED BY A PRESSURE GRADIENT (PRESSURE DIFFUSION)

A typical example for pressure diffusion is the use of an ultracentrifuge for the separation of macromolecules. Consider a small cylindrical cell containing a binary liquid mixture and rotating at a constant angular velocity Ω in an ultracentrifuge. The centrifugal force exerted on a unit mass of species i in a mixture is given by

$$\widehat{F}_i = \Omega^2 r, \tag{8.59}$$

where r is the radial distance from the axis of rotation. Substitution of Eq. (8.59) into Eq. (8.45) yields

$$cRT\mathbf{d}_i = cRT\sum_{k=1}^{\mathcal{N}-1}\Gamma_{ik}\nabla x_k + (c_i\overline{V}_i - \omega_i)\nabla P \tag{8.60}$$

For an isothermal system ($\nabla T = 0$) under steady-state conditions ($\mathbf{j}_i = 0$), Eq. (8.49) indicates that $\mathbf{d}_i = 0$. Thus, the r-component of Eq. (8.60) for a binary system is written as

$$cRT\left(1 + x_i\frac{d\ln\gamma_i}{dx_i}\right)\frac{dx_i}{dr} + (c_i\overline{V}_i - \omega_i)\frac{\partial P}{\partial r} = 0 \tag{8.61}$$

The equation of motion is expressed as

$$\rho \frac{D\mathbf{v}}{Dt} = -\nabla P - \nabla \cdot \tau + \rho \widehat{\mathbf{F}} \tag{8.62}$$

Noting that v_r and v_z are zero, the r-component of the equation of motion gives

$$0 = -\frac{\partial P}{\partial r} + \rho \Omega^2 r \tag{8.63}$$

Substitution of Eq. (8.63) into Eq. (8.61) gives

$$\left(1 + x_i \frac{d \ln \gamma_i}{d x_i}\right) \frac{d x_i}{d r} = (\omega_i - c_i \overline{V}_i) \frac{M \Omega^2 r}{RT}, \tag{8.64}$$

where M is the molecular weight of the mixture. For the separation to take place, mass fraction must be different from volume fraction so that $\omega_i - c_i \overline{V}_i \neq 0$. For an ideal mixture, i.e., $\gamma_i = 1$, Eq. (8.64) reduces to

$$\frac{d x_i}{d r} = (\omega_i - c_i \overline{V}_i) \frac{M \Omega^2 r}{RT} \tag{8.65}$$

Integration of Eq. (8.65) yields the concentration profile.

8.3.3 DIFFUSION INDUCED BY AN ELECTROSTATIC POTENTIAL GRADIENT

In the case of transport of ionic species in electrolyte solutions, electrostatic potential gradient comes into play. Electrical force per unit mole is given by

$$\widetilde{\mathbf{F}}_i = -z_i \mathbf{F} \nabla \psi, \tag{8.66}$$

where z_i is the ionic charge (or valence), $\mathbf{F}$ is Faraday's constant ($96,485.3 \, C/mol$), and ψ is the electrostatic potential (V). The electrostatic potential indicates the amount of work needed to move a unit charge from a reference point to a specific point against an electric field. The electrical force per unit mass, $\widehat{\mathbf{F}}_i$, is given by

$$\widehat{\mathbf{F}}_i = -\frac{z_i \mathbf{F}}{M_i} \nabla \psi \tag{8.67}$$

Substitution of Eq. (8.67) into the third term on the right side of Eq. (8.45) gives

$$\rho_i \left(\widehat{\mathbf{F}}_i - \sum_{k=1}^{\mathcal{N}} \omega_k \widehat{\mathbf{F}}_k\right) = -c_i \mathbf{F} \nabla \psi \left(z_i - M_i \sum_{k=1}^{\mathcal{N}} \frac{\omega_k z_k}{M_k}\right) \tag{8.68}$$

Noting that $\omega_k / M_k = x_k / M$, Eq. (8.68) takes the form

$$\rho_i \left(\widehat{\mathbf{F}}_i - \sum_{k=1}^{\mathcal{N}} \omega_k \widehat{\mathbf{F}}_k\right) = -c_i \mathbf{F} \nabla \psi \left(z_i - \frac{M_i}{M} \sum_{k=1}^{\mathcal{N}} x_k z_k\right) \tag{8.69}$$

The electroneutrality principle states that the number of positive and negative charges in a mixture must be the same.[1] In other words, the sum of all charges must be zero, i.e.,

$$\sum_{k=1}^{\mathcal{N}} x_k z_k = 0, \tag{8.70}$$

---

[1] The electroneutrality principle does not hold near charged surfaces.

so that Eq. (8.69) simplifies to

$$\rho_i \left(\widehat{\mathbf{F}}_i - \sum_{k=1}^{\mathcal{N}} \omega_k \widehat{\mathbf{F}}_k \right) = -\mathbf{F} c_i z_i \nabla \psi \tag{8.71}$$

Substitution of Eq. (8.71) into Eq. (8.45) and expressing $\mathbf{d}_i$ with the help of Eq. (3.77) lead to

$$\sum_{\substack{k=1 \\ k \neq i}}^{\mathcal{N}} \frac{x_i \mathbf{J}_k^* - x_k \mathbf{J}_i^*}{\mathcal{D}_{ik}} = c \sum_{k=1}^{\mathcal{N}-1} \Gamma_{ik} \nabla x_k + \frac{(c_i \overline{V}_i - \omega_i)}{RT} \nabla P + \left(\frac{\mathbf{F}}{RT} \right) c_i z_i \nabla \psi \tag{8.72}$$

The left side of Eq. (8.72) is expanded as

$$\sum_{\substack{k=1 \\ k \neq i}}^{\mathcal{N}} \frac{x_i \mathbf{J}_k^* - x_k \mathbf{J}_i^*}{\mathcal{D}_{ik}} = x_i \sum_{\substack{k=1 \\ k \neq i}}^{\mathcal{N}} \frac{\mathbf{J}_k^*}{\mathcal{D}_{ik}} - \mathbf{J}_i^* \sum_{\substack{k=1 \\ k \neq i}}^{\mathcal{N}} \frac{x_k}{\mathcal{D}_{ik}} \tag{8.73}$$

For a dilute (the dominant component is usually water) solution, i.e., $x_i \ll 1$, it is plausible to assume that

$$\mathbf{J}_i^* \sum_{\substack{k=1 \\ k \neq i}}^{\mathcal{N}} \frac{x_k}{\mathcal{D}_{ik}} \gg x_i \sum_{\substack{k=1 \\ k \neq i}}^{\mathcal{N}} \frac{\mathbf{J}_k^*}{\mathcal{D}_{ik}} \tag{8.74}$$

In addition, defining the ionic diffusion coefficient in water as

$$\frac{1}{\mathcal{D}_{iw}} = \sum_{\substack{k=1 \\ k \neq i}}^{\mathcal{N}} \frac{x_k}{\mathcal{D}_{ik}} \tag{8.75}$$

simplifies Eq. (8.73) to

$$\sum_{\substack{k=1 \\ k \neq i}}^{\mathcal{N}} \frac{x_i \mathbf{J}_k^* - x_k \mathbf{J}_i^*}{\mathcal{D}_{ik}} \simeq -\frac{\mathbf{J}_i^*}{\mathcal{D}_{iw}} \tag{8.76}$$

In the absence of pressure diffusion, substitution of Eq. (8.76) into (8.72) gives the *Nernst–Planck equation*:

$$\boxed{\mathbf{J}_i^* = -\mathcal{D}_{iw} \nabla c_i - \left(\frac{\mathbf{F}}{RT} \right) c_i z_i \mathcal{D}_{iw} \nabla \psi} \qquad i = 1, 2, \ldots, \mathcal{N}-1 \tag{8.77}$$

PROBLEMS

8.1 Consider absorption of species 1 from a ternary gas mixture into a nonvolatile liquid as described in Example 8.2. Calculate the molar flux of species 1 using the following data:

$$P = 1\,\text{atm} \qquad T = 298\,\text{K} \qquad \mathcal{D}_{12} = 0.32\,\text{cm}^2/\text{s} \qquad \mathcal{D}_{13} = 0.58\,\text{cm}^2/\text{s} \qquad \delta = 0.15\,\text{cm}$$

$$y_{1_o} = 0.12 \qquad y_{1_\delta} = 0.45 \qquad y_{2_\delta} = 0.17 \qquad y_{3_\delta} = 0.38$$

(Answer: $-5.816 \times 10^{-5}\,\text{mol/cm}^2.\text{s}$)

8.2 Consider steady-state diffusion of species 1 and 2 at 330K and 1atm through a stagnant gas (species 3) film of thickness 0.15cm. The compositions of the species at the film boundaries are given in the table below:

	Mole Fraction	
Species	$z = 0$ cm	$z = 0.15$ cm
1	0.00	0.15
2	0.28	0.00
3	0.72	0.85

If the MS diffusion coefficients are given as

$$\text{Đ}_{12} = 0.15\,\text{cm}^2/\text{s} \qquad \text{Đ}_{13} = 0.10\,\text{cm}^2/\text{s} \qquad \text{Đ}_{23} = 0.23\,\text{cm}^2/\text{s}$$

calculate the molar fluxes of species 1 and 2.

(Answer: $N_1 = -3.294 \times 10^{-6}\,\text{mol/cm}^2.\text{s}$, $N_2 = 1.698 \times 10^{-5}\,\text{mol/cm}^2.\text{s}$)

8.3 Ammonia (1) is diffusing from a gas mixture containing ammonia and air (3) into water (2) at 0.20265 bar and 328.15 K.[2] Assume that the diffusion takes place through a stagnant gas layer of 1 mm thickness. At one point in the apparatus, the gas contains 3% ammonia by volume, and the concentration of ammonia in the water is so low that the partial pressure of ammonia over the solution may be neglected at the position under consideration. The bulk gas is dry. Allowing for water vaporization, calculate the rate of diffusion of ammonia by using the following data:

$$P_2^{vap} = 0.07359\,\text{bar} \qquad \text{Đ}_{12} = 147\,\text{mm}^2/\text{s} \qquad \text{Đ}_{13} = 107.5\,\text{mm}^2/\text{s} \qquad \text{Đ}_{23} = 124.5\,\text{mm}^2/\text{s}$$

Take $z = 0$ as the interface and $z = \delta$ as the bulk gas phase.

(Answer: $N_1 = -0.0211\,\text{mol/m}^2.\text{s}$, $N_2 = 0.4136\,\text{mol/m}^2.\text{s}$)

8.4 A falling liquid film consisting of acetone (1) and benzene (2) is brought into contact with a downward flowing turbulent gas mixture of acetone, benzene, and helium (3). Calculate the molar fluxes of acetone and benzene for the following conditions:[3]

$$P = 1.013\,\text{bar} \qquad T = 301.1\,\text{K} \qquad \delta = 1.34\,\text{mm}$$

$$\text{Đ}_{12} = 4\,\text{mm}^2/\text{s} \qquad \text{Đ}_{13} = 41\,\text{mm}^2/\text{s} \qquad \text{Đ}_{23} = 39\,\text{mm}^2/\text{s}$$

$$y_{1_o} = 0.082 \qquad y_{2_o} = 0.118 \qquad y_{1_\delta} = 0.116 \qquad y_{2_\delta} = 0.030$$

(Answer: $N_1 = 0.0134\,\text{mol/m}^2.\text{s}$, $N_2 = 0.0642\,mol/\text{m}^2.\text{s}$)

8.5 Calculate the condensation rates of ammonia (1) and water vapor (2) in the presence of inert hydrogen (3) for the following conditions:[4]

$$P = 3.404\,\text{bar} \qquad T = 366.38\,\text{K} \qquad \delta = 10\,\text{mm}$$

$$\text{Đ}_{12} = 29.4\,\text{mm}^2/\text{s} \qquad \text{Đ}_{13} = 113\,\text{mm}^2/\text{s} \qquad \text{Đ}_{23} = 130\,\text{mm}^2/\text{s}$$

$$y_{1_o} = 0.455 \qquad y_{2_o} = 0.195 \qquad y_{1_\delta} = 0.3 \qquad y_{2_\delta} = 0.4$$

(Answer: $N_1 = -0.0388\,\text{mol/m}^2.\text{s}$, $N_2 = -0.1793\,\text{mol/m}^2.\text{s}$)

---

[2] This problem is taken from Krishna (1979).

[3] This problem is taken from Krishna (1979).

[4] This problem is taken from Krishna (1979).

8.6 The following data are provided for a ternary mixture of helium (1), sulfur hexafluoride (2), and oxygen (3) at 1bar and 310K (Tai and Chang, 1979):

$$Đ_{12} = 43.534\,\text{mm}^2/\text{s} \qquad Đ_{13} = 79.150\,\text{mm}^2/\text{s} \qquad Đ_{23} = 9.993\,\text{mm}^2/\text{s}$$

$$\delta = 0.3\,\text{mm} \qquad y_{1_o} = 0 \qquad y_{2_o} = 0.25 \qquad y_{1_\delta} = 1 \qquad y_{2_\delta} = 0$$

$$M_1 = 4.003\,\text{g/mol} \qquad M_2 = 146.06\,\text{g/mol} \qquad M_3 = 31.999\,\text{g/mol}$$

a) Calculate the molar fluxes (in $\text{mol/m}^2.\text{s}$) of the species using Eq. (8.22).

b) Calculate the molar fluxes (in $\text{mol/m}^2.\text{s}$) of the species using Eq. (8.23).

(Answer: a) $N_1 = -23.43$, $N_2 = 0.211$, $N_3 = 1.97\,\text{mol/m}^2.\text{s}$ b) $N_1 = -14.975$, $N_2 = 0.787$, $N_3 = 3.614$)

8.7 For the distillation of a ternary mixture of acetic acid (1), water (2), and methanol (3) at 1 atm and 371.25K, Krishna (2017) provided the following data:

$$Đ_{12} = 24.5\,\text{mm}^2/\text{s} \qquad Đ_{13} = 15\,\text{mm}^2/\text{s} \qquad Đ_{23} = 30.4\,\text{mm}^2/\text{s}$$

$$\delta = 1\,\text{mm} \qquad y_{1_o} = 0.64 \qquad y_{2_o} = 0.20 \qquad y_{1_\delta} = 0.3386 \qquad y_{2_\delta} = 0.33078$$

$$\Delta\widetilde{H}_1^{vap} = 23.5\,\text{kJ/mol} \qquad \Delta\widetilde{H}_2^{vap} = 40.7\,\text{kJ/mol} \qquad \Delta\widetilde{H}_3^{vap} = 35.43\,\text{kJ/mol}$$

a) Calculate the molar fluxes (in $\text{mol/m}^2.\text{s}$) of the species.

b) Calculate the molar fluxes (in $\text{mol/m}^2.\text{s}$) by assuming equimolar counterdiffusion.

(Answer: a) $N_1 = 0.23264$, $N_2 = -0.08203$, $N_3 = -0.06007\,\text{mol/m}^2.\text{s}$ b) $N_1 = 0.1879$, $N_2 = -0.106$, $N_3 = -0.0819\,\text{mol/m}^2.\text{s}$)

8.8 For equimolar counterdiffusion of a ternary gas mixture, Toor (1957) provided the following equations:

$$\beta_1(1-\beta_2)\Lambda_1 + \beta_2(1-\beta_1)\Lambda_2 = (1-\beta_2)(y_{1_o}-y_{1_\delta}) + (1-\beta_1)(y_{2_o}-y_{2_\delta}) \tag{1}$$

$$(1-\beta_2)\Lambda_1 + (1-\beta_1)\Lambda_2 = \ln\left[\frac{\dfrac{y_{1_\delta}}{\Lambda_1} - \dfrac{y_{2_\delta}}{\Lambda_2} - \dfrac{\beta_1-\beta_2}{(1-\beta_2)\Lambda_1 + (1-\beta_1)\Lambda_2}}{\dfrac{y_{1_o}}{\Lambda_1} - \dfrac{y_{2_o}}{\Lambda_2} - \dfrac{\beta_1-\beta_2}{(1-\beta_2)\Lambda_1 + (1-\beta_1)\Lambda_2}}\right], \tag{2}$$

where the dimensionless quantities are defined by Eq. (8.17). Simultaneous solution of Eqs. (1) and (2) yields molar fluxes.

a) Derive Eqs. (1) and (2).

b) Resolve part (b) of Problem 8.7 by using Eqs. (1) and (2). As pointed out by Krishna (2017), Eqs. (1) and (2) may result in multiple solutions depending on the starting guess values for Λ_1 and Λ_2. Assuming that an approximate solution is a straight line connecting the appropriate boundary points and using the values at $z = 0$, Eqs. (22) and (23) of Problem 8.10 give the initial guess values as

$$\Lambda_1^{(0)} = \frac{Đ_{23}\Omega y_{1_o} - y_{1_\delta} + y_{1_o}}{(\beta_1/\beta_2)y_{1_o} + y_{2_o} + \beta_1 y_{3_o}} \tag{3}$$

$$\Lambda_2^{(0)} = \frac{Đ_{13}\Omega y_{2_o} - y_{2_\delta} + y_{2_o}}{y_{1_o} + (\beta_2/\beta_1)y_{2_o} + \beta_1 y_{3_o}} \tag{4}$$

(Answer: $N_1 = 0.1879\,\text{mol/m}^2.\text{s}$, $N_2 = -0.106\,\text{mol/m}^2.\text{s}$, $N_3 = -0.0819\,\text{mol/m}^2.\text{s}$)

8.9 Let Θ be a square matrix of order $(\mathcal{N}-1)$ with components

$$\Theta_{ii} = \frac{\mathbf{N}_i}{c\,\mathcal{D}_{i\mathcal{N}}} + \sum_{\substack{k=1 \\ k\neq i}}^{\mathcal{N}} \frac{\mathbf{N}_k}{c\,\mathcal{D}_{ik}} \qquad \text{and} \qquad \Theta_{ik} = \left(\frac{\mathbf{N}_i}{c\,\mathcal{D}_{i\mathcal{N}}} - \frac{\mathbf{N}_i}{c\,\mathcal{D}_{ik}}\right) \quad i\neq k, \tag{1}$$

and Φ be a $(\mathcal{N}-1)$ column vector with components

$$\Phi_i = \frac{\mathbf{N}_i}{c\,\mathcal{D}_{i\mathcal{N}}}, \tag{2}$$

a) Show that Eq. (8.8) is expressed in matrix notation as

$$[\nabla x] = [\Theta]\,[x] + [\Phi], \tag{3}$$

which is a system of linear ODEs with constant coefficients.

b) Krishna and Standart (1976) showed that the solution of Eq. (3) is given by

$$(x - x_o) = \underbrace{\exp\left[[\Theta]\,\xi - [I]\right]\left[\exp[\Theta] - [I]\right]^{-1}}_{[F]}(x_\delta - x_o), \tag{4}$$

where $[I]$ is an identity matrix. Taylor and Krishna (1993) showed that

$$[F] = \left[\frac{\exp(\lambda_1\xi)-1}{\exp(\lambda_1)-1}\right]\frac{\left[[\Theta]-\lambda_2[I]\right]}{\lambda_1-\lambda_2} + \left[\frac{\exp(\lambda_2\xi)-1}{\exp(\lambda_2)-1}\right]\frac{\left[[\Theta]-\lambda_1[I]\right]}{\lambda_2-\lambda_1}, \tag{5}$$

where λ_1 and λ_2 are the distinct eigenvalues of the matrix $[\Theta]$. Resolve Problem 8.5 by using this procedure.

8.10 For a ternary gas mixture, instead of using the MS equations given by Eqs. (8.15) and (8.16), Amundson et al. (2003) inverted these equations for the case of equimolar counterdiffusion as follows:

a) Starting with the set of equations in the form

$$c\frac{dy_1}{dz} = -\left(\frac{y_2}{\mathcal{D}_{12}} + \frac{y_3}{\mathcal{D}_{13}}\right)N_1 + \frac{y_1}{\mathcal{D}_{12}}N_2 + \frac{y_1}{\mathcal{D}_{13}}N_3 \tag{1}$$

$$c\frac{dy_2}{dz} = \frac{y_2}{\mathcal{D}_{12}}N_1 - \left(\frac{y_1}{\mathcal{D}_{12}} + \frac{y_3}{\mathcal{D}_{23}}\right)N_2 + \frac{y_2}{\mathcal{D}_{23}}N_3 \tag{2}$$

$$0 = N_1 + N_2 + N_3 \tag{3}$$

use Cramer's rule as explained in Section C.5 in Appendix C to obtain

$$\begin{pmatrix} N_1 \\ N_2 \\ N_3 \end{pmatrix} = -\frac{c}{\Delta} \begin{pmatrix} \dfrac{1-y_1}{\mathcal{D}_{23}} & -\dfrac{y_1}{\mathcal{D}_{13}} & -\dfrac{y_1}{\mathcal{D}_{12}} \\ -\dfrac{y_2}{\mathcal{D}_{23}} & \dfrac{1-y_2}{\mathcal{D}_{13}} & -\dfrac{y_2}{\mathcal{D}_{12}} \\ -\dfrac{y_3}{\mathcal{D}_{23}} & -\dfrac{y_3}{\mathcal{D}_{13}} & \dfrac{1-y_3}{\mathcal{D}_{12}} \end{pmatrix} \cdot \begin{pmatrix} \dfrac{dy_1}{dz} \\ \dfrac{dy_2}{dz} \\ \dfrac{dy_3}{dz} \end{pmatrix}, \tag{4}$$

where

$$\Delta = \frac{y_1\mathcal{D}_{23} + y_2\mathcal{D}_{13} + y_3\mathcal{D}_{12}}{\mathcal{D}_{12}\mathcal{D}_{13}\mathcal{D}_{23}} \tag{5}$$

b) Multiply Eq. (4) by the diagonal matrix

$$
\begin{pmatrix}
Đ_{23} & 0 & 0 \\
0 & Đ_{13} & 0 \\
0 & 0 & Đ_{12}
\end{pmatrix}
\tag{6}
$$

to obtain

$$
Đ_{23} N_1 = -\frac{c}{\Delta}\left[(1-y_1)\frac{dy_1}{dz} - \frac{Đ_{23}}{Đ_{13}}y_1\frac{dy_2}{dz} - \frac{Đ_{23}}{Đ_{12}}y_1\frac{dy_3}{dz}\right]
\tag{7}
$$

$$
Đ_{13} N_2 = -\frac{c}{\Delta}\left[-\frac{Đ_{13}}{Đ_{23}}y_2\frac{dy_1}{dz} + (1-y_2)\frac{dy_2}{dz} - \frac{Đ_{13}}{Đ_{12}}y_2\frac{dy_3}{dz}\right]
\tag{8}
$$

$$
Đ_{12} N_3 = -\frac{c}{\Delta}\left[-\frac{Đ_{12}}{Đ_{23}}y_3\frac{dy_1}{dz} - \frac{Đ_{12}}{Đ_{13}}y_3\frac{dy_2}{dz} + (1-y_3)\frac{dy_3}{dz}\right]
\tag{9}
$$

c) Show that the addition of Eqs. (7)–(9) and rearrangement give

$$
\frac{N_1}{Đ_{12}Đ_{13}} + \frac{N_2}{Đ_{12}Đ_{23}} + \frac{N_3}{Đ_{13}Đ_{23}} = c\left(\frac{1}{Đ_{23}}\frac{dy_1}{dz} + \frac{1}{Đ_{13}}\frac{dy_2}{dz} + \frac{1}{Đ_{12}}\frac{dy_3}{dz}\right)
\tag{10}
$$

d) Integrate Eq. (10) from $z = 0$ to $z = \delta$ to obtain

$$
\frac{N_1}{Đ_{12}Đ_{13}} + \frac{N_2}{Đ_{12}Đ_{23}} + \frac{N_3}{Đ_{13}Đ_{23}} = c\frac{\Omega}{\delta},
\tag{11}
$$

where

$$
\Omega = \frac{y_{1\delta} - y_{1_o}}{Đ_{23}} + \frac{y_{2\delta} - y_{2_o}}{Đ_{13}} + \frac{y_{3\delta} - y_{3_o}}{Đ_{12}}
\tag{12}
$$

e) First substitute Eq. (11) into Eq. (10) to obtain

$$
\frac{1}{Đ_{23}}\frac{dy_1}{dz} + \frac{1}{Đ_{13}}\frac{dy_2}{dz} + \frac{1}{Đ_{12}}\frac{dy_3}{dz} = \frac{\Omega}{\delta}
\tag{13}
$$

and then use Eq. (13) in the molar flux expressions given by Eq. (4) to show that

$$
N_1 = -\frac{c}{\Delta}\left(\frac{1}{Đ_{23}}\frac{dy_1}{dz} - \frac{\Omega}{\delta}y_1\right)
\tag{14}
$$

$$
N_2 = -\frac{c}{\Delta}\left(\frac{1}{Đ_{13}}\frac{dy_2}{dz} - \frac{\Omega}{\delta}y_2\right)
\tag{15}
$$

$$
N_3 = -\frac{c}{\Delta}\left(\frac{1}{Đ_{12}}\frac{dy_3}{dz} - \frac{\Omega}{\delta}y_3\right)
\tag{16}
$$

f) In terms of the dimensionless quantities

$$
\xi = \frac{z}{\delta} \qquad \Lambda_1 = \frac{N_1\delta}{cĐ_{12}} \qquad \Lambda_2 = \frac{N_2\delta}{cĐ_{12}} \qquad \Lambda_3 = \frac{N_3\delta}{cĐ_{12}}
\tag{21}
$$

show that Eqs. (14)–(16) transform into

$$
-\frac{dy_1}{d\xi} + Đ_{23}\Omega y_1 = \Lambda_1\left[\left(\frac{Đ_{23}}{Đ_{13}}\right)y_1 + y_2 + \left(\frac{Đ_{12}}{Đ_{13}}\right)y_3\right]
\tag{22}
$$

$$-\frac{dy_2}{d\xi} + Đ_{13}\Omega y_2 = \Lambda_2 \left[y_1 + \left(\frac{Đ_{13}}{Đ_{23}}\right) y_2 + \left(\frac{Đ_{12}}{Đ_{23}}\right) y_3 \right] \tag{23}$$

$$-\frac{dy_3}{d\xi} + Đ_{12}\Omega y_3 = \Lambda_3 \left[\left(\frac{Đ_{12}}{Đ_{13}}\right) y_1 + \left(\frac{Đ_{12}}{Đ_{23}}\right) y_2 + \left(\frac{Đ_{12}^2}{Đ_{13}Đ_{23}}\right) y_3 \right] \tag{24}$$

What is the advantage of using Eqs. (22)–(24) over Eqs. (1)–(3)?

8.11 Consider equimolar counterdiffusion in a ternary gas mixture of H_2 (1), N_2(2), and CO_2 (3) at 1 atm and 308.35 K. Krishna (2017) provided the following data:

$$Đ_{12} = 8.33 \times 10^{-5}\,m^2/s \qquad Đ_{13} = 6.8 \times 10^{-5}\,m^2/s \qquad Đ_{23} = 1.68 \times 10^{-5}\,m^2/s$$

$$\delta = 1\,mm \qquad y_{1_o} = 0 \qquad y_{2_o} = 0.50086 \qquad y_{1_\delta} = 0.25061 \qquad y_{2_\delta} = 0.49982$$

Calculate the molar fluxes of the species.

(Answer: $N_1 = -0.749\,mol/m^2.s$, $N_2 = 0.328\,mol/m^2.s$, $N_3 = 0.421\,mol/m^2.s$)

8.12 Consider the case when the semi-infinite medium assumption in Example 6.2 does not hold. Thus, the governing equation and its associated initial and boundary conditions are given as

$$\frac{\partial c_A}{\partial t} = D_{AB}\frac{\partial^2 c_A}{\partial z^2} \tag{1}$$

$$\text{at} \quad t = 0 \qquad c_A = 0 \tag{2}$$

$$\text{at} \quad z = 0 \qquad c_A = c_{A_o} \tag{3}$$

$$\text{at} \quad z = L \qquad \frac{\partial c_A}{\partial z} = 0 \tag{4}$$

a) Show that the solution is

$$c_A = c_{A_o}\left\{ 1 - \frac{2}{\pi}\sum_{n=0}^{\infty}\frac{1}{2n+1}\exp\left[-\frac{(2n+1)^2\pi^2 D_{AB}t}{4L^2}\right]\sin\left[\frac{(2n+1)\pi z}{2L}\right] \right\} \tag{5}$$

b) Instead of a binary mixture, let us consider a ternary system. In matrix notation, the governing equations are expressed in the form

$$\frac{\partial}{\partial t}\begin{pmatrix} c_1 \\ c_2 \end{pmatrix} = \begin{pmatrix} \mathcal{D}_{11}^* & \mathcal{D}_{12}^* \\ \mathcal{D}_{21}^* & \mathcal{D}_{22}^* \end{pmatrix}\frac{\partial^2}{\partial z^2}\begin{pmatrix} c_1 \\ c_2 \end{pmatrix} \tag{6}$$

or

$$\frac{\partial}{\partial t}[c] = [\mathcal{D}^*]\frac{\partial^2}{\partial z^2}[c] \tag{7}$$

As stated by Eq. (C.39) in Appendix C, a nonsingular square matrix $[\mathcal{D}^*]$ can be expressed in the form of

$$[\mathcal{D}^*] = [P][A][P]^{-1}, \tag{8}$$

where $[P]$ is a square matrix of eigenvectors and $[A]$ is the diagonal matrix with the eigenvalues on the diagonal. Thus, the matrix $[A]$ is

$$[A] = \begin{pmatrix} \lambda_1 & 0 \\ 0 & \lambda_2 \end{pmatrix}, \tag{9}$$

where the eigenvalues are given by

$$\lambda_1 = \frac{\mathcal{D}_{11}^* + \mathcal{D}_{22}^* + \sqrt{(\mathcal{D}_{11}^* - \mathcal{D}_{22}^*)^2 + 4\mathcal{D}_{12}^* \mathcal{D}_{21}^*}}{2} \tag{10}$$

$$\lambda_2 = \frac{\mathcal{D}_{11}^* + \mathcal{D}_{22}^* - \sqrt{(\mathcal{D}_{11}^* - \mathcal{D}_{22}^*)^2 + 4\mathcal{D}_{12}^* \mathcal{D}_{21}^*}}{2} \tag{11}$$

On the other hand, the matrix $[P]$ is given by

$$[P] = \begin{pmatrix} 1 & \dfrac{\mathcal{D}_{12}^*}{\lambda_2 - \mathcal{D}_{11}^*} \\ \dfrac{\lambda_1 - \mathcal{D}_{11}^*}{\mathcal{D}_{12}^*} & 1 \end{pmatrix} \tag{12}$$

Hence, the inverse of the matrix $[P]$ is

$$[P]^{-1} = \frac{\mathcal{D}_{11}^* - \lambda_2}{\lambda_1 - \lambda_2} \begin{pmatrix} 1 & \dfrac{\mathcal{D}_{12}^*}{\mathcal{D}_{11}^* - \lambda_2} \\ \dfrac{\mathcal{D}_{11}^* - \lambda_1}{\mathcal{D}_{12}^*} & 1 \end{pmatrix} \tag{13}$$

Substitute Eq. (8) into Eq. (7) to obtain

$$\frac{\partial}{\partial t}[c] = [P][A][P]^{-1} \frac{\partial^2}{\partial z^2}[c] \tag{14}$$

c) Show that the multiplication of Eq. (14) by $[P]^{-1}$ from the left side yields

$$\frac{\partial}{\partial t}[P]^{-1}[c] = [A]\frac{\partial^2}{\partial z^2}[P]^{-1}[c] \tag{15}$$

d) Show that defining another concentration variable φ in the form

$$[\varphi] = [P]^{-1}[c] \tag{16}$$

transforms Eq. (15) into

$$\frac{\partial}{\partial t}[\varphi] = [A]\frac{\partial^2}{\partial z^2}[\varphi] \tag{17}$$

or

$$\frac{\partial}{\partial t}\begin{pmatrix} \varphi_1 \\ \varphi_2 \end{pmatrix} = \begin{pmatrix} \lambda_1 & 0 \\ 0 & \lambda_2 \end{pmatrix} \frac{\partial^2}{\partial z^2}\begin{pmatrix} \varphi_1 \\ \varphi_2 \end{pmatrix} \tag{18}$$

Note that Eq. (18) results in two uncoupled equations with the following initial and boundary conditions:

$$\text{at} \quad t = 0 \quad [\varphi] = [0] \tag{19}$$

$$\text{at} \quad z = 0 \quad [\varphi] = [\varphi_o] \tag{20}$$

$$\text{at} \quad z = L \quad \frac{\partial}{\partial z}[\varphi] = [0] \tag{21}$$

This procedure of decoupling the governing equations was first suggested by Cussler (2009).

e) With the help of Eq. (5), show that the solutions are expressed as

$$\varphi_1 = \varphi_{1_o} K_1 \tag{22}$$

$$\varphi_2 = \varphi_{2_o} K_2, \tag{23}$$

where

$$K_1 = 1 - \frac{2}{\pi} \sum_{n=0}^{\infty} \frac{1}{2n+1} \exp\left[-\frac{(2n+1)^2 \pi^2 \lambda_1 t}{4L^2}\right] \sin\left[\frac{(2n+1)\pi z}{2L}\right] \tag{24}$$

$$K_2 = 1 - \frac{2}{\pi} \sum_{n=0}^{\infty} \frac{1}{2n+1} \exp\left[-\frac{(2n+1)^2 \pi^2 \lambda_2 t}{4L^2}\right] \sin\left[\frac{(2n+1)\pi z}{2L}\right] \tag{25}$$

f) Use Eq. (16) to show that

$$\varphi_1 = \Omega c_1 + \frac{\mathcal{D}_{12}^*}{\lambda_1 - \lambda_2} c_2 \quad \text{and} \quad \varphi_2 = -\frac{\mathcal{D}_{21}^*}{\lambda_1 - \lambda_2} c_1 + \Omega c_2, \tag{26}$$

where

$$\Omega = \frac{\mathcal{D}_{11}^* - \lambda_2}{\lambda_1 - \lambda_2} \tag{27}$$

g) Show that the use of Eq. (26) in Eqs. (22) and (23) leads to

$$\Omega c_1 + \frac{\mathcal{D}_{12}^*}{\lambda_1 - \lambda_2} c_2 = \left(\Omega c_{1_o} + \frac{\mathcal{D}_{12}^*}{\lambda_1 - \lambda_2} c_{2_o}\right) K_1 \tag{28}$$

$$-\frac{\mathcal{D}_{21}^*}{\lambda_1 - \lambda_2} c_1 + \Omega c_2 = \left(-\frac{\mathcal{D}_{21}^*}{\lambda_1 - \lambda_2} c_{1_o} + \Omega c_{2_o}\right) K_2 \tag{29}$$

h) From Eqs. (28) and (29), show that the concentrations are expressed as

$$\begin{pmatrix} c_1 \\ c_2 \end{pmatrix} = \begin{pmatrix} \Omega & \dfrac{\mathcal{D}_{12}^*}{\lambda_1 - \lambda_2} \\ -\dfrac{\mathcal{D}_{21}^*}{\lambda_1 - \lambda_2} & \Omega \end{pmatrix}^{-1} \begin{pmatrix} \left(\Omega c_{1_o} + \dfrac{\mathcal{D}_{12}^*}{\lambda_1 - \lambda_2} c_{2_o}\right) K_1 \\ \left(-\dfrac{\mathcal{D}_{21}^*}{\lambda_1 - \lambda_2} c_{1_o} + \Omega c_{2_o}\right) K_2 \end{pmatrix} \tag{30}$$

REFERENCES

Amundson, N. R., T. W. Pan and V. I. Paulsen. 2003. Diffusing with Stefan and Maxwell. *AIChE J.* 49(4):813–30.

Arnold, K. R. and H. L. Toor. 1967. Unsteady diffusion in ternary gas mixtures. *AIChE J.* 13:909–14.

Benítez, J. 2009. *Principles and Modern Applications of Mass Transfer Operations*, 2nd edn. Hoboken: Wiley.

Bird R. B., W. E. Stewart and E. N. Lightfoot. 2007. *Transport Phenomena*, 2nd edn. New York: Wiley.

Carty, R. and T. Schrodt. 1975. Concentration profiles in ternary gaseous diffusion. *Ind. Eng. Chem. Fundam.* 14(3):276–78.

Chapman, S. and T. G. Cowling. 1970. *The Mathematical Theory of Non-Uniform Gases*, 3rd edn. Cambridge: Cambridge University Press.

Curtiss, C. F. and R. B. Bird. 1999. Multicomponent diffusion. *Ind. Eng. Chem. Res.* 38:2515–22; errata, 2001. 40:1791.

Cussler, E. L. 2009. *Diffusion – Mass Transfer in Fluid Systems*, 3rd edn. Cambridge: Cambridge University Press.

Duncan, J. B. and H. L. Toor. 1962. An experimental study of three component gas diffusion. *AIChE J.* 8(1):38–41.

Hsu, H. W. and R. B. Bird. 1960. Multicomponent diffusion problems. *AIChE J.* 6(3):516–24.

Krishna, R. 1981. An alternative linearized theory of multicomponent mass transfer. *Chem. Eng. Sci.* 36:219–22.

Krishna, R. 2016. Diffusing uphill with James Clerk Maxwell and Josef Stefan. *Curr. Opin. Chem. Eng.* 12:106–19.

Krishna, R. 2017. Highlighting multiplicity in the Gilliland solution to the Maxwell-Stefan equations describing diffusion distillation. *Chem. Eng. Sci.* 164:63–70.

Krishna, R. and G. L. Standart. 1976. A multicomponent film model incorporating a general matrix method of solution to the Maxwell-Stefan equations. *AIChE J.* 22(2):383–89.

Rao, Y. K. 1979. Diffusion-limited heterogeneous processes. *Can. Metall. Quart.* 18:379–81.

Tai, R. C. and H. K. Chang. 1979. A mathematical study of non-equimolar ternary gas diffusion. *B. Math. Biol.* 41:591–606.

Taylor, R. and R. Krishna. 1993. *Multicomponent Mass Transfer*. New York: Wiley.

Toor, H. L. 1957. Diffusion in three-component gas mixtures. *AIChE J.* 3(2):198–207.

9 Approximate Solution of the Species Continuity Equation

Solution of the species continuity equation gives the concentration profile as a function of position and time. When the governing equation(s) for mass transfer appears as a partial differential equation (PDE), the solution usually requires tedious and complex analytical and/or numerical techniques. In most experimental studies related to mass transfer, the measured quantity is not the local concentration but either the average or bulk concentration. As a result, in engineering analysis, once the concentration distribution is obtained, comparison of the experimental and theoretical results requires the average (or bulk) concentration to be determined. The practical question to ask at this stage is: "Is it possible to obtain the average concentration in a simpler way without solving the governing PDE?"

Instead of solving for the local concentration, an alternative approach is to obtain the average concentration by integrating the governing equation over either the area or the volume of the system. Since integration eliminates position dependence, the averaging procedure paves the way to an equation simpler to solve by reducing the number of independent variables by one. The averaged equation, however, not only contains the average concentration but also the local concentration and/or its gradient, both evaluated on the system boundaries. This is the price one must pay for such simplification. To proceed further, local concentration and/or its gradient on the system boundaries must be related to the average concentration. This task is accomplished by the use of Hermite polynomials.

In this chapter, first mathematical preliminaries for the two-point Hermite expansion are provided, and then the averaging technique is applied to various mass transfer problems and compared with the exact solutions. The problems considered here are taken from Özyilmaz (1996) and Dalgiç (2008).

9.1 TWO-POINT HERMITE EXPANSION

Mennig et al. (1983) used a two-point Hermite interpolation formula to solve linear initial and boundary value problems. They derived the Hermite expansion in two different forms. The first one is in integro-differential form represented by

$$\int_a^b f(x)\,dx = \sum_{n=0}^{a} C_n(\alpha,\beta)(b-a)^{n+1} \left.\frac{d^n f(x)}{dx^n}\right|_{x=a}$$
$$+ \sum_{n=0}^{\beta} C_n(\beta,\alpha)(-1)^n (b-a)^{n+1} \left.\frac{d^n f(x)}{dx^n}\right|_{x=b}, \tag{9.1}$$

which expresses the integral $\int_a^b f(x)\,dx$ as a linear combination of $f(a)$, $f(b)$, and their derivatives. The second formula is in purely differential form represented by

$$f(x)|_{x=b} - f(x)|_{x=a} = \sum_{n=0}^{a} C_n(\alpha,\beta)(b-a)^{n+1} \left.\frac{d^{n+1} f(x)}{dx^{n+1}}\right|_{x=a}$$
$$+ \sum_{n=0}^{\beta} C_n(\beta,\alpha)(-1)^n (b-a)^{n+1} \left.\frac{d^{n+1} f(x)}{dx^{n+1}}\right|_{x=b} \tag{9.2}$$

Table 9.1

List of Hermite Coefficients $C_n(\alpha, \beta)$

α	β	$C_0(\alpha,\beta)$	$C_1(\alpha,\beta)$	$C_2(\alpha,\beta)$	$C_3(\alpha,\beta)$	$C_4(\alpha,\beta)$
0	0	1/2				
0	1	1/3				
0	2	1/4				
0	3	1/5				
0	4	1/6				
1	0	2/3	1/6			
1	1	2/4	1/12			
1	2	2/5	1/20			
1	3	2/6	1/30			
1	4	2/7	1/42			
2	0	3/4	3/12	1/24		
2	1	3/5	3/20	1/60		
2	2	3/6	3/30	1/120		
2	3	3/7	3/42	1/210		
2	4	3/8	3/56	1/336		
3	0	4/5	6/20	4/60	1/120	
3	1	4/6	6/30	4/120	1/360	
3	2	4/7	6/42	4/210	1/840	
3	3	4/8	6/56	4/336	1/1,680	
3	4	4/9	6/72	4/504	1/1024	
4	0	5/6	10/30	10/120	5/360	1/720
4	1	5/7	10/42	10/210	5/840	1/2,520
4	2	5/8	10/56	10/336	5/1,680	1/6,720
4	3	5/9	10/72	10/504	5/3,024	1/15,120
4	4	5/10	10/90	10/720	5/5,040	1/30,240

Source: (Mennig et al., 1983)

The coefficients $C_n(\alpha, \beta)$ that appear in Eqs. (9.1) and (9.2) are called *Hermite coefficients*, and some values of $C_n(\alpha, \beta)$ given by Mennig et al. are listed in Table 9.1.

Approximate expressions representing

$$I = \frac{1}{b-a} \int_a^b f(x)\, dx \tag{9.3}$$

can be obtained by first substituting coefficients $C_n(\alpha, \beta)$ into Eqs. (9.1) and (9.2) and then combining them. Depending on the values of α and β, the results are given in Tables 9.2–9.5.

9.2 DRUG RELEASE FROM A SLAB

A long slab of thickness L, length H, and width W is initially at a uniform concentration of c_{A_o}. At $t = 0$, while the surface at $z = 0$ is exposed to fluid having a bulk concentration of $c_{A_{b_1}}$, the surface at $z = L$ is exposed to fluid having a bulk concentration of $c_{A_{b_2}}$. The mass transfer coefficients between the fluids and the surfaces located at $z = 0$ and $z = L$ are k_{c_1} and k_{c_2}, respectively. The schematic representation of the system is shown in Figure 9.1. It is required to determine the variation in average concentration with time.

Table 9.2

Two-Point Hermite Expansions for $\alpha = 0$ and $\beta = 0$

$$I = \frac{1}{2}\left[f(x)|_{x=a} + f(x)|_{x=b}\right] \qquad (A)$$

$$I = f(x)|_{x=a} + \frac{b-a}{4}\left(\frac{df}{dx}\bigg|_{x=a} + \frac{df}{dx}\bigg|_{x=b}\right) \qquad (B)$$

$$I = f(x)|_{x=b} - \frac{b-a}{4}\left(\frac{df}{dx}\bigg|_{x=a} + \frac{df}{dx}\bigg|_{x=b}\right) \qquad (C)$$

Table 9.3

Two-Point Hermite Expansions for $\alpha = 1$ and $\beta = 0$

$$I = \frac{2}{3}f(x)|_{x=a} + \frac{1}{3}f(x)|_{x=b} + \frac{b-a}{6}\frac{df}{dx}\bigg|_{x=a} \qquad (A)$$

$$I = \frac{5}{12}f(x)|_{x=a} + \frac{7}{12}f(x)|_{x=b} - \frac{b-a}{12}\frac{df}{dx}\bigg|_{x=b} - \frac{(b-a)^2}{24}\frac{df}{dx}\bigg|_{x=a} \qquad (B)$$

$$I = f(x)|_{x=a} + \frac{7(b-a)}{18}\frac{df}{dx}\bigg|_{x=a} + \frac{b-a}{9}\frac{df}{dx}\bigg|_{x=b} + \frac{(b-a)^2}{18}\frac{d^2f}{dx^2}\bigg|_{x=a} \qquad (C)$$

$$I = f(x)|_{x=b} - \frac{5(b-a)}{18}\frac{df}{dx}\bigg|_{x=a} - \frac{2(b-a)}{9}\frac{df}{dx}\bigg|_{x=b} - \frac{(b-a)^2}{9}\frac{d^2f}{dx^2}\bigg|_{x=a} \qquad (D)$$

Table 9.4

Two-Point Hermite Expansions for $\alpha = 0$ and $\beta = 1$

$$I = \frac{1}{3}f(x)|_{x=a} + \frac{2}{3}f(x)|_{x=b} - \frac{b-a}{6}\frac{df}{dx}\bigg|_{x=b} \qquad (A)$$

$$I = \frac{7}{12}f(x)|_{x=a} + \frac{5}{12}f(x)|_{x=b} + \frac{b-a}{12}\frac{df}{dx}\bigg|_{x=a} - \frac{(b-a)^2}{24}\frac{df}{dx}\bigg|_{x=b} \qquad (B)$$

$$I = f(x)|_{x=a} + \frac{2(b-a)}{9}\frac{df}{dx}\bigg|_{x=a} + \frac{5(b-a)}{18}\frac{df}{dx}\bigg|_{x=b} - \frac{(b-a)^2}{9}\frac{d^2f}{dx^2}\bigg|_{x=b} \qquad (C)$$

$$I = f(x)|_{x=b} - \frac{b-a}{9}\frac{df}{dx}\bigg|_{x=a} - \frac{7(b-a)}{18}\frac{df}{dx}\bigg|_{x=b} + \frac{(b-a)^2}{18}\frac{d^2f}{dx^2}\bigg|_{x=b} \qquad (D)$$

For $L/W \ll 1$ and $L/H \ll 1$, the equation of continuity for species A, Eq. (A) in Table 6.1, takes the form

$$\frac{\partial c_A}{\partial t} = \mathcal{D}_{AB}\frac{\partial^2 c_A}{\partial z^2} \qquad (9.4)$$

Table 9.5

Two-Point Hermite Expansions for $\alpha = 1$ and $\beta = 1$

$$I = \frac{1}{3} f(x)|_{x=a} + \frac{2}{3} f(x)|_{x=b} - \frac{b-a}{6} \left.\frac{df}{dx}\right|_{x=b} \tag{A}$$

$$I = \frac{7}{12} f(x)|_{x=a} + \frac{5}{12} f(x)|_{x=b} + \frac{b-a}{12} \left.\frac{df}{dx}\right|_{x=a} - \frac{(b-a)^2}{24} \left.\frac{df}{dx}\right|_{x=b} \tag{B}$$

$$I = f(x)|_{x=a} + \frac{2(b-a)}{9} \left.\frac{df}{dx}\right|_{x=a} + \frac{5(b-a)}{18} \left.\frac{df}{dx}\right|_{x=b} - \frac{(b-a)^2}{9} \left.\frac{d^2f}{dx^2}\right|_{x=b} \tag{C}$$

$$I = f(x)|_{x=b} - \frac{b-a}{9} \left.\frac{df}{dx}\right|_{x=a} - \frac{7(b-a)}{18} \left.\frac{df}{dx}\right|_{x=b} + \frac{(b-a)^2}{18} \left.\frac{d^2f}{dx^2}\right|_{x=b} \tag{D}$$

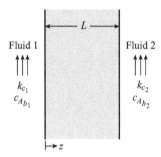

Figure 9.1   Drug release from a slab.

with the following initial and boundary conditions:

$$\text{at} \quad t = 0 \qquad c_A = c_{A_o} \tag{9.5}$$

$$\text{at} \quad z = 0 \qquad \mathcal{D}_{AB} \frac{\partial c_A}{\partial z} = \frac{k_{c_1}}{K_A} \left(c_A - K_A c_{A_{b_1}} \right) \tag{9.6}$$

$$\text{at} \quad z = L \qquad -\mathcal{D}_{AB} \frac{\partial c_A}{\partial z} = \frac{k_{c_2}}{K_A} \left(c_A - K_A c_{A_{b_2}} \right), \tag{9.7}$$

where K_A is the partition coefficient. Introduction of the dimensionless quantities

$$\theta = \frac{c_A - K_A c_{A_{b_1}}}{c_{A_o} - K_A c_{A_{b_1}}} \qquad \tau = \frac{\mathcal{D}_{AB} t}{L^2} \qquad \xi = \frac{z}{L}$$

$$\text{Bi}_{M_1} = \frac{k_{c_1} L}{K_A \mathcal{D}_{AB}} \qquad \text{Bi}_{M_2} = \frac{k_{c_2} L}{K_A \mathcal{D}_{AB}} \qquad \Omega = \text{Bi}_{M_2} K_A \left(\frac{c_{A_{b_1}} - c_{A_{b_2}}}{c_{A_o} - K_A c_{A_{b_1}}} \right) \tag{9.8}$$

reduces Eqs. (9.4)–(9.7) to

$$\frac{\partial \theta}{\partial \tau} = \frac{\partial^2 \theta}{\partial \xi^2} \tag{9.9}$$

$$\text{at} \quad \tau = 0 \qquad \theta = 1 \tag{9.10}$$

$$\text{at} \quad \xi = 0 \qquad \frac{\partial \theta}{\partial \xi} = \text{Bi}_{M_1} \theta \tag{9.11}$$

$$\text{at} \quad \xi = 1 \qquad -\frac{\partial \theta}{\partial \xi} = \text{Bi}_{M_2} \theta + \Omega \tag{9.12}$$

9.2.1 ANALYTICAL SOLUTION

Since the boundary condition at $\xi = 1$ is nonhomogeneous, the dimensionless concentration distribution is proposed in the form

$$\theta(\tau,\xi) = \theta_\infty(\xi) + \theta_t(\tau,\xi) \tag{9.13}$$

so that Eq. (9.9) is split into two differential equations: $\theta_\infty(\xi)$ and $\theta_t(\tau,\xi)$, being the steady-state and transient solutions, respectively. Using the procedure given in Example E.9, the solution is

$$\theta = -\frac{\Omega}{\Lambda}(1 + \mathrm{Bi_{M_1}}\,\xi) - \sum_{n=1}^{\infty} C_n\, e^{-\lambda_n^2 \tau} \left[\cos(\lambda_n \xi) + \frac{\mathrm{Bi_{M_1}}}{\lambda_n} \sin(\lambda_n \xi) \right], \tag{9.14}$$

where

$$\Lambda = \mathrm{Bi_{M_1}} + \mathrm{Bi_{M_2}} + \mathrm{Bi_{M_1}}\,\mathrm{Bi_{M_2}} \tag{9.15}$$

The coefficients C_n are given by

$$C_n = \frac{2}{X_n}\left(\mathrm{Bi_{M_2}^2} + \lambda_n^2\right)\left[\mathrm{Bi_{M_1}}(\cos\lambda_n - 1) - \lambda_n \sin\lambda_n + \Omega Y_n \right], \tag{9.16}$$

where

$$X_n = \mathrm{Bi_{M_1}}\,\mathrm{Bi_{M_2}}\,\Lambda + \left(\mathrm{Bi_{M_1}} + \mathrm{Bi_{M_2}} + \mathrm{Bi_{M_1}^2} + \mathrm{Bi_{M_2}^2}\right)\lambda_n^2 + \lambda_n^4 \tag{9.17}$$

$$Y_n = \frac{\mathrm{Bi_{M_1}^2}\,\lambda_n \cos\lambda_n - \sin\lambda_n\left(\lambda_n^2\,\mathrm{Bi_{M_1}} + \lambda_n^2 + \mathrm{Bi_{M_1}}\right)}{\Lambda\,\lambda_n} \tag{9.18}$$

The eigenvalues λ_n are the roots of the following transcendental equation:

$$\tan\lambda_n = \frac{\lambda_n\left(\mathrm{Bi_{M_1}} + \mathrm{Bi_{M_2}}\right)}{\lambda_n^2 - \mathrm{Bi_{M_1}}\,\mathrm{Bi_{M_2}}} \tag{9.19}$$

The first ten eigenvalues for different combinations of Biot numbers are given in Table 9.6.

Table 9.6
The Eigenvalues for Different Combinations of Biot Numbers

	λ_n		
n	$\mathrm{Bi_{M_1}} = 1,\ \mathrm{Bi_{M_2}} = 0.1$	$\mathrm{Bi_{M_1}} = 5,\ \mathrm{Bi_{M_2}} = 1$	$\mathrm{Bi_{M_1}} = 10,\ \mathrm{Bi_{M_2}} = 1$
1	0.9293	1.7523	1.8753
2	3.4523	4.2406	4.5073
3	6.4532	7.0417	7.3549
4	9.5396	9.9888	10.2923
5	12.6528	13.0100	13.2869
6	15.7771	16.0716	16.3189
7	18.9071	19.1570	19.3775
8	22.0404	22.2570	22.4546
9	25.1757	25.3667	25.5445
10	28.3124	28.4831	28.6450

The average concentration is defined by

$$\langle c_A \rangle = \frac{1}{L} \int_0^L c_A \, dz \tag{9.20}$$

In terms of the dimensionless quantities, Eq. (9.20) takes the form

$$\langle \theta \rangle = \frac{\langle c_A \rangle - K_A c_{A_{b_1}}}{c_{A_o} - K_A c_{A_{b_1}}} = \int_0^1 \theta \, d\xi \tag{9.21}$$

Substitution of Eq. (9.14) into Eq. (9.21) and integration lead to

$$\langle \theta \rangle_{exact} = -\frac{\Omega}{2\Lambda}(2 + \mathrm{Bi_{M_1}}) - \sum_{n=1}^{\infty} \frac{C_n}{\lambda_n} e^{-\lambda_n^2 \tau} \left[\sin \lambda_n - \frac{\mathrm{Bi_{M_1}}}{\lambda_n}(\cos \lambda_n - 1) \right] \tag{9.22}$$

9.2.2 APPROXIMATE SOLUTION BY AREA AVERAGING

Area averaging is performed by integrating Eq. (9.9) in the direction of mass transfer, i.e., z-direction. For this purpose, Eq. (9.9) is multiplied by $d\xi$ and integrated from $\xi = 0$ to $\xi = 1$. The result is

$$\int_0^1 \frac{\partial \theta}{\partial \tau} \, d\xi = \int_0^1 \frac{\partial^2 \theta}{\partial \xi^2} \, d\xi \tag{9.23}$$

or

$$\frac{d}{d\tau} \int_0^1 \theta \, d\xi = \frac{\partial \theta}{\partial \xi} \Big|_{\xi=1} - \frac{\partial \theta}{\partial \xi} \Big|_{\xi=0} \tag{9.24}$$

Substitution of Eq. (9.21) into the left side and the boundary conditions defined by Eqs. (9.11) and (9.12) into the right side of Eq. (9.24) gives

$$\frac{d\langle \theta \rangle}{d\tau} = -\left(\mathrm{Bi_{M_2}} \, \theta|_{\xi=1} + \mathrm{Bi_{M_1}} \, \theta|_{\xi=0} + \Omega \right) \tag{9.25}$$

To proceed further, it is necessary to express $\theta|_{\xi=1}$ and $\theta|_{\xi=0}$ in terms of the average concentration.

The Hermite expansion of $\langle \theta \rangle$, defined by Eq. (9.21), for $\alpha = 1$ and $\beta = 0$ using Eq. (A) in Table 9.3 results in

$$\langle \theta \rangle = \int_0^1 \theta \, d\xi = \frac{2}{3} \theta|_{\xi=0} + \frac{1}{3} \theta|_{\xi=1} + \frac{1}{6} \frac{\partial \theta}{\partial \xi} \Big|_{\xi=0} \tag{9.26}$$

On the other hand, the Hermite expansion of $\langle \theta \rangle$ for $\alpha = 0$ and $\beta = 1$ using Eq. (A) in Table 9.4 yields

$$\langle \theta \rangle = \int_0^1 \theta \, d\xi = \frac{1}{3} \theta|_{\xi=0} + \frac{2}{3} \theta|_{\xi=1} - \frac{1}{6} \frac{\partial \theta}{\partial \xi} \Big|_{\xi=1} \tag{9.27}$$

Substitution of the boundary conditions defined by Eqs. (9.11) and (9.12) into Eqs. (9.26) and (9.27), respectively, and the simultaneous solution of the resulting equations yield

$$\theta|_{\xi=0} = \frac{6}{\omega}\left(2 + \text{Bi}_{M_2}\right)\langle\theta\rangle + \frac{2\Omega}{\omega} \tag{9.28}$$

$$\theta|_{\xi=1} = \frac{6}{\omega}\left(2 + \text{Bi}_{M_1}\right)\langle\theta\rangle - \frac{\Omega}{\omega}\left(4 + \text{Bi}_{M_1}\right), \tag{9.29}$$

where

$$\omega = \left(4 + \text{Bi}_{M_1}\right)\left(4 + \text{Bi}_{M_2}\right) - 4 \tag{9.30}$$

Substitution of Eqs. (9.28) and (9.29) into Eq. (9.25) gives

$$\frac{d\langle\theta\rangle}{d\tau} + \frac{12}{\Lambda}\langle\theta\rangle = -\frac{6}{\omega}\left(2 + \text{Bi}_{M_1}\right)\Omega \tag{9.31}$$

The initial condition associated with Eq. (9.31) is

$$\text{at} \quad \tau = 0 \quad \langle\theta\rangle = 1 \tag{9.32}$$

The solution of Eq. (9.31) gives the average dimensionless concentration as

$$\langle\theta\rangle_{approx.} = -\frac{\Omega}{2\Lambda}\left(2 + \text{Bi}_{M_1}\right) + \left[1 + \frac{\Omega}{2\Lambda}\left(2 + \text{Bi}_{M_1}\right)\right]\exp\left(-\frac{12\Lambda}{\omega}\tau\right) \tag{9.33}$$

9.2.3 COMPARISON OF RESULTS

A comparison of the analytical solution, Eq. (9.22), with the approximate one, Eq. (9.33), for $\Omega = 1$ and different combinations of Biot numbers is given in Table 9.7. When the Biot number is small, concentration distribution within the slab is almost uniform. As the Biot number increases, concentration distribution within the slab starts to develop. The term Ω takes into account the difference between the bulk concentrations.

As can be seen from the values given in Table 9.7, the approximate values are very close to the exact ones. Since the dimensionless average concentration, $\langle\theta\rangle$, is defined as

$$\langle\theta\rangle = \frac{\langle c_A\rangle - K_A c_{A_{b_1}}}{c_{A_o} - K_A c_{A_{b_1}}} \tag{9.34}$$

Note that $\langle\theta\rangle$ takes negative values when $\langle c_A\rangle < K_A c_{A_{b_1}}$, which occurs for large values of τ.

Since different alternatives exist for the Hermite expansion depending on the choice of α and β values, the legitimate question to ask at this point is, how to pick suitable α and β values? The boundary conditions of the problem obviously impose a constraint in choosing α and β values. In addition, the limiting cases of the approximate solution should be investigated. For example, when $\tau \to \infty$, Eqs. (9.22) and (9.33) both reduce to

$$\langle\theta\rangle_\infty = -\frac{\Omega}{2\Lambda}\left(2 + \text{Bi}_{M_1}\right) \tag{9.35}$$

This implies that the analytical and approximate solutions are identical when the system reaches steady-state. Although this does not necessarily imply that the values of α and β used in the Hermite expansion are the correct choice, the chance of them being correct is fairly high.

The dimensionless time needed to reach steady-state, τ_∞, and the dimensionless average concentration under steady conditions, $\langle\theta\rangle_\infty$, are given in Table 9.8. As the Biot number increases, the external (fluid) resistance to mass transfer decreases. As a result, the system reaches steady conditions in a shorter time.

Table 9.7

Numerical Results of Eqs. (9.22) and (9.33) for Different Combinations of Bi_M

τ	$Bi_{M_1} = 1, Bi_{M_2} = 0.1$		$Bi_{M_1} = 5, Bi_{M_2} = 1$		$Bi_{M_1} = 10, Bi_{M_2} = 1$	
	$\langle\theta\rangle_{exact}$	$\langle\theta\rangle_{approx.}$	$\langle\theta\rangle_{exact}$	$\langle\theta\rangle_{approx.}$	$\langle\theta\rangle_{exact}$	$\langle\theta\rangle_{approx.}$
0.00	1.0000	1.0000	1.0000	1.0000	1.0000	1.0000
0.01	0.9799	0.9804	0.9454	0.9582	0.9258	0.9518
0.10	0.8124	0.8120	0.6218	0.6371	0.5670	0.5919
0.20	0.6420	0.6396	0.3717	0.3742	0.3119	0.3134
0.30	0.4856	0.4817	0.1891	0.1836	0.1344	0.1232
0.50	0.2103	0.2044	-0.0437	-0.0546	-0.0778	-0.0952
0.70	-0.0213	-0.0286	-0.1697	-0.1798	-0.1828	-0.1969
1.00	-0.3018	-0.3099	-0.2591	-0.2655	-0.2499	-0.2575
1.25	-0.4859	-0.4942	-0.2907	-0.2946	-0.2708	-0.2748
1.50	-0.6343	-0.6424	-0.3054	-0.3076	-0.2795	-0.2815
2.00	-0.8502	-0.8572	-0.3154	-0.3161	-0.2847	-0.2851

Table 9.8

The Values of τ_∞ and $\langle\theta\rangle_\infty$ as a Function of Biot Numbers

Bi_{M_1}	Bi_{M_2}	τ_∞	$\langle\theta\rangle_\infty$
1	0.1	12.3	-1.250
5	1	2.9	-0.318
10	1	2.6	-0.286

9.2.4 LIMITING CASE FOR EQUAL BULK CONCENTRATIONS

When the bulk concentrations are the same, the term Ω equals zero, and Eq. (9.22) simplifies to

$$\langle\theta\rangle_{exact} = -\sum_{n=1}^{\infty} \frac{C_n^*}{\lambda_n} e^{-\lambda_n^2 \tau} \left[\sin\lambda_n - \frac{Bi_{M_1}}{\lambda_n}(\cos\lambda_n - 1)\right], \tag{9.36}$$

where

$$C_n^* = \frac{2}{X_n}\left(Bi_{M_2}^2 + \lambda_n^2\right)\left[Bi_{M_1}(\cos\lambda_n - 1) - \lambda_n \sin\lambda_n\right] \tag{9.37}$$

On the other hand, the approximate solution given by Eq. (9.33) reduces to

$$\langle\theta\rangle_{approx.} = \exp\left(-\frac{12\Lambda}{\omega}\tau\right) \tag{9.38}$$

9.3 DIFFUSION INTO A SLAB FROM A LIMITED VOLUME OF SOLUTION

9.3.1 ANALYTICAL SOLUTION

This problem is analyzed in Section 6.6, and the fractional uptake is given by Eq. (6.212), i.e.,

$$\boxed{\left(\frac{\mathbb{N}_A}{\mathbb{N}_{A_\infty}}\right)_{exact} = 1 - 2\sum_{n=1}^{\infty}\frac{\Omega(1+\Omega)}{1+\Omega+\Omega^2\lambda_n^2}e^{-\lambda_n^2\tau},} \tag{9.39}$$

Table 9.9

The Eigenvalues as a Function of Ω

	λ_n		
n	$\Omega = 1$	$\Omega = 10$	$\Omega = 50$
1	2.0288	1.6320	1.5834
2	4.9132	4.7335	4.7166
3	7.9787	7.8667	7.8565
4	11.0855	11.0047	10.9974
5	14.2074	14.1442	14.1386
6	17.3364	17.2845	17.2799
7	20.4692	20.4252	20.4213
8	23.6043	23.5662	23.5628
9	26.7409	26.7073	26.7043
10	29.8786	29.8485	29.8458

where the eigenvalues are the roots of the following transcendental equation:

$$\tan \lambda_n = -\Omega \lambda_n \tag{9.40}$$

The first ten eigenvalues for various values of Ω are given in Table 9.9.

9.3.2 APPROXIMATE SOLUTION BY AREA AVERAGING

The average concentration is defined by

$$\langle c \rangle = \frac{\displaystyle\int_0^L c \, dz}{\displaystyle\int_0^L dz} = \frac{1}{L} \int_0^L c \, dz = \int_0^1 c \, d\xi, \tag{9.41}$$

where $\xi = z/L$. Dividing Eq. (9.41) by Kc_{s_0} yields the average dimensionless concentration as

$$\boxed{\langle \theta \rangle = \frac{\langle c \rangle}{Kc_{s_0}} = \int_0^1 \theta \, d\xi} \tag{9.42}$$

The solute uptake of the slab is

$$\mathbb{N}_A = 2AL \langle c \rangle = 2ALKc_{s_0} \langle \theta \rangle \tag{9.43}$$

The maximum amount of solute transferred into the slab is given by Eq. (6.211) as

$$\mathbb{N}_{A_\infty} = 2ALKc_{s_0} \left(\frac{1+\Omega}{\Omega} \right) \tag{9.44}$$

Therefore, the fractional uptake is given by

$$\boxed{\frac{\mathbb{N}_A}{\mathbb{N}_{A_\infty}} = \left(\frac{1+\Omega}{\Omega} \right) \langle \theta \rangle} \tag{9.45}$$

Area averaging is performed by integrating Eq. (6.184) in the direction of mass transfer, i.e., z-direction. For this purpose, Eq. (6.184) is multiplied by $d\xi$ and integrated from $\xi = 0$ to $\xi = 1$. The result is

$$\int_0^1 \frac{\partial \theta}{\partial \tau} d\xi = \int_0^1 \frac{\partial^2 \theta}{\partial \xi^2} d\xi \tag{9.46}$$

or

$$\frac{d}{d\tau} \int_0^1 \theta \, d\xi = \left.\frac{\partial \theta}{\partial \xi}\right|_{\xi=1} - \left.\frac{\partial \theta}{\partial \xi}\right|_{\xi=0} \tag{9.47}$$

Substitution of Eq. (9.42) into the left side and the boundary condition defined by Eq. (6.187) into the right side of Eq. (9.47) gives

$$\boxed{\frac{d \langle \theta \rangle}{d\tau} = \left.\frac{\partial \theta}{\partial \xi}\right|_{\xi=1}} \tag{9.48}$$

Combination of Eq. (9.48) with Eq. (6.185) results in

$$-\frac{d \langle \theta \rangle}{d\tau} = \Omega \frac{d\theta_s}{d\tau} \tag{9.49}$$

The solution of Eq. (9.49) using the initial condition of

$$\text{at} \quad \tau = 0 \quad \langle \theta \rangle = 0 \quad \text{and} \quad \theta_s = 1 \tag{9.50}$$

leads to

$$\langle \theta \rangle = \Omega(1 - \theta_s) \qquad \Rightarrow \qquad \theta_s = 1 - \frac{\langle \theta \rangle}{\Omega} \tag{9.51}$$

To proceed one step further, it is necessary to express $\partial \theta / \partial \xi|_{\xi=1}$ in terms of the dimensionless average concentration, $\langle \theta \rangle$. The Hermite expansion for $\alpha = 1$ and $\beta = 0$, Eq. (A) in Table 9.3, gives

$$\int_0^1 \theta \, d\xi = \langle \theta \rangle = \frac{2}{3} \theta|_{\xi=0} + \frac{1}{3} \theta|_{\xi=1} + \frac{1}{6} \left.\frac{\partial \theta}{\partial \xi}\right|_{\xi=0} \tag{9.52}$$

On the other hand, the Hermite expansion for $\alpha = 0$ and $\beta = 1$, Eq. (A) in Table 9.4, yields

$$\int_0^1 \theta \, d\xi = \langle \theta \rangle = \frac{1}{3} \theta|_{\xi=0} + \frac{2}{3} \theta|_{\xi=1} - \frac{1}{6} \left.\frac{\partial \theta}{\partial \xi}\right|_{\xi=1} \tag{9.53}$$

The use of the boundary conditions defined by Eqs. (6.6–10) and (6.6–11) reduces Eqs. (9.52) and (9.53) to

$$\langle \theta \rangle = \frac{2}{3} \theta|_{\xi=0} + \frac{1}{3} \theta_s \tag{9.54}$$

$$\langle \theta \rangle = \frac{1}{3} \theta|_{\xi=0} + \frac{2}{3} \theta_s - \frac{1}{6} \left.\frac{\partial \theta}{\partial \xi}\right|_{\xi=1} \tag{9.55}$$

Elimination of $\theta|_{\xi=0}$ between Eqs. (9.54) and (9.55) gives

$$\left.\frac{\partial \theta}{\partial \xi}\right|_{\xi=1} = 3 (\theta_s - \langle \theta \rangle) \tag{9.56}$$

Substitution of Eq. (9.51) into Eq. (9.56) leads to

$$\left.\frac{\partial \theta}{\partial \xi}\right|_{\xi=1} = 3 \left[1 - \left(\frac{1+\Omega}{\Omega} \right) \langle \theta \rangle \right] \tag{9.57}$$

Table 9.10

Fractional Uptakes Calculated from Eqs. (9.39) and (9.60) with Ω as a Parameter

	$\Omega = 1$		$\Omega = 10$		$\Omega = 50$	
τ	**Exact**	**Approx.**	**Exact**	**Approx.**	**Exact**	**Approx.**
0.1	0.553	0.451	0.382	0.281	0.362	0.264
0.2	0.712	0.699	0.533	0.483	0.510	0.458
0.3	0.810	0.835	0.643	0.628	0.619	0.601
0.4	0.874	0.909	0.727	0.733	0.704	0.706
0.5	0.916	0.950	0.791	0.808	0.770	0.783
0.6	0.945	0.973	0.840	0.862	0.821	0.841
0.7	0.963	0.985	0.877	0.901	0.860	0.883
0.8	0.976	0.992	0.906	0.929	0.891	0.914
0.9	0.984	0.995	0.928	0.949	0.915	0.936
1.0	0.989	0.998	0.945	0.963	0.934	0.953

Substitution of Eq. (9.57) into Eq. (9.48) results in the linear differential equation

$$\frac{d\langle\theta\rangle}{d\tau} + 3\left(\frac{1+\Omega}{\Omega}\right)\langle\theta\rangle = 3, \tag{9.58}$$

which is subject to the initial condition defined by Eq. (9.50). The solution is given by

$$\langle\theta\rangle = \frac{\Omega}{1+\Omega}\left\{1 - \exp\left[-3\left(\frac{1+\Omega}{\Omega}\right)\tau\right]\right\} \tag{9.59}$$

so that the fractional uptake is expressed with the help of Eq. (9.45) as

$$\boxed{\left(\frac{\mathbb{N}_A}{\mathbb{N}_{A_\infty}}\right)_{approx.} = 1 - \exp\left[-3\left(\frac{1+\Omega}{\Omega}\right)\tau\right]} \tag{9.60}$$

9.3.3 COMPARISON OF RESULTS

The exact and approximate uptake values are tabulated in Table 9.10 and also presented in Figure 9.2 for various values of Ω. Note that the term Ω represents the ratio of the solution volume to the product of the slab volume and the partition coefficient relating concentrations of species A at the solid–fluid interface under equilibrium conditions. While the approximate solution slightly underestimates the exact solution for small values of τ, the reverse is true when τ is large.

9.4 CONVECTIVE MASS TRANSPORT BETWEEN TWO PARALLEL PLATES WITH A WALL REACTION

An incompressible Newtonian fluid flows between two large parallel plates separated by a distance B under the action of a constant pressure gradient as shown in Figure 9.3. While a first-order irreversible chemical reaction takes place at the upper plate, the lower plate is impermeable to mass transfer of species. The system is isothermal, and it is continuously fed at $z = 0$ with a dilute solution chemical reactant of uniform concentration c_{A_o}. It is required to determine the bulk concentration of species as a function of the axial direction under steady conditions.

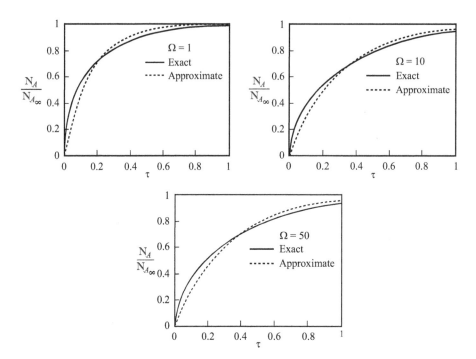

Figure 9.2   Comparison of the analytical and approximate fractional uptake values as a function of τ with Ω as a parameter.

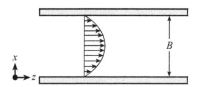

Figure 9.3   Convective mass transport and reaction between two parallel plates.

The fully developed velocity profile is given by

$$v_z = \frac{(\mathcal{P}_o - \mathcal{P}_L)B^2}{2\mu L}\left[\frac{x}{B} - \left(\frac{x}{B}\right)^2\right],$$ (9.61)

where $\mathcal{P}$ is the modified pressure defined by

$$\mathcal{P} = P + \rho g x$$ (9.62)

When the Peclet number is large, the conservation of chemical species under steady conditions takes the form

$$\frac{(\mathcal{P}_o - \mathcal{P}_L)B^2}{2\mu L}\left[\frac{x}{B} - \left(\frac{x}{B}\right)^2\right]\frac{\partial c_A}{\partial z} = \mathcal{D}_{AB}\frac{\partial^2 c_A}{\partial x^2}$$ (9.63)

The boundary conditions associated with Eq. (9.63) are

$$\text{at} \quad z = 0 \qquad c_A = c_{A_o}$$ (9.64)

$$\text{at} \quad x = 0 \qquad \frac{\partial c_A}{\partial x} = 0$$ (9.65)

$$\text{at} \quad x = B \qquad -\mathcal{D}_{AB}\frac{\partial c_A}{\partial x} = k_1'' c_A$$ (9.66)

Introduction of the dimensionless variables

$$\theta = \frac{c_A}{c_{A_o}} \qquad \xi = \frac{x}{B} \qquad \eta = \frac{2\mu L \mathcal{D}_{AB} z}{(\mathcal{P}_o - \mathcal{P}_L) B^4} \qquad \Lambda = \frac{k_1'' B}{\mathcal{D}_{AB}} \tag{9.67}$$

reduces Eqs. (9.63)–(9.66) to the forms

$$\left(\xi - \xi^2\right) \frac{\partial \theta}{\partial \eta} = \frac{\partial^2 \theta}{\partial \xi^2} \tag{9.68}$$

$$\text{at} \quad \eta = 0 \qquad \theta = 1 \tag{9.69}$$

$$\text{at} \quad \xi = 0 \qquad \frac{\partial \theta}{\partial \xi} = 0 \tag{9.70}$$

$$\text{at} \quad \xi = 1 \qquad -\frac{\partial \theta}{\partial \xi} = \Lambda \theta \tag{9.71}$$

9.4.1 ANALYTICAL SOLUTION

Representing the solution as a product of two functions of the form

$$\theta(\xi, \eta) = F(\eta) G(\xi) \tag{9.72}$$

reduces Eq. (9.68) to

$$\frac{1}{F} \frac{dF}{d\eta} = \frac{1}{(\xi - \xi^2) G} \frac{d^2 G}{d\xi^2} = -\lambda^2, \tag{9.73}$$

which results in two ordinary differential equations:

$$\frac{dF}{d\eta} + \lambda^2 F = 0 \qquad \Rightarrow \qquad F = C_1 e^{-\lambda^2 \eta} \tag{9.74}$$

$$\frac{d^2 G}{d\xi^2} + \lambda^2 \left(\xi - \xi^2\right) G = 0 \tag{9.75}$$

Equation (9.75) is a Sturm–Liouville equation with a weight function of $\left(\xi - \xi^2\right)$, and the boundary conditions associated with it are

$$\text{at} \quad \xi = 0 \qquad \frac{dG}{d\xi} = 0 \tag{9.76}$$

$$\text{at} \quad \xi = 1 \qquad -\frac{dG}{d\xi} = \Lambda G \tag{9.77}$$

The use of the transformations

$$Z = \frac{\lambda}{4} (2\xi - 1)^2 \qquad \text{and} \qquad W = \frac{G}{\sqrt{Z}} e^{\frac{Z}{2} - \frac{\lambda}{8}} \tag{9.78}$$

reduces Eq. (9.75) to

$$Z \frac{d^2 W}{dZ^2} + \left(\frac{3}{2} - Z\right) \frac{dW}{dZ} - \left(\frac{12 - \lambda}{16}\right) W = 0 \tag{9.79}$$

Equation (9.79) is Kummer's equation, and the solution is given by

$$W = C_2 M \left(\frac{12 - \lambda}{16}, \frac{3}{2}, Z\right) + \frac{C_3}{\sqrt{Z}} M \left(\frac{4 - \lambda}{16}, \frac{1}{2}, Z\right) \tag{9.80}$$

Hence, the expression for $G(\xi)$ takes the form

$$G(\xi) = e^{-\frac{\lambda}{2}(\xi-1)\xi} \left\{ C_4(2\xi-1)M\left[\frac{12-\lambda}{16}, \frac{3}{2}, \frac{\lambda(2\xi-1)^2}{4}\right] + C_5 M\left[\frac{4-\lambda}{16}, \frac{1}{2}, \frac{\lambda(2\xi-1)^2}{4}\right] \right\}$$

(9.81)

The use of the boundary condition given by Eq. (9.76) yields

$$G(\xi) = C_4 e^{-\frac{\lambda}{2}(\xi-1)\xi} \left\{ (2\xi-1)M\left[\frac{12-\lambda}{16}, \frac{3}{2}, \frac{\lambda(2\xi-1)^2}{4}\right] + SM\left[\frac{4-\lambda}{16}, \frac{1}{2}, \frac{\lambda(2\xi-1)^2}{4}\right] \right\},$$

(9.82)

where

$$S = \frac{12(\lambda-4)M\left(\frac{12-\lambda}{16}, \frac{3}{2}, \frac{\lambda}{4}\right) + (\lambda-12)\lambda M\left(\frac{28-\lambda}{16}, \frac{5}{2}, \frac{\lambda}{4}\right)}{3\lambda\left[4M\left(\frac{4-\lambda}{16}, \frac{1}{2}, \frac{\lambda}{4}\right) + (\lambda-4)M\left(\frac{20-\lambda}{16}, \frac{3}{2}, \frac{\lambda}{4}\right)\right]}$$

(9.83)

On the other hand, the use of the boundary condition given by Eq. (9.77) gives the following transcendental equation for the eigenvalues:

$$12S(\lambda_n - 2\Lambda)M\left(\frac{4-\lambda_n}{16}, \frac{1}{2}, \frac{\lambda_n}{4}\right) + 12\left[\lambda_n - 2(2+\Lambda)\right]M\left(\frac{12-\lambda_n}{16}, \frac{3}{2}, \frac{\lambda_n}{4}\right)$$
$$= -3\lambda_n(\lambda_n - 4)SM\left(\frac{20-\lambda_n}{16}, \frac{3}{2}, \frac{\lambda_n}{4}\right) - \lambda_n(\lambda_n - 12)M\left(\frac{28-\lambda_n}{16}, \frac{5}{2}, \frac{\lambda_n}{4}\right) \quad (9.84)$$

The first ten eigenvalues for various values of Λ are given in Table 9.11. Thus, the solution is expressed in the form

$$\theta(\xi, \eta) = \sum_{n=1}^{\infty} C_n e^{-\lambda_n^2 \eta} G_n(\xi)$$

(9.85)

Table 9.11
The Eigenvalues as a Function of Λ

n	λ_n		
	$\Lambda = 0.1$	$\Lambda = 0.5$	$\Lambda = 1.0$
1	0.7601	1.5886	2.0837
2	9.1261	9.3925	9.6706
3	17.1960	17.3740	17.5723
4	25.2269	25.3650	25.5244
5	33.2448	33.3602	33.4952
6	41.2567	41.3568	41.4751
7	49.2653	49.3544	49.4604
8	57.2718	57.3525	57.4489
9	65.2770	65.3510	65.4398
10	73.2812	73.3497	73.4323

Application of Eq. (9.69) gives the constants C_n as

$$C_n = \frac{\int_0^1 (\xi - \xi^2)\, G_n(\xi)\, d\xi}{\int_0^1 (\xi - \xi^2)\, G_n^2(\xi)\, d\xi} \tag{9.86}$$

The bulk concentration, c_b, is defined by

$$c_{A_b} = \frac{\int_0^H \int_0^B c_A v_z\, dx dy}{\int_0^H \int_0^B v_z\, dx dy}, \tag{9.87}$$

where H is the width of the plate. In terms of the dimensionless quantities, Eq. (9.87) takes the form

$$\theta_b = \frac{c_{A_b}}{c_{A_o}} = \frac{\int_0^1 \theta\, (\xi - \xi^2)\, d\xi}{\int_0^1 (\xi - \xi^2)\, d\xi} = 6 \int_0^1 \theta\, (\xi - \xi^2)\, d\xi \tag{9.88}$$

Substitution of Eq. (9.85) into Eq. (9.88) and integration give the dimensionless bulk concentration as

$$\theta_{b,exact} = 6 \sum_{n=1}^{\infty} C_n e^{-\lambda_n^2 \eta} \int_0^1 (\xi - \xi^2)\, G_n(\xi)\, d\xi \tag{9.89}$$

9.4.2 APPROXIMATE SOLUTION BY AREA AVERAGING

Multiplication of Eq. (9.68) by $d\xi$ and integration from $\xi = 0$ to $\xi = 1$ give

$$\int_0^1 (\xi - \xi^2) \frac{\partial \theta}{\partial \eta}\, d\xi = \int_0^1 \frac{\partial^2 \theta}{\partial \xi^2}\, d\xi \tag{9.90}$$

or

$$\frac{d}{d\eta} \int_0^1 \theta\, (\xi - \xi^2)\, d\xi = \left. \frac{\partial \theta}{\partial \xi} \right|_{\xi=1} - \left. \frac{\partial \theta}{\partial \xi} \right|_{\xi=0} \tag{9.91}$$

Substitution of Eq. (9.98) into the left side and the boundary conditions defined by Eqs. (9.70) and (9.71) into the right side of Eq. (9.91) yields

$$\boxed{\frac{1}{6} \frac{d\theta_b}{d\eta} = -\Lambda\, \theta|_{\xi=1}} \tag{9.92}$$

To proceed further, it is necessary to express $\theta|_{\xi=1}$ in terms of θ_b.

The Hermite expansion for $\alpha = 0$ and $\beta = 0$, Eq. (B) in Table 9.2, gives

$$\int_0^1 \theta\, (\xi - \xi^2)\, d\xi = \frac{1}{4} \left. \frac{\partial\, [\theta\, (\xi - \xi^2)]}{\partial \xi} \right|_{\xi=1} + \frac{1}{4} \left. \frac{\partial\, [\theta\, (\xi - \xi^2)]}{\partial \xi} \right|_{\xi=0} \tag{9.93}$$

On the other hand, the Hermite expansion for $\alpha = 1$ and $\beta = 1$, Eq. (B) in Table 9.5, gives

$$\int_0^1 \theta\left(\xi - \xi^2\right) d\xi = \frac{1}{3}\left[\theta\left(\xi - \xi^2\right)\right]_{\xi=0} + \frac{2}{3}\left[\theta\left(\xi - \xi^2\right)\right]_{\xi=1} - \frac{1}{6} \left.\frac{\partial\left[\theta\left(\xi - \xi^2\right)\right]}{\partial\xi}\right|_{\xi=1}$$

$$+ \frac{1}{72}\left\{ \left.\frac{\partial^2\left[\theta\left(\xi - \xi^2\right)\right]}{\partial\xi^2}\right|_{\xi=1} - \left.\frac{\partial^2\left[\theta\left(\xi - \xi^2\right)\right]}{\partial\xi^2}\right|_{\xi=0} \right\} \quad (9.94)$$

Substitution of the boundary conditions defined by Eqs. (9.70) and (9.71) into Eqs. (9.93) and (9.94) and the simultaneous solution of the resulting equations yield

$$\theta|_{\xi=1} = \left[\frac{16}{3\left(6 + \Lambda\right)}\right]\theta_b \quad (9.95)$$

The use of Eq. (9.95) in Eq. (9.92) yields

$$\frac{d\theta_b}{d\eta} + \left(\frac{32\Lambda}{6 + \Lambda}\right)\theta_b = 0, \quad (9.96)$$

which is subject to the following boundary condition:

$$\text{at} \quad \eta = 0 \quad \theta_b = 1 \quad (9.97)$$

The solution of Eq. (9.96) is given by

$$\theta_{b,approx.} = \exp\left[-\left(\frac{32\Lambda}{6 + \Lambda}\right)\eta\right] \quad (9.98)$$

Table 9.12

Dimensionless Bulk Concentration Values with Λ as a Parameter

τ	$\Lambda = 0.1$		$\Lambda = 0.5$		$\Lambda = 1.0$	
	$\theta_{b,exact}$	$\theta_{b,approx.}$	$\theta_{b,exact}$	$\theta_{b,approx.}$	$\theta_{b,exact}$	$\theta_{b,approx.}$
0.00	1.0000	1.0000	1.0000	1.0000	1.0000	1.0000
0.02	0.9884	0.9896	0.9487	0.9520	0.9106	0.9126
0.04	0.9770	0.9792	0.9018	0.9062	0.8341	0.8329
0.06	0.9725	0.9690	0.8573	0.8627	0.7646	0.7601
0.08	0.9560	0.9589	0.8151	0.8213	0.7010	0.6937
0.10	0.9437	0.9489	0.7750	0.7818	0.6427	0.6331
0.12	0.9328	0.9390	0.7368	0.7442	0.5892	0.5778
0.14	0.9221	0.9292	0.7005	0.7085	0.5402	0.5273
0.16	0.9115	0.9195	0.6661	0.6745	0.4953	0.4812
0.18	0.9010	0.9099	0.6333	0.6421	0.4541	0.4392
0.20	0.8906	0.9004	0.6021	0.6112	0.4163	0.4008

9.4.3 COMPARISON OF RESULTS

The exact and approximate dimensionless bulk concentrations are tabulated in Table 9.12 for various values of the Thiele modulus, Λ, which represents the ratio of the rate of surface reaction to the rate of diffusion. The exact and approximate results are almost identical, the largest deviation being around 4% when $\Lambda = 1.0$ and $\eta = 0.2$. As the Thiele modulus increases, the rate of surface reaction becomes more dominant than the rate of diffusion. As a result, species are consumed faster with a concomitant decrease in the bulk concentration, θ_b.

REFERENCES

Dalgiç, M. 2008. Solutions of the equations of change by the averaging technique. MS Thesis. Ankara, Turkey: Middle East Technical University.

Mennig, J., T. Auerbach and W. Hälg. 1983. Two point Hermite approximations for the solution of linear initial value and boundary value problems. *Comput. Methods Appl. Mech. Eng.* 39:199–224.

Özyilmaz, M. 1996. Solutions of transport phenomena problems by averaging technique. MS Thesis. Ankara, Turkey: Middle East Technical University.

A Vector and Tensor Algebra

Quantities that have only magnitude are called *scalars*, such as pressure, temperature, concentration, volume, time, and mass. Scalars can also be regarded as zero-order tensors. A *vector* is a quantity that associates a scalar with each coordinate direction. This definition implies that each vector has a magnitude and a direction. Velocity, force, momentum, and acceleration are all vector quantities. Vectors can also be regarded as first-order tensors. A *second-order tensor* is a quantity that associates a vector with each coordinate direction or a quantity that associates a scalar with each ordered pair of coordinate directions. Shear stress, vorticity, and rate of strain (or shear rate) are some examples of second-order tensors.

A.1 THE OPERATIONS ON VECTORS

A vector has a magnitude and a direction[1]; the magnitude of the vector $\mathbf{v}$ is designated by $|\mathbf{v}|$. Equality of two vectors $\mathbf{v}$ and $\mathbf{w}$ implies that $|\mathbf{v}| = |\mathbf{w}|$, and they point in the same direction. The vectors $\mathbf{v}$ and $-\mathbf{v}$ have the same magnitude $|\mathbf{v}|$, but point in opposite directions, i.e., the angle between them is $180°$. Various operations on vectors, namely, addition, scalar multiplication, scalar (or dot) product, and vector (or cross) product are briefly explained below.

A.1.1 ADDITION

Two vectors $\mathbf{v}$ and $\mathbf{w}$ are added according to the *parallelogram law* of addition as shown in Figure A.1-a. Repeated application of the parallelogram law determines the sum of any number of vectors. Subtraction of vectors is carried out on the same lines as their addition. The vector difference $\mathbf{v} - \mathbf{w}$ is expressed as

$$\mathbf{v} - \mathbf{w} = \mathbf{v} + (-\mathbf{w}) \tag{A.1}$$

and reduces the operation of subtraction to one of addition as shown in Figure A.1-b. Vector addition satisfies the following algebraic rules:

Commutative	$\mathbf{v} + \mathbf{w} = \mathbf{w} + \mathbf{v}$
Associative	$\mathbf{u} + (\mathbf{v} + \mathbf{w}) = (\mathbf{u} + \mathbf{v}) + \mathbf{w}$
Identity	$\mathbf{v} + \mathbf{0} = \mathbf{v}$
Inverse	$\mathbf{v} + (-\mathbf{v}) = \mathbf{0}$

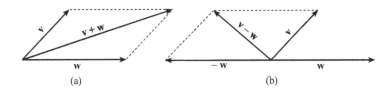

(a) (b)

Figure A.1 (a) Addition of vectors; (b) subtraction of vectors.

---

[1] The *zero vector* is an exception. It has zero length and an arbitrary direction.

347

A.1.2 SCALAR MULTIPLICATION

Let α be a scalar (real number) and $\mathbf{v}$ a vector. Scalar multiplication $\alpha\mathbf{v}$ is defined to be another vector of length $|\alpha|\,|\mathbf{v}|$; the direction of $\alpha\mathbf{v}$ is the same as that of $\mathbf{v}$ if $\alpha > 0$ and in the opposite direction if $\alpha < 0$. Scalar multiplication satisfies the following algebraic rules:

$$
\begin{array}{ll}
\text{Associative} & \alpha\,(\beta\mathbf{v}) = (\alpha\beta)\,\mathbf{v} \\
\text{Identity} & 1\,\mathbf{v} = \mathbf{v} \\
\text{Distributive} & \alpha\,(\mathbf{v}+\mathbf{w}) = \alpha\,\mathbf{v}+\alpha\,\mathbf{w} \\
\text{Distributive} & (\alpha+\beta)\,\mathbf{v} = \alpha\,\mathbf{v}+\beta\,\mathbf{v}
\end{array}
$$

A.1.3 SCALAR (OR DOT) PRODUCT

The scalar product of two vectors $\mathbf{v}$ and $\mathbf{w}$ is defined as the product of the magnitudes of the two vectors times the cosine of the angle between the vectors, i.e.,

$$
\boxed{\mathbf{v}\cdot\mathbf{w} = |\mathbf{v}|\,|\mathbf{w}|\cos\theta} \tag{A.2}
$$

As the name implies, $\mathbf{v}\cdot\mathbf{w}$ is a scalar quantity.

Consider the vectors $\mathbf{v}$ and $\mathbf{w}$ as shown in Figure A.2. The cosine of the angle between these two vectors can be expressed as

$$
\cos\theta = \frac{\overline{OA}}{|\mathbf{w}|} = \frac{\overline{OB}}{|\mathbf{v}|} \tag{A.3}
$$

The use of Eq. (A.3) in Eq. (A.2) gives

$$
\mathbf{v}\cdot\mathbf{w} = |\mathbf{v}|\,\overline{OA} = |\mathbf{w}|\,\overline{OB} \tag{A.4}
$$

Note that

$$
\overline{OA} = \text{Projection of } \mathbf{w} \text{ in the direction of } \mathbf{v}
$$

$$
\overline{OB} = \text{Projection of } \mathbf{v} \text{ in the direction of } \mathbf{w}
$$

Thus, Eq. (A.4) implies that the scalar product is the magnitude of $\mathbf{v}$ multiplied by the projection of $\mathbf{w}$ on $\mathbf{v}$ or the magnitude of $\mathbf{w}$ multiplied by the projection of $\mathbf{v}$ on $\mathbf{w}$. The scalar product of a vector with itself is just the square of the magnitude of the vector, i.e.,

$$
\mathbf{v}\cdot\mathbf{v} = |\mathbf{v}|^2 \quad\Rightarrow\quad \boxed{|\mathbf{v}| = \sqrt{\mathbf{v}\cdot\mathbf{v}}} \tag{A.5}
$$

The rules governing the scalar product are as follows:

$$
\begin{array}{ll}
\text{Commutative} & \mathbf{v}\cdot\mathbf{w} = \mathbf{w}\cdot\mathbf{v} \\
\text{Not associative} & \mathbf{u}\,(\mathbf{v}\cdot\mathbf{w}) \neq (\mathbf{u}\cdot\mathbf{v})\,\mathbf{w} \\
\text{Distributive} & \mathbf{u}\cdot(\mathbf{v}+\mathbf{w}) = \mathbf{u}\cdot\mathbf{v}+\mathbf{u}\cdot\mathbf{w}
\end{array}
$$

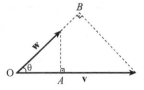

Figure A.2 The scalar product of two vectors.

A.1.4 VECTOR (OR CROSS) PRODUCT

The vector product of two vectors $\mathbf{v}$ and $\mathbf{w}$ is a vector defined by

$$\boxed{\mathbf{v} \times \mathbf{w} = |\mathbf{v}|\,|\mathbf{w}|\sin\theta\,\mathbf{n},} \tag{A.6}$$

where $\mathbf{n}$ is a vector of unit length. The direction of $\mathbf{n}$ is determined by the right-hand rule, i.e., when the index finger points in the direction of $\mathbf{v}$ and the middle finger points in the direction of $\mathbf{w}$, the thumb points in the direction of $\mathbf{n}$. The magnitude of the vector $\mathbf{v} \times \mathbf{w}$ is the area of the parallelogram formed by the vectors $\mathbf{v}$ and $\mathbf{w}$. The rules governing the vector product are as follows:

Not commutative	$\mathbf{v} \times \mathbf{w} \neq \mathbf{w} \times \mathbf{v}$
Not associative	$\mathbf{u} \times (\mathbf{v} \times \mathbf{w}) \neq (\mathbf{u} \times \mathbf{v}) \times \mathbf{w}$
Distributive	$(\mathbf{u} + \mathbf{v}) \times \mathbf{w} = \mathbf{u} \times \mathbf{w} + \mathbf{v} \times \mathbf{w}$

A.2 BASIS AND BASIS VECTORS

Consider a set $S = \{\mathbf{v}_1, \mathbf{v}_2, \mathbf{v}_3\}$ of three vectors. The expression

$$\sum_{i=1}^{3} \alpha_i \mathbf{v}_i = \alpha_1 \mathbf{v}_1 + \alpha_2 \mathbf{v}_2 + \alpha_3 \mathbf{v}_3, \tag{A.7}$$

where $\{\alpha_1, \alpha_2, \alpha_3\}$ is a set of scalars, is called a *linear combination* of the elements of S. These three vectors are said to be *linearly independent* when

$$\sum_{i=1}^{3} \alpha_i \mathbf{v}_i = 0 \tag{A.8}$$

holds if and only if $\alpha_1 = \alpha_2 = \alpha_3 = 0$. When one of the scalars is different from zero, then the vectors are *linearly dependent*. Geometrically, three vectors are linearly independent if they are not all parallel to one plane.

A set $S = \{\mathbf{e}_1, \mathbf{e}_2, \mathbf{e}_3\}$ of three vectors forms a *basis* if it meets either of the following criteria:

- $\mathbf{e}_1$, $\mathbf{e}_2$, $\mathbf{e}_3$ are linearly independent.
- Any vector $\mathbf{v}$ can be written as a linear combination of $\mathbf{e}_1$, $\mathbf{e}_2$, $\mathbf{e}_3$ such that

$$\mathbf{v} = v_1\mathbf{e}_1 + v_2\mathbf{e}_2 + v_3\mathbf{e}_3 = \sum_{i=1}^{3} v_i\mathbf{e}_i, \tag{A.9}$$

where v_1, v_2, v_3 are called the *components* of the vector $\mathbf{v}$ and $\mathbf{e}_1$, $\mathbf{e}_2$, $\mathbf{e}_3$ are called the *basis vectors*.

A basis $(\mathbf{e}_1, \mathbf{e}_2, \mathbf{e}_3)$ is said to be *orthonormal* if each element in the set is a unit vector, i.e.,

$$\mathbf{e}_1 \cdot \mathbf{e}_1 = \mathbf{e}_2 \cdot \mathbf{e}_2 = \mathbf{e}_3 \cdot \mathbf{e}_3 = 1 \tag{A.10}$$

and the elements are orthogonal to one another at every point, i.e.,

$$\mathbf{e}_i \cdot \mathbf{e}_j = 0 \quad \text{for} \quad i \neq j \tag{A.11}$$

The basis vectors $(\mathbf{e}_1, \mathbf{e}_2, \mathbf{e}_3)$ in the *Cartesian* (or *rectangular*) *coordinate* system are orthonormal, i.e., they are of unit length and mutually orthogonal. Moreover, they point in the same direction at two different locations. This implies

$$\mathbf{e}_i(x, y, z) = \mathbf{e}_i(x^*, y^*, z^*) \quad \text{for} \quad i = 1, 2, 3 \tag{A.12}$$

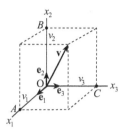

Figure A.3   The projections of a vector on the Cartesian coordinate axes x_1, x_2, and x_3.

In other words, Cartesian basis vectors are independent of position.

In Cartesian coordinates, each vector can be written as a linear combination of the basis vectors as[2]

$$\mathbf{v} = v_1\mathbf{e}_1 + v_2\mathbf{e}_2 + v_3\mathbf{e}_3 = \sum_{i=1}^{3} v_i\mathbf{e}_i \qquad (A.13)$$

The v_i are called the *Cartesian components* of vector $\mathbf{v}$, and they are scalars, whereas the $v_i\mathbf{e}_i$ are vectors[3], which when added together vectorially give $\mathbf{v}$ as shown in Figure A.3. Note that the components are simply the projections of the vector $\mathbf{v}$ along the coordinate axes x_1, x_2, and x_3, i.e.,

$$v_1 = \overline{OA} = \mathbf{v} \cdot \mathbf{e}_1 \qquad v_2 = \overline{OB} = \mathbf{v} \cdot \mathbf{e}_2 \qquad v_3 = \overline{OC} = \mathbf{v} \cdot \mathbf{e}_3 \qquad (A.14)$$

A.3   SUMMATION CONVENTION[4]

When a subscript or superscript (index) is repeated in a given term of an expression, then summation over that index is implied. Using the summation convention, Eq. (A.13) can be expressed as

$$\mathbf{v} = v_i\mathbf{e}_i \qquad (A.15)$$

with the understanding that i goes from 1 to 3 since it is repeated. A repeated index is called a *dummy index* because the expression is independent of the letter used for the repeated index. An index that is not repeated is called a *free index*.

The scalar product of two basis vectors of unit length is given by

$$\mathbf{e}_i \cdot \mathbf{e}_j = \delta_{ij}, \qquad (A.16)$$

where δ_{ij}, the *Kronecker delta*, is defined by

$$\delta_{ij} = \begin{cases} 1 & \text{if} & i = j \\ 0 & \text{if} & i \neq j \end{cases} \qquad (A.17)$$

On the other hand, the vector product of two basis vectors of unit length is given by

$$\mathbf{e}_i \times \mathbf{e}_j = \varepsilon_{ijk}\,\mathbf{e}_k, \qquad (A.18)$$

---

[2]Cartesian basis vectors are also designated as $(\mathbf{i}, \mathbf{j}, \mathbf{k})$.

[3]Remember that a vector associates a scalar with each coordinate direction.

[4]Also known as the *Einstein summation convention*.

where ε_{ijk} is called the *alternating unit tensor* (or *permutation symbol*). It is defined as

$$\varepsilon_{ijk} = \begin{cases} 0 & \text{when any two of the indices are equal} \\ +1 & \text{when } (i,j,k) \text{ are } (1,2,3) \text{ or an even permutation of } (1,2,3) \\ -1 & \text{when } (i,j,k) \text{ are an odd permutation of } (1,2,3) \end{cases} \tag{A.19}$$

If (i, j, k) are an even permutation of $(1, 2, 3)$, then (i, j, k) require an even number of inversions to be placed in the same order as $(1, 2, 3)$. The sign convention can be remembered by marking the numbers $(1, 2, 3)$ on a circle. Then any even permutation will be in cyclic order, i.e., it will go around the circle in the same sense as $(1, 2, 3)$, $(2, 3, 1)$, or $(3, 1, 2)$. An odd permutation will go in the reverse direction, i.e., $(1, 3, 2)$, $(3, 2, 1)$, or $(2, 1, 3)$.

The following relations involving the Kronecker delta and alternating unit tensor are useful in proving some vector identities:

$$\varepsilon_{ijk}\,\varepsilon_{mjk} = 2\,\delta_{im} \tag{A.20}$$

$$\varepsilon_{ijk}\,\varepsilon_{mnk} = \delta_{im}\,\delta_{jn} - \delta_{in}\,\delta_{jm} \tag{A.21}$$

Using summation convention, various operations on vectors are carried out as follows:

Vector addition $\qquad \mathbf{v} + \mathbf{w} = v_i\mathbf{e}_i + w_i\mathbf{e}_i = (v_i + w_i)\,\mathbf{e}_i$

Scalar multiplication $\qquad \alpha\,\mathbf{v} = (\alpha\mathbf{v_i})\,\mathbf{e}_i$

Scalar product $\qquad \mathbf{v} \cdot \mathbf{w} = (v_i\mathbf{e}_i) \cdot (w_j\mathbf{e}_j) = v_iw_j\underbrace{(\mathbf{e}_i \cdot \mathbf{e}_j)}_{\delta_{ij}} = v_iw_i$

Vector product $\qquad \mathbf{v} \times \mathbf{w} = (v_i\mathbf{e}_i) \times (w_j\mathbf{e}_j) = v_iw_j(\mathbf{e}_i \times \mathbf{e}_j) = \varepsilon_{ijk}v_iw_j\mathbf{e}_k$

A.4 SECOND-ORDER TENSORS

Using the summation convention, a second-order tensor $\mathbf{T}$ is defined by

$$\mathbf{T} = T_{ij}\mathbf{e}_i\mathbf{e}_j, \tag{A.22}$$

where the T_{ij}'s are called the *components* of the tensor $\mathbf{T}$ and can be displayed as a matrix in the form

$$T_{ij} = \begin{pmatrix} T_{11} & T_{12} & T_{13} \\ T_{21} & T_{22} & T_{23} \\ T_{31} & T_{32} & T_{33} \end{pmatrix} \tag{A.23}$$

When two vector quantities are written side by side without any multiplication sign between them, the result is a second-order tensor called a *dyadic product*. The term $\mathbf{e}_i\mathbf{e}_j$ in Eq. (A.22) is a dyadic product of basis vectors of unit length.

A second-order tensor $\mathbf{T}$ transforms a vector into another vector such that

$$\mathbf{T} \cdot \mathbf{v} = (T_{ij}\mathbf{e}_i\mathbf{e}_j) \cdot (v_k\mathbf{e}_k) = T_{ij}v_k\underbrace{(\mathbf{e}_j \cdot \mathbf{e}_k)}_{\delta_{jk}}\mathbf{e}_i = (T_{ik}v_k)\mathbf{e}_i \tag{A.24}$$

On the other hand,

$$\mathbf{v} \cdot \mathbf{T} = (v_k\mathbf{e}_k) \cdot (T_{ij}\mathbf{e}_i\mathbf{e}_j) = T_{ij}v_k\underbrace{(\mathbf{e}_k \cdot \mathbf{e}_i)}_{\delta_{ki}}\mathbf{e}_j = (T_{ij}v_i)\mathbf{e}_j \tag{A.25}$$

Thus,

$$\mathbf{T} \cdot \mathbf{v} \neq \mathbf{v} \cdot \mathbf{T} \tag{A.26}$$

The following are several special kinds of second-order tensors encountered in transport of mass, momentum, and energy:

- A *unit tensor* or an *identity tensor* $\mathbf{I}$

$$\boxed{\mathbf{I} = \delta_{ij}\mathbf{e}_i\mathbf{e}_j} \tag{A.27}$$

transforms every vector into itself, i.e.,

$$\mathbf{I} \cdot \mathbf{v} = \mathbf{v} \cdot \mathbf{I} = \mathbf{v} \tag{A.28}$$

- The *transpose* of $\mathbf{T}$, $\mathbf{T}^{\mathrm{T}}$, is defined as follows:

$$\boxed{\mathbf{T} \cdot \mathbf{v} = \mathbf{v} \cdot \mathbf{T}^{\mathrm{T}}} \tag{A.29}$$

If a second-order tensor $\mathbf{T}$ and its components are defined as

$$\mathbf{T} = T_{ij}\mathbf{e}_i\mathbf{e}_j \qquad \text{with} \qquad T_{ij} = \begin{pmatrix} T_{11} & T_{12} & T_{13} \\ T_{21} & T_{22} & T_{23} \\ T_{31} & T_{32} & T_{33} \end{pmatrix} \tag{A.30}$$

then the transpose of $\mathbf{T}$, $\mathbf{T}^{\mathrm{T}}$, is given by

$$\mathbf{T}^{\mathrm{T}} = T_{ji}\mathbf{e}_i\mathbf{e}_j \qquad \text{with} \qquad T_{ji} = \begin{pmatrix} T_{11} & T_{21} & T_{31} \\ T_{12} & T_{22} & T_{32} \\ T_{13} & T_{23} & T_{33} \end{pmatrix} \tag{A.31}$$

If $\mathbf{T}$ and $\mathbf{U}$ are any two second-order tensors, then

$$\boxed{(\mathbf{T} \cdot \mathbf{U})^{\mathrm{T}} = \mathbf{U}^{\mathrm{T}} \cdot \mathbf{T}^{\mathrm{T}}} \tag{A.32}$$

- A second-order tensor $\mathbf{T}$ is said to be *symmetric* if

$$\mathbf{T} = \mathbf{T}^{\mathrm{T}} \qquad \text{or} \qquad T_{ij} = T_{ji} \tag{A.33}$$

Therefore, the number of independent components of a symmetric tensor is 6.

- A second-order tensor is said to be *skew-symmetric* (or antisymmetric) if

$$\mathbf{T} = -\mathbf{T}^{\mathrm{T}} \qquad \text{or} \qquad T_{ij} = -T_{ji} \tag{A.34}$$

Since the diagonal elements (T_{ii}) are all zero according to Eq. (A.34), the number of independent components of a skew-symmetric tensor is 3.

A.4.1 TRACE OF A TENSOR

An operation "tr" that assigns to each second-order tensor $\mathbf{T}$ a number $\mathrm{tr}(\mathbf{T})$ is called a *trace* if it obeys the following rules:

$$\begin{aligned} \mathrm{tr}(\mathbf{T} + \mathbf{S}) &= \mathrm{tr}(\mathbf{T}) + \mathrm{tr}(\mathbf{S}) \\ \mathrm{tr}(\alpha\mathbf{T}) &= \alpha\,\mathrm{tr}(\mathbf{T}) \\ \mathrm{tr}(\mathbf{v}\mathbf{w}) &= \mathbf{v} \cdot \mathbf{w} \end{aligned} \tag{A.35}$$

With the help of these rules, the trace of a second-order tensor is given by

$$
\mathrm{tr}(\mathbf{T}) = \mathrm{tr}(T_{mn}\mathbf{e}_m\mathbf{e}_n) = T_{mn}\,\mathrm{tr}(\mathbf{e}_m\mathbf{e}_n) = T_{mn}\underbrace{(\mathbf{e}_m \cdot \mathbf{e}_n)}_{\delta_{mn}}
$$

$$
= T_{11} + T_{22} + T_{33}
$$

(A.36)

Therefore, the trace of a second-order tensor is the sum of the diagonal components of a matrix.

A.4.2   INVARIANTS OF A TENSOR

Note that a scalar may be formed from a single vector $\mathbf{v}$ by the product $\mathbf{v} \cdot \mathbf{v}$. In the case of a second-order tensor $\mathbf{T}$, three independent scalars, called the *invariants* of the tensor $\mathbf{T}$, can be formed as follows:

$$
\mathrm{I_T} = \mathrm{tr}(\mathbf{T}) \quad = T_{ii}
$$

$$
\mathrm{II_T} = \mathrm{tr}(\mathbf{T}^2) \quad = \mathrm{tr}(\mathbf{T} \cdot \mathbf{T}) = T_{ij}T_{ji}
$$

(A.37)

$$
\mathrm{III_T} = \mathrm{tr}(\mathbf{T}^3) \quad = T_{ij}T_{jk}T_{ki}
$$

Any combination of these invariants is also an invariant.

A.5   VECTOR AND TENSOR DIFFERENTIAL OPERATIONS

The vector differential operator ∇, known as *del* or *nabla*, is defined in the Cartesian coordinate system as

$$
\nabla = \frac{\partial}{\partial x_i}\mathbf{e}_i = \frac{\partial}{\partial x}\mathbf{e}_x + \frac{\partial}{\partial y}\mathbf{e}_y + \frac{\partial}{\partial z}\mathbf{e}_z
$$

(A.38)

Keep in mind that Cartesian basis vectors are independent of position.

A.5.1   GRADIENT OF A SCALAR FIELD

The gradient of a scalar field α is a vector field denoted by $\nabla\alpha$. In the Cartesian coordinate system, it is expressed as

$$
\nabla\alpha = \frac{\partial\alpha}{\partial x_i}\mathbf{e}_i = \frac{\partial\alpha}{\partial x}\mathbf{e}_x + \frac{\partial\alpha}{\partial y}\mathbf{e}_y + \frac{\partial\alpha}{\partial z}\mathbf{e}_z
$$

(A.39)

The components of $\nabla\alpha$ represent the rate of change of the scalar field with respect to each coordinate direction. The gradient operation has the following properties:

Not commutative	$\nabla\alpha \neq \alpha\nabla$
Not associative	$(\nabla\alpha)\beta \neq \nabla(\alpha\beta)$
Distributive	$\nabla(\alpha+\beta) = \nabla\alpha + \nabla\beta$

A.5.2   DIVERGENCE OF A VECTOR FIELD

The divergence of a vector field $\mathbf{v}$ is a scalar field denoted by $\nabla \cdot \mathbf{v}$. In the Cartesian coordinate system, it is expressed as

$$
\nabla \cdot \mathbf{v} = \frac{\partial}{\partial x_i}\mathbf{e}_i \cdot (v_j\mathbf{e}_j) = \frac{\partial v_j}{\partial x_i}\underbrace{(\mathbf{e}_i \cdot \mathbf{e}_j)}_{\delta_{ij}} = \frac{\partial v_i}{\partial x_i}
$$

$$
= \frac{\partial v_x}{\partial x} + \frac{\partial v_y}{\partial y} + \frac{\partial v_z}{\partial z}
$$

(A.40)

The divergence operation has the following properties:

Not commutative $\nabla \cdot \mathbf{v} \neq \mathbf{v} \cdot \nabla$

Not associative $\nabla \cdot (s\mathbf{v}) \neq (\nabla s) \cdot \mathbf{v}$

Distributive $\nabla \cdot (\mathbf{v} + \mathbf{w}) = \nabla \cdot \mathbf{v} + \nabla \cdot \mathbf{w}$

A.5.3   CURL OF A VECTOR FIELD

The curl of a vector field $\mathbf{v}$ is also a vector field denoted by $\nabla \times \mathbf{v}$. The vector product between the ∇ operator and the vector $\mathbf{v}$ is expressed as

$$\nabla \times \mathbf{v} = \frac{\partial}{\partial x_i} \mathbf{e}_i \times (v_j \mathbf{e}_j) = \frac{\partial v_j}{\partial x_i} (\mathbf{e}_i \times \mathbf{e}_j) = \varepsilon_{ijk} \frac{\partial v_j}{\partial x_i} \mathbf{e}_k \tag{A.41}$$

Summation over the indices i, j, and k leads to 27 terms. The curl operation has the following properties:

Not commutative $\nabla \times \mathbf{v} \neq \mathbf{v} \times \nabla$

Not associative $\nabla \times (s\mathbf{v}) \neq (\nabla s) \times \mathbf{v}$

Distributive $\nabla \times (\mathbf{v} + \mathbf{w}) = \nabla \times \mathbf{v} + \nabla \times \mathbf{w}$

A.5.4   GRADIENT OF A VECTOR FIELD

The gradient of a vector field $\mathbf{v}$ is a second-order tensor field denoted by $\nabla \mathbf{v}$. In the Cartesian coordinate system, it is expressed as

$$\boxed{\nabla \mathbf{v} = \frac{\partial v_j}{\partial x_i} \mathbf{e}_i \mathbf{e}_j} \tag{A.42}$$

The transpose of $\nabla \mathbf{v}$ is

$$\boxed{(\nabla \mathbf{v})^{\mathrm{T}} = \frac{\partial v_i}{\partial x_j} \mathbf{e}_i \mathbf{e}_j} \tag{A.43}$$

Note that the trace of the gradient of a vector field is the divergence of a vector field, i.e.,

$$\mathrm{tr}(\nabla \mathbf{v}) = \nabla \cdot \mathbf{v} \tag{A.44}$$

A.5.5   LAPLACIAN OF A SCALAR FIELD

In the Cartesian coordinate system, the divergence of the gradient of a scalar field α is given by

$$\nabla \cdot \nabla \alpha = \nabla^2 \alpha = \frac{\partial}{\partial x_i} \mathbf{e}_i \cdot \frac{\partial \alpha}{\partial x_j} \mathbf{e}_j = \frac{\partial^2 \alpha}{\partial x_i \partial x_j} \underbrace{(\mathbf{e}_i \cdot \mathbf{e}_j)}_{\delta_{ij}} = \frac{\partial^2 \alpha}{\partial x_i \partial x_i}$$

$$= \frac{\partial^2 \alpha}{\partial x^2} + \frac{\partial^2 \alpha}{\partial y^2} + \frac{\partial^2 \alpha}{\partial z^2} \tag{A.45}$$

$\nabla \cdot \nabla = \nabla^2$ is called the *Laplacian* operator.

A.5.6 SOME USEFUL IDENTITIES

Some of the useful identities involving vector and tensor differential operations are given below:

$$
\begin{aligned}
\nabla \cdot \alpha \mathbf{v} &= \alpha \left(\nabla \cdot \mathbf{v} \right) + \mathbf{v} \cdot \nabla \alpha \\
\nabla \cdot \alpha \mathbf{I} &= \nabla \alpha \\
\nabla \cdot \mathbf{vw} &= \mathbf{v} \cdot \nabla \mathbf{w} + \mathbf{w} \left(\nabla \cdot \mathbf{v} \right) \\
\nabla \times \alpha \mathbf{v} &= \nabla \alpha \times \mathbf{v} + \alpha \left(\nabla \times \mathbf{v} \right) \\
\nabla \cdot \alpha \mathbf{T} &= \nabla \alpha \cdot \mathbf{T} + \alpha \left(\nabla \cdot \mathbf{T} \right)
\end{aligned}
\tag{A.46}
$$

A.6 VECTOR AND TENSOR ALGEBRA IN CURVILINEAR COORDINATES

Besides Cartesian coordinates, the two most commonly used coordinate systems are *cylindrical* and *spherical coordinates*. In these two curvilinear coordinate systems, however, the basis vectors are dependent on position.

The cylindrical coordinate system is shown in Figure A.4. For cylindrical coordinates, the variables (r, θ, z) are related to the Cartesian coordinates (x, y, z) as follows:

$$
\begin{array}{ll}
x = r\cos\theta & r = \sqrt{x^2 + y^2} \\
y = r\sin\theta & \theta = \arctan(y/x) \\
z = z & z = z
\end{array}
\tag{A.47}
$$

The ranges of the variables (r, θ, z) are

$$
0 \leq r \leq \infty \qquad 0 \leq \theta \leq 2\pi \qquad -\infty \leq z \leq \infty
\tag{A.48}
$$

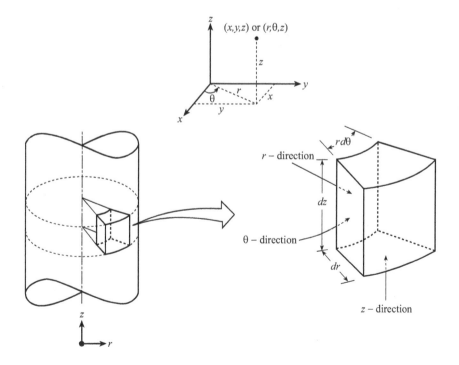

Figure A.4 The cylindrical coordinate system.

The relationships between the basis vectors of the Cartesian and cylindrical coordinate systems are expressed in the forms

$$\begin{aligned}
\mathbf{e}_x &= \cos\theta\,\mathbf{e}_r - \sin\theta\,\mathbf{e}_\theta \\
\mathbf{e}_y &= \sin\theta\,\mathbf{e}_r + \cos\theta\,\mathbf{e}_\theta \\
\mathbf{e}_z &= \mathbf{e}_z
\end{aligned} \tag{A.49}$$

and

$$\begin{aligned}
\mathbf{e}_r &= \cos\theta\,\mathbf{e}_x + \sin\theta\,\mathbf{c}_y \\
\mathbf{e}_\theta &= -\sin\theta\,\mathbf{e}_x + \cos\theta\,\mathbf{e}_y \\
\mathbf{e}_z &= \mathbf{e}_z
\end{aligned} \tag{A.50}$$

The spherical coordinate system is shown in Figure A.5. For spherical coordinates, the variables (r,θ,ϕ) are related to the Cartesian coordinates (x,y,z) as follows:

$$\begin{aligned}
x &= r\sin\theta\cos\phi & r &= \sqrt{x^2+y^2+z^2} \\
y &= r\sin\theta\sin\phi & \theta &= \arctan\left(\sqrt{x^2+y^2}/z\right) \\
z &= r\cos\theta & \phi &= \arctan(y/x)
\end{aligned} \tag{A.51}$$

The relationships between the basis vectors of the Cartesian and spherical coordinate systems are expressed in the forms

$$\begin{aligned}
\mathbf{e}_x &= \sin\theta\cos\phi\,\mathbf{e}_r + \cos\theta\cos\phi\,\mathbf{e}_\theta - \sin\phi\,\mathbf{e}_\phi \\
\mathbf{e}_y &= \sin\theta\sin\phi\,\mathbf{e}_r + \cos\theta\sin\phi\,\mathbf{e}_\theta + \cos\phi\,\mathbf{e}_\phi \\
\mathbf{e}_z &= \cos\theta\,\mathbf{e}_r - \sin\theta\,\mathbf{e}_\theta + \cos\phi\,\mathbf{e}_\phi
\end{aligned} \tag{A.52}$$

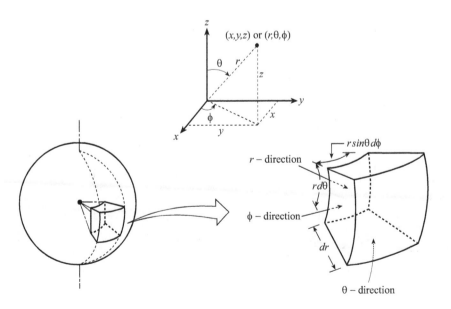

Figure A.5 The spherical coordinate system.

and

$$
\begin{aligned}
\mathbf{e}_r &= \sin\theta\cos\phi\,\mathbf{e}_x + \sin\theta\sin\phi\,\mathbf{e}_y + \cos\theta\,\mathbf{e}_z \\
\mathbf{e}_\theta &= \cos\theta\cos\phi\,\mathbf{e}_x + \cos\theta\sin\phi\,\mathbf{e}_y - \sin\theta\,\mathbf{e}_z \\
\mathbf{e}_\phi &= -\sin\phi\,\mathbf{e}_x + \cos\phi\,\mathbf{e}_y
\end{aligned}
\tag{A.53}
$$

A.6.1 DOT AND CROSS PRODUCT OPERATIONS

Vectors and tensors can be decomposed into components with respect to curvilinear coordinates just as with respect to Cartesian coordinates, and the various dot and cross product operations are performed in a similar way as shown below:

$$
\begin{aligned}
\mathbf{v}\cdot\mathbf{w} &= v_i w_i = v_1 w_1 + v_2 w_2 + v_3 w_3 \\
&= \begin{cases}
v_x w_x + v_y w_y + v_z w_z & \text{Cartesian} \\
v_r w_r + v_\theta w_\theta + v_z w_z & \text{Cylindrical} \\
v_r w_r + v_\theta w_\theta + v_\phi w_\phi & \text{Spherical}
\end{cases}
\end{aligned}
\tag{A.54}
$$

$$
\begin{aligned}
\mathbf{v}\times\mathbf{w} &= (v_2 w_3 - v_3 w_2)\mathbf{e}_1 - (v_1 w_3 - v_3 w_1)\mathbf{e}_2 + (v_1 w_2 - v_2 w_1)\mathbf{e}_3 \\
&= \begin{cases}
(v_y w_z - v_z w_y)\mathbf{e}_x - (v_x w_z - v_z w_x)\mathbf{e}_y + (v_x w_y - v_y w_x)\mathbf{e}_z & \text{Cartesian} \\
(v_\theta w_z - v_z w_\theta)\mathbf{e}_r - (v_r w_z - v_z w_r)\mathbf{e}_\theta + (v_r w_\theta - v_\theta w_r)\mathbf{e}_z & \text{Cylindrical} \\
(v_\theta w_\phi - v_\phi w_\theta)\mathbf{e}_r - (v_r w_\phi - v_\phi w_r)\mathbf{e}_\theta + (v_r w_\theta - v_\theta w_r)\mathbf{e}_\phi & \text{Spherical}
\end{cases}
\end{aligned}
\tag{A.55}
$$

A.6.2 DIFFERENTIAL OPERATIONS

In Cartesian coordinates, the gradient of a scalar field α is defined by Eq. (A.39), i.e.,

$$
\boxed{\nabla\alpha = \frac{\partial\alpha}{\partial x}\mathbf{e}_x + \frac{\partial\alpha}{\partial y}\mathbf{e}_y + \frac{\partial\alpha}{\partial z}\mathbf{e}_z}
\tag{A.56}
$$

In cylindrical and spherical coordinates, basis vectors are dependent on coordinate direction. Thus, the gradient of a scalar field α in these coordinate systems is given by

$$
\boxed{
\nabla\alpha = \begin{cases}
\dfrac{\partial\alpha}{\partial r}\mathbf{e}_r + \dfrac{1}{r}\dfrac{\partial\alpha}{\partial\theta}\mathbf{e}_\theta + \dfrac{\partial\alpha}{\partial z}\mathbf{e}_z & \text{Cylindrical} \\[2ex]
\dfrac{\partial\alpha}{\partial r}\mathbf{e}_r + \dfrac{1}{r}\dfrac{\partial\alpha}{\partial\theta}\mathbf{e}_\theta + \dfrac{1}{r\sin\theta}\dfrac{\partial\alpha}{\partial\phi}\mathbf{e}_\phi & \text{Spherical}
\end{cases}
}
\tag{A.57}
$$

The divergence of a vector field $\mathbf{v}$ in the different coordinate systems is given by

$$
\boxed{
\nabla\cdot\mathbf{v} = \begin{cases}
\dfrac{\partial v_x}{\partial x} + \dfrac{\partial v_y}{\partial y} + \dfrac{\partial v_z}{\partial z} & \text{Cartesian} \\[2ex]
\dfrac{1}{r}\dfrac{\partial}{\partial r}(r v_r) + \dfrac{1}{r}\dfrac{\partial v_\theta}{\partial\theta} + \dfrac{\partial v_z}{\partial z} & \text{Cylindrical} \\[2ex]
\dfrac{1}{r^2}\dfrac{\partial}{\partial r}(r^2 v_r) + \dfrac{1}{r\sin\theta}\dfrac{\partial}{\partial\theta}(v_\theta\sin\theta) + \dfrac{1}{r\sin\theta}\dfrac{\partial v_\phi}{\partial\phi} & \text{Spherical}
\end{cases}
}
\tag{A.58}
$$

The Laplacian of a scalar field α in the different coordinate systems is expressed as

$$\nabla^2 \alpha = \begin{cases} \dfrac{\partial^2 \alpha}{\partial x^2} + \dfrac{\partial^2 \alpha}{\partial y^2} + \dfrac{\partial^2 \alpha}{\partial z^2} & \text{Cartesian} \\[3ex] \dfrac{1}{r}\dfrac{\partial}{\partial r}\left(r\dfrac{\partial \alpha}{\partial r}\right) + \dfrac{1}{r^2}\dfrac{\partial^2 \alpha}{\partial \theta^2} + \dfrac{\partial^2 \alpha}{\partial z^2} & \text{Cylindrical} \\[3ex] \dfrac{1}{r^2}\dfrac{\partial}{\partial r}\left(r^2\dfrac{\partial \alpha}{\partial r}\right) + \dfrac{1}{r^2 \sin\theta}\dfrac{\partial}{\partial \theta}\left(\sin\theta\dfrac{\partial \alpha}{\partial \theta}\right) + \dfrac{1}{r^2 \sin^2\theta}\dfrac{\partial^2 \alpha}{\partial \phi^2} & \text{Spherical} \end{cases}$$

(A.59)

A.7 VECTOR AND TENSOR INTEGRAL THEOREMS

A.7.1 GREEN'S TRANSFORMATION

If V is a closed region in space enclosed by a surface A, then for a scalar α

$$\int_V \nabla \alpha\, dV = \int_A \lambda \alpha\, dA,$$

(A.60)

where λ is the outwardly directed unit normal vector to A.

Similarly, for any vector $\mathbf{v}$

$$\int_V (\nabla \cdot \mathbf{v})\, dV = \int_A (\lambda \cdot \mathbf{v})\, dA,$$

(A.61)

which is known as the *divergence (Gauss's) theorem.*

A.7.2 THE LEIBNIZ FORMULA

The Leibniz formula in its simplest form is expressed as

$$\frac{d}{dt}\int_a^b f(x,t)\, dx = \int_a^b \frac{\partial f}{\partial t}\, dx,$$

(A.62)

which implies that the order of integration and differentiation can be interchanged if and only if the limits of integration are constant.

If the limits of integration in Eq. (A.62) are dependent on t, then the Leibniz formula takes the form

$$\frac{d}{dt}\int_{a(t)}^{b(t)} f(x,t)\, dx = \int_{a(t)}^{b(t)} \frac{\partial f}{\partial t}\, dx + f\left[b(t),t\right]\frac{db}{dt} - f\left[a(t),t\right]\frac{da}{dt}$$

(A.63)

Note that if $f = f(x)$, then Eq. (A.63) reduces to

$$\frac{d}{dt}\int_{a(t)}^{b(t)} f(x)\, dx = f\left[b(t)\right]\frac{db}{dt} - f\left[a(t)\right]\frac{da}{dt}$$

(A.64)

In general, Eq. (A.63) can be extended to three dimensions as follows:

$$\frac{d}{dt}\int_{V(t)} f\, dV = \int_{V(t)} \frac{\partial f}{\partial t}\, dV + \int_{A(t)} f\,(\mathbf{w}\cdot\lambda)\, dA,$$

(A.65)

where $f(x,y,z,t)$ is a scalar function of position and time, $A(t)$ is the area enclosing $V(t)$, λ is the outwardly directed unit normal to the surface $A(t)$, and $\mathbf{w}$ is the velocity of the surface $A(t)$.

B Order of Magnitude (Scale) Analysis

Order of magnitude or *scale analysis* is a powerful tool for those interested in mathematical modeling. The purpose is to get an idea about the approximate magnitudes of the terms appearing in the governing equation(s). In this way, only the terms having, more or less, the same order of magnitude are kept in the equation, and the remaining ones are eliminated. As a result, the ratios of the terms kept in the governing equation are dimensionless terms having an order of magnitude of unity. Astarita (1997) stated that

"Very often more than nine-tenths of what one can ever hope to know about a problem can be obtained from this tool, without actually solving the problem; the remaining one-tenth requires painstaking algebra and/or lots of computer time, it adds very little to our understanding of the problem, and if we have not done the first part right, all that the algebra and the computer will produce will be a lot of nonsense. Of course, when nonsense comes out of a computer people have a lot of respect for it, and that is exactly the problem."

The pioneering works on the topic are those by Whitaker (1976, 1988) and Bejan (1984). Order of magnitude analysis should not be confused with dimensional analysis.

The first step in order of magnitude analysis is to define the region of interest over which the analysis will be performed. For example, consider a function $f(x)$ in the region $0 \leq x \leq L$. The order of magnitude of this function, designated by $O(f)$, is defined as the average of the absolute value of the function over this interval, i.e.,

$$O(f) \sim \frac{1}{L} \int_0^L |f| \, dx \tag{B.1}$$

Similarly, if a function $g(x, y)$ is defined over a surface occupying $0 \leq x \leq L$ and $0 \leq y \leq H$, then

$$O(g) \sim \frac{1}{LH} \int_0^H \int_0^L |g| \, dx dy \tag{B.2}$$

Order of magnitude of the derivative df/dx in the region $0 \leq x \leq L$ is given by

$$O\left(\frac{df}{dx}\right) \sim \frac{1}{L} \int_0^L \left|\frac{df}{dx}\right| dx \tag{B.3}$$

Order of magnitude analysis is not concerned with the sign. Thus, Eq. (B.3) can be expressed as

$$O\left(\frac{df}{dx}\right) \sim \frac{1}{L} \int_0^L \left(\frac{df}{dx}\right) dx = \frac{f(L) - f(0)}{L} \tag{B.4}$$

If $f(x)$ is a reasonably smooth function, it is plausible to assume that

$$O[f(L)] \sim O[f(0)] \sim O(f) \tag{B.5}$$

Hence, the order of magnitude of the derivative is

$$O\left(\frac{df}{dx}\right) \sim \frac{O(f)}{L} \tag{B.6}$$

The order of magnitude of the second derivative follows the same lines, i.e.,

$$O\left(\frac{d^2 f}{dx^2}\right) \sim \frac{1}{L}\int_0^L \left(\frac{d^2 f}{dx^2}\right) dx = \frac{1}{L}\int_0^L \frac{d}{dx}\left(\frac{df}{dx}\right) dx = \frac{1}{L}\left(\frac{df}{dx}\bigg|_{x=L} - \frac{df}{dx}\bigg|_{x=0}\right) \quad (B.7)$$

With the help of Eq. (B.6), one can claim

$$O\left(\frac{df}{dx}\bigg|_{x=L}\right) \sim O\left(\frac{df}{dx}\bigg|_{x=0}\right) \sim O\left(\frac{df}{dx}\right) = \frac{O(f)}{L} \quad (B.8)$$

Thus, Eq. (B.7) gives the order of magnitude of the second derivative as

$$\boxed{O\left(\frac{d^2 f}{dx^2}\right) \sim \frac{O(f)}{L^2}} \quad (B.9)$$

In carrying out order of magnitude analysis, one should be aware of the following rules:

- Consider the addition or subtraction of two terms

$$f = g \pm h \quad (B.10)$$

If the order of magnitude of one term, say g, is greater than the order of magnitude of the other term, i.e., $O(g) > O(h)$, then the order of magnitude of the result is dictated by the dominant term. Hence

$$O(f) \sim O(g) \quad (B.11)$$

In other words, 100 ± 1 is equal to 100!

- Consider the addition or subtraction of two terms given by Eq. (B.10). If these terms are of the same order of magnitude, i.e., $O(g) \sim O(h)$, then the result is also of the same order of magnitude given by

$$O(f) \sim O(g) \sim O(h) \quad (B.12)$$

- Consider the product of two terms

$$f = gh \quad (B.13)$$

The order of magnitude of the result is equal to the product of the orders of magnitude of the two factors, i.e.,

$$O(f) \sim O(g)O(h) \quad (B.14)$$

- Consider the ratio of two terms

$$f = \frac{g}{h} \quad (B.15)$$

The order of magnitude of the result is equal to the ratio of the orders of magnitude of the two factors, i.e.,

$$O(f) \sim \frac{O(g)}{O(h)} \quad (B.16)$$

Example B.1 Consider diffusion of gaseous species A into a solid slab (species B). Initially, the solid slab is free of species A. If the diffusion coefficient is $8 \times 10^{-7}\,\text{cm}^2/\text{s}$, how long will it take for species A to penetrate 1.5 mm into the solid slab? The governing equation for this unsteady-state diffusion process is given by

$$\frac{\partial c_A}{\partial t} = \mathcal{D}_{AB}\frac{\partial^2 c_A}{\partial x^2} \quad (1)$$

Solution

The order of magnitude of the terms can be expressed as

$$O\left(\frac{\partial c_A}{\partial t}\right) \sim \frac{c_A^*}{t} \tag{2}$$

$$O\left(\mathcal{D}_{AB}\frac{\partial^2 c_A}{\partial x^2}\right) \sim \frac{\mathcal{D}_{AB}\, c_A^*}{\delta^2}, \tag{3}$$

where c_A^* is the concentration of species A on the surface of the solid slab and δ is the penetration depth of species A.

The terms in the governing equation should have the same order of magnitude as long as Eq. (1) represents the diffusion process. Thus,

$$O\left(\frac{\partial c_A}{\partial t}\right) \sim O\left(\mathcal{D}_{AB}\frac{\partial^2 c_A}{\partial x^2}\right) \tag{4}$$

or

$$\frac{c_A^*}{t} \sim \frac{\mathcal{D}_{AB}\, c_A^*}{\delta^2} \qquad \Rightarrow \qquad t = \frac{\delta^2}{\mathcal{D}_{AB}} = \frac{(0.15)^2}{8 \times 10^{-7}} = 28,125\,\text{s} = 7.8\,\text{h}$$

REFERENCES

Astarita, G. 1997. Dimensional analysis, scaling, and orders of magnitude. *Chem. Eng. Sci.* 52(24):4681-89.

Bejan, A. 1984. *Convection Heat Transfer.* New York: Wiley.

Whitaker, S. 1976. *Elementary Heat Transfer Analysis.* New York: Pergamon Press.

Whitaker, S. 1988. Levels of simplification: The use of assumptions, restrictions, and constraints in engineering analysis. *Chem. Eng. Ed.* 22(2):104-8.

C Matrices

C.1 BASIC MATRIX OPERATIONS

A rectangular array of elements or functions is called a *matrix*. If the array has m rows and n columns, it is called a matrix of order (m,n) or an $m \times n$ matrix and is expressed in the form

$$[A] = \begin{pmatrix} A_{11} & A_{12} & A_{13} & \dots & A_{1n} \\ A_{21} & A_{22} & A_{23} & \dots & A_{2n} \\ \dots & \dots & \dots & \dots & \dots \\ A_{m1} & A_{m2} & A_{m3} & \dots & A_{mn} \end{pmatrix} \tag{C.1}$$

The numbers or functions A_{ij} are called the elements of a matrix. Equation (C.1) is also expressed as

$$[A] = (A_{ij}), \tag{C.2}$$

in which the subscripts i and j represent the row and the column of the matrix, respectively.

A matrix having only one row is called a *row matrix* (or *row vector*) while a matrix having only one column is called a *column matrix* (or *column vector*). When the number of rows and the number of columns are the same, i.e., $m = n$, the matrix is called a *square matrix* or a matrix of order n (or m).

The fundamental algebraic operations involving matrices can be briefly summarized as follows:

- Two matrices $[A] = (A_{ij})$ and $[B] = (B_{ij})$ of the same order are equal if and only if $A_{ij} = B_{ij}$.
- If $[A] = (A_{ij})$ and $[B] = (B_{ij})$ have the same order, the sum of $[A]$ and $[B]$ is defined as

$$[A] + [B] = (A_{ij} + B_{ij}) \tag{C.3}$$

Matrix addition satisfies the following algebraic rules:

$$\text{Commutative} \quad [A] + [B] = [B] + [A]$$
$$\text{Associative} \quad [A] + ([B] + [C]) = ([A] + [B]) + [C]$$

- If $[A] = (A_{ij})$ and $[B] = (B_{ij})$ have the same order, the difference between $[A]$ and $[B]$ is defined as

$$[A] - [B] = (A_{ij} - B_{ij}) \tag{C.4}$$

- If $[A] = (A_{ij})$ and λ is any number, the product of $[A]$ by λ is defined as

$$\lambda [A] = [A] \lambda = (\lambda A_{ij}) \tag{C.5}$$

- The product of two matrices $[A]$ and $[B]$, $[A][B]$, is defined only if the number of columns in $[A]$ is equal to the number of rows in $[B]$. For example, if $[A]$ is of order $(4,2)$ and $[B]$ is of order $(2,3)$, then the product $[A][B]$ is

$$[A][B] = \begin{pmatrix} A_{11} & A_{12} \\ A_{21} & A_{22} \\ A_{31} & A_{32} \\ A_{41} & A_{42} \end{pmatrix} \cdot \begin{pmatrix} B_{11} & B_{12} & B_{13} \\ B_{21} & B_{22} & B_{23} \end{pmatrix}$$

$$= \begin{pmatrix} A_{11}B_{11}+A_{12}B_{21} & A_{11}B_{12}+A_{12}B_{22} & A_{11}B_{13}+A_{12}B_{23} \\ A_{21}B_{11}+A_{22}B_{21} & A_{21}B_{12}+A_{22}B_{22} & A_{21}B_{13}+A_{22}B_{23} \\ A_{31}B_{11}+A_{32}B_{21} & A_{31}B_{12}+A_{32}B_{22} & A_{31}B_{13}+A_{32}B_{23} \\ A_{41}B_{11}+A_{42}B_{21} & A_{41}B_{12}+A_{42}B_{22} & A_{41}B_{13}+A_{42}B_{23} \end{pmatrix} \quad \text{(C.6)}$$

In general, if a matrix of order (m,r) is multiplied by a matrix of order (r,n), the product is a matrix of order (m,n). Symbolically, this may be expressed as

$$(m,r) \times (r,n) = (m,n) \quad \text{(C.7)}$$

- A matrix $[A]$ can be multiplied by itself if and only if it is a square matrix. The product $[A][A]$ can be expressed as $[A]^2$.

- The rules governing the matrix multiplication are as follows:

Not commutative $[A][B] \neq [B][A]$

Associative $[A]([B][C]) = ([A][B])[C]$

Distributive $\begin{cases} [A]([B]+[C]) = [A][B]+[A][C] \\ ([B]+[C])[A] = [B][A]+[C][A] \end{cases}$

C.2   DETERMINANTS

For each square matrix $[A]$, it is possible to associate a scalar quantity called the determinant of $[A]$, $\det[A]$. If the matrix $[A]$ in Eq. (C.1) is a square matrix of order n, then the determinant of $[A]$ is given by

$$\det[A] = \begin{vmatrix} A_{11} & A_{12} & A_{13} & \cdots & A_{1n} \\ A_{21} & A_{22} & A_{23} & \cdots & A_{2n} \\ \cdots & \cdots & \cdots & \cdots & \cdots \\ A_{n1} & A_{n2} & A_{n3} & \cdots & A_{nn} \end{vmatrix} \quad \text{(C.8)}$$

If the row and column containing an element A_{ij} in a square matrix $[A]$ are deleted, the determinant of the remaining square array is called the *minor* of A_{ij} and denoted by M_{ij}. The cofactor of A_{ij}, denoted by A_{ij}^c, is then defined by the relation

$$A_{ij}^c = (-1)^{i+j} M_{ij} \quad \text{(C.9)}$$

Thus, if the sum of the row and column indices of an element is even, the cofactor and the minor of that element are identical; otherwise, they differ in sign.

The determinant of a square matrix $[A]$ can be calculated by the following formula:

$$\det[A] = \begin{cases} \displaystyle\sum_{k=1}^{n} A_{ik}A_{ik}^c & \text{For any row } i \\ \\ \displaystyle\sum_{k=1}^{n} A_{kj}A_{kj}^c & \text{For any column } j \end{cases} \quad \text{(C.10)}$$

Therefore, the determinants of 2×2 and 3×3 matrices are given by

$$\begin{vmatrix} A_{11} & A_{12} \\ A_{21} & A_{22} \end{vmatrix} = A_{11}A_{22} - A_{12}A_{21} \quad \text{(C.11)}$$

and

$$\begin{vmatrix} A_{11} & A_{12} & A_{13} \\ A_{21} & A_{22} & A_{23} \\ A_{31} & A_{32} & A_{33} \end{vmatrix} = A_{11}A_{22}A_{33} + A_{12}A_{23}A_{31} + A_{13}A_{21}A_{32}$$

$$- A_{11}A_{23}A_{32} - A_{12}A_{21}A_{33} - A_{13}A_{22}A_{31} \quad \text{(C.12)}$$

C.2.1 SOME PROPERTIES OF DETERMINANTS

- If all elements in a row or column are zero, the determinant is zero, i.e.,

$$\begin{vmatrix} A_{11} & A_{12} & A_{13} \\ A_{21} & A_{22} & A_{23} \\ 0 & 0 & 0 \end{vmatrix} = 0 \qquad \begin{vmatrix} 0 & A_{12} & A_{13} \\ 0 & A_{22} & A_{23} \\ 0 & A_{32} & A_{33} \end{vmatrix} = 0 \quad \text{(C.13)}$$

- The value of a determinant is not altered when the rows are changed to columns and the columns to rows, i.e., when the rows and columns are interchanged.
- The interchange of any two columns or any two rows of a determinant changes the sign of the determinant.
- If two columns or two rows of a determinant are identical, the determinant is equal to zero.
- If each element in any column or row of a determinant is expressed as the sum of two quantities, the determinant can be expressed as the sum of two determinants of the same order, i.e.,

$$\begin{vmatrix} A_{11}+D_1 & A_{12} & A_{13} \\ A_{21}+D_2 & A_{22} & A_{23} \\ A_{31}+D_3 & A_{32} & A_{33} \end{vmatrix} = \begin{vmatrix} A_{11} & A_{12} & A_{13} \\ A_{21} & A_{22} & A_{23} \\ A_{31} & A_{32} & A_{33} \end{vmatrix} + \begin{vmatrix} D_1 & A_{12} & A_{13} \\ D_2 & A_{22} & A_{23} \\ D_3 & A_{32} & A_{33} \end{vmatrix} \quad \text{(C.14)}$$

- Adding the same multiple of each element of one row to the corresponding element of another row does not change the value of the determinant. The same holds true for the columns.

$$\begin{vmatrix} A_{11} & A_{12} & A_{13} \\ A_{21} & A_{22} & A_{23} \\ A_{31} & A_{32} & A_{33} \end{vmatrix} = \begin{vmatrix} (A_{11}+\lambda A_{12}) & A_{12} & A_{13} \\ (A_{21}+\lambda A_{22}) & A_{22} & A_{23} \\ (A_{31}+\lambda A_{32}) & A_{32} & A_{33} \end{vmatrix} \quad \text{(C.15)}$$

- If all the elements in any column or row are multiplied by any factor, the determinant is multiplied by that factor, i.e.,

$$\begin{vmatrix} \lambda A_{11} & A_{12} & A_{13} \\ \lambda A_{21} & A_{22} & A_{23} \\ \lambda A_{31} & A_{32} & A_{33} \end{vmatrix} = \lambda \begin{vmatrix} A_{11} & A_{12} & A_{13} \\ A_{21} & A_{22} & A_{23} \\ A_{31} & A_{32} & A_{33} \end{vmatrix} \quad \text{(C.16)}$$

$$\begin{vmatrix} (1/\lambda)A_{11} & A_{12} & A_{13} \\ (1/\lambda)A_{21} & A_{22} & A_{23} \\ (1/\lambda)A_{31} & A_{32} & A_{33} \end{vmatrix} = \frac{1}{\lambda} \begin{vmatrix} A_{11} & A_{12} & A_{13} \\ A_{21} & A_{22} & A_{23} \\ A_{31} & A_{32} & A_{33} \end{vmatrix} \quad \text{(C.17)}$$

C.3 TYPES OF MATRICES

C.3.1 TRANSPOSE OF A MATRIX

The matrix obtained from $[A]$ by interchanging rows and columns is called the *transpose* of $[A]$ and is denoted by $[A]^{\text{T}}$. The transpose of the product $[A][B]$ is the product of the transposes in the form

$$([A][B])^{\text{T}} = [B]^{\text{T}}[A]^{\text{T}} \quad \text{(C.18)}$$

C.3.2   UNIT MATRIX

The *unit matrix* $[\mathrm{I}]$ of order n is the square $n \times n$ matrix having ones in its principal diagonal and zeros elsewhere, i.e.,

$$[\mathrm{I}] = \begin{pmatrix} 1 & 0 & \ldots & 0 \\ 0 & 1 & \ldots & 0 \\ \ldots & \ldots & \ldots & \ldots \\ 0 & 0 & \ldots & 1 \end{pmatrix} \tag{C.19}$$

For any matrix

$$[\mathrm{A}][\mathrm{I}] = [\mathrm{I}][\mathrm{A}] = [\mathrm{A}] \tag{C.20}$$

A square matrix $[\mathrm{A}]$ is said to be an *orthogonal matrix* if

$$[\mathrm{A}][\mathrm{A}]^{\mathrm{T}} = [\mathrm{I}] \tag{C.21}$$

C.3.3   SYMMETRIC AND SKEW-SYMMETRIC MATRICES

A square matrix $[\mathrm{A}]$ is said to be *symmetric* if

$$[\mathrm{A}] = [\mathrm{A}]^{\mathrm{T}} \quad \Rightarrow \quad A_{ij} = A_{ji} \tag{C.22}$$

A square matrix $[\mathrm{A}]$ is said to be *skew-symmetric* (or *antisymmetric*) if

$$[\mathrm{A}] = -[\mathrm{A}]^{\mathrm{T}} \quad \Rightarrow \quad A_{ij} = -A_{ji} \tag{C.23}$$

Equation (C.23) implies that the diagonal elements of a skew-symmetric matrix are all zero.

C.3.4   SINGULAR MATRIX

A square matrix $[\mathrm{A}]$ for which the determinant $|\mathrm{A}|$ of its elements is zero is termed a *singular* matrix. If $|\mathrm{A}| \neq 0$, then $[\mathrm{A}]$ is *nonsingular*.

C.3.5   TRACE OF A MATRIX

The trace of a square matrix $[\mathrm{A}]$ of order n is the sum of the diagonal elements, i.e.,

$$\mathrm{tr}[\mathrm{A}] = \sum_{i=1}^{n} A_{ii} \tag{C.24}$$

C.3.6   INVERSE OF A MATRIX

If the determinant of a square matrix $[\mathrm{A}]$ does not vanish, i.e., a nonsingular matrix, it then possesses an *inverse* (or *reciprocal*) matrix $[\mathrm{A}]^{-1}$ such that

$$[\mathrm{A}][\mathrm{A}]^{-1} = [\mathrm{A}]^{-1}[\mathrm{A}] = [\mathrm{I}] \tag{C.25}$$

The inverse of a matrix $[\mathrm{A}]$ is defined by

$$[\mathrm{A}]^{-1} = \frac{\mathrm{adj}[\mathrm{A}]}{\det[\mathrm{A}]}, \tag{C.26}$$

where $\mathrm{adj}[\mathrm{A}]$ is called the *adjoint* of $[\mathrm{A}]$. It is obtained from a square matrix $[\mathrm{A}]$ by replacing each element by its cofactor and then interchanging rows and columns.

The inverse of the product $[A][B]$ is the product of the inverses in the form

$$([A][B])^{-1} = [B]^{-1}[A]^{-1} \tag{C.27}$$

Also note that

$$\left([A]^{-1}\right)^T = \left([A]^T\right)^{-1} \tag{C.28}$$

A square matrix in which all the elements are zeros other than the main diagonal is called a *diagonal matrix*, i.e.,

$$[D] = \begin{pmatrix} D_1 & 0 & 0 & 0 \\ 0 & D_2 & 0 & 0 \\ 0 & 0 & D_3 & 0 \\ 0 & 0 & 0 & D_4 \end{pmatrix} \tag{C.29}$$

The inverse of a diagonal matrix is

$$[D]^{-1} = \begin{pmatrix} 1/D_1 & 0 & 0 & 0 \\ 0 & 1/D_2 & 0 & 0 \\ 0 & 0 & 1/D_3 & 0 \\ 0 & 0 & 0 & 1/D_4 \end{pmatrix} \tag{C.30}$$

• **Sherman–Morrison formula**

If a matrix $[B]$ is expressed in the form of

$$[B] = [A] - [u][v]^T, \tag{C.31}$$

where $[A]$ is a nonsingular $n \times n$ matrix and $[u]$ and $[v]$ are column n-vectors, the formula given by Sherman and Morrison (1950) provides an explicit formula for the inverse of a matrix $[B]$ in the form

$$\boxed{[B]^{-1} = \left\{ [I] + \frac{1}{1 - [v]^T \left([A]^{-1}[u]\right)} \left([A]^{-1}[u]\right)[v]^T \right\}[A]^{-1},} \tag{C.32}$$

where $[I]$ is an identity matrix. When $[A] = [I]$, Eq. (C.32) simplifies to

$$[B]^{-1} = [I] + \frac{[u][v]^T}{1 - [v]^T[u]} \tag{C.33}$$

C.4   EIGENVALUES AND EIGENVECTORS OF A MATRIX

As stated in Appendix A (Section A.4), a second-order tensor $\mathbf{T}$ transforms a vector $\mathbf{v}$ into another vector $\mathbf{w}$ such that

$$\mathbf{T} \cdot \mathbf{v} = \mathbf{w} \tag{C.34}$$

The directions of $\mathbf{v}$ and $\mathbf{w}$ are obviously different from each other. Now consider a special case in which $\mathbf{w} = \lambda \mathbf{v}$, where λ is a scalar. Hence, Eq. (C.34) becomes

$$\mathbf{T} \cdot \mathbf{v} = \lambda \mathbf{v}, \tag{C.35}$$

which implies that the result of the operation $\mathbf{T} \cdot \mathbf{v}$ is given by

$$\mathbf{T} \cdot \mathbf{v} = \begin{cases} \text{Another vector in the direction of } \mathbf{v} & \text{if } \lambda > 0 \\ \text{Another vector in the opposite direction of } \mathbf{v} & \text{if } \lambda < 0 \end{cases} \tag{C.36}$$

In either case, the magnitude of the resulting vector will change depending on the value of λ. The vector will be shrunk when the absolute value of λ varies between 0 and 1 or will be stretched when the absolute value of λ is greater than 1.

Now consider the equation

$$[\mathrm{A}][\mathrm{v}] = \lambda[\mathrm{v}], \tag{C.37}$$

where $[\mathrm{A}]$ is a nonsingular $n \times n$ matrix, $[\mathrm{v}]$ is a column n-vector, and λ is a scalar. Any value of λ for which Eq. (C.37) has a solution is called an *eigenvalue* (or *characteristic value*) of the matrix $[\mathrm{A}]$. The eigenvalues can be found by solving the so-called *characteristic equation* given in the form

$$\det([\mathrm{A}] - \lambda[\mathrm{I}]) = 0 \tag{C.38}$$

The column n-vector $[\mathrm{v}]$ corresponding to each eigenvalue is called an *eigenvector*.

C.4.1 SOME PROPERTIES OF EIGENVALUES AND EIGENVECTORS

- The sum of the eigenvalues of a matrix equals the trace of the matrix.
- The product of the eigenvalues of a matrix equals the determinant of the matrix.
- Let $[\mathrm{v}]$ be the eigenvector associated with the eigenvalue λ of the square matrix $[\mathrm{A}]$:

  (*i*) The eigenvalue of the inverse matrix $[\mathrm{A}]^{-1}$ is $1/\lambda$, with the same eigenvector $[\mathrm{v}]$.

  (*ii*) For $k > 0$, the eigenvalue of the matrix $[\mathrm{A}]^k$ is λ^k, with the same eigenvector $[\mathrm{v}]$.

- A nonsingular square matrix $[\mathrm{A}]$ can be expressed in the form of

$$[\mathrm{A}] = [\mathrm{P}][\mathrm{D}][\mathrm{P}]^{-1}, \tag{C.39}$$

where $[\mathrm{P}]$ is a square matrix of eigenvectors and $[\mathrm{D}]$ is the diagonal matrix with the eigenvalues on the diagonal.

C.5 SOLUTION OF ALGEBRAIC EQUATIONS – CRAMER'S RULE

Consider the system of n nonhomogeneous algebraic equations

$$\begin{aligned} A_{11}x_1 + A_{12}x_2 + \ldots + A_{1n}x_n &= C_1 \\ A_{21}x_1 + A_{22}x_2 + \ldots + A_{2n}x_n &= C_2 \\ \cdots\cdots\cdots\cdots\cdots\cdots\cdots\cdots\cdots &= \cdots \\ A_{n1}x_1 + A_{n2}x_2 + \ldots + A_{nn}x_n &= C_n, \end{aligned} \tag{C.40}$$

in which the coefficients A_{ij} and the constants C_i are independent of $x_1, x_2, \ldots, x_n$ but are otherwise arbitrary. In matrix notation, Eq. (C.40) is expressed as

$$\begin{pmatrix} A_{11} & A_{12} & \cdots & A_{1n} \\ A_{21} & A_{22} & \cdots & A_{2n} \\ \cdots & \cdots & \cdots & \cdots \\ A_{n1} & A_{n2} & \cdots & A_{nn} \end{pmatrix} \begin{pmatrix} x_1 \\ x_2 \\ \cdots \\ x_n \end{pmatrix} = \begin{pmatrix} C_1 \\ C_2 \\ \cdots \\ C_n \end{pmatrix} \tag{C.41}$$

or

$$[\mathrm{A}][\mathrm{x}] = [\mathrm{C}] \tag{C.42}$$

Cramer's rule states that if the determinant of matrix $[A]$ does not vanish, the system of algebraic linear equations has a solution given by

$$x_j = \frac{\det[A_j]}{\det[A]},$$ (C.43)

where $\det[A_j]$ stands for the determinant of the substituted matrix that is obtained by replacing the jth column of $\det[A]$ by the column of C's, i.e.,

$$\det[A_j] = \begin{vmatrix} A_{11} & A_{12} & \cdots & C_1 & \cdots & A_{1n} \\ A_{21} & A_{22} & \cdots & C_2 & \cdots & A_{2n} \\ \cdots & \cdots & \cdots & \cdots & \cdots & \cdots \\ A_{n1} & A_{n2} & \cdots & C_n & \cdots & A_{nn} \end{vmatrix}$$ (C.44)

C.6 MATRIX OPERATIONS USING MATHCAD

The Mathcad worksheet given below shows the basic matrix operations.

ORIGIN:= 1

Matrix Multiplication

$$A := \begin{pmatrix} 2 & 3 & -4 & 1 \\ 0 & -1 & -2 & 5 \\ 8 & -6 & -1 & 1 \end{pmatrix} \qquad B := \begin{pmatrix} 3 & -2 \\ 6 & 5 \\ 0 & -3 \\ 8 & 2 \end{pmatrix}$$

$$A \cdot B = \begin{pmatrix} 32 & 25 \\ 34 & 11 \\ -4 & -41 \end{pmatrix}$$

Transpose of a Matrix

$$A := \begin{pmatrix} 1 & 2 & 3 & 4 \\ 5 & 6 & 7 & 8 \end{pmatrix}$$

$$A^T = \begin{pmatrix} 1 & 5 \\ 2 & 6 \\ 3 & 7 \\ 4 & 8 \end{pmatrix}$$

Inverse of a Matrix

$$A := \begin{pmatrix} 3 & -4 & 1 \\ -1 & -2 & 5 \\ -6 & -1 & 1 \end{pmatrix}$$

$$A^{-1} = \begin{pmatrix} 0.026 & 0.026 & -0.158 \\ -0.254 & 0.079 & -0.14 \\ -0.096 & 0.237 & -0.088 \end{pmatrix} \qquad A^{-1} \rightarrow \begin{pmatrix} \dfrac{1}{38} & \dfrac{1}{38} & \dfrac{3}{19} \\ \dfrac{29}{114} & \dfrac{3}{38} & \dfrac{8}{57} \\ \dfrac{11}{114} & \dfrac{9}{38} & \dfrac{5}{57} \end{pmatrix}$$

Mathcad worksheet on matrix operations.

Eigenvalues and Eigenvectors

$$A := \begin{pmatrix} 2 & 1 & 0 \\ 1 & 2 & 1 \\ 0 & 1 & 2 \end{pmatrix}$$

$$M := \text{eigenvals}(A) \rightarrow \begin{pmatrix} \sqrt{2} + 2 \\ 2 \\ 2 - \sqrt{2} \end{pmatrix}$$

$$\text{eigenvec}(A, M_1) \rightarrow \begin{pmatrix} 1 \\ \sqrt{2} \\ 1 \end{pmatrix} \qquad \text{eigenvec}(A, M_2) \rightarrow \begin{pmatrix} -1 \\ 0 \\ 1 \end{pmatrix} \qquad \text{eigenvec}(A, M_3) \rightarrow \begin{pmatrix} 1 \\ -\sqrt{2} \\ 1 \end{pmatrix}$$

$$P := \begin{pmatrix} 1 & -1 & 1 \\ \sqrt{2} & 0 & -\sqrt{2} \\ 1 & 1 & 1 \end{pmatrix} \qquad D := \begin{pmatrix} \sqrt{2} + 2 & 0 & 0 \\ 0 & 2 & 0 \\ 0 & 0 & 2 - \sqrt{2} \end{pmatrix}$$

$$P \cdot D \cdot P^{-1} = \begin{pmatrix} 2 & 1 & 0 \\ 1 & 2 & 1 \\ 0 & 1 & 2 \end{pmatrix}$$

Mathcad worksheet on matrix operations.

REFERENCE

Sherman, J., and W. J. Morrison. 1950. Adjustment of an inverse matrix corresponding to a change in one element of a given matrix. *Ann. Math. Statist.* 21(1):124–27.

D Ordinary Differential Equations

A differential equation containing ordinary derivatives is called an *ordinary differential equation* (ODE). The *order* of a differential equation is the order of the highest derivative in the equation. A differential equation is *linear* when (1) every dependent variable and every derivative involved occur to the first degree only and (2) neither products nor powers of dependent variables nor products of dependent variables with differentials exist.

D.1 FIRST-ORDER ODEs

First-order ODEs for which solutions may be obtained by analytical methods are classified as (1) separable equations, (2) exact equations, (3) homogeneous equations, (4) linear equations, and (5) Bernoulli equations.

D.1.1 SEPARABLE EQUATION

An equation of the form

$$f_1(x)g_1(y)\,dx + f_2(x)g_2(y)\,dy = 0 \tag{D.1}$$

is called a *separable equation*. Dividing Eq. (D.1) by $g_1(y)f_2(x)$ results in

$$\frac{f_1(x)}{f_2(x)}\,dx + \frac{g_2(y)}{g_1(y)}\,dy = 0 \tag{D.2}$$

Integration of Eq. (D.2) gives

$$\int \frac{f_1(x)}{f_2(x)}\,dx + \int \frac{g_2(y)}{g_1(y)}\,dy = C, \tag{D.3}$$

where C is an integration constant.

D.1.2 EXACT EQUATION

The expression $M(x,y)\,dx + N(x,y)\,dy$ is called an *exact differential*[1] if there exists some $\phi = \phi(x,y)$ for which this expression is replaced by the total differential $d\phi(x,y)$, i.e.,

$$M(x,y)\,dx + N(x,y)\,dy = d\phi(x,y) \tag{D.4}$$

A necessary and sufficient condition for the expression $M(x,y)\,dx + N(x,y)\,dy$ to be expressed as a total differential is that

$$\frac{\partial M(x,y)}{\partial y} = \frac{\partial N(x,y)}{\partial x} \tag{D.5}$$

If $M(x,y)\,dx + N(x,y)\,dy$ is an exact differential, then the differential equation

$$M(x,y)\,dx + N(x,y)\,dy = 0 \tag{D.6}$$

is called an *exact differential equation*. Since an exact differential can be expressed in the form of a total differential $d\phi$, then

$$M(x,y)\,dx + N(x,y)\,dy = d\phi(x,y) = 0 \tag{D.7}$$

---

[1] In thermodynamics, an exact differential is called a *state function*.

and the solution can easily be obtained as

$$\phi(x, y) = C, \tag{D.8}$$

where C is a constant.

D.1.3 HOMOGENEOUS EQUATION

A function $f(x, y)$ is said to be *homogeneous of degree n* if

$$f(\lambda x, \lambda y) = \lambda^n f(x, y) \tag{D.9}$$

for all λ. For an equation,

$$M(x, y)\, dx + N(x, y)\, dy = 0 \tag{D.10}$$

if M and N are homogeneous of the same degree, the transformation

$$y(x) = u x \tag{D.11}$$

makes the equation separable.

LINEAR EQUATION

An equation of the form

$$\frac{dy(x)}{dx} + p(x)\, y(x) = q(x) \tag{D.12}$$

is called a *linear equation*. To solve Eq. (D.12), the first step is to find an *integrating factor*, $\mu(x)$, which is defined by

$$\mu(x) = e^{\int p(x)\, dx} \qquad \Rightarrow \qquad \frac{d\mu(x)}{dx} = p(x)\, \mu(x) \tag{D.13}$$

Multiplication of Eq. (D.12) by the integrating factor and rearrangement give

$$\frac{d}{dx}\left[\mu(x)\, y(x) \right] = q(x)\, \mu(x) \tag{D.14}$$

Integration of Eq. (D.14) gives the solution as

$$y = \frac{1}{\mu(x)} \int q(x)\, \mu(x)\, dx + \frac{C}{\mu(x)}, \tag{D.15}$$

where C is an integration constant.

D.1.4 BERNOULLI EQUATION

A *Bernoulli equation* has the form

$$\frac{dy(x)}{dx} + p(x)\, y(x) = q(x)\, y(x)^n \qquad n \neq 0, 1 \tag{D.16}$$

The transformation

$$u(x) = y(x)^{1-n} \tag{D.17}$$

reduces the Bernoulli equation to a linear equation, Eq. (D.12).

D.2 SECOND-ORDER ODEs

A general second-order linear differential equation with constant coefficients is written as

$$a_o \frac{d^2 y}{dx^2} + a_1 \frac{dy}{dx} + a_2 y = R(x) \tag{D.18}$$

If $R(x) = 0$, the equation

$$a_o \frac{d^2 y}{dx^2} + a_1 \frac{dy}{dx} + a_2 y = 0 \tag{D.19}$$

is called a *homogeneous equation*.

D.2.1 SOLUTION OF A HOMOGENEOUS EQUATION

The second-order homogeneous ODE with constant coefficients can be solved by proposing a solution of the form

$$y = e^{\lambda x}, \tag{D.20}$$

where λ is a constant. Substitution of Eq. (D.20) into Eq. (D.19) gives

$$a_o \lambda^2 + a_1 \lambda + a_2 = 0, \tag{D.21}$$

which is known as the *characteristic* or *auxiliary equation*. Solution of the given differential equation depends on the roots of the characteristic equation.

• **Distinct real roots**

When the roots of Eq. (D.21), λ_1 and λ_2, are real and distinct, the solution is

$$\boxed{y = C_1 e^{\lambda_1 x} + C_2 e^{\lambda_2 x}} \tag{D.22}$$

• **Repeated real roots**

When the roots of Eq. (D.21), λ_1 and λ_2, are real and equal to each other, i.e., $\lambda_1 = \lambda_2 = \lambda$, the solution is

$$\boxed{y = (C_1 + C_2 x) e^{\lambda x}} \tag{D.23}$$

• **Conjugate complex roots**

When the roots of Eq. (D.21), λ_1 and λ_2, are complex and conjugate, i.e., $\lambda_{1,2} = a \pm ib$, the solution is

$$\boxed{y = e^{ax} \left[C_1 \cos(bx) + C_2 \sin(bx) \right]} \tag{D.24}$$

D.2.2 SOLUTION OF A NONHOMOGENOUS EQUATION

Consider a general second-order ODE given by

$$\frac{d^2 y(x)}{dx^2} + p(x) \frac{dy(x)}{dx} + q(x) y(x) = R(x) \tag{D.25}$$

If one solution of the homogeneous equation is known, i.e., say $y = y_1(x)$, then the complete solution is given by (Murray, 1924)

$$\boxed{y = C_1 y_1(x) + C_2 y_1(x) \int \frac{e^{-\int p(x)dx}}{y_1(x)^2} dx + y_1(x) \int \frac{e^{-\int p(x)dx}}{y_1(x)^2} \left[\int^x y_1(u) R(u) e^{\int p(u)du} \right] dx,} \tag{D.26}$$

where C_1 and C_2 are constants.

D.2.3 BESSEL'S EQUATION

An ODE given in the general form

$$\frac{d}{dx}\left(x^p \frac{dy}{dx}\right) + (ax^j + bx^k)y = 0 \qquad j > k \tag{D.27}$$

with either $k = p - 2$ or $b = 0$ is known as *Bessel's equation*. The solution to Bessel's equation depends on whether the term a is positive or negative.

- **Solution for $a > 0$**

In this case, the solution is given by

$$y = \begin{cases} x^{\alpha\beta}\left[C_1 J_n(\Omega x^\alpha) + C_2 J_{-n}(\Omega x^\alpha)\right] & n \neq \text{integer} \\[2ex] x^{\alpha\beta}\left[C_1 J_n(\Omega x^\alpha) + C_2 Y_n(\Omega x^\alpha)\right] & n = \text{integer}, \end{cases} \tag{D.28}$$

where C_1 and C_2 are constants; the terms α, β, n, and Ω are defined by

$$\boxed{\alpha = \frac{2 - p + j}{2} \qquad \beta = \frac{1 - p}{2 - p + j} \qquad n = \frac{\sqrt{(1 - p)^2 - 4b}}{2 - p + j}} \tag{D.29}$$

$$\boxed{\Omega = \frac{\sqrt{a}}{\alpha}} \tag{D.30}$$

The term $J_n(x)$ is known as the *Bessel function of the first kind of order n* and is given by

$$\boxed{J_n(x) = \sum_{i=0}^{\infty} \frac{(-1)^i (x/2)^{2i+n}}{i!\,\Gamma(i + n + 1)}} \tag{D.31}$$

When n is not an integer, the functions $J_n(x)$ and $J_{-n}(x)$ are linearly independent solutions of Bessel's equation.[2] When n is an integer, however, these two functions are no longer linearly independent. In this case, $J_{-n}(x)$ is replaced with $Y_n(x)$, *Weber's Bessel function of the second kind of order n*, defined by

$$\boxed{Y_n(x) = \frac{J_n(x)\cos(n\pi) - J_{-n}(x)}{\sin(n\pi)}} \tag{D.32}$$

- **Solution for $a < 0$**

In this case, the solution is given by

$$y = \begin{cases} x^{\alpha\beta}\left[C_1 I_n(\Omega x^\alpha) + C_2 I_{-n}(\Omega x^\alpha)\right] & n \neq \text{integer} \\[2ex] x^{\alpha\beta}\left[C_1 I_n(\Omega x^\alpha) + C_2 K_n(\Omega x^\alpha)\right] & n = \text{integer}, \end{cases} \tag{D.33}$$

where C_1 and C_2 are constants; the terms α, β, and n are defined by Eq. (D.29), and Ω is defined by

$$\boxed{\Omega = -i\frac{\sqrt{a}}{\alpha}} \tag{D.34}$$

---

[2] $J_{-n}(x)$ is obtained by simply replacing n in Eq. (D.31) with $-n$.

The term $I_n(x)$ is known as the *modified Bessel function of the first kind of order n* and is given by

$$I_n(x) = \sum_{i=0}^{\infty} \frac{(x/2)^{2i+n}}{i!\,\Gamma(i+n+1)} \tag{D.35}$$

When n is not an integer, the functions $I_n(x)$ and $I_{-n}(x)$ are linearly independent solutions of Bessel's equation.[3] When n is an integer, however, the functions $I_n(x)$ and $I_{-n}(x)$ become linearly dependent. In this case, $I_{-n}(x)$ is replaced with $K_n(x)$, the *modified Bessel function of the second kind of order n*, defined by

$$K_n(x) = \frac{\pi}{2} \frac{I_{-n}(x) - I_n(x)}{\sin(n\pi)} \tag{D.36}$$

The properties of Bessel functions are summarized in Table D.1.

D.3 SPECIAL CASES OF SECOND-ORDER DIFFERENTIAL EQUATIONS

The following differential equations are frequently encountered in steady-state mass transfer problems:

$$\nabla^2 \theta - \lambda^2 \theta = 0 \tag{D.37}$$

$$\nabla^2 \theta + \lambda^2 \theta = 0, \tag{D.38}$$

where θ is a dimensionless concentration and λ is a dimensionless number.

D.3.1 CARTESIAN COORDINATE SYSTEM

- The one-dimensional form of Eq. (D.37) in a Cartesian coordinate system is

$$\frac{d^2\theta}{d\xi^2} - \lambda^2 \theta = 0 \tag{D.39}$$

where ξ is a dimensionless coordinate. The solution of Eq. (D.39) is given by

$$\theta = C_1 e^{\lambda\xi} + C_2 e^{-\lambda\xi}, \tag{D.40}$$

where C_1 and C_2 are constants. Using the identities

$$\cosh\lambda x = \frac{e^{\lambda x} + e^{-\lambda x}}{2} \qquad \text{and} \qquad \sinh\lambda x = \frac{e^{\lambda x} - e^{-\lambda x}}{2} \tag{D.41}$$

Eq. (D.40) can also be expressed in the form

$$\theta = C_1^* \sinh(\lambda\xi) + C_2^* \cosh(\lambda\xi), \tag{D.42}$$

where C_1^* and C_2^* are constants different from C_1 and C_2.

- The one-dimensional form of Eq. (D.38) in a Cartesian coordinate system is

$$\frac{d^2\theta}{d\xi^2} + \lambda^2 \theta = 0 \tag{D.43}$$

The solution of Eq. (D.43) is given by

$$\theta = C_1 \sin(\lambda\xi) + C_2 \cos(\lambda\xi) \tag{D.44}$$

The exponential, hyperbolic, and trigonometric functions are plotted in Figure D.1.

---

[3] $I_{-n}(x)$ is obtained by simply replacing n in Eq. (D.35) with $-n$.

Table D.1
Properties of the Bessel Functions

Behavior Near the Origin

$$J_o(0) = I_o(0) = 1$$

$$-Y_n(0) = K_n(0) = \infty \qquad \text{for all } n$$

$$J_n(0) = I_n(0) = 0 \qquad \text{for } n > 0$$

$J_n(x)$ and $I_n(x)$ are the only physically permissible solutions at the origin.

Bessel Functions of Negative Order ($n = $ integer)

$$J_{-n}(\lambda x) = (-1)^n J_n(\lambda x) \qquad\qquad Y_{-n}(\lambda x) = (-1)^n Y_n(\lambda x)$$

$$I_{-n}(\lambda x) = I_n(\lambda x) \qquad\qquad K_{-n}(\lambda x) = K_n(\lambda x)$$

Recurrence Formulas

$$J_n(\lambda x) = \frac{\lambda x}{2n}\left[J_{n+1}(\lambda x) + J_{n-1}(\lambda x)\right] \qquad Y_n(\lambda x) = \frac{\lambda x}{2n}\left[Y_{n+1}(\lambda x) + Y_{n-1}(\lambda x)\right]$$

$$I_n(\lambda x) = -\frac{\lambda x}{2n}\left[I_{n+1}(\lambda x) - I_{n-1}(\lambda x)\right] \qquad K_n(\lambda x) = \frac{\lambda x}{2n}\left[K_{n+1}(\lambda x) - K_{n-1}(\lambda x)\right]$$

Integral Properties

$$\int \lambda x^n J_{n-1}(\lambda x)\, dx = x^n J_n(\lambda x) \qquad\qquad \int \lambda x^n Y_{n-1}(\lambda x)\, dx = x^n Y_n(\lambda x)$$

$$\int \lambda x^n I_{n-1}(\lambda x)\, dx = x^n I_n(\lambda x) \qquad\qquad \int \lambda x^n K_{n-1}(\lambda x)\, dx = -x^n K_n(\lambda x)$$

Differential Relations

$$\frac{d}{dx}J_n(\lambda x) = \lambda J_{n-1}(\lambda x) - \frac{n}{x}J_n(\lambda x) = -\lambda J_{n+1}(\lambda x) + \frac{n}{x}J_n(\lambda x)$$

$$\frac{d}{dx}Y_n(\lambda x) = \lambda Y_{n-1}(\lambda x) - \frac{n}{x}Y_n(\lambda x) = -\lambda Y_{n+1}(\lambda x) + \frac{n}{x}Y_n(\lambda x)$$

$$\frac{d}{dx}I_n(\lambda x) = \lambda I_{n-1}(\lambda x) - \frac{n}{x}I_n(\lambda x) = \lambda I_{n+1}(\lambda x) + \frac{n}{x}I_n(\lambda x)$$

$$\frac{d}{dx}K_n(\lambda x) = -\lambda K_{n-1}(\lambda x) - \frac{n}{x}K_n(\lambda x) = -\lambda K_{n+1}(\lambda x) + \frac{n}{x}K_n(\lambda x)$$

Bessel Functions of Fractional Order

$$J_{1/2}(x) = \sqrt{\frac{2}{\pi x}}\sin x \qquad\qquad I_{1/2}(x) = \sqrt{\frac{2}{\pi x}}\sinh x$$

$$J_{3/2}(x) = \sqrt{\frac{2}{\pi x}}\left(\frac{\sin x}{x} - \cos x\right) \qquad I_{3/2}(x) = \sqrt{\frac{2}{\pi x}}\left(\cosh x - \frac{\sinh x}{x}\right)$$

D.3.2   CYLINDRICAL COORDINATE SYSTEM

- The one-dimensional form of Eq. (D.37) in a cylindrical coordinate system is

$$\frac{1}{\xi}\frac{d}{d\xi}\left(\xi\frac{d\theta}{d\xi}\right) - \lambda^2\theta = 0, \tag{D.45}$$

where ξ is a dimensionless radial coordinate. Comparison of Eq. (D.45) with Eq. (D.27) indicates that

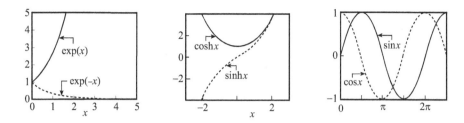

Figure D.1 Behavior of exponential, hyperbolic, and trigonometric functions.

$$p = 1 \qquad j = 1 \qquad a = -\lambda^2 \qquad b = 0 \tag{D.46}$$

Therefore, Eq. (D.45) is Bessel's equation, and the use of Eqs. (D.29), (D.33), and (D.34) gives the solution as

$$\boxed{\theta = C_1 I_o(\lambda \xi) + C_2 K_o(\lambda \xi)} \tag{D.47}$$

- The one-dimensional form of Eq. (D.38) in a cylindrical coordinate system is

$$\frac{1}{\xi} \frac{d}{d\xi} \left(\xi \frac{d\theta}{d\xi} \right) + \lambda^2 \theta = 0 \tag{D.48}$$

Comparison of Eq. (D.48) with Eq. (D.27) indicates that

$$p = 1 \qquad j = 1 \qquad a = \lambda^2 \qquad b = 0 \tag{D.49}$$

Therefore, Eq. (D.48) is Bessel's equation, and the use of Eqs. (D.28)–(D.30) gives the solution as

$$\boxed{\theta = C_1 J_o(\lambda \xi) + C_2 Y_o(\lambda \xi)} \tag{D.50}$$

The behavior of Bessel functions is shown in Figure D.2.

D.3.3 SPHERICAL COORDINATE SYSTEM

- The one-dimensional form of Eq. (D.37) in a spherical coordinate system is

$$\frac{1}{\xi^2} \frac{d}{d\xi} \left(\xi^2 \frac{d\theta}{d\xi} \right) - \lambda^2 \theta = 0, \tag{D.51}$$

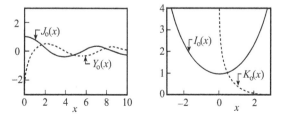

Figure D.2 Behavior of Bessel functions.

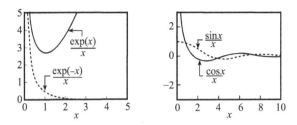

Figure D.3   Behavior of the functions in Eqs. (D.54) and (D.57).

where ξ is a dimensionless radial coordinate. The transformation in the form

$$\theta = \frac{u}{\xi} \tag{D.52}$$

converts Eq. (D.51) to a Cartesian coordinate system, i.e.,

$$\frac{d^2u}{d\xi^2} - \lambda^2 u = 0 \tag{D.53}$$

Thus, the solution is expressed as

$$\boxed{\theta = C_1 \frac{e^{\lambda\xi}}{\xi} + C_2 \frac{e^{-\lambda\xi}}{\xi}} \quad \text{or} \quad \boxed{\theta = C_1^* \frac{\sinh(\lambda\xi)}{\xi} + C_2^* \frac{\cosh(\lambda\xi)}{\xi}} \tag{D.54}$$

• The one-dimensional form of Eq. (D.38) in a spherical coordinate system is

$$\frac{1}{\xi^2} \frac{d}{d\xi}\left(\xi^2 \frac{d\theta}{d\xi}\right) + \lambda^2 \theta = 0 \tag{D.55}$$

The transformation given by Eq. (D.52) converts Eq. (D.55) to

$$\frac{d^2u}{d\xi^2} + \lambda^2 u = 0 \tag{D.56}$$

Therefore, the solution is

$$\boxed{\theta = C_1 \frac{\sin(\lambda\xi)}{\xi} + C_2 \frac{\cos(\lambda\xi)}{\xi}} \tag{D.57}$$

The behavior of the functions appearing in the solutions is shown in Figure D.3.

REFERENCE

Murray, D. A. 1924. *Introductory Course in Differential Equations*. New York: Longmans, Green & Co.

E Partial Differential Equations

E.1 PRELIMINARIES

E.1.1 CLASSIFICATION OF PARTIAL DIFFERENTIAL EQUATIONS

As a function of two independent variables, x and y, the most general form of a second-order linear partial differential equation (PDE) has the form

$$A(x,y)\frac{\partial^2 u}{\partial x^2} + 2B(x,y)\frac{\partial^2 u}{\partial x \partial y} + C(x,y)\frac{\partial^2 u}{\partial y^2} + D(x,y)\frac{\partial u}{\partial x}$$

$$+ E(x,y)\frac{\partial u}{\partial y} + F(x,y)u = G(x,y) \tag{E.1}$$

It is assumed that the coefficient functions and the given function G are real-valued and twice continuously differentiable on a region $\mathbb{R}$ of the x,y plane. When $G = 0$, the equation is *homogeneous*; otherwise the equation is *nonhomogeneous*.

The criterion, $B^2 - AC$, that will indicate whether the second-order equation is a graph of a parabola, ellipse, or hyperbola is called the *discriminant*, Δ, i.e.,

$$\Delta = B^2 - AC \begin{cases} > 0 & \text{Hyperbolic PDE} \\ = 0 & \text{Parabolic PDE} \\ < 0 & \text{Elliptic PDE} \end{cases} \tag{E.2}$$

E.1.2 ORTHOGONAL FUNCTIONS

Let $f(x)$ and $g(x)$ be real-valued functions defined on the interval $a \leq x \leq b$. The *inner product*[1] of $f(x)$ and $g(x)$ with respect to $w(x)$ is defined by

$$\langle f,g \rangle = \int_a^b w(x) f(x) g(x)\, dx, \tag{E.3}$$

in which the *weight function* $w(x)$ is considered positive on the interval (a,b).

The inner product has the following properties:

$$\langle f,g \rangle = \langle g,f \rangle \tag{E.4}$$

$$\langle f,g+h \rangle = \langle f,g \rangle + \langle f,h \rangle \tag{E.5}$$

$$\langle \alpha f,g \rangle = \alpha \langle f,g \rangle \qquad \alpha \text{ is a scalar} \tag{E.6}$$

When $\langle f,g \rangle = 0$ on (a,b), $f(x)$ is *orthogonal* to $g(x)$ with respect to the weight function $w(x)$ on (a,b), and when $\langle f,f \rangle = 1$, $f(x)$ is an *orthonormal* function. In the special case where $w(x) = 1$ for $a \leq x \leq b$, $f(x)$ and $g(x)$ are said to be *simply orthogonal*.

A sequence of functions $\{f_n\}_{n=0}^{\infty}$ is an *orthogonal set* of functions if

$$\langle f_n, f_m \rangle = \begin{cases} 0 & \text{if} \quad n \neq m \\ \text{Nonzero} & \text{if} \quad n = m \end{cases} \tag{E.7}$$

---

[1] Note that the scalar (or dot) product is a special case of an inner product.

The orthogonal set is a linearly independent set. When

$$\langle f_n, f_m \rangle = \begin{cases} 0 & \text{if} \quad n \neq m \\ 1 & \text{if} \quad n = m \end{cases} \tag{E.8}$$

such a set is called an *orthonormal set*.

E.1.3 SECOND-ORDER SELF-ADJOINT DIFFERENTIAL EQUATIONS

Consider a second-order ordinary differential equation (ODE) of the form

$$a_o(x) \frac{d^2 y}{dx^2} + a_1(x) \frac{dy}{dx} + a_2(x) y = 0 \tag{E.9}$$

To make the coefficient of the second-order derivative unity, dividing Eq. (E.9) by $a_o(x)$ yields

$$\frac{d^2 y}{dx^2} + \frac{a_1(x)}{a_o(x)} \frac{dy}{dx} + \frac{a_2(x)}{a_o(x)} y = 0 \tag{E.10}$$

The *integrating factor* $\mu(x)$ is defined by

$$\boxed{\mu(x) = e^{\int \frac{a_1(x)}{a_o(x)} dx}} \tag{E.11}$$

Differentiation of Eq. (E.11) with respect to x gives

$$\frac{d\mu(x)}{dx} = \frac{a_1(x)}{a_o(x)} \mu(x) \tag{E.12}$$

Multiplication of Eq. (E.10) by the integrating factor gives

$$\mu(x) \frac{d^2 y}{dx^2} + \frac{a_1(x)}{a_o(x)} \mu(x) \frac{dy}{dx} + q(x) y = 0, \tag{E.13}$$

where $q(x)$ is defined by

$$q(x) = \frac{a_2(x)}{a_o(x)} \mu(x) \tag{E.14}$$

The use of Eq. (E.12) in Eq. (E.13) gives

$$\mu(x) \frac{d^2 y}{dx^2} + \frac{d\mu(x)}{dx} \frac{dy}{dx} + q(x) y = 0, \tag{E.15}$$

which can be rearranged as

$$\boxed{\frac{d}{dx} \left[\mu(x) \frac{dy}{dx} \right] + q(x) y = 0} \tag{E.16}$$

A second-order differential equation in this form is said to be in *self-adjoint form*.

Example E.1 To express the following differential equation in self-adjoint form

$$(x^2 - 1) \frac{d^2 y}{dx^2} + x \frac{dy}{dx} + (x+3) y = 0 \tag{1}$$

the first step is to make the coefficient of the second-order derivative unity. Thus, dividing Eq. (1) by $(x^2 - 1)$ gives

$$\frac{d^2y}{dx^2} + \frac{x}{x^2-1}\frac{dy}{dx} + \left(\frac{x+3}{x^2-1}\right)y = 0 \tag{2}$$

The integrating factor is

$$\mu(x) = e^{\int \frac{x}{x^2-1}dx} = \sqrt{x^2-1} \tag{3}$$

Multiplication of Eq. (2) by $\mu(x)$ gives

$$\sqrt{x^2-1}\frac{d^2y}{dx^2} + \frac{x}{\sqrt{x^2-1}}\frac{dy}{dx} + \frac{x+3}{\sqrt{x^2-1}}y = 0 \tag{4}$$

Note that Eq. (4) can be rearranged as

$$\frac{d}{dx}\left(\sqrt{x^2-1}\frac{dy}{dx}\right) + \frac{x+3}{\sqrt{x^2-1}}y = 0 \tag{5}$$

E.1.4   STURM–LIOUVILLE PROBLEM

The linear and homogeneous second-order equation

$$\boxed{\frac{1}{w(x)}\frac{d}{dx}\left[p(x)\frac{dy}{dx}\right] + q(x)y = -\lambda y} \tag{E.17}$$

on some interval $a \leq x \leq b$ satisfying boundary conditions of the forms

$$\alpha_1 y(a) + \alpha_2 \left.\frac{dy}{dx}\right|_{x=a} = 0 \tag{E.18}$$

$$\beta_1 y(b) + \beta_2 \left.\frac{dy}{dx}\right|_{x=b} = 0, \tag{E.19}$$

where $\alpha_1, \alpha_2, \beta_1, \beta_2$ are given constants; $p(x)$, $q(x)$, $w(x)$ are given functions that are differentiable; and λ is an unspecified parameter independent of x, is called the *Sturm–Liouville equation*.

The values of λ for which the problem given by Eqs. (E.17)–(E.19) has a nontrivial solution, i.e., a solution other than $y = 0$, are called the *eigenvalues*. The corresponding solutions are the *eigenfunctions*. Eigenfunctions corresponding to different eigenvalues are orthogonal with respect to the weight function $w(x)$. All the eigenvalues are positive. In particular, $\lambda = 0$ is not an eigenvalue.

Example E.2   Consider the differential equation given by Eq. (D.48)

$$\frac{1}{\xi}\frac{d}{d\xi}\left(\xi\frac{d\theta}{d\xi}\right) + \lambda_n^2\theta = 0 \qquad n = 1, 2, 3, \ldots \tag{1}$$

with the following boundary conditions:

$$\xi = 0 \qquad \frac{d\theta}{d\xi} = 0$$

$$\tag{2}$$

$$\xi = 1 \qquad \theta = 0$$

Note that Eq. (1) is in the form of a Sturm–Liouville equation, Eq. (E.17), with the weight function ξ. For each eigenvalue λ_n, the corresponding eigenfunction $\theta_n(\xi)$, i.e., the solution of Eq. (1), is given by Eq. (D.50) as

$$\theta_n(\xi) = C_1 J_o(\lambda_n \xi) + C_2 Y_o(\lambda_n \xi), \tag{3}$$

which holds over the interval $0 \leq \xi \leq 1$. Since $Y_o(0) = -\infty$, C_2 must be zero. Application of the boundary condition at $\xi = 1$ gives the following transcendental equation:

$$J_o(\lambda_n) = 0 \qquad n = 1, 2, 3, \ldots \tag{4}$$

Solution of Eq. (4) gives the eigenvalues, λ_n. The corresponding eigenfunctions, $J_o(\lambda_n \xi)$, are orthogonal to each other with respect to the weight function ξ, i.e.,

$$\int_0^1 \xi J_o(\lambda_n \xi) J_o(\lambda_m \xi) \, d\xi = \begin{cases} 0 & \text{if} \quad n \neq m \\ \text{Nonzero} & \text{if} \quad n = m \end{cases} \tag{5}$$

• Method of Stodola and Vianello

The method of Stodola and Vianello (Bird et al., 1987; Hildebrand, 1976) is an iterative procedure that makes use of successive approximation to estimate the value of λ in Eq. (E.17) with appropriate homogeneous boundary conditions at $x = a$ and $x = b$ when $q(x) = 0$. The procedure is as follows:

1. Assume a trial function for $y_1(x)$ that satisfies the boundary conditions $x = a$ and $x = b$.
2. On the right side of Eq. (E.17), replace $y(x)$ by $y_1(x)$.
3. Solve the resulting differential equation, and express the solution in the form

$$y(x) = \lambda f_1(x) \tag{E.20}$$

4. Repeat step (2) with a second trial function $y_2(x)$ defined by

$$y_2(x) = f_1(x) \tag{E.21}$$

5. Solve the resulting differential equation, and express the solution in the form

$$y(x) = \lambda f_2(x) \tag{E.22}$$

6. Continue the process as long as desired. The nth approximation to the smallest permissible value of λ is given by

$$\lambda_1^n = \frac{\displaystyle\int_a^b w(x) f_n(x) y_n(x) \, dx}{\displaystyle\int_a^b w(x) \left[f_n(x) \right]^2 dx} \tag{E.23}$$

E.1.5 FOURIER SERIES

Let $f(x)$ be an arbitrary function defined on $a \leq x \leq b$, and let $\{\phi_n\}_{n=1}^{\infty}$ be an orthogonal set of functions over the same interval with weight function $w(x)$. Let us assume that $f(x)$ can be represented by an infinite series of the form

$$f(x) = \sum_{n=1}^{\infty} C_n \phi_n(x) \tag{E.24}$$

The series $\sum C_n \phi_n(x)$ is called the *Fourier series* of $f(x)$, and the coefficients C_n are called the *Fourier coefficients* of $f(x)$ with respect to the orthogonal functions $\phi_n(x)$.

To determine the Fourier coefficients, multiply both sides of Eq. (E.24) by $w(x)\phi_m(x)$, and integrate from $x = a$ to $x = b$, i.e.,

$$\int_a^b f(x)\,w(x)\,\phi_m(x)\,dx = \sum_{n=1}^{\infty} C_n \int_a^b \phi_n(x)\,\phi_m(x)\,w(x)\,dx \tag{E.25}$$

Because of the orthogonality, all the integrals on the right side of Eq. (E.25) are zero except when $n = m$. Therefore, the summation drops out, and Eq. (E.25) takes the form

$$\boxed{C_n = \frac{\displaystyle\int_a^b f(x)\,w(x)\,\phi_n(x)\,dx}{\displaystyle\int_a^b \phi_n^2(x)\,w(x)\,dx}} \tag{E.26}$$

Some of the useful integration formulas used in the evaluation of Fourier coefficients are given in Tables E.1–E.3.

Table E.1
Integrals Involving the sine Function

Integral	$\lambda_n = n\pi$	$\lambda_n = (2n+1)\pi/2$
$\int_0^1 \sin(\lambda_n \xi)\,d\xi$	$\begin{array}{ll} 0 & \text{if } n=0 \\ [1-(-1)^n]/\lambda_n & \text{if } n\neq 0 \end{array}$	$1/\lambda_n$
$\int_0^1 \sin^2(\lambda_n \xi)\,d\xi$	$\begin{array}{ll} 0 & \text{if } n=0 \\ 1/2 & \text{if } n\neq 0 \end{array}$	$1/2$
$\int_0^1 \xi \sin(\lambda_n \xi)\,d\xi$	$\begin{array}{ll} 0 & \text{if } n=0 \\ -(-1)^n/\lambda_n & \text{if } n\neq 0 \end{array}$	$(-1)^n/\lambda_n^2$
$\int_0^1 \xi^2 \sin(\lambda_n \xi)\,d\xi$	$\begin{array}{ll} 0 & \text{if } n=0 \\ -\dfrac{2+(\lambda_n^2-2)(-1)^n}{\lambda_n^3} & \text{if } n\neq 0 \end{array}$	$\dfrac{2(-1)^n}{\lambda_n^2} - \dfrac{2}{\lambda_n^3}$

Table E.2
Integrals Involving the cosine Function

Integral	$\lambda_n = n\pi$	$\lambda_n = (2n+1)\pi/2$
$\int_0^1 \cos(\lambda_n \xi)\,d\xi$	$\begin{array}{ll} 1 & \text{if } n=0 \\ 0 & \text{if } n\neq 0 \end{array}$	$(-1)^n/\lambda_n$
$\int_0^1 \cos^2(\lambda_n \xi)\,d\xi$	$\begin{array}{ll} 1 & \text{if } n=0 \\ 1/2 & \text{if } n\neq 0 \end{array}$	$1/2$
$\int_0^1 \xi \cos(\lambda_n \xi)\,d\xi$	$\begin{array}{ll} 1/2 & \text{if } n=0 \\ [(-1)^n - 1]/\lambda_n^2 & \text{if } n\neq 0 \end{array}$	$\dfrac{(-1)^n}{\lambda_n} - \dfrac{1}{\lambda_n^2}$
$\int_0^1 \xi^2 \cos(\lambda_n \xi)\,d\xi$	$\begin{array}{ll} 1/3 & \text{if } n=0 \\ 2(-1)^n/\lambda_n^2 & \text{if } n\neq 0 \end{array}$	$(-1)^n(\lambda_n^2 - 2)/\lambda_n^3$

Table E.3

Integrals Involving the Bessel Function of the First Kind

$$\int x^{n+1} J_n(\lambda x)\, dx = \frac{x^{n+1}}{\lambda} J_{n+1}(\lambda x)$$

$$\int x J_n^2(\lambda x)\, dx = \frac{x^2}{2}\left[J_n^2(\lambda x) + J_{n+1}^2(\lambda x)\right] - \frac{nx}{\lambda} J_n(\lambda x) J_{n+1}(\lambda x)$$

$$\int x^{n+3} J_n(\lambda x)\, dx = \left[\frac{x^{n+3}}{\lambda} - \frac{4(n+1)\,x^{n+1}}{\lambda^3}\right] J_{n+1}(\lambda x) + \frac{2x^{n+2}}{\lambda^2} J_n(\lambda x)$$

Example E.3 Let us express the Fourier series of $f(\xi) = \xi^2$ with respect to $J_o(\lambda_n \xi)$, i.e.,

$$\xi^2 = \sum_{n=1}^{\infty} C_n J_o(\lambda_n \xi), \tag{1}$$

where the eigenvalues are the roots of the following transcendental equation:

$$J_o(\lambda_n) = 0 \qquad n = 1,2,3,\ldots \tag{2}$$

Example E.2 indicates that $J_o(\lambda_n \xi)$ are orthogonal to each other with respect to the weight function ξ. Multiplication of Eq. (1) by $\xi J_o(\lambda_m \xi)\, d\xi$ and integration from $\xi = 0$ to $\xi = 1$ give

$$\int_0^1 \xi^3 J_o(\lambda_m \xi)\, d\xi = \sum_{n=1}^{\infty} C_n \int_0^1 \xi J_o(\lambda_n \xi) J_o(\lambda_m \xi)\, d\xi \tag{3}$$

The integral on the right side of Eq. (3) is zero when $n \neq m$ and nonzero when $n = m$. Therefore, when $n = m$ the summation drops out, and Eq. (3) reduces to the form

$$\int_0^1 \xi^3 J_o(\lambda_n \xi)\, d\xi = C_n \int_0^1 \xi J_o^2(\lambda_n \xi)\, d\xi \tag{4}$$

Evaluation of the integrals and making use of Eq. (2) yield

$$C_n = \left(\frac{2}{\lambda_n} - \frac{8}{\lambda_n^3}\right) \frac{1}{J_1(\lambda_n)} \tag{5}$$

E.2   ANALYTICAL SOLUTION OF PDEs

Various analytical methods are available to solve PDEs. In the determination of the solution method to be used, the structure of the equation is not the sole factor that should be taken into consideration as in the case for ODEs. The boundary conditions are almost as important as the equation itself.

E.2.1 SEPARATION OF VARIABLES

The method of separation of variables requires the PDE to be homogeneous[2] and the boundary conditions to be defined over a limited interval. Furthermore, the boundary conditions must be homogeneous in at least one dimension.

Example E.4 A parabolic PDE in a Cartesian coordinate system and its associated initial and boundary conditions are given as

$$
\begin{aligned}
&\frac{\partial \theta}{\partial \tau} = \frac{\partial^2 \theta}{\partial \xi^2} \\
&\tau = 0 \qquad \theta = 1 \\
&\xi = 0 \qquad \frac{\partial \theta}{\partial \xi} = 0 \\
&\xi = 1 \qquad -\frac{\partial \theta}{\partial \xi} = \Lambda \theta
\end{aligned}
\tag{1}
$$

The terms θ, τ, ξ, and Λ represent dimensionless concentration, dimensionless time, dimensionless coordinate, and a dimensionless number, respectively. Since $0 \leq \xi \leq 1$ and the PDE as well as the boundary conditions is linear and homogeneous, the solution can be obtained by using the separation of variables method.

The separation of variables method assumes that the solution can be represented as a product of two functions of the form

$$
\theta(\tau, \xi) = F(\tau) G(\xi)
\tag{2}
$$

Substitution of Eq. (2) into the governing differential equation and rearrangement give

$$
\frac{1}{F} \frac{dF}{d\tau} = \frac{1}{G} \frac{d^2 G}{d\xi^2}
\tag{3}
$$

While the left side of Eq. (3) is a function of τ only, the right side is dependent only on ξ. This is possible only if both sides of Eq. (3) are equal to a constant, say $-\lambda^2$, i.e.,

$$
\frac{1}{F} \frac{dF}{d\tau} = \frac{1}{G} \frac{d^2 G}{d\xi^2} = -\lambda^2
\tag{4}
$$

Equation (4) results in two ODEs. The equation for F is given by

$$
\frac{dF}{d\tau} + \lambda^2 F = 0
\tag{5}
$$

The solution of Eq. (5) is

$$
F(\tau) = C_1 e^{-\lambda^2 \tau},
\tag{6}
$$

where C_1 is a constant. The reason for choosing a negative constant in Eq. (4), i.e., $-\lambda^2$, is obvious from this solution. The solution decays to zero as $\tau \to \infty$ (steady-state case). The choice of a positive constant would give a solution that becomes infinite as $\tau \to \infty$.

---

[2]A linear differential equation or a linear boundary condition is said to be homogeneous if, when satisfied by a function f, it is also satisfied by βf, where β is an arbitrary constant.

On the other hand, the equation for G is

$$\frac{d^2G}{d\xi^2} + \lambda^2 G = 0 \tag{7}$$

and it is subject to the boundary conditions

$$\text{at} \quad \xi = 0 \qquad \frac{dG}{d\xi} = 0 \tag{8}$$

$$\text{at} \quad \xi = 1 \qquad -\frac{dG}{d\xi} = \Lambda G \tag{9}$$

Note that Eq. (7) is a Sturm–Liouville equation with a weight function of unity. The solution of Eq. (7) is given by[3]

$$G(\xi) = C_2 \sin(\lambda \xi) + C_3 \cos(\lambda \xi), \tag{10}$$

where C_2 and C_3 are constants. The use of Eq. (8) gives $C_2 = 0$. The same conclusion can be reached by noting that the problem is symmetric around the ξ axis, and hence the solution must be expressed in terms of even functions.[4] Application of Eq. (9) gives

$$-\Big[-C_3\lambda \sin(\lambda\xi)\Big]_{\xi=1} = \Lambda \Big[C_3 \cos(\lambda\xi)\Big]_{\xi=1} \tag{11}$$

Simplification of Eq. (11) leads to the following transcendental equation:

$$\boxed{\lambda_n \tan \lambda_n = \Lambda} \qquad n = 1, 2, 3, \ldots \tag{12}$$

where the roots of Eq. (12) are the eigenvalues, λ_n. Note that n does not start from zero since $\lambda_o = 0$ is not an eigenvalue for $\Lambda \neq 0$. The corresponding eigenfunctions are given by

$$G_n(\xi) = C_3 \cos(\lambda_n \xi) \tag{13}$$

Substitution of Eqs. (6) and (13) into Eq. (2) gives

$$\theta_n(\tau, \xi) = C_n e^{-\lambda_n^2 \tau} \cos(\lambda_n \xi), \tag{14}$$

where $C_n = C_1 C_3$.

If θ_1 and θ_2 are the solutions satisfying the linear and homogeneous PDE and the boundary conditions, then the linear combination of the solutions, i.e., $\alpha_1 \theta_1 + \alpha_2 \theta_2$, also satisfies the PDE and the boundary conditions. Therefore, the complete solution is

$$\theta = \sum_{n=1}^{\infty} C_n e^{-\lambda_n^2 \tau} \cos(\lambda_n \xi) \tag{15}$$

---

[3]The reason for choosing a constant as $-\lambda^2$ and not $-\lambda$ in Eq. (4) is simply for convenience in writing the solution. Taking $-\lambda$ as a constant would give the solution in the form

$$G(\xi) = C_2 \sin(\sqrt{\lambda}\xi) + C_3 \cos(\sqrt{\lambda}\xi)$$

[4]A function $f(x)$ is said to be an *odd function* if $f(-x) = -f(x)$ and an *even function* if $f(-x) = f(x)$. While sine is an odd function, cosine is an even function.

The unknown coefficients C_n can be determined by using the initial condition, i.e.,

$$1 = \sum_{n=1}^{\infty} C_n \cos(\lambda_n \xi) \tag{16}$$

Since the eigenfunctions are simply orthogonal, multiplication of Eq. (16) by $\cos(\lambda_m \xi)\, d\xi$ and integration from $\xi = 0$ to $\xi = 1$ give

$$\int_0^1 \cos(\lambda_m \xi)\, d\xi = \sum_{n=1}^{\infty} C_n \int_0^1 \cos(\lambda_n \xi) \cos(\lambda_m \xi)\, d\xi \tag{17}$$

The integral on the right side of Eq. (17) is zero when $n \neq m$ and nonzero when $n = m$. Therefore, the summation drops out when $n = m$, and Eq. (17) reduces to the form

$$\int_0^1 \cos(\lambda_n \xi)\, d\xi = C_n \int_0^1 \cos^2(\lambda_n \xi)\, d\xi \tag{18}$$

Evaluation of the integrals results in

$$C_n = \frac{4\sin\lambda_n}{2\lambda_n + \sin(2\lambda_n)} \tag{19}$$

Thus, the solution becomes

$$\boxed{\theta = 4\sum_{n=1}^{\infty} \frac{\sin\lambda_n}{2\lambda_n + \sin(2\lambda_n)}\, e^{-\lambda_n^2 \tau} \cos(\lambda_n \xi)} \tag{20}$$

Example E.5 A parabolic PDE in a Cartesian coordinate system and its associated initial and boundary conditions are given as

$$\boxed{\begin{aligned}
\frac{\partial \theta}{\partial \tau} &= \frac{\partial^2 \theta}{\partial \xi^2} \\[2mm]
\tau = 0 \qquad & \theta = \xi \\[2mm]
\xi = 0 \qquad & \theta = 0 \\[2mm]
\xi = 1 \qquad & -\frac{\partial \theta}{\partial \xi} = \Lambda\theta
\end{aligned}} \tag{1}$$

The use of the method of separation of variables in which the solution is sought in the form

$$\theta(\tau, \xi) = F(\tau)\, G(\xi) \tag{2}$$

reduces the governing PDE to

$$\frac{1}{F}\frac{dF}{d\tau} = \frac{1}{G}\frac{d^2G}{d\xi^2} = -\lambda^2 \tag{3}$$

Equation (3) results in two ODEs of the form

$$\frac{dF}{d\tau} + \lambda^2 F = 0 \qquad \Rightarrow \qquad F(\tau) = C_1 e^{-\lambda^2 \tau} \tag{4}$$

$$\frac{d^2 G}{d\xi^2} + \lambda^2 G = 0 \qquad \Rightarrow \qquad G(\xi) = C_2 \sin(\lambda \xi) + C_3 \cos(\lambda \xi) \tag{5}$$

Application of the boundary condition at $\xi = 0$ gives $C_3 = 0$. The boundary condition at $\xi = 1$ leads to the following transcendental equation:

$$\boxed{\lambda_n \cot \lambda_n + \Lambda = 0} \qquad n = 1, 2, 3, \ldots \tag{6}$$

The general solution is the summation of all possible solutions, i.e.,

$$\theta = \sum_{n=1}^{\infty} C_n e^{-\lambda_n^2 \tau} \sin(\lambda_n \xi) \tag{7}$$

The unknown coefficients C_n can be determined by using the initial condition. The result is

$$C_n = \frac{\displaystyle\int_0^1 \xi \sin(\lambda_n \xi)\, d\xi}{\displaystyle\int_0^1 \sin^2(\lambda_n \xi)\, d\xi} = \frac{4}{\lambda_n} \left[\frac{\sin \lambda_n - \lambda_n \cos \lambda_n}{2\lambda_n - \sin(2\lambda_n)} \right] \tag{8}$$

Equation (8) can be further simplified with the help of Eq. (6) to

$$C_n = 4(1 + \Lambda) \frac{\sin \lambda_n}{\lambda_n \left[2\lambda_n - \sin(2\lambda_n) \right]} \tag{9}$$

Thus, the solution is expressed as

$$\boxed{\theta = 4(1 + \Lambda) \sum_{n=1}^{\infty} \frac{\sin \lambda_n}{\lambda_n \left[2\lambda_n - \sin(2\lambda_n) \right]} e^{-\lambda_n^2 \tau} \sin(\lambda_n \xi)} \tag{10}$$

As can be seen from Examples E.4 and E.5, sine and cosine functions frequently appear in the solution of parabolic PDEs in Cartesian coordinates. Some useful formulas involving sine and cosine functions are given in Table E.4.

Table E.4

Some Identities for sine and cosine Functions

Function	$\lambda_n = n\pi$	$\lambda_n = (2n+1)\pi/2$
$\sin \lambda_n$	0	$(-1)^n$
$\cos \lambda_n$	$(-1)^n$	0

Example E.6 A parabolic PDE in a cylindrical coordinate system and its associated initial and boundary conditions are given as

$$\frac{\partial \theta}{\partial \tau} = \frac{1}{\xi} \frac{\partial}{\partial \xi} \left(\xi \frac{\partial \theta}{\partial \xi} \right) - \Lambda^2 \theta$$

$$\begin{aligned} \tau = 0 & \quad \theta = \xi^2 \\ \xi = 0 & \quad \theta = 0 \\ \xi = 1 & \quad \theta = 0 \end{aligned}$$

(1)

Representing the solution as a product of two functions of the form

$$\theta(\tau, \xi) = F(\tau) G(\xi)$$

(2)

reduces the governing PDE to

$$\frac{1}{F} \frac{dF}{d\tau} + \Lambda^2 = \frac{1}{G\xi} \frac{d}{d\xi} \left(\xi \frac{dG}{d\xi} \right) = -\lambda^2,$$

(3)

which results in two ODEs:

$$\frac{dF}{d\tau} + (\lambda^2 + \Lambda^2)F = 0 \qquad \Rightarrow \qquad F(\tau) = C_1 e^{-(\lambda^2 + \Lambda^2)\tau}$$

(4)

$$\frac{d}{d\xi} \left(\xi \frac{dG}{d\xi} \right) + \lambda^2 \xi G = 0 \qquad \Rightarrow \qquad G(\xi) = C_2 J_o(\lambda \xi) + C_3 Y_o(\lambda \xi)$$

(5)

The boundary conditions for $G(\xi)$ are

$$\text{at} \quad \xi = 0 \qquad G = 0$$

(6)

$$\text{at} \quad \xi = 1 \qquad G = 0$$

(7)

Since $Y_o(0) = -\infty$, $C_3 = 0$. Application of Eq. (7) yields

$$C_2 J_o(\lambda) = 0$$

(8)

For a nontrivial solution, the eigenvalues, λ_n, are the roots of the following transcendental equation:

$$J_o(\lambda_n) = 0 \qquad n = 1, 2, 3, \dots$$

(9)

The corresponding eigenfunctions, $J_o(\lambda_n \xi)$, are orthogonal to each other with respect to the weight function ξ.

The general solution is the summation of all possible solutions, i.e.,

$$\theta = \sum_{n=1}^{\infty} C_n e^{-(\lambda_n^2 + \Lambda^2)\tau} J_o(\lambda_n \xi)$$

(10)

The unknown coefficients C_n can be determined by using the initial condition, i.e.,

$$\xi^2 = \sum_{n=1}^{\infty} C_n J_o(\lambda_n \xi)$$

(11)

Multiplication of Eq. (11) by $\xi J_o(\lambda_m \xi) d\xi$ and integration from $\xi = 0$ to $\xi = 1$ give

$$\int_0^1 \xi^3 J_o(\lambda_m \xi) d\xi = \sum_{n=1}^{\infty} C_n \int_0^1 \xi J_o(\lambda_n \xi) J_o(\lambda_m \xi) d\xi$$

(12)

The integral on the right side of Eq. (12) is zero when $n \neq m$ and nonzero when $n = m$. Therefore, the summation drops out when $n = m$, and Eq. (12) reduces to the form

$$\int_0^1 \xi^3 J_o(\lambda_n \xi)\, d\xi = C_n \int_0^1 \xi J_o^2(\lambda_n \xi)\, d\xi \tag{13}$$

Evaluation of the integrals with the help of the formulas given in Table E.3 and the use of Eq. (9) give

$$C_n = \left(\frac{1}{\lambda_n} - \frac{4}{\lambda_n^3} \right) \frac{2}{J_1(\lambda_n)} \tag{14}$$

Hence, the solution is expressed as

$$\theta = 2 \sum_{n=1}^{\infty} \left(\frac{1}{\lambda_n} - \frac{4}{\lambda_n^3} \right) e^{-(\lambda_n^2 + \Lambda^2)\tau} \frac{J_o(\lambda_n \xi)}{J_1(\lambda_n)} \tag{15}$$

Example E.7   A parabolic PDE in a spherical coordinate system and its associated initial and boundary conditions are given as

$$\frac{\partial \theta}{\partial \tau} = \frac{1}{\xi^2} \frac{\partial}{\partial \xi} \left(\xi^2 \frac{\partial \theta}{\partial \xi} \right)$$

$$\tau = 0 \qquad \theta = 1$$

$$\xi = 0 \qquad \frac{\partial \theta}{\partial \xi} = 0 \tag{1}$$

$$\xi = 1 \qquad -\frac{\partial \theta}{\partial \xi} = \Lambda \theta$$

The transformation

$$\theta(\tau, \xi) = \frac{u(\tau, \xi)}{\xi} \tag{2}$$

converts the spherical coordinate system into the Cartesian coordinate system. Thus, Eq. (1) becomes

$$\frac{\partial u}{\partial \tau} = \frac{\partial^2 u}{\partial \xi^2}$$

$$\tau = 0 \qquad u = \xi$$

$$\xi = 0 \qquad u = 0 \tag{3}$$

$$\xi = 1 \qquad -\frac{\partial u}{\partial \xi} = (\Lambda - 1) u$$

Note that Eq. (3) is similar to Eq. (1) of Example E.5 with a slight difference in the boundary condition at $\xi = 1$. Thus, replacing Λ by $\Lambda - 1$ in Eqs. (10) and (6) of Example E.5 results in

$$u = 4\Lambda \sum_{n=1}^{\infty} \frac{\sin \lambda_n}{\lambda_n \left[2\lambda_n - \sin(2\lambda_n) \right]} e^{-\lambda_n^2 \tau} \sin(\lambda_n \xi), \tag{4}$$

where

$$\boxed{\lambda_n \cot \lambda_n = 1 - \Lambda} \qquad n = 1, 2, 3, \dots \tag{5}$$

Substitution of Eq. (4) into Eq. (2) gives the solution as

$$\boxed{\theta = 4\Lambda \sum_{n=1}^{\infty} \frac{\sin \lambda_n}{\lambda_n \left[2\lambda_n - \sin(2\lambda_n)\right]} e^{-\lambda_n^2 \tau} \frac{\sin(\lambda_n \xi)}{\xi}} \tag{6}$$

Example E.8 An elliptic PDE in a cylindrical coordinate system and its associated boundary conditions are given as

$$\frac{1}{\xi} \frac{\partial}{\partial \xi} \left(\xi \frac{\partial \theta}{\partial \xi} \right) + \frac{\partial^2 \theta}{\partial \eta^2} = 0$$

$$\xi = 0 \qquad \frac{\partial \theta}{\partial \xi} = 0$$

$$\xi = 1 \qquad \frac{\partial \theta}{\partial \xi} = \alpha = \text{constant} \tag{1}$$

$$\eta = 0 \qquad \theta = 0$$

$$\eta = \beta \qquad \frac{\partial \theta}{\partial \eta} = 0$$

While the boundary conditions in the η-direction are homogeneous, the boundary condition at $\xi = 1$ is nonhomogeneous. Application of the separation of variables method and proposing the solution as a product of two functions of the form

$$\theta(\tau, \xi) = F(\xi) G(\eta) \tag{2}$$

reduce the governing PDE to

$$\frac{1}{\xi F} \frac{d}{d\xi} \left(\xi \frac{dF}{d\xi} \right) = -\frac{1}{G} \frac{d^2 G}{d\eta^2} \tag{3}$$

While the left side of Eq. (3) is a function of ξ only, the right side is dependent only on η. This is possible only if both sides of Eq. (3) are equal to a constant. The separation constant should be chosen such that the boundary value problem of the homogeneous direction leads to the Sturm–Liouville equation. Since η is the homogeneous direction, choosing a positive sign for the separation constant, λ^2, gives the Sturm–Liouville equation,[5] i.e.,

$$\frac{1}{\xi F} \frac{d}{d\xi} \left(\xi \frac{dF}{d\xi} \right) = -\frac{1}{G} \frac{d^2 G}{d\eta^2} = \lambda^2 \tag{4}$$

The equation for G is

$$\frac{d^2 G}{d\eta^2} + \lambda^2 G = 0 \tag{5}$$

---

[5] If Eq. (3) is expressed as

$$-\frac{1}{\xi F} \frac{d}{d\xi} \left(\xi \frac{dF}{d\xi} \right) = \frac{1}{G} \frac{d^2 G}{d\eta^2}$$

then a negative sign should be chosen for the separation constant.

and it is subject to the boundary conditions

$$
\text{at} \quad \eta = 0 \qquad G = 0 \tag{6}
$$

$$
\text{at} \quad \eta = \beta \qquad \frac{dG}{d\eta} = 0 \tag{7}
$$

The solution of Eq. (5) is given by

$$
G(\xi) = C_1 \sin(\lambda \eta) + C_2 \cos(\lambda \eta), \tag{8}
$$

where C_1 and C_2 are constants. The use of Eq. (6) gives $C_2 = 0$. Application of Eq. (7) gives

$$
\cos(\lambda \beta) = 0 \quad \Rightarrow \quad \boxed{\lambda_n \beta = \left(n + \frac{1}{2}\right)\pi \quad n = 0,1,2,\ldots} \tag{9}
$$

The equation for F is

$$
\frac{1}{\xi}\frac{d}{d\xi}\left(\xi \frac{dF}{d\xi}\right) - \lambda_n^2 F = 0 \tag{10}
$$

The solution of Eq. (10) is given by Eq. (D.47) as

$$
F = C_3 I_o(\lambda_n \xi) + C_4 K_o(\lambda_n \xi) \tag{11}
$$

Since $K_o(\lambda_n \xi)$ is unbounded, C_4 must be zero. Thus, the solution becomes

$$
\theta = \sum_{n=0}^{\infty} C_n I_o(\lambda_n \xi) \sin(\lambda_n \eta) \tag{12}
$$

The unknown coefficients C_n can be determined by using the boundary condition at $\xi = 1$, i.e.,

$$
\alpha = \sum_{n=0}^{\infty} C_n \lambda_n I_1(\lambda_n) \sin(\lambda_n \eta) \tag{13}
$$

Multiplication of Eq. (13) by $\sin(\lambda_m \eta)\,d\eta$ and integration from $\eta = 0$ to $\eta = \beta$ give

$$
C_n = \frac{\alpha \displaystyle\int_0^\beta \sin(\lambda_n \eta)\,d\eta}{\lambda_n I_1(\lambda_n) \displaystyle\int_0^\beta \sin^2(\lambda_n \eta)\,d\eta} \tag{14}
$$

Evaluation of the integrals leads to

$$
C_n = \frac{2\alpha}{\beta \lambda_n^2 I_1(\lambda_n)} \tag{15}
$$

Hence, the solution is given by

$$
\boxed{\theta = \frac{2\alpha}{\beta}\sum_{n=0}^{\infty}\frac{1}{\lambda_n^2 I_1(\lambda_n)} I_o(\lambda_n \xi)\sin(\lambda_n \eta)} \tag{16}
$$

• Principle of Superposition

The method of separation of variables cannot be used if the PDE and/or the boundary conditions are nonhomogeneous. One-dimensional unsteady-state problems with several nonhomogeneities may be split into two simpler problems, one steady-state and one transient, which can be added together (or superimposed) to give the solution to the original problem. The steady-state problem includes the nonhomogeneous term(s) in the PDE as well as the nonhomogeneous boundary condition(s). This makes the transient problem consisting of a homogeneous PDE subject to homogeneous boundary conditions. The superposition principle is only applicable to linear problems. The following example clarifies this technique.

Example E.9 A parabolic PDE in a Cartesian coordinate system and its associated initial and boundary conditions are given as

$$\frac{\partial \theta}{\partial \tau} = \frac{\partial^2 \theta}{\partial \xi^2} + \Lambda$$

$$
\begin{aligned}
\tau = 0 & \quad \theta = 1 \\
\xi = 0 & \quad \theta = 0 \\
\xi = 1 & \quad \theta = 0
\end{aligned}
$$

(1)

Since the PDE is nonhomogeneous, the solution is proposed in the form

$$\theta(\tau, \xi) = \theta_\infty(\xi) + \theta_t(\tau, \xi),$$ (2)

in which θ_∞ is the solution of the steady-state problem given by

$$\frac{d^2 \theta_\infty}{d\xi^2} + \Lambda = 0$$ (3)

with the following boundary conditions:

$$\text{at} \quad \xi = 0 \quad \theta_\infty = 0$$ (4)
$$\text{at} \quad \xi = 1 \quad \theta_\infty = 0$$ (5)

The solution of Eq. (3) is

$$\theta_\infty = \frac{\Lambda}{2}(\xi - \xi^2)$$ (6)

The use of Eq. (6) in Eq. (2) gives

$$\theta(\tau, \xi) = \frac{\Lambda}{2}(\xi - \xi^2) + \theta_t(\tau, \xi)$$ (7)

Substitution of Eq. (7) into Eq. (1) leads to the following governing equation for the transient problem together with the initial and the boundary conditions:

$$\frac{\partial \theta_t}{\partial \tau} = \frac{\partial^2 \theta_t}{\partial \xi^2}$$ (8)

$$\text{at} \quad \tau = 0 \quad \theta_t = 1 - \frac{\Lambda}{2}(\xi - \xi^2)$$ (9)
$$\text{at} \quad \xi = 0 \quad \theta_t = 0$$ (10)
$$\text{at} \quad \xi = 1 \quad \theta_t = 0,$$ (11)

which can be solved by the method of separation of variables.

Representing the solution as a product of two functions of the form

$$\theta_t(\tau, \xi) = F(\tau)G(\xi) \tag{12}$$

reduces Eq. (8) to

$$\frac{1}{F}\frac{dF}{d\tau} = \frac{1}{G}\frac{d^2G}{d\xi^2} = -\lambda^2, \tag{13}$$

which results in two ODEs:

$$\frac{dF}{d\tau} + \lambda^2 F = 0 \quad \Rightarrow \quad F(\tau) = C_1 e^{-\lambda^2\tau} \tag{14}$$

$$\frac{d^2G}{d\xi^2} + \lambda^2 G = 0 \quad \Rightarrow \quad G(\xi) = C_2\sin(\lambda\xi) + C_3\cos(\lambda\xi) \tag{15}$$

The boundary conditions for $G(\xi)$ are

$$\text{at} \quad \xi = 0 \quad G = 0 \tag{16}$$

$$\text{at} \quad \xi = 1 \quad G = 0 \tag{17}$$

The use of Eq. (16) gives $C_3 = 0$. Application of the boundary condition defined by Eq. (17) gives

$$\sin\lambda = 0 \quad \Rightarrow \quad \boxed{\lambda_n = n\pi} \quad n = 1, 2, \ldots \tag{18}$$

Therefore, the transient solution is

$$\theta_t = \sum_{n=1}^{\infty} C_n e^{-n^2\pi^2\tau}\sin(n\pi\xi) \tag{19}$$

The unknown coefficients C_n can be determined by using the initial condition, Eq. (9), with the result

$$C_n = \frac{\int_0^1\left[1 - \frac{\Lambda}{2}(\xi - \xi^2)\right]\sin(n\pi\xi)\,d\xi}{\int_0^1 \sin^2(n\pi\xi)\,d\xi} = \frac{2\left[1 - (-1)^n\right]}{n\pi}\left(1 - \frac{\Lambda}{n^2\pi^2}\right) \tag{20}$$

Note that

$$C_n = \begin{cases} \dfrac{4}{n\pi}\left(1 - \dfrac{\Lambda}{n^2\pi^2}\right) & n = 1, 3, 5, \ldots \\ 0 & n = 2, 4, 6, \ldots \end{cases} \tag{21}$$

Therefore, the transient solution is given by

$$\theta_t = \frac{4}{\pi}\sum_{n=1,3,5}^{\infty}\frac{1}{n}\left(1 - \frac{\Lambda}{n^2\pi^2}\right)e^{-n^2\pi^2\tau}\sin(n\pi\xi) \tag{22}$$

Substitution of the steady-state and transient solutions, Eqs. (6) and (22), into Eq. (2) gives the solution as

$$\boxed{\theta = \frac{\Lambda}{2}(\xi - \xi^2) + \frac{4}{\pi}\sum_{n=1,3,5}^{\infty}\frac{1}{n}\left(1 - \frac{\Lambda}{n^2\pi^2}\right)e^{-n^2\pi^2\tau}\sin(n\pi\xi)} \tag{23}$$

E.2.2 SIMILARITY SOLUTION

This method is also known as the *method of combination of variables*. The basis of this method is to combine the two independent variables in a new single variable so as to transform the given PDE into a second-order ODE.

Similarity solutions are a special class of solutions used to solve parabolic second-order PDEs when there is no geometric length scale in the problem, i.e., the domain must be either semi-infinite or infinite. Moreover, the initial condition should match the boundary condition at infinity.

Example E.10 A parabolic PDE in a Cartesian coordinate system and its associated initial and boundary conditions are given as

$$\frac{\partial \theta}{\partial t} = \mathcal{D}_{AB} \frac{\partial^2 \theta}{\partial z^2}$$

$$\begin{array}{ll} t = 0 & \theta = 0 \\ z = 0 & \theta = 1 \\ z = \infty & \theta = 0 \end{array} \tag{1}$$

The solution is sought in the form

$$\theta = \theta(\eta), \tag{2}$$

where the dimensionless similarity variable η combines the independent variables, t and z, in the form

$$\eta = \frac{z}{2\sqrt{\mathcal{D}_{AB}t}} \tag{3}$$

The chain rule of differentiation gives

$$\frac{\partial \theta}{\partial t} = \frac{d\theta}{d\eta} \frac{\partial \eta}{\partial t} = -\frac{1}{2} \frac{\eta}{t} \frac{d\theta}{d\eta} \tag{4}$$

$$\frac{\partial^2 \theta}{\partial z^2} = \frac{d^2\theta}{d\eta^2} \left(\frac{\partial \eta}{\partial z}\right)^2 + \frac{d\theta}{d\eta} \frac{\partial^2 \eta}{\partial z^2} = \frac{1}{4\mathcal{D}_{AB}t} \frac{d^2\theta}{d\eta^2} \tag{5}$$

Substitution of Eqs. (4) and (5) into the PDE results in the following second-order ODE:

$$\frac{d^2\theta}{d\eta^2} + 2\eta \frac{d\theta}{d\eta} = 0 \tag{6}$$

The boundary conditions associated with Eq. (6) are

$$\begin{array}{lll} \text{at} & \eta = 0 & \theta = 1 \\ \text{at} & \eta = \infty & \theta = 0 \end{array} \tag{7}$$

The integrating factor for Eq. (6) is

$$\mu = e^{\int 2\eta \, d\eta} = e^{\eta^2} \tag{8}$$

Multiplication of Eq. (6) by the integrating factor yields[6]

$$\frac{d}{d\eta}\left(e^{\eta^2}\frac{d\theta}{d\eta}\right)=0,\tag{9}$$

which implies that

$$\frac{d\theta}{d\eta}=C_1 e^{-\eta^2}\tag{10}$$

Integration of Eq. (10) gives

$$\theta=C_1\int_0^\eta e^{-u^2}du+C_2,\tag{11}$$

where u is a dummy variable of integration. Application of the boundary condition at $\eta=0$ gives $C_2=1$. On the other hand, application of the boundary condition at $\eta=1$ gives

$$C_1=-\frac{1}{\displaystyle\int_0^\infty e^{-u^2}du}=-\frac{2}{\sqrt{\pi}}\tag{12}$$

Therefore, the solution becomes

$$\begin{aligned}\theta &= 1-\frac{2}{\sqrt{\pi}}\int_0^\eta e^{-u^2}du=1-\mathrm{erf}(\eta)=\mathrm{erfc}(\eta)\\ &= 1-\mathrm{erf}\left(\frac{z}{2\sqrt{\mathcal{D}_{AB}t}}\right)=\mathrm{erfc}\left(\frac{z}{2\sqrt{\mathcal{D}_{AB}t}}\right),\end{aligned}\tag{13}$$

where $\mathrm{erf}(x)$ and $\mathrm{erfc}(x)$ represent the *error* and *complementary error* functions, respectively. These functions are defined by

$$\boxed{\mathrm{erf}(x)=\frac{2}{\sqrt{\pi}}\int_0^x e^{-u^2}du}\quad\text{and}\quad\boxed{\mathrm{erfc}(x)=1-\mathrm{erf}(x)=\frac{2}{\sqrt{\pi}}\int_x^\infty e^{-u^2}du}\tag{14}$$

The error and complementary error functions are plotted in Figure E.1. Some useful formulas involving error and complementary error functions are given in Table E.5.

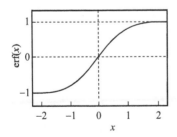 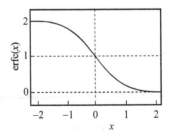

Figure E.1 Plots of the error and complementary error functions.

---

[6]The advantage of including the term 2 in the denominator of the similarity variable η in Eq. (3) can be seen here. Without it, the result would have been

$$\frac{d}{d\eta}\left(e^{\eta^2/2}\frac{d\theta}{d\eta}\right)$$

Table E.5

Some Properties of Error and Complementary Error Functions

$$\text{erf}(-x) = -\text{erf}(x) \qquad\qquad \text{erfc}(-x) = 2 - \text{erfc}(x)$$

$$\text{erf}(x) = \frac{2}{\sqrt{\pi}} x \quad \text{if } x \ll 1 \qquad\qquad \text{erf}(x) = \frac{1}{\sqrt{\pi}} \frac{e^{-x^2}}{x} \quad \text{if } x \gg 1$$

$$\frac{d}{dx}\text{erf}(\beta x) = \frac{2\beta}{\sqrt{\pi}} e^{-\beta^2 x^2} \qquad\qquad \frac{d}{dx}\text{erfc}(\beta x) = -\frac{2\beta}{\sqrt{\pi}} e^{-\beta^2 x^2}$$

$$\int \text{erf}(\beta x)\, dx = x\,\text{erf}(\beta x) + \frac{1}{\beta\sqrt{\pi}} e^{-\beta^2 x^2} \qquad\qquad \int \text{erfc}(\beta x)\, dx = x\,\text{erfc}(\beta x) - \frac{1}{\beta\sqrt{\pi}} e^{-\beta^2 x^2}$$

$$\int x\,\text{erf}(\beta x)\, dx = \frac{1}{2} x^2\,\text{erf}(\beta x) - \frac{1}{4\beta^2}\text{erf}(\beta x) + \frac{x}{2\beta\sqrt{\pi}} e^{-\beta^2 x^2}$$

$$\int x\,\text{erfc}(\beta x)\, dx = \frac{1}{2} x^2\,\text{erfc}(\beta x) + \frac{1}{4\beta^2}\text{erf}(\beta x) - \frac{x}{2\beta\sqrt{\pi}} e^{-\beta^2 x^2}$$

E.2.3 THE LAPLACE TRANSFORM TECHNIQUE

The Laplace transformation method is extensively used in the solution of unsteady-state problems as well as steady multidimensional problems in which one of the domains is semi-infinite. The Laplace transformation is generally applied to the time variable, t, in the form

$$\mathcal{L}[F(t)] = \overline{F}(s) = \int_0^\infty e^{-st} F(t)\, dt \qquad\qquad (E.27)$$

Transformation of the equation from the t-domain to the s-domain converts time derivatives into algebraic functions of position and s. Thus, the PDE is reduced to an ODE leading to an equation much easier to solve in the s-domain. The most difficult task, however, is to invert the solution back to the t-domain. The inverse Laplace transform is given by

$$F(t) = \mathcal{L}^{-1}\left[\overline{F}(s)\right] \qquad\qquad (E.28)$$

Some properties of the Laplace transform

• **Linear property**

$$\mathcal{L}[\alpha F(t) + \beta G(t)] = \alpha \mathcal{L}[F(t)] + \beta \mathcal{L}[G(t)], \qquad\qquad (E.29)$$

where α and β are scalars.

• **Transform of derivatives**

$$\mathcal{L}\left[\frac{dF(t)}{dt}\right] = s\mathcal{L}[F(t)] - F(0) \qquad\qquad (E.30)$$

$$\mathcal{L}\left[\frac{d^2 F(t)}{dt^2}\right] = s^2 \mathcal{L}[F(t)] - s F(0) - \left.\frac{dF}{dt}\right|_{t=0} \qquad\qquad (E.31)$$

• **Shifting properties**

$$\mathcal{L}\left[e^{\mp at} F(t)\right] = \overline{F}(s \pm a) \qquad\qquad (E.32)$$

If

$$\mathcal{L}[F(t)] = \overline{F}(s) \qquad \text{and} \qquad G(t) = \begin{cases} F(t-a) & t > a \\ 0 & t < a \end{cases} \tag{E.33}$$

then

$$\mathcal{L}[G(t)] = e^{-as} \overline{F}(s) \tag{E.34}$$

• **Convolution theorem**

If

$$\mathcal{L}^{-1}[\overline{F}(s)] = F(t) \qquad \text{and} \qquad \mathcal{L}^{-1}[\overline{G}(s)] = G(t) \tag{E.35}$$

then

$$\begin{aligned} \mathcal{L}^{-1}[\overline{F}(s)\overline{G}(s)] &= F(t) * G(t) \\ &= \int_0^t F(t^*) G(t-t^*) dt^* = \int_0^t F(t-t^*) G(t^*) dt^* \end{aligned} \tag{E.36}$$

• **Asymptotic behavior**

$$\lim_{t \to 0} F(t) = \mathcal{L}^{-1}\left[\lim_{s \to \infty} s\overline{F}(s)\right] \tag{E.37}$$

$$\lim_{t \to \infty} F(t) = \mathcal{L}^{-1}\left[\lim_{s \to 0} s\overline{F}(s)\right] \tag{E.38}$$

The Dirac delta function

The *Dirac delta function*,[7] $\delta(x)$, is infinitely peaked at $x = 0$ with the total area of unity. In mathematical terms, it is defined by

$$\delta(x) = \begin{cases} \infty & x = 0 \\ 0 & \text{Otherwise} \end{cases} \tag{E.39}$$

with

$$\int_{-\infty}^{\infty} \delta(x) dx = 1 \tag{E.40}$$

The value of x at which the Dirac delta function becomes infinite can be controlled by substituting $x - x_o$ for x. Thus

$$\delta(x - x_o) = \begin{cases} \infty & x = x_o \\ 0 & \text{Otherwise} \end{cases} \tag{E.41}$$

Let us consider the integral

$$I = \int_{-\infty}^{\infty} f(x) \delta(x) dx \tag{E.42}$$

for any function $f(x)$. Since $\delta(x)$ vanishes everywhere except at $x = 0$,

$$f(x) \delta(x) = f(0) \delta(x) \tag{E.43}$$

The use of Eq. (E.43) in Eq. (E.42) yields

$$\int_{-\infty}^{\infty} f(x) \delta(x) dx = f(0) \underbrace{\int_{-\infty}^{\infty} \delta(x) dx}_{1} = f(0) \tag{E.44}$$

---

[7]The Dirac delta function should not be confused with the Kronecker delta function! It has the inverse dimension of its argument.

In other words, $\int \delta(x)\,dx$ can be interpreted as an "operator" that evaluates the value of a function at $x = 0$. The generalization of Eq. (E.44) is expressed as

$$\boxed{\int_{-\infty}^{\infty} f(x)\,\delta(x - x_o)\,dx = f(x_o)} \tag{E.45}$$

Inversion of the Laplace transform

Inversion from the s-domain to the t-domain is time-consuming and requires lot of algebraic manipulations. The use of Laplace transform tables available from many sources, such as Crank (1975), Carslaw and Jaeger (1959), Churchill (1972), Oberhettinger and Badii (1973), Gradshteyn and Ryzhik (2007), and Hahn and Ozisik (2012), greatly simplifies the inversion. Table E.6 has been compiled from these sources.

Table E.6
Inverse Laplace Transform Table

$\overline{F}(s)$	$F(t)$	
$\dfrac{1}{s}$	1	(1)
$\dfrac{1}{s^2}$	t	(2)
$\dfrac{1}{s^n}\ (n > 0)$	$\dfrac{t^{n-1}}{\Gamma(n)}$	(3)
$\dfrac{1}{s \mp a}$	$e^{\pm at}$	(4)
$\dfrac{\sqrt{\pi}}{2\sqrt{s^3}}$	$\sqrt{t}$	(5)
$\sqrt{\dfrac{\pi}{s}}$	$\dfrac{1}{\sqrt{t}}$	(6)
$\dfrac{n!}{(s-a)^{n+1}}$	$t^n e^{at}$	(7)
$\dfrac{a}{s^2 + a^2}$	$\sin at$	(8)
$\dfrac{s}{s^2 + a^2}$	$\cos at$	(9)
1	$\delta(t)$	(10)
e^{-as}	$\delta(t - a)$	(11)
$\dfrac{e^{-as}}{s}$	$H(t - a)$	(12)
$\dfrac{e^{-a/s}}{s}$	$J_o(2\sqrt{at})$	(13)

(Continued)

Table E.6 (*Continued*)
Inverse Laplace Transform Table

$\overline{F}(s)$	$F(t)$	
$\dfrac{e^{-a\sqrt{s}}}{\sqrt{s}}$	$\dfrac{e^{-a^2/4t}}{\sqrt{\pi t}}$	(14)
$e^{-a\sqrt{s}}$	$\dfrac{a}{2\sqrt{\pi t^3}}\, e^{-a^2/4t}$	(15)
$\dfrac{1-e^{-a\sqrt{s}}}{s}$	$\operatorname{erf}\left(\dfrac{a}{2\sqrt{t}}\right)$	(16)
$\dfrac{e^{-a\sqrt{s}}}{s}$	$\operatorname{erfc}\left(\dfrac{a}{2\sqrt{t}}\right)$	(17)
$\dfrac{e^{-a\sqrt{s}}}{s^{3/2}}$	$2\sqrt{\dfrac{t}{\pi}}\, e^{-a^2/4t} - a\operatorname{erfc}\left(\dfrac{a}{2\sqrt{t}}\right)$	(18)
$\dfrac{e^{-a\sqrt{s}}}{\sqrt{s}\,(\sqrt{s}+b)}$	$e^{b^2 t + ab}\operatorname{erfc}\left(b\sqrt{t}+\dfrac{a}{2\sqrt{t}}\right)$	(19)
$\dfrac{b\,e^{-a\sqrt{s}}}{s(\sqrt{s}+b)}$	$-e^{b^2 t + ab}\operatorname{erfc}\left(b\sqrt{t}+\dfrac{a}{2\sqrt{t}}\right) + \operatorname{erfc}\left(\dfrac{a}{2\sqrt{t}}\right)$	(20)
$\dfrac{J_o(ix\sqrt{s})}{s\,J_o(ia\sqrt{s})}$	$1-2\displaystyle\sum_{n=1}^{\infty}\dfrac{e^{-\lambda_n^2 t/a^2}J_o(\lambda_n x/a)}{\lambda_n J_1(\lambda_n)}$ $\quad\lambda_n$ roots of $J_o(\lambda_n)=0$	(21)
$\ln\left(\dfrac{s+a}{s+b}\right)$	$\dfrac{1}{t}\left(e^{-bt}-e^{-at}\right)$	(22)
$\ln\left(\dfrac{s^2+a^2}{s^2}\right)$	$\dfrac{2}{t}\left(1-\cos at\right)$	(23)
$\ln\left(\dfrac{s^2-a^2}{s^2}\right)$	$\dfrac{2}{t}\left(1-\cosh at\right)$	(24)
$K_o\left(a\sqrt{s}\right)$	$\dfrac{1}{2t}\,e^{-\frac{a^2}{4t}}$	(25)
$\dfrac{1}{\sqrt{s}}K_1\left(a\sqrt{s}\right)$	$\dfrac{1}{a}\,e^{-\frac{a^2}{4t}}$	(26)
$\dfrac{\sinh xs}{s\sinh as}$	$\dfrac{x}{a}+\dfrac{2}{\pi}\displaystyle\sum_{n=1}^{\infty}\dfrac{(-1)^n}{n}\cos\lambda_n t\sin\lambda_n x$ $\quad\lambda_n=\dfrac{n\pi}{a}$	(27)
$\dfrac{\sinh xs}{s\cosh as}$	$\dfrac{4}{\pi}\displaystyle\sum_{n=1}^{\infty}\dfrac{(-1)^n}{(2n-1)}\sin\lambda_n t\sin\lambda_n x$ $\quad\lambda_n=\dfrac{(2n-1)\pi}{2a}$	(28)
$\dfrac{\cosh xs}{s\sinh as}$	$\dfrac{t}{a}+\dfrac{2}{\pi}\displaystyle\sum_{n=1}^{\infty}\dfrac{(-1)^n}{n}\sin\lambda_n t\cos\lambda_n x$ $\quad\lambda_n=\dfrac{n\pi}{a}$	(29)
$\dfrac{\sinh x\sqrt{s}}{\sqrt{s}\cosh a\sqrt{s}}$	$\dfrac{2}{a}\displaystyle\sum_{n=1}^{\infty}(-1)^{n-1}e^{-\lambda_n^2 t}\sin\lambda_n x$ $\quad\lambda_n=\dfrac{(2n-1)\pi}{2a}$	(30)
$\dfrac{\cosh x\sqrt{s}}{\sqrt{s}\sinh a\sqrt{s}}$	$\dfrac{1}{a}+\dfrac{2}{a}\displaystyle\sum_{n=1}^{\infty}(-1)^n e^{-\lambda_n^2 t}\cos\lambda_n x$ $\quad\lambda_n=\dfrac{n\pi}{a}$	(31)

(*Continued*)

Table E.6 (*Continued*)
Inverse Laplace Transform Table

$\bar{F}(s)$	$F(t)$		
$\dfrac{\sinh x \sqrt{s}}{s \sinh a \sqrt{s}}$	$\dfrac{x}{a} + \dfrac{2}{\pi} \displaystyle\sum_{n=1}^{\infty} \dfrac{(-1)^n}{n} e^{-\lambda_n^2 t} \sin \lambda_n x$	$\lambda_n = \dfrac{n\pi}{a}$	(32)
$\dfrac{\cosh x \sqrt{s}}{s \cosh a \sqrt{s}}$	$1 + \dfrac{4}{\pi} \displaystyle\sum_{n=1}^{\infty} \dfrac{(-1)^n}{(2n-1)} e^{-\lambda_n^2 t} \cos \lambda_n x$	$\lambda_n = \dfrac{(2n-1)\pi}{2a}$	(33)
$\dfrac{\sinh x \sqrt{s}}{s^2 \sinh a \sqrt{s}}$	$\dfrac{xt}{a} + \dfrac{2}{a} \displaystyle\sum_{n=1}^{\infty} \dfrac{(-1)^n}{\lambda_n^3} (1 - e^{-\lambda_n^2 t}) \sin \lambda_n x$	$\lambda_n = \dfrac{n\pi}{a}$	(34)
$\dfrac{\cosh x \sqrt{s}}{s^2 \cosh a \sqrt{s}}$	$\dfrac{x^2 - a^2}{2} + t - \dfrac{2}{a} \displaystyle\sum_{n=1}^{\infty} \dfrac{(-1)^n}{\lambda_n^3} e^{-\lambda_n^2 t} \cos \lambda_n x$	$\lambda_n = \dfrac{(2n-1)\pi}{2a}$	(35)

In addition to using Laplace transform tables, the *Heaviside partial fractions expansion theorem* is a useful method for inverting the Laplace transform. According to this theorem:

- If $Q(s)$ is a polynomial of degree n and $P(s)$ is of degree $(n-1)$ or less, and if roots of $Q(s) = 0$ are real and distinct, then

$$\mathcal{L}^{-1}\left\{ \frac{P(s)}{Q(s)} \right\} = \sum_{m=1}^{n} \frac{P(s_m)}{Q'(s_m)} e^{s_m t}, \tag{E.46}$$

where s_m are the roots of $Q(s) = 0$ and $Q' = dQ/ds$.
- If $Q(s)$ is of the form

$$Q(s) = (s - s_1)^{m_1} (s - s_2)^{m_2} \ldots (s - s_n)^{m_n} \tag{E.47}$$

and $P(s)$ is of degree $(\sum_{j=1}^{n} m_j) - 1$ or less, then

$$\mathcal{L}^{-1}\left\{ \frac{P(s)}{Q(s)} \right\} = \sum_{k=1}^{n} \sum_{\ell=1}^{m_k} \frac{\phi_{k\ell}(s_k)}{(m_k - \ell)!(\ell - 1)!} t^{m_k - \ell} e^{s_k t}, \tag{E.48}$$

in which

$$\phi_{k\ell}(s) = \frac{d^{\ell-1}}{ds^{\ell-1}} \left[\frac{P(s)}{Q_k(s)} \right], \tag{E.49}$$

where

$$Q_k(s) = \frac{Q(s)}{(s - s_k)^{m_k}} \tag{E.50}$$

Some useful identities used in the application of the Heaviside method are given in Table E.7.

Table E.7
Some Identities for Hyperbolic Functions

$\sinh(ix) = i\sin x$	$\cosh(ix) = \cos x$
$\tanh(ix) = i\tan x$	$\coth h(ix) = -i\cot x$
$\operatorname{sec}h(ix) = \sec x$	$\operatorname{csc}h(ix) = -i\csc x$

Example E.11   A parabolic PDE in a Cartesian coordinate system and its associated initial and boundary conditions are given as

$$\frac{\partial \theta}{\partial \tau} = \frac{\partial^2 \theta}{\partial \xi^2}$$

$$\begin{array}{ll} \tau = 0 & \theta = 0 \\ \xi = 0 & \theta = 1 \\ \xi = 1 & \theta = 0 \end{array} \tag{1}$$

The Laplace transform of the given PDE is

$$s\overline{\theta} = \frac{d^2\overline{\theta}}{d\xi^2} \tag{2}$$

where

$$\overline{\theta} = \int_0^\infty e^{-s\tau}\,\theta\,d\tau \tag{3}$$

The solution of Eq. (3) is given by

$$\overline{\theta} = C_1 \cosh(\xi\sqrt{s}) + C_2 \sinh(\xi\sqrt{s}) \tag{4}$$

Using the boundary conditions in the Laplace domain, i.e.,

$$\text{at}\quad \xi = 0 \qquad \overline{\theta} = \frac{1}{s} \tag{5}$$

$$\text{at}\quad \xi = 1 \qquad \overline{\theta} = 0 \tag{6}$$

the constants are evaluated as

$$C_1 = -\frac{\cosh\sqrt{s}}{s\sinh\sqrt{s}} \quad\text{and}\quad C_2 = \frac{1}{s} \tag{7}$$

so that the solution in the Laplace domain becomes

$$\overline{\theta} = \frac{\sinh\left[(1-\xi)\sqrt{s}\right]}{s\sinh\sqrt{s}} \tag{8}$$

Using Eq. (32) from Table E.6, the inverse Laplace transform becomes

$$\theta = 1 - \xi + \frac{2}{\pi}\sum_{n=1}^{\infty}\frac{(-1)^n}{n}e^{-n^2\pi^2\tau}\sin\left[n\pi(1-\xi)\right] \tag{9}$$

Using the identity

$$\sin\left[n\pi(1-\xi)\right] = -(-1)^n \sin(n\pi\xi) \tag{10}$$

Eq. (9) simplifies to

$$\theta = 1 - \xi - \frac{2}{\pi}\sum_{n=1}^{\infty}\frac{1}{n}e^{-n^2\pi^2\tau}\sin(n\pi\xi) \tag{11}$$

Example E.12   A parabolic PDE and its associated initial and boundary conditions are given as

$$\frac{\partial\theta}{\partial\tau} = \frac{\partial^2\theta}{\partial\xi^2}$$

$$\tau = 0 \qquad \theta = 1$$

$$\xi = 0 \qquad \frac{\partial\theta}{\partial\xi} = 0 \tag{1}$$

$$\xi = 1 \qquad \theta = 0$$

The Laplace transform of the PDE leads to the following ODE:

$$\frac{d^2\overline{\theta}}{d\xi^2} - s\overline{\theta} = -1 \tag{2}$$

The boundary conditions in the Laplace domain are

$$\text{at}\quad \xi = 0 \qquad \frac{d\overline{\theta}}{d\xi} = 0 \tag{3}$$

$$\text{at}\quad \xi = 1 \qquad \overline{\theta} = 0 \tag{4}$$

The solution of Eq. (2) is given by

$$\overline{\theta} = \frac{1}{s} - \frac{\cosh(\xi\sqrt{s})}{s\cosh\sqrt{s}} \tag{5}$$

Using Eqs. (1) and (33) from Table E.6, the inverse Laplace transform becomes

$$\theta = -\frac{4}{\pi}\sum_{n=1}^{\infty}\frac{(-1)^n}{2n-1}e^{-\left[\frac{(2n-1)\pi}{2}\right]^2\tau}\cos\left[\left(\frac{2n-1}{2}\right)\pi\xi\right] \tag{6}$$

Using

$$m = n - 1 \tag{7}$$

Eq. (6) becomes

$$\theta = \frac{2}{\pi}\sum_{m=0}^{\infty}\frac{(-1)^m}{m+\frac{1}{2}}e^{-\left(m+\frac{1}{2}\right)^2\pi^2\tau}\cos\left[\left(m+\frac{1}{2}\right)\pi\xi\right] \tag{8}$$

● Short time solution (τ is small)

Short time solutions ($\tau \to 0$) correspond to large values of s in the Laplace domain, i.e., $s \to \infty$. Thus, hyperbolic terms in Eq. (5) are approximated in terms of the exponential functions as

$$\cosh(\xi \sqrt{s}) = \frac{e^{\xi \sqrt{s}} + e^{-\xi \sqrt{s}}}{2} \simeq \frac{e^{\xi \sqrt{s}}}{2} \tag{9}$$

$$\cosh \sqrt{s} = \frac{e^{\sqrt{s}} + e^{-\sqrt{s}}}{2} \simeq \frac{e^{\sqrt{s}}}{2} \tag{10}$$

Substitution of Eqs. (9) and (10) into Eq. (5) leads to

$$\overline{\theta} = \frac{1}{s} - \frac{e^{-(1-\xi)\sqrt{s}}}{s} \tag{11}$$

Using Eqs. (1) and (17) from Table E.6, the inverse Laplace transform becomes

$$\boxed{\theta = 1 - \mathrm{erfc}\left(\frac{1-\xi}{2\sqrt{\tau}}\right) = \mathrm{erf}\left(\frac{1-\xi}{2\sqrt{\tau}}\right)} \tag{12}$$

Example E.13   A parabolic PDE in a Cartesian coordinate system and its associated initial and boundary conditions are given as

$$\frac{\partial \theta}{\partial \tau} = \frac{\partial^2 \theta}{\partial \xi^2} - \Lambda \theta$$

$$\begin{array}{ll} \tau = 0 & \theta = 0 \\ \xi = 0 & \theta = 0 \\ \xi = 1 & \theta = 1 \end{array} \tag{1}$$

The Laplace transform of the PDE leads to the following ODE:

$$\frac{d^2\overline{\theta}}{d\xi^2} - (\Lambda + s)\,\overline{\theta} = 0 \tag{2}$$

The boundary conditions in the Laplace domain are

$$\text{at} \quad \xi = 0 \qquad \overline{\theta} = 0 \tag{3}$$

$$\text{at} \quad \xi = 1 \qquad \overline{\theta} = \frac{1}{s} \tag{4}$$

The solution of Eq. (2) is given by

$$\overline{\theta} = \frac{\sinh(\xi \sqrt{\Lambda + s})}{s \sinh \sqrt{\Lambda + s}} \tag{5}$$

Since the inverse Laplace transform of Eq. (5) is not readily available from Table E.6, let us rearrange Eq. (5) as the product of two terms:

$$\theta = \mathcal{L}^{-1}\left[\frac{\Lambda + s}{s} \frac{\sinh(\xi \sqrt{\Lambda + s})}{(\Lambda + s) \sinh \sqrt{\Lambda + s}}\right] = \mathcal{L}^{-1}\left[\overline{F}(s)\overline{G}(s, \xi)\right], \tag{6}$$

where

$$\overline{F}(s) = \frac{\Lambda + s}{s} = \frac{\Lambda}{s} + 1 \qquad \text{and} \qquad \overline{G}(s,\xi) = \frac{\sinh(\xi\sqrt{\Lambda + s})}{(\Lambda + s)\sinh\sqrt{\Lambda + s}} \tag{7}$$

Using Eqs. (1) and (10) from Table E.6, the inverse Laplace transform of $\overline{F}(s)$ is

$$F(\tau) = \Lambda + \delta(\tau) \tag{8}$$

Using Eq. (32) from Table E.6 together with the shifting property, Eq. (E.32), the inverse Laplace transform of $\overline{G}(s,\xi)$ is

$$G(\tau,\xi) = \left[\xi + \frac{2}{\pi}\sum_{n=1}^{\infty}\frac{(-1)^n}{n}e^{-n^2\pi^2\tau}\sin(n\pi\xi)\right]e^{-\Lambda\tau} \tag{9}$$

Application of the convolution theorem gives

$$\theta = \int_0^\tau \left[\Lambda + \delta(\tau^*)\right]G(\tau - \tau^*,\xi)\,d\tau^* \tag{10}$$

Using the property of the Dirac delta function given by Eq. (E.45) yields

$$\theta = \Lambda\int_0^\tau G(\tau - \tau^*,\xi)\,d\tau^* + G(\tau,\xi) \tag{11}$$

Substitution of Eq. (9) into Eq. (11) and carrying out the integration give the solution as

$$\boxed{\theta = \xi + 2\sum_{n=1}^{\infty}\frac{(-1)^n}{n\pi(n^2\pi^2 + \Lambda)}\left[\Lambda + n^2\pi^2 e^{-(n^2\pi^2 + \Lambda)\tau}\right]\sin(n\pi\xi)} \tag{12}$$

Example E.14 A parabolic PDE in a Cartesian coordinate system and its associated initial and boundary conditions are given as

$$\frac{\partial\theta}{\partial t} = \mathcal{D}_{AB}\frac{\partial^2\theta}{\partial z^2} - k\theta$$

$$\begin{array}{ll} t = 0 & \theta = 0 \\ z = 0 & \theta = 1 \\ z = \infty & \theta = 0 \end{array} \tag{1}$$

The Laplace transform of the PDE leads to the following ODE:

$$\frac{d^2\overline{\theta}}{dz^2} - \left(\frac{k+s}{\mathcal{D}_{AB}}\right)\overline{\theta} = 0 \tag{2}$$

The boundary conditions in the Laplace domain are

$$\text{at} \quad z = 0 \qquad \overline{\theta} = \frac{1}{s} \tag{3}$$

$$\text{at} \quad z = \infty \qquad \overline{\theta} = 0 \tag{4}$$

The solution of Eq. (2) is

$$\overline{\theta} = \frac{1}{s}e^{-\frac{z}{\sqrt{\mathcal{D}_{AB}}}\sqrt{s+k}} \tag{5}$$

Since the inverse Laplace transform of Eq. (5) is not readily available from Table E.6, let us rearrange Eq. (5) as the product of two terms:

$$\theta = \mathcal{L}^{-1}\left[\frac{1}{s}e^{-\frac{z}{\sqrt{\mathcal{D}_{AB}}}\sqrt{s+k}}\right] = \mathcal{L}^{-1}\left[\overline{F}(s)\,\overline{G}(s,z)\right], \tag{6}$$

where

$$\overline{F}(s) = \frac{1}{s} \quad \text{and} \quad \overline{G}(s,z) = e^{-\frac{z}{\sqrt{\mathcal{D}_{AB}}}\sqrt{s+k}} \tag{7}$$

Using Eq. (1) from Table E.6, the inverse Laplace transform of $\overline{F}(s)$ is

$$F(t) = 1 \tag{8}$$

Using Eq. (15) from Table E.6 together with the shifting property, Eq. (E.32), the inverse Laplace transform of $\overline{G}(s,z)$ is

$$G(t,z) = \frac{z}{2\sqrt{\pi \mathcal{D}_{AB}}}\frac{1}{\sqrt{t^3}}e^{-\left(\frac{z^2}{4\mathcal{D}_{AB}t}+kt\right)} \tag{9}$$

Application of the convolution theorem gives

$$\theta = \frac{z}{2\sqrt{\pi \mathcal{D}_{AB}}}\int_0^t \frac{1}{\sqrt{t^{*3}}}e^{-\left(\frac{z^2}{4\mathcal{D}_{AB}t^*}+kt^*\right)}dt^* \tag{10}$$

Making use of the substitutions

$$\alpha^2 = \frac{z^2}{4\mathcal{D}_{AB}} \quad \text{and} \quad \beta^2 = k \tag{11}$$

Eq. (10) takes the form

$$\theta = \frac{\alpha}{\sqrt{\pi}}\int_0^t \frac{1}{\sqrt{t^{*3}}}e^{-\left(\frac{\alpha^2}{t^*}+\beta^2 t^*\right)}dt^* \tag{12}$$

Let us rearrange Eq. (12) as

$$\theta = \frac{1}{\sqrt{\pi}}\int_0^t \left(\frac{\alpha}{\sqrt{t^{*3}}}+\frac{\beta}{\sqrt{t^*}}-\frac{\beta}{\sqrt{t^*}}\right)e^{-\left(\frac{\alpha^2}{t^*}+\beta^2 t^*\right)}dt^* \tag{13}$$

• **Case** (*i*)

Equation (13) can be expressed as

$$\theta = \underbrace{\frac{1}{\sqrt{\pi}}\int_0^t \left(\frac{\alpha}{\sqrt{t^{*3}}}+\frac{\beta}{\sqrt{t^*}}\right)e^{-\left(\frac{\alpha^2}{t^*}+\beta^2 t^*\right)}dt^*}_{I}-\frac{\beta}{\sqrt{\pi}}\int_0^t \frac{1}{\sqrt{t^*}}e^{-\left(\frac{\alpha^2}{t^*}+\beta^2 t^*\right)}dt^* \tag{14}$$

To evaluate the term I, let us make the substitution

$$u = \frac{\alpha}{\sqrt{t^*}}-\beta\sqrt{t^*} \tag{15}$$

Thus

$$u^2 = \frac{\alpha^2}{t^*}+\beta^2 t^* - 2\alpha\beta \quad \text{and} \quad du = -\frac{1}{2}\left(\frac{\alpha}{\sqrt{t^{*3}}}+\frac{\beta}{\sqrt{t^*}}\right)dt^* \tag{16}$$

The term I now becomes

$$I = e^{-2\alpha\beta} \frac{2}{\sqrt{\pi}} \int_{\frac{\alpha}{\sqrt{t}} - \beta\sqrt{t}}^{\infty} e^{-u^2} du = e^{-2\alpha\beta} \, \text{erfc}\left(\frac{\alpha}{\sqrt{t}} - \beta\sqrt{t}\right) \tag{17}$$

• **Case** (*ii*)

Equation (13) can also be expressed as

$$\theta = \underbrace{\frac{1}{\sqrt{\pi}} \int_0^t \left(\frac{\alpha}{\sqrt{t^{*3}}} - \frac{\beta}{\sqrt{t^*}}\right) e^{-\left(\frac{\alpha^2}{t^*} + \beta^2 t^*\right)} dt^* + \frac{\beta}{\sqrt{\pi}} \int_0^t \frac{1}{\sqrt{t^*}} e^{-\left(\frac{\alpha^2}{t^*} + \beta^2 t^*\right)} dt^*}_{II} \tag{18}$$

To evaluate the term II, let us make the substitution

$$\bar{u} = \frac{\alpha}{\sqrt{t^*}} + \beta\sqrt{t^*} \tag{19}$$

Thus

$$\bar{u}^2 = \frac{\alpha^2}{t^*} + \beta^2 t^* + 2\alpha\beta \quad \text{and} \quad d\bar{u} = -\frac{1}{2}\left(\frac{\alpha}{\sqrt{t^{*3}}} - \frac{\beta}{\sqrt{t^*}}\right) dt^* \tag{20}$$

The term II now becomes

$$II = e^{2\alpha\beta} \frac{2}{\sqrt{\pi}} \int_{\frac{\alpha}{\sqrt{t}} + \beta\sqrt{t}}^{\infty} e^{-\bar{u}^2} d\bar{u} = e^{2\alpha\beta} \, \text{erfc}\left(\frac{\alpha}{\sqrt{t}} + \beta\sqrt{t}\right) \tag{21}$$

Addition of Eqs. (14) and (18) leads to

$$\theta = \frac{1}{2}(I + II) \tag{22}$$

Substitution of Eqs. (17) and (21) into Eq. (22) gives

$$\theta = \frac{1}{2} e^{-2\alpha\beta} \, \text{erfc}\left(\frac{\alpha}{\sqrt{t}} - \beta\sqrt{t}\right) + \frac{1}{2} e^{2\alpha\beta} \, \text{erfc}\left(\frac{\alpha}{\sqrt{t}} + \beta\sqrt{t}\right) \tag{23}$$

or

$$\boxed{\theta = \frac{1}{2} e^{-\sqrt{\frac{k}{\mathcal{D}_{AB}}} z} \, \text{erfc}\left(\frac{z}{\sqrt{4\mathcal{D}_{AB}t}} - \sqrt{kt}\right) + \frac{1}{2} e^{\sqrt{\frac{k}{\mathcal{D}_{AB}}} z} \, \text{erfc}\left(\frac{z}{\sqrt{4\mathcal{D}_{AB}t}} + \sqrt{kt}\right)} \tag{24}$$

E.2.4 THE FOURIER TRANSFORM TECHNIQUE

While the Laplace transformation is applicable for semi-infinite domains, the Fourier transformation is used for infinite domains. The *Fourier transformation* is defined by

$$\boxed{\mathcal{F}\{F(x)\} = \widehat{F}(\omega) = \int_{-\infty}^{\infty} F(x) e^{-i\omega x} dx} \tag{E.51}$$

Transformation from the *x*-domain to the *ω*-domain converts position derivatives into algebraic functions of time and *ω*, leading to an equation much easier to solve in the *ω*-domain. Once the solution is obtained in the ω-domain, it should be inverted back to the x-domain by using the following formula:

$$F(x) = \mathcal{F}^{-1}\left[\widehat{F}(\omega)\right] = \frac{1}{2\pi}\int_{-\infty}^{\infty}\widehat{F}(\omega)\,e^{i\omega x}d\omega \tag{E.52}$$

Some properties of the Fourier transform

• Linear property

$$\mathcal{F}\{\alpha F(x) + \beta G(x)\} = \alpha\mathcal{F}\{F(x)\} + \beta\mathcal{F}\{G(x)\}, \tag{E.53}$$

where α and β are scalars.

• Transform of derivatives

$$\mathcal{F}\left[\frac{dF(x)}{dx}\right] = i\omega\widehat{F}(\omega) \tag{E.54}$$

$$\mathcal{F}\left[\frac{d^2F(x)}{dx^2}\right] = (i\omega)^2\widehat{F}(\omega) = -\omega^2\widehat{F}(\omega) \tag{E.55}$$

• Shifting properties

$$\mathcal{F}^{-1}\left[\widehat{F}(\omega - a)\right] = e^{iax}F(x) \tag{E.56}$$

$$\mathcal{F}^{-1}\left[e^{-ia\omega}\widehat{F}(\omega)\right] = F(x - a) \tag{E.57}$$

• Transform of the Dirac delta function

$$\mathcal{F}\left[\delta(x - a)\right] = e^{-ia\omega} \tag{E.58}$$

• Convolution theorem

If

$$\mathcal{F}^{-1}\left[\widehat{F}(\omega)\right] = F(x) \qquad \text{and} \qquad \mathcal{F}^{-1}\left[\widehat{G}(\omega)\right] = G(x) \tag{E.59}$$

then

$$\begin{aligned}\mathcal{F}^{-1}\left[\widehat{F}(\omega)\,\widehat{G}(\omega)\right] &= F(x) * G(x) \\ &= \int_{-\infty}^{\infty}F(x - u)\,G(u)\,du = \int_{-\infty}^{\infty}F(u)\,G(x - u)\,du\end{aligned} \tag{E.60}$$

Example E.15   A parabolic PDE in a Cartesian coordinate system and its associated initial and boundary conditions are given as

$$\frac{\partial c_A}{\partial t} = \mathcal{D}_{AB}\frac{\partial^2 c_A}{\partial z^2}$$

$$\begin{array}{ll} t = 0 & c_A = m\,\delta(z) \\ z = \pm\infty & c_A = 0 \end{array} \tag{1}$$

Taking the Fourier transform of the governing equation gives the following linear first-order ODE:

$$\frac{d\widehat{c}_A}{dt} = -\mathcal{D}_{AB}\,\omega^2\,\widehat{c}_A, \tag{2}$$

where

$$\widehat{c}_A = \mathcal{F}(c_A) = \int_{-\infty}^{\infty} c_A e^{-i\omega z} dz \tag{3}$$

The solution of Eq. (2) is

$$\widehat{c}_A = C e^{-\mathcal{D}_{AB}\omega^2 t}, \tag{4}$$

where C is a constant. The Fourier transform of the initial condition is

$$t = 0 \qquad \widehat{c}_A = m \tag{5}$$

Thus, $C = m$, and the solution in the ω-domain becomes

$$\widehat{c}_A = m e^{-\mathcal{D}_{AB}\omega^2 t} \tag{6}$$

According to Eq. (E.52), the inverse Fourier transform of Eq. (6) is

$$c_A = \frac{m}{2\pi} \int_{-\infty}^{\infty} e^{-\mathcal{D}_{AB}\omega^2 t} e^{i\omega z} d\omega = \frac{m}{2\pi} \int_{-\infty}^{\infty} e^{-\mathcal{D}_{AB}\omega^2 t + i\omega z} d\omega \tag{7}$$

From integral tables

$$\int_{-\infty}^{\infty} e^{-p^2 x^2 + qx} dx = \frac{\sqrt{\pi}}{p} e^{\frac{q^2}{4p^2}} \tag{8}$$

If we let

$$x = \omega \qquad q = zi \qquad p^2 = \mathcal{D}_{AB}t \tag{9}$$

Eq. (8) becomes

$$\int_{-\infty}^{\infty} e^{-\mathcal{D}_{AB}\omega^2 t + i\omega z} d\omega = \frac{\sqrt{\pi}}{\sqrt{\mathcal{D}_{AB}t}} e^{-\frac{z^2}{4\mathcal{D}_{AB}t}} \tag{10}$$

Substitution of Eq. (10) into Eq. (7) gives the solution as

$$\boxed{c_A = \frac{m}{2\sqrt{\pi\mathcal{D}_{AB}t}} e^{-\frac{z^2}{4\mathcal{D}_{AB}t}}} \tag{11}$$

E.3 DUHAMEL'S THEOREM

Duhamel's theorem is used to solve unsteady-state mass transfer problems with time-dependent boundary conditions. It is applicable when the initial condition is zero. Let us consider the PDE

$$\frac{\partial \theta}{\partial \tau} = \frac{\partial^2 \theta}{\partial \xi^2} \tag{E.61}$$

subject to the following initial and boundary conditions:

$$\text{at} \quad \tau = 0 \qquad \theta = 0 \tag{E.62}$$

$$\text{at} \quad \xi = 0 \qquad \theta = f(\tau) \tag{E.63}$$

$$\text{at} \quad \xi = \infty \qquad \theta = 0 \tag{E.64}$$

The first step in the application of Duhamel's theorem is to form an auxiliary problem by letting the time-dependent boundary condition equal unity, i.e.,

$$\frac{\partial \varphi}{\partial \tau} = \frac{\partial^2 \varphi}{\partial \xi^2} \tag{E.65}$$

$$\text{at} \quad \tau = 0 \qquad \varphi = 0 \tag{E.66}$$

$$\text{at} \quad \xi = 0 \qquad \varphi = 1 \tag{E.67}$$

$$\text{at} \quad \xi = \infty \qquad \varphi = 0, \tag{E.68}$$

where $\varphi(\tau, \xi)$ is the dependent variable of the auxiliary problem. Once the solution is obtained for $\varphi(\tau, \xi)$, the solution for $\theta(\tau, \xi)$ is given by

$$\theta(\tau, \xi) = \int_0^\tau f(u) \frac{\partial \varphi(\tau - u, \xi)}{\partial \tau} \, du, \tag{E.69}$$

where u is a dummy variable.

Example E.16 A parabolic PDE in a Cartesian coordinate system and its associated initial and boundary conditions are given as

$$\frac{\partial \theta}{\partial \tau} = \frac{\partial^2 \theta}{\partial \xi^2}$$

$$\begin{aligned} \text{at} \quad \tau = 0 \quad & \theta = 0 \\ \text{at} \quad \xi = 0 \quad & \theta = e^{-\beta \tau} \\ \text{at} \quad \xi = 1 \quad & \theta = 0 \end{aligned} \tag{1}$$

The auxiliary problem is

$$\frac{\partial \varphi}{\partial \tau} = \frac{\partial^2 \varphi}{\partial \xi^2}$$

$$\begin{aligned} \text{at} \quad \tau = 0 \quad & \varphi = 0 \\ \text{at} \quad \xi = 0 \quad & \varphi = 1 \\ \text{at} \quad \xi = 1 \quad & \varphi = 0 \end{aligned} \tag{2}$$

The solution of the auxiliary problem can be obtained from Example E.11 as

$$\varphi = 1 - \xi - \frac{2}{\pi} \sum_{n=1}^\infty \frac{1}{n} e^{-n^2 \pi^2 \tau} \sin(n\pi\xi) \tag{3}$$

Application of Eq. (E.69) gives

$$\theta = 2\pi \sum_{n=1}^\infty n \sin(n\pi\xi) \int_0^\tau e^{-\beta u} e^{-n^2 \pi^2 (\tau - u)} \, du \tag{4}$$

or

$$\theta = 2\pi e^{-\beta \tau} \sum_{n=1}^\infty \frac{n}{n^2 \pi^2 - \beta} \left[1 - e^{-(n^2 \pi^2 - \beta)\tau} \right] \sin(n\pi\xi) \tag{5}$$

E.4 SOLUTION OF PDEs BY MATHCAD

E.4.1 DETERMINATION OF EIGENVALUES

Once the analytical solution of a given PDE is obtained, calculation of the numerical values of the dependent variable requires eigenvalues to be known. Eigenvalues, on the other hand, are usually obtained from the solution of a transcendental equation.

The built-in function **root**$(f(x), x)$ solves one of the roots of an equation

$$f(x) = 0 \qquad \text{(E.70)}$$

An initial guess value for x is needed. The Mathcad subroutine Roots(N) shown in Figure E.2 calculates the eigenvalues of any given transcendental equation. In Figure E.2, the first ten roots of the transcendental equation

$$J_o(\lambda_n)Y_o(\kappa\lambda_n) - Y_o(\lambda_n)J_o(\kappa\lambda_n) = 0 \qquad \text{(E.71)}$$

are calculated for $\kappa = 1.5$.

E.4.2 NUMERICAL SOLUTION OF PARABOLIC PDEs

• Cartesian coordinate system

Let us consider the dimensionless PDE in a Cartesian coordinate system

$$\frac{\partial \theta}{\partial \tau} = \frac{\partial^2 \theta}{\partial \xi^2} \qquad \text{(E.72)}$$

subject to the following initial and boundary conditions:

$$\text{at} \quad \tau = 0 \qquad \theta = 1 \qquad \text{(E.73)}$$

$$\text{at} \quad \xi = 0 \qquad \frac{\partial \theta}{\partial \xi} = 0 \qquad \text{(E.74)}$$

$$\text{at} \quad \xi = 1 \qquad \theta = 0 \qquad \text{(E.75)}$$

The built-in function **Pdesolve**$(u, x, xrange, t, trange)$ solves the given PDE. The arguments of **Pdesolve** are given as

$u = $ dependent variable

$x = $ independent position variable

$xrange = $ a *two*-element column vector containing the real boundary values for x

$t = $ independent time variable

$trange = $ a *two*-element column vector containing the real boundary values for t

In this specific case, x goes from 0 to 1, and t goes from 0 to any desired dimensionless time value, say 2. The Mathcad worksheet is shown in Figure E.3. The following rules apply in the solution of PDEs:

- Functions must be defined explicitly in terms of their variables. For example, use $\theta(x, t)$, not just θ. Also keep in mind that the order of the arguments of functions must be (x, t) and not (t, x).
- The partial derivatives are typed using subscript notation, i.e., typing a period ".". For example, the second partial derivative of θ with respect to x is written as $\theta_{xx}(x, t)$. Since Mathcad does not allow Greek symbols to be used as subscripts, τ and ξ are replaced by t and x, respectively, in the worksheet.
- **Pdesolve** must be used in a "Solve Block."
- Equations must be defined using Boolean equals.
- Second partial derivatives are not allowed on the left side of the equation(s), i.e., you cannot type the equation as

$$\theta_{xx}(x, t) = \theta_t(x, t)$$

```
ORIGIN:= 1

κ := 1.5

f(λ) := J0(λ)·Y0(κ·λ) − Y0(λ)·J0(κ·λ)

Roots(N) := | a ← 10^-3
            | rtDifference ← 0
            | rt ← rtDifference
            | Δλ ← 10^-6
            | for j ∈ 1..N
            |   | a ← a + rtDifference
            |   | fl ← f(a)
            |   | fr ← f(a + Δλ)
            |   | while fl·fr > 0
            |   |   | fl ← f(a)
            |   |   | b ← a + Δλ
            |   |   | fr ← f(b)
            |   |   | a ← b
            |   | rt ← root(f(a), a)
            |   | a ← a − Δλ
            |   | sol_j ← rt
            |   | rtDifference ← sol_j  if j = 1
            |   | rtDifference ← (sol_j − sol_j−1)·0.1  if j > 1
            | sol
```

N represents the number of roots

Roots(10) =

	1
1	6.27024
2	12.55978
3	18.84515
4	25.12943
5	31.41328
6	37.6969
7	43.9804
8	50.26383
9	56.54719
10	62.83053

Figure E.2 Mathcad worksheet for subroutine roots (N).

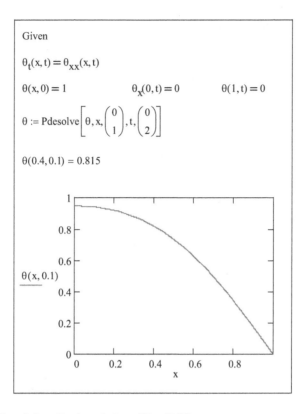

Figure E.3 Mathcad worksheet for the solution of Eq. (E.72).

• Cylindrical coordinate system

Let us consider the dimensionless PDE in a cylindrical coordinate system

$$\frac{\partial \theta}{\partial \tau} = \frac{1}{\xi} \frac{\partial}{\partial \xi} \left(\xi \frac{\partial \theta}{\partial \xi} \right) \tag{E.76}$$

subject to the following initial and boundary conditions:

$$\text{at} \quad \tau = 0 \qquad \theta = 1 \tag{E.77}$$

$$\text{at} \quad \xi = 0 \qquad \frac{\partial \theta}{\partial \xi} = 0 \tag{E.78}$$

$$\text{at} \quad \xi = 1 \qquad \frac{\partial \theta}{\partial \xi} = -\Lambda \theta \tag{E.79}$$

In Eq. (E.76), the presence of ξ in the denominator causes a singularity at the center of the cylinder, i.e., $\xi = 0$. Note that the right side of Eq. (E.76) is expressed as

$$\frac{1}{\xi} \frac{\partial}{\partial \xi} \left(\xi \frac{\partial \theta}{\partial \xi} \right) = \frac{1}{\xi} \frac{\partial \theta}{\partial \xi} + \frac{\partial^2 \theta}{\partial \xi^2} \tag{E.80}$$

At $\xi = 0$, the first term of the right side of Eq. (E.80) is

$$\lim_{\xi \to 0} \left(\frac{\partial \theta / \partial \xi}{\xi} \right) = \frac{0}{0} \tag{E.81}$$

Application of L'Hôpital's rule, i.e., differentiation of the numerator and the denominator separately, yields

$$\lim_{\xi \to 0} \left(\frac{\partial \theta / \partial \xi}{\xi} \right) = \lim_{\xi \to 0} \left(\frac{\partial^2 \theta / \partial \xi^2}{1} \right) = \frac{\partial^2 \theta}{\partial \xi^2} \tag{E.82}$$

Thus, at $\xi = 0$, the governing equation becomes

$$\frac{\partial \theta}{\partial \tau} = 2 \frac{\partial^2 \theta}{\partial \xi^2} \tag{E.83}$$

The Mathcad worksheet of the problem is shown in Figure E.4. Note that τ and ξ are replaced by t and r, respectively.

• Spherical coordinate system

Let us consider the dimensionless PDE in a spherical coordinate system

$$\frac{\partial \theta}{\partial \tau} = \frac{1}{\xi^2} \frac{\partial}{\partial \xi} \left(\xi^2 \frac{\partial \theta}{\partial \xi} \right) \tag{E.84}$$

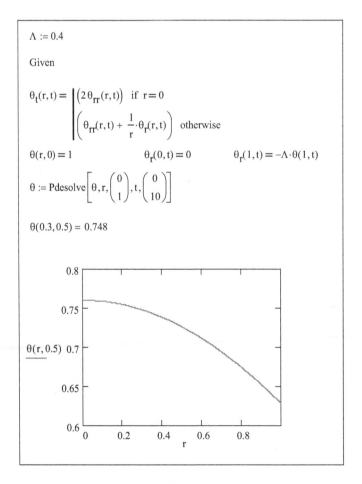

Figure E.4   Mathcad worksheet for the solution of Eq. (E.76) for $\Lambda = 0.4$.

subject to the following initial and boundary conditions:

$$\text{at} \quad \tau = 0 \qquad \theta = 1 \tag{E.85}$$

$$\text{at} \quad \xi = 0 \qquad \frac{\partial \theta}{\partial \xi} = 0 \tag{E.86}$$

$$\text{at} \quad \xi = 1 \qquad \frac{\partial \theta}{\partial \xi} = -\Lambda \theta \tag{E.87}$$

The presence of ξ^2 in the denominator of Eq. (E.84) causes a singularity at the center, i.e., $\xi = 0$. Note that the right side of Eq. (E.84) is expressed as

$$\frac{1}{\xi^2} \frac{\partial}{\partial \xi} \left(\xi^2 \frac{\partial \theta}{\partial \xi} \right) = \frac{2}{\xi} \frac{\partial \theta}{\partial \xi} + \frac{\partial^2 \theta}{\partial \xi^2} \tag{E.88}$$

At $\xi = 0$, the first term of the right side of Eq. (E.88) is

$$\lim_{\xi \to 0} 2 \left(\frac{\partial \theta / \partial \xi}{\xi} \right) = \frac{0}{0} \tag{E.89}$$

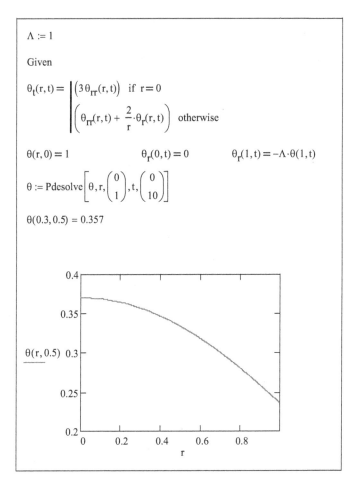

Figure E.5 Mathcad worksheet for the solution of Eq. (E.84) for $\Lambda = 1$.

Application of L'Hôpital's rule yields

$$\lim_{\xi \to 0} 2 \left(\frac{\partial \theta / \partial \xi}{\xi} \right) = \lim_{\xi \to 0} 2 \left(\frac{\partial^2 \theta / \partial \xi^2}{1} \right) = 2 \frac{\partial^2 \theta}{\partial \xi^2} \tag{E.90}$$

Thus, at $\xi = 0$, the governing equation becomes

$$\frac{\partial \theta}{\partial \tau} = 3 \frac{\partial^2 \theta}{\partial \xi^2} \tag{E.91}$$

The Mathcad worksheet of the problem is shown in Figure E.5. Note that τ and ξ are replaced by t and r, respectively.

REFERENCES

Bird, R. B., R. C. Armstrong and O. Hassager. 1987. *Dynamics of Polymeric Liquids*, Volume 1: Fluid Dynamics, 2nd edn. New York: Wiley.

Carslaw, H. S. and J. C. Jaeger. 1959. *Conduction of Heat in Solids*, 2nd edn. London: Oxford University Press.

Churchill, R. V. 1972. *Operational Mathematics*, 3rd edn. New York: McGraw-Hill.

Crank, J. 1975. *The Mathematics of Diffusion*, 2nd edn. London: Oxford University Press.

Gradshteyn, I. S. and I. M. Ryzhik. 2007. *Table of Integrals, Series, and Products*, 7th edn. New York: Academic Press.

Hahn, D. W. and M. N. Ozisik. 2012. *Heat Conduction*, 3 rd edn. Hoboken: Wiley.

Hildebrand, F. B. 1976. *Advanced Calculus for Applications*, 2nd edn. Englewood Cliffs: Prentice-Hall.

Oberhettinger, F. and L. Badii. 1973. *Tables of Laplace Transforms*. Berlin: Springer.

F Critical Constants and Acentric Factors

Compiled from

1. NIST (National Institute of Standards and Technology) Chemistry WebBook
   https://www.nist.gov/chemistry

2. Korea Thermophysical Properties Data Bank (KDB)
   https://www.cheric.org/research/kdb

Name	Formula	Molecular Weight	T_c (K)	P_c (bar)	$\widetilde{V}_c$ (cm^3/mol)	ω
Elements						
Argon	Ar	39.948	150.86	48.98	75	-0.004
Bromine	Br$_2$	159.808	588.0	103.4	127	0.108
Chlorine	Cl$_2$	70.906	416.96	79.77	122.93	0.090
Helium	He	4.003	5.2	2.27	57.47	-0.387
Hydrogen	H$_2$	2.016	33.18	13.0	64.94	-0.216
Iodine	I$_2$	253.809	819.0	116.5	155	0.229
Neon	Ne	20.180	44.4	27.6	42	-0.029
Nitrogen	N$_2$	28.013	126.19	33.98	89.45	0.039
Oxygen	O$_2$	31.999	154.58	50.43	73.53	0.025
Hydrocarbons						
Acetylene	C$_2$H$_2$	26.037	308.3	61.38	112.2	0.190
Benzene	C$_6$H$_6$	78.112	562.0	48.9	256	0.212
n-Butane	C$_4$H$_{10}$	58.122	425.0	38.0	255	0.199
Cumene	C$_9$H$_{12}$	120.192	631.0	32.1	431.03	0.326
Cyclohexane	C$_6$H$_{12}$	84.160	554.0	40.7	308	0.212
Cyclopentane	C$_5$H$_{10}$	70.133	511.7	45.1	259	0.196
n-Decane	C$_{10}$H$_{22}$	142.282	617.8	21.1	624	0.489
Ethane	C$_2$H$_6$	30.069	305.3	49.0	147	0.099
Ethylbenzene	C$_8$H$_{10}$	106.165	617.0	36.4	374	0.302
Ethylene	C$_2$H$_4$	28.053	282.5	50.6	131.1	0.089
n-Heptane	C$_7$H$_{16}$	100.202	540.0	27.4	428	0.349
1-Heptene	C$_7$H$_{14}$	98.186	537.3	29.2	409	0.358
n-Hexane	C$_6$H$_{14}$	86.175	507.6	30.2	368	0.299
1-Hexene	C$_6$H$_{14}$	84.160	504.0	32.1	355.1	0.285
Isobutane	C$_4$H$_{10}$	58.122	407.7	36.5	259	0.183
Isopentane	C$_5$H$_{12}$	72.149	461.0	33.8	306	0.227
Methane	CH$_4$	16.043	190.6	46.1	98.6	0.011
Naphthalene	C$_{10}$H$_8$	128.171	748.0	41.0	407	0.302
n-Octane	C$_8$H$_{18}$	114.229	568.9	24.9	492	0.398
1-Octene	C$_8$H$_{16}$	112.213	567.0	26.8	468	0.386
n-Pentane	C$_5$H$_{12}$	72.149	469.8	33.6	311	0.251
Propane	C$_3$H$_8$	44.096	369.9	42.5	200	0.153
Propylene	C$_3$H$_6$	42.080	365.2	46.0	184.6	0.144
Toluene	C$_7$H$_8$	92.138	593.0	41.0	316	0.263
o-Xylene	C$_8$H$_{10}$	106.17	631.0	37.0	370	0.310

Name	Formula	Molecular Weight	T_c (K)	P_c (bar)	$\widetilde{V}_c$ (cm^3/mol)	ω
Inorganic Compounds						
Ammonia	NH_3	17.031	405.4	113.0	72.0	0.250
Carbon dioxide	CO_2	44.010	304.18	73.80	91.9	0.239
Carbon disulfide	CS_2	76.141	552.0	79.0	173	0.109
Carbon monoxide	CO	28.010	134.45	34.99	90.09	0.066
Hydrogen chloride	HCl	36.461	324.68	82.56	81	0.133
Hydrogen cyanide	HCN	27.025	456.7	53.9	139	0.388
Hydrogen sulfide	H_2S	34.081	373.3	89.70	98.04	0.081
Nitric oxide	NO	30.006	180.0	64.8	58	0.588
Nitrous oxide	N_2O	44.013	309.56	72.38	95.5	0.165
Sulfur dioxide	SO_2	64.064	430.34	78.8	122	0.256
Sulfur trioxide	SO_3	80.063	491.0	82.0	127	0.481
Water	H_2O	18.016	647.0	220.64	55.87	0.344
Organic Compounds						
Acetaldehyde	C_2H_4O	44.053	466.0	55.7	154.08	0.303
Acetic acid	$C_2H_4O_2$	60.052	593.0	57.81	171.23	0.447
Acetone	C_3H_6O	58.079	508.0	48.0	215.98	0.304
Acetonitrile	C_2H_3N	41.052	545.0	48.7	173	0.327
Aniline	C_6H_7N	93.127	698.8	53.1	287.36	0.384
n-Butanol	$C_4H_{10}O$	74.122	562.0	45.0	274	0.593
Carbon tetrachloride	CCl_4	153.823	556.36	44.93	276.24	0.193
Chlorobenzene	C_6H_5Cl	112.557	632.35	45.19	308.64	0.249
Chloroform	$CHCl_3$	119.378	537.0	53.29	243.31	0.218
Diethyl ether	$C_4H_{10}O$	74.122	467.0	36.0	274	0.281
Dimethyl ether	C_2H_6O	46.068	401.0	54.0	164	0.200
Ethanol	C_2H_6O	46.068	514.0	63.0	168	0.644
Ethyl acetate	$C_4H_8O_2$	88.105	530.0	38.82	286.37	0.362
Ethylene oxide	C_2H_4O	44.053	468.9	72.33	140.25	0.202
Formaldehyde	CH_2O	30.026	408.0	65.9	115	0.253
n-Heptanol	$C_7H_{16}O$	116.203	632.6	30.6	435	0.560
Isobutanol	$C_4H_{10}O$	74.122	547.8	42.95	274	0.592
Isopropanol	C_3H_8O	60.096	508.3	47.64	222	0.665
Methanol	CH_4O	32.042	512.5	80.84	117	0.556
Methyl acetate	$C_3H_6O_2$	74.079	506.55	47.50	228	0.326
Methyl ethyl ketone	C_4H_8O	72.107	536.78	42.07	267	0.320
Phenol	C_6H_6O	94.113	694.2	61.30	229	0.438
n-Propanol	C_3H_8O	60.096	536.8	51.69	218	0.623

G Physical Properties of Water

Density[1]

$$\rho = (999.83952 + 16.945176\,t - 7.9870401 \times 10^{-3}t^2 - 47.170461 \times 10^{-6}t^3$$
$$+ 105.56302 \times 10^{-9}t^4 - 280.54253 \times 10^{-12}t^5)/(1 + 16.879850 \times 10^{-3}t)$$

where ρ is in kg/m^3 and t is in °C.

Viscosity[2]

$$\mu \times 10^6 = \sum_{i=1}^{4} a_i \left(\frac{T}{300}\right)^{b_i}$$

where μ is in Pa.s and T is in K. The values of a_i and b_i are given as

i	a_i	b_i
1	280.68	−1.9
2	511.45	−7.7
3	61.131	−19.6
4	0.45903	−40.0

Vapor Pressure[3]

$$\log P^{vap} = A - \frac{B}{C+T}$$

where P^{vap} is in bar and T is in K. The parameters A, B, and C are given as

A	B	C	Temperature (K)
5.40221	1838.675	−31.737	273–303
5.20389	1733.926	−39.485	304–333
5.0768	1659.793	−45.854	334–363
5.08354	1663.125	−45.622	364–373
3.55959	643.748	−198.043	379–573

---

[1]Kell, G. S. 1975. Thermal expansivity, and compressibility of liquid water from 0°C to 150°C: Correlations and tables for atmospheric pressure and saturation reviewed and expressed on 1968 temperature scale. *J. Phys. Chem. Ref. Data* 20(1):97–105.

[2]Patek, J., J. Hruby, J. Klomfar, M. Souckova and A. H. Harvey. 2009. Reference correlations for thermophysical properties of liquid water at 0.1 MPa. *J. Phys. Chem. Ref. Data* 38(1):21–9.

[3]NIST (National Institute of Standards and Technology) Chemistry WebBook (*https://www.nist.gov/chemistry*).

H Mathcad Subroutines

H.1 MULTICOMPONENT – WILSON

The subroutine named "Multicomponent – Wilson" calculates the thermodynamic factor using Eq. (3.97) as shown in Figure H.1. Prior to calling this subroutine, specification of the number of species (N) and the calculation of Λ values are necessary.

$$
\Gamma := \left| \begin{array}{l}
\text{for } i \in 1..N \\[4pt]
\quad S_i \leftarrow \displaystyle\sum_{j=1}^{N} \left(x_j \cdot \Lambda_{i,j}\right) \\[10pt]
\text{for } i \in 1..N \\
\quad \text{for } j \in 1..N \\[4pt]
\quad\quad Q_{i,j} \leftarrow \dfrac{-\Lambda_{i,j}}{S_i} - \dfrac{\Lambda_{j,i}}{S_j} + \displaystyle\sum_{k=1}^{N} \left[\dfrac{x_k \cdot \Lambda_{k,i} \cdot \Lambda_{k,j}}{\left(S_k\right)^2} \right] \\[12pt]
\text{for } i \in 1..(N-1) \\
\quad \text{for } j \in 1..(N-1) \\[4pt]
\quad\quad \Gamma_{i,j} \leftarrow \delta(i,j) + x_i \cdot \left(Q_{i,j} - Q_{i,N}\right) \\[8pt]
\Gamma
\end{array} \right.
$$

Figure H.1 Subroutine "Multicomponent – Wilson."

H.2 MULTICOMPONENT – NRTL

The subroutine named "Multicomponent – NRTL" calculates the thermodynamic factor using Eq. (3.102) as shown in Figure H.2. Prior to calling this subroutine, specification of the number of species (N) and the calculation of τ and G values are necessary.

H.3 ROOT

The subroutine named "Root" calculates the roots of Eq. (3.106) as shown in Figure H.3. If the equation has three distinct real roots, then root(p,q,r)$_1$ and root(p,q,r)$_2$ give the largest and the smallest roots, respectively. If the equation has a single real root, the other two being complex conjugate, root(p,q,r)$_1$ and root(p,q,r)$_2$ give the same real root.

H.4 MIXTURE

The subroutine named "Mixture" is shown in Figure H.4. It calculates the compressibility factor, Z, as well as the dimensionless parameters A and B for the mixture using the Peng–Robinson equation of state. Prior to calling this subroutine, subroutine "Root" must be called, and the critical properties as well as the number of species (N) must be specified.

$$\Gamma := \begin{vmatrix} \text{for } i \in 1..N \\ \quad \begin{vmatrix} S_i \leftarrow \sum_{j=1}^{N} \left(x_j \cdot G_{j,i} \right) \\ C_i \leftarrow \sum_{j=1}^{N} \left(x_j \cdot G_{j,i} \cdot \tau_{j,i} \right) \end{vmatrix} \\ \text{for } i \in 1..N \\ \quad \text{for } j \in 1..N \\ \quad \quad \varepsilon_{i,j} \leftarrow \dfrac{G_{i,j} \cdot \left(\tau_{i,j} - \dfrac{C_j}{S_j} \right)}{S_j} \\ \text{for } i \in 1..N \\ \quad \text{for } j \in 1..N \\ \quad \quad Q_{i,j} \leftarrow \varepsilon_{i,j} + \varepsilon_{j,i} - \sum_{k=1}^{N} \dfrac{x_k \cdot \left(G_{i,k} \cdot \varepsilon_{j,k} + G_{j,k} \cdot \varepsilon_{i,k} \right)}{S_k} \\ \text{for } i \in 1..(N-1) \\ \quad \text{for } j \in 1..(N-1) \\ \quad \quad \Gamma_{i,j} \leftarrow \delta(i,j) + x_i \cdot \left(Q_{i,j} - Q_{i,N} \right) \\ \Gamma \end{vmatrix}$$

Figure H.2   Subroutine "Multicomponent-NRTL."

$$\text{root}(p,q,r) := \begin{vmatrix} v \leftarrow \begin{pmatrix} r \\ q \\ p \\ 1 \end{pmatrix} \\ x \leftarrow \text{polyroots}(v) \\ \text{for } i \in 1..3 \\ \quad x_i \leftarrow 0 \ \text{if } \text{Im}(x_i) \neq 0 \\ x1 \leftarrow \max(x) \\ y \leftarrow \min(x) \\ x2 \leftarrow \begin{vmatrix} \max(x) \ \text{if } y = 0 \\ y \ \text{otherwise} \end{vmatrix} \\ \begin{pmatrix} x1 \\ x2 \end{pmatrix} \end{vmatrix}$$

Figure H.3   Subroutine "Root."

$$M := \quad \text{for } i \in 1..N$$

$$Tr_i \leftarrow \frac{T}{Tc_i}$$

$$Pr_i \leftarrow \frac{P}{Pc_i}$$

$$\alpha_i \leftarrow \left[1 + \left[0.37464 + 1.54226 \cdot \omega_i - 0.26992 \cdot \left(\omega_i\right)^2 \right] \cdot \left(1 - \sqrt{Tr_i} \right) \right]^2$$

$$A_{i,i} \leftarrow 0.45724 \cdot \left[\frac{Pr_i}{\left(Tr_i\right)^2} \right] \cdot \alpha_i$$

$$B_i \leftarrow 0.07780 \cdot \left(\frac{Pr_i}{Tr_i} \right)$$

$$\text{for } i \in 1..N$$

$$\text{for } j \in 1..N$$

$$A_{i,j} \leftarrow 1 - k_{i,j} \cdot \sqrt{A_{i,i} \cdot A_{j,j}}$$

$$Amix \leftarrow \sum_{i=1}^{N} \sum_{j=1}^{N} \left(x_i \cdot x_j \cdot A_{i,j} \right)$$

$$Bmix \leftarrow \sum_{i=1}^{N} \left(x_i \cdot B_i \right)$$

$$p \leftarrow -1 + Bmix$$

$$q \leftarrow Amix - 2 \cdot Bmix - 3 \cdot Bmix^2$$

$$r \leftarrow -Amix \cdot Bmix + Bmix^2 + Bmix^3$$

$$Z \leftarrow root(p,q,r)_1$$

$$\begin{pmatrix} Z \\ A \\ B \\ Amix \\ Bmix \end{pmatrix}$$

$$Z := M_1 \qquad A := M_2 \qquad B := M_3 \qquad Amix := M_4 \qquad Bmix := M_5$$

Figure H.4 Subroutine "Mixture."

Suggested Books on Mass Transfer for Further Reading

Benítez, J. 2016. *Principles and Modern Applications of Mass Transfer Operations*, 3rd edn. Hoboken: Wiley.

Bird R. B., W. E. Stewart and E. N. Lightfoot. 2007. *Transport Phenomena*, 2nd edn. New York: Wiley.

Carslaw, H. S. and J. C. Jaeger. 1959. *Conduction of Heat in Solids*, 2nd edn. London: Oxford University Press.

Crank, J. 1975. *The Mathematics of Diffusion*, 2nd edn. London: Oxford University Press.

Cussler, E. L. 2009. *Diffusion – Mass Transfer in Fluid Systems*, 3rd edn. Cambridge: Cambridge University Press.

Deen, W. M. 2012. *Analysis of Transport Phenomena*, 2nd edn. New York: Oxford University Press.

Demirel, Y. 2014. *Nonequilibrium Thermodynamics – Transport and Rate Processes in Physical, Chemical and Biological Systems*, 3rd edn. Amsterdam: Elsevier.

Middleman, S. 1998. *An Introduction to Mass and Heat Transfer*. New York: Wiley.

Sherwood, T. K., R. L. Pigford and C. R. Wilke. 1975. *Mass Transfer*. New York: McGraw-Hill.

Skelland, A. H. P. 1974. *Diffusional Mass Transfer*. New York: Wiley.

Slattery, J. C. 1999. *Advanced Transport Phenomena*. Cambridge: Cambridge University Press.

Taylor, R. and R. Krishna. 1993. *Multicomponent Mass Transfer*. New York: Wiley.

Wankat, P. C. 2012. *Separation Process Engineering*, 3 rd edn. Upper Saddle River: Prentice-Hall.

Wesselingh, J. A. and R. Krishna. 2006. *Mass Transfer in Multicomponent Mixtures*. Delft: VSSD.

J Constants and Conversion Factors

J.1 PHYSICAL CONSTANTS

Gas constant (R)
$$\begin{cases} = 82.05\,\text{cm}^3.\text{atm/mol.K} \\ = 0.08205\,\text{m}^3.\text{atm/kmol.K} \\ = 1.987\,\text{cal/mol.K} \\ = 8.314\,\text{J/mol.K} \\ = 8.314 \times 10^{-6}\,\text{MPa.m}^3/\text{mol.K} \\ = 8.314 \times 10^{-3}\,\text{kPa.m}^3/\text{mol.K} \\ = 8.314 \times 10^{-5}\,\text{bar.m}^3/\text{mol.K} \\ = 8.314 \times 10^{-2}\,\text{bar.L/mol.K} \\ = 8.314 \times 10^{-2}\,\text{bar.m}^3/\text{kmol.K} \\ = 83.14\,\text{bar.cm}^3/\text{mol.K} \end{cases}$$

Acceleration of gravity (g)
$$\begin{cases} = 9.8067\,\text{m/s}^2 \\ = 32.1740\,\text{ft/s}^2 \end{cases}$$

Avogadro's number $\qquad 6.0221415 \times 10^{23}$ entities (atoms or molecules)/mol

J.2 CONVERSION FACTORS

Density
$1\,\text{kg/m}^3 = 10^{-3}\,\text{g/cm}^3 = 10^{-3}\,\text{kg/L}$
$1\,\text{kg/m}^3 = 0.06243\,\text{lb/ft}^3$

Energy, Heat, Work
$1\,\text{J} = 1\,\text{W.s} = 1\,\text{N.m} = 10^{-3}\,\text{kJ} = 10^{-5}\,\text{bar.m}^3 = 10\,\text{bar.cm}^3$
$1\,\text{cal} = 4.184\,\text{J}$
$1\,\text{kJ} = 2.7778 \times 10^{-4}\,\text{kW.h} = 0.94783\,\text{Btu}$

Heat capacity
$1\,\text{kJ/kg.K} = 0.239\,\text{cal/g.K}$
$1\,\text{kJ/kg.K} = 0.239\,\text{Btu/lb.}^\circ\text{R}$

Force
$1\,\text{N} = 1\,\text{kg.m/s}^2 = 10^5\,\text{g.cm/s}^2 \text{ (dyne)}$
$1\,\text{N} = 0.2248\,\text{lbf} = 7.23275\,\text{lb.ft/s}^2 \text{ (poundals)}$

Length
$1\,\text{m} = 100\,\text{cm} = 10^6\,\mu\text{m} = 10^9\,\text{nm}$
$1\,\text{m} = 39.370\,\text{in} = 3.2808\,\text{ft}$

Mass
$1\,\text{kg} = 1,000\,\text{g}$
$1\,\text{kg} = 2.2046\,\text{lb}$

Power
$1\,\text{W} = 1\,\text{J/s} = 10^{-3}\,\text{kW}$
$1\,\text{kW} = 3412.2\,\text{Btu/h} = 1.341\,\text{hp}$

Pressure

$1\,\mathrm{Pa} = 1\mathrm{N/m^2}$
$1\,\mathrm{kPa} = 10^3\mathrm{Pa} = 10^{-3}\mathrm{MPa}$
$1\,\mathrm{bar} = 10^5\mathrm{Pa} = 100\,\mathrm{kPa} = 0.98692\,\mathrm{atm}$
$1\,\mathrm{atm} = 1.01325\,\mathrm{bar} = 101.325\,\mathrm{kPa} = 760\,\mathrm{mmHg}$
$1\,\mathrm{atm} = 14.696\,\mathrm{lbf/in^2}$

Temperature

$1\,\mathrm{K} = 1.8\,^\circ\mathrm{R}$
$T(^\circ\mathrm{F}) = 1.8\,T(^\circ\mathrm{C}) + 32$

Volume

$1\,\mathrm{m^3} = 1{,}000\,\mathrm{L}$
$1\,\mathrm{m^3} = 6.1022 \times 10^4\,\mathrm{in^3} = 35.313\,\mathrm{ft^3} = 264.17\,\mathrm{gal}$

Index